Digital Orthopedics

图书在版编目（CIP）数据

数字骨科学 = Digital Orthopedics : 英文 / 裴国献主编. —北京: 人民卫生出版社, 2019
ISBN 978-7-117-25996-5

Ⅰ. ①数… Ⅱ. ①裴… Ⅲ. ①数字技术-应用-骨科学-英文 Ⅳ. ①R68-39

中国版本图书馆CIP数据核字（2019）第097001号

人卫智网	www.ipmph.com	医学教育、学术、考试、健康，购书智慧智能综合服务平台
人卫官网	www.pmph.com	人卫官方资讯发布平台

数字骨科学（英文版）

主　　编:裴国献
出版发行:人民卫生出版社（中继线 010-59780011）
地　　址:北京市朝阳区潘家园南里 19 号
邮　　编:100021
E - mail:pmph @ pmph.com
购书热线:010-59787592　010-59787584　010-65264830
印　　刷:人卫印务（北京）有限公司
经　　销:新华书店
开　　本:889×1194　1/16　印张:29
字　　数:960 千字
版　　次:2019 年 6 月第 1 版　2019 年 6 月第 1 版第 1 次印刷
标准书号:ISBN 978-7-117-25996-5
定　　价:398.00 元

打击盗版举报电话:010-59787491　E-mail:WQ @ pmph.com
（凡属印装质量问题请与本社市场营销中心联系退换）

Guoxian Pei

Editor

Digital Orthopedics

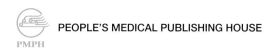

PEOPLE'S MEDICAL PUBLISHING HOUSE

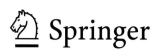

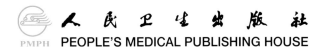

PEOPLE'S MEDICAL PUBLISHING HOUSE

Website: http://www.pmph.com/

Book Title: Digital Orthopedics

Contact address: No. 19, Pan Jia Yuan Nan Li, Chaoyang District, Beijing 100021, P.R. China, phone/fax: 8610 5978 7427, E-mail: pmph@pmph.com

First published: 2019
ISBN: 978-7-117-25996-5
Cataloguing in Publication Data:
A catalogue record for this book is available from the CIP-Database China.

ISBN 978-7-117-25996-5

Printed in The People's Republic of China

Acquisitions Editor: Ni WEN
Editor in Charge: Ni WEN
Cover Design: Xi LI
Book Design: Qiuzhai LI

Informative Abstract

The book is the second edition of *Digital Orthopaedics.* The edition is divided into three parts, which deal with the basis, research, and applications of digital orthopedics, with a total of 18 chapters. Based on the first edition, the second edition adds "CAD and CAM," "additive manufacturing technology," "reverse engineering technology," and other new technologies which have been developed rapidly over the years and have been actually applied clinically. The biggest feature of the edition, as a whole, is its introduction of application research, actual application, and latest development of digital orthopedics in clinical medicine over the years. These include research of 3D visualized application of digital tissue flap and peripheral nerves; application of 3D-printed orthopedic models; application of navigation template; application of computer-aided navigation orthopedic technique in fracture repair, spine surgery, hip surgery, knee-joint replacement, and bone tumor surgery; and actual application of robots in traumatic orthopedics, spine surgery, and joint surgical operation. The content of the book is novel and complete, fully presents the latest developments of digital orthopedic techniques, and is applicable to orthopedists, postgraduates, medical postgraduates, and iconography personnel for reading and reference.

Preface

The development of digital medicine has promoted the rapid development of digital technology in orthopedics. Over the past 20 years, digital orthopedic techniques have considerably developed. In 2006, we presented the concept of "digital orthopedics," wherein we classified, refined, and promoted the digital technical attributes of the field of orthopedics with great variety and broad content, achieving a higher and faster digital technology development. Digital orthopaedics is a new interdisciplinary subject which combines digital technology with orthopaedics. It involves anatomy, stereogeometry, biomechanics, materials science, information science, electronics and mechanical engineering. Digital orthopaedics has a wide range. Any technology used in orthopaedic research, diagnosis, treatment, rehabilitation and orthopaedic education by digital means belongs to the scope of digital orthopaedics. The application of digital orthopaedic technology will certainly promote the digitalization, individualization, visualization, virtualization, precision and intellectualization of orthopaedic diagnosis and treatment in the future, and further achieve standardization and standardization. "Digital orthopedics," as an important branch and composition of orthopedics, has become one of the subspecialties which developed most rapidly and has the highest level of new technical content in orthopedics with huge development prospect.

In 2008, we compiled and published Chinese version of *Digital Orthopaedics*. In the past decade, digital orthopaedics has developed rapidly. New technologies such as 3D printing technology, VR, AR, MR, robotics technology and artificial intelligence emerge in endlessly, which promote the individualization and precision of Orthopaedic Surgery Diagnosis and treatment, and lead and promote the further development of orthopaedics. In order to introduce the latest theories, knowledge, and technology of digital orthopedics in a timely manner and to promote its clinical application more effectively, relevant experts were asked to compile the English edition of *Digital Orthopaedics*, which is the first monograph of digital orthopeadics in the world. In order to expand the readership, the Chinese version of the book will be published in China at the same time.

The edition is divided into three parts, which deal with the basis, research, and applications of digital orthopedics, with a total of 18 chapters. Based on the first Chinese edition, this book adds "CAD and CAM," "additive manufacturing technology," "reverse engineering technology," and other technologies which have been developed rapidly over the years and have been actually applied clinically. The biggest feature of the edition, as a whole, is its introduction of application research, actual application, and latest development of digital orthopedics in clinical medicine over the years. These include research of 3D visualized application of digital flap, muscle flap and bone flap, perforator flap, and peripheral nerves; application of 3D-printed orthopedic models; design and application of surgery navigation template, preoperative planning, and virtual surgery of computer-aided orthopedics; application of augmented reality technology in digital orthopedics; application of computer-aided navigation orthopedic technique in fracture repair, spine surgery, hip surgery, knee-joint replacement, and bone tumor surgery; and actual application of robots in traumatic orthopedics, spine surgery, and joint surgical operation. Application of these new technologies expands the range of orthopedic surgery, promotes its quality, and fully embodies the latest treatment concept and requirement of individuation, precision and intellectualization surgery in orthopedics, which is an important direction of orthopedic development.

This monograph systematically introduces digital orthopedic techniques and their latest development over the recent years and represents the current technological level in the field. Digital Orthopedics is a interdisciplinary subject. Therefore, this systematic, novel, practical, and authoritative monograph is authored by biomechanics, materials science, 3D printing, fundamental research, and clinical orthopedic doctors and has a relatively strong reference value. Upon submission of the book for publication, I want to give my special thanks to all editors and Dr. Zhang Shuaishuai who have contributed hard labor, Thanks to Wen Ni, editor in charge of this book and Hu Bin, editor of Asian Division of Springer Publishing Group, for his good guidance and full support. For any error of the book, corrections are welcomed for its revision.

Xi'an, China
November 2018

Foreword for the English version of *Digital Orthopaedics*

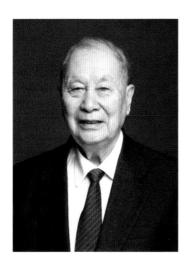

"The first person to eat crab must be a warrior." Ten years ago, Professor Guoxian Pei, editor in chief of this monograph, dared to put forward the new concept of "digital orthopedics." "What's learned from books is superficial after all. It is crucial to have it personally tested somehow." He organized an excellent team to practice what he preached and be the first to set an example. Supported by the People's Medical Publishing House academic team, his monograph *Digital Orthopaedics* was edited and published in 2009. In 2011, he established the first national academic "Digital Orthopaedics Group" of the Medical Engineering Society of the Chinese Medical Association and served as its team leader. *Digital orthopedics* has become one of the subspecialties in orthopedics which developed most rapidly and has the highest level of new technology, with great prospects for development.

"Only leave the ingenuity to pass through the ages." In order to promote the clinical application of digital orthopedic technology, he organized relevant experts to write this English version of *Digital Orthopaedics*. In addition, the English version (*Digital Orthopaedics*) of this book, which was also the first international monograph related to digital orthopedics, was published internationally by the world-famous publishing group Springer.

"Learn widely from other's strong points and develop a new way; mold and educate persons through the ages and have a style of one's own." Based on the first edition, the second edition adds contents such as "computer-aided design (CAD) and computer-aided manufacturing (CAM)," "additive manufacturing technology," "reverse engineering technology," "3D print technology," and "technology combined with robots." It focuses on introducing the clinical research and actual application of digital orthopedic technology in recent years. It clarifies that to advance with the times, embracing new technology is important for orthopedic development.

"Taishan Mountain can be so high because it does not reject any soil; river and sea can be so deep because it does not reject the trickles." The authors of this monograph come from all over the country and various schools of thought, and they innovate and develop in interdisciplinary zones. The completion of this book is a grand event achieved by the scholars of medical biomechanics, materials science, and computer technology related to fundamental research after clinical orthopedic physicians put forward the problems in urgent need of being improved. "The person in the tower close to the water catches the moonlight first." "The duck knows first when the river becomes warm in spring." I am lucky to have read the manuscript of the English version of *Digital Orthopaedics*, which I congratulate the author, and I'm glad to write its preface!

Guangzhou, China
November 2018

Shigui Zhong

Foreword

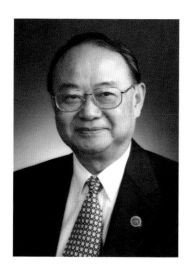

Since the twenty-first century, computer-aided design (CAD) and computer-aided manufacturing (CAM), image technology, reverse engineering, 3D printing, finite element analysis, surgical navigation, virtual simulation, robotic surgery, and other digital technologies continue to expand the scope and depth in clinical application, which constantly changes the basic appearance of modern medicine and promotes modern medicine into the digital era. In the past few decades, the development of digital medical technology and concept has penetrated into all fields of medicine, promoting the rapid development of technology, equipment, and concept of various basic and clinical branches of medical science, as well as hospital construction and management, and promoting the development of medical science toward modern medicine characterized by "precision, individualization, minimally invasive and remote mode." Among them, a large number of basic researchers, clinical experts, and engineering technicians engaged in orthopedic digital medicine at home and abroad have cooperated with each other to introduce digital medical technology into the field of orthopedics and formed a unique digital orthopedic technology and concept under constant exploration.

Digital Orthopedics, based on the clinical needs of orthopedics, relying on advanced digital technology such as the computer, involves many disciplines such as biomechanics, human anatomy, mechanical engineering, and so on. It is the crystallization of the collective wisdom of multidisciplinary experts who closely integrate clinical and digital orthopedic technology. The clinical application of digital orthopedic technology is advancing the orthopedic surgical technology and diagnostic technology to a new level.

Domestic digital medical technology, especially the development of digital orthopedic technology, has developed rapidly and continuously improved in the past few decades. It's important position in the field of orthopedics has been irreplaceable. It has promoted the precision and remote progress of surgical design, navigation, consultation, and operation and has improved the diagnosis and treatment of intractable trauma, tumor, and deformity. The medical application of 3D printing technology can satisfy the personalized needs of diagnosis and treatment in orthopedics. The application of bio-3D printing in orthopedic research opens up a new way for the regeneration and repair of bone, cartilage, muscle, and ligament damages. The application of digital surgical guides has greatly improved the accuracy of orthopedic surgery and embodied the development direction of individualized orthopedic medical technology. Surgical robots play an important role in the difficult and delicate operation of orthopedic surgery. They not only reduce the burden of surgeons but also enhance the efficiency and success of surgery. There are many other applications, such as reverse engineering technology, three-dimensional image technology of bone tissue, and image fusion technology, in preoperative planning, intraoperative operation, and postoperative management. Computer virtual surgery makes virtual reality technology and biomechanical feedback technology simulate the operation process vividly. It can not only improve the success rate of operation but also train young doctors in surgical skills more quickly and effectively and improve the efficiency and quality of personnel training.

With the improvement of people's living standards and the gradual improvement of food and clothing, the four important elements of people's lives are evolving into five elements: clothing, food, housing, transportation, and medicine. People's demand for medical services is increasing day by day. This brings us both opportunities and great challenges. At present, there are still many problems in the field of digital orthopedic medicine in China. Medical and engineering technicians at all levels do not understand each other's needs, and there is still a shortage of personnel who can grasp the knowledge and skills of both medical and engineering fields. Although some research institutes have been set up and some theoretical works have been published, they are still not mature enough, and many aspects are still in the initial stage. However, the twenty-first century is bound to be a new era of great development of digital medical technology, which forms a huge gap between subjective ability and objective needs.

The publication of the English version of *Digital Orthopedics* will contribute to the introduction and popularization of new achievements, knowledge, and communication between doctors and workers in the field of digital orthopedics. Thanks to the engineering and medical experts for their hard work in writing this book!

Academician of Chinese Academy of Engineering,
Tenured Professor and Honorary President of The Ninth People's
Hospital Affiliated to Shanghai Jiao Tong University School of Medicine,
Shanghai, China
November 2018

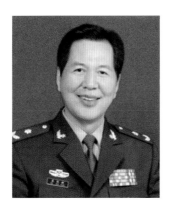

Guoxian Pei, born in October 1954, in Linying, Henan, is a medical doctor, chief physician, professor of military professional skill (Grade II) and civil service (Grade I), and tutor of doctors and postgraduates. He now acts as director of Xijing Orthopaedic Hospital, Fourth Military Medical University, and Army Orthopaedic Institute and chief editor of *Chinese Journal of Orthopaedic Trauma*. He has successively acted as member of the discipline appraisal group of the fifth Academic Degree Commission of the State Council and of the subject matter expert group of national biological material and tissue and organ repair; assessment expert of the National Award for Science and Technology Progress, National Natural Science Foundation of China, and Chinese Medical Science and Technology Award; secretary-general of the first session of the international Composite Tissue Allotransplantation Committee; director of the Asian Association for Dynamic Osteosynthesis; leader of the Digital Orthopaedics Group of the Medical Engineering Society of the Chinese Medical Association; chairman of the seventh Committee of Microsurgery Society of the Chinese Medical Association and other academic positions; and a pioneer of limb allotransplantation and digital orthopedics in China.

A famous orthopedic expert in China, for over 40 years, Professor Guoxian Pei has been engaged in the medical research of clinical bone regeneration after trauma and established many new theories and new technologies on severe limb injury and trauma treatment, formed a relatively complete theory and clinical treatment system, and obtained many innovative results internationally and in Asia. Internationally, he initiatively reported the success of simultaneous amputation and replantation of arms and legs and created "double-bridge skin flap transplantation," a new repair technology for severe lower extremity trauma, resulting in fewer amputations. He pioneered limb allotransplantation and successfully carried out the first and second hand allotransplantation surgeries in Asia (the third and fourth in the world), which were evaluated as "Top Ten News of China Medicine Technology" in 2000. He is one of the pioneers of domestic bone regeneration medical researchers, and, internationally, presented and successfully developed the new theory of "synchronized building of blood vessel, nerve, and tissue- engineered tissue and organ." He is the first man who proposed the concept of "digital orthopedics," and took the lead and established the Digital Orthopaedics Group of the Medical Engineering Society of the Chinese Medical Association; he led the team to initiatively carry out implantation of 3D-printed metal prosthesis and orthopedic robot surgery in China. He compiled 16 monographs and published 36 SCIs as the first author and corresponding author. He presided over 21 major projects, such as major projects in "863 Program" and "973 Program" and projects of NSFC, military outstanding fund for young and middle-aged talents, and major military funds. He obtained 15 achievement awards, including one second prize of the State Science and Technology Progress Award, three first prizes of the Provincial (Military) Science and Technology Progress Award, one first prize of the Natural Science Award of Ministry of Education, and two Military Major Scientific and Technical Awards and six national invention patents. He was successively recognized as belonging to "The First Batch of National Young and Middle-Aged Star of Medical Science and Technology" and "The First Batch of Person Selected for New Century Talents Project" and was acknowledged as "National Young and Middle-Aged Scientific and Technical Expert with Outstanding Contributions," among other titles. In 2000, he was awarded the "Military Scientific and Technical Star." In 2001, he was acknowledged as belonging to the first batch of "Academician Alternatives" by the General Logistics Department. In 2002, he was awarded the "Military Significant Contribution Award on Professional Skill." In 2003, he was awarded "Type I Post Allowance of Excellent Military Talent." In 2006, he was approved by the Organization Department of the CPC Central Committee as "senior expert contacted directly by the Central Government." In 2014, he led the orthopedic team and won the award of "Three-Star Talent Innovation Team" issued by the General Logistics Department.

Contents

Part I

Basis of Digital Orthopeadics

G. X. Pei and Y. Z. Zhang

1   The Establishment of Digital Orthopedics

Since the 1970s, anatomy and clinical practice have greatly influenced the field of clinical medical research, resulting in the development of many new surgical methods. The simulation of surgical procedures has been used for clinical training, teaching, and operation design. Traditional clinical teaching is completely based on the two-dimensional plane, which can be intuitive. However, a three-dimensional dynamic display has been used recently, allowing visualization of the vascular tissue, nerve tissue, and anatomical structures.

"Visual Human Plan" (1989) first promoted the emergence and development of digital medical imaging using modern information technology in medical disciplines. This was a new frontier that had a far-reaching impact on the development of science and technology. Digital technology uses dynamic three-dimensional images to supplement traditional two-dimensional medical images. For example, a computed tomography (CT) image is a three-dimensional reconstruction in rows, which can accurately show the complex structure of biological tissue. CT allows for arbitrary rotation and slicing in observation and procedures; it also can measure a three-dimensional structure for reconstructions, including the length, area, volume, and angles, thus providing precise anatomic parameters. Such imaging can be used for clinical diagnosis, auxiliary surgery, and surgical simulation, among others [1].

Zhong Shizhen, a professor at the Southern Medical University (formerly the First Military Medical University), launched a "virtual Chinese human" model as part of his research on the human body. This provided the necessary foundation for China's "Digital Human" and digital anatomy in general, in which three-dimensional anatomy is created from the two-dimensional. The development of digital anatomy has rapidly improved traditional teaching, training, and operation designs. The technology of digital medicine has provided a new development platform for clinical medicine with three-dimensional anatomy and clinical training simulations. Virtual human technology and digital anatomy have expanded into a variety of fields, including bone science. Using digital virtual technology, bone science and clinical research can be organically combined with digital technology, creating a new, multidisciplinary branch of bone science—digital bone science.

The concept of digital orthopedics is based on digital medicine. Digital technology, digital medical equipment, computer network platforms, and medical professional software provided the basis for a digital, three-dimensional orthopedic anatomy atlas. In addition to the treatment of patients, orthopedic data acquisition, storage, transmission, and processing into digital orthopedic databases have allowed us to achieve two other goals: information and resource sharing. Orthopedic surgeons can consult the digital database for the latest technical information, then share their experiences and achievements to improve the data. Also through the computer network, the technology can be used in teaching to demonstrate techniques and establish an orthopedic simulation classroom.

2   The Scope of Digital Orthopedics

The rapid development of computer technology, image processing technology, and medical physics have improved medical diagnosis and treatment in all fields of medicine. Surgeons use digital orthopedics along with modern diagnostic imaging, surgical techniques, and advanced materials to ensure a patient's safety and accurately perform minimally invasive surgery. The computer navigation system is a new advancement in the field of digital medicine, allowing for speed, accuracy, and flexibility in minimally invasive and

G. X. Pei (✉)
The First Affiliated Hospital of Air Force
Medical University, Xi'an, China

Y. Z. Zhang
The Affiliated Hospital of Inner Mongolia
Medical University, Hohhot, China

© Springer Nature B.V. and People's Medical Publishing House 2018
G. Pei (ed.), *Digital Orthopedics*, https://doi.org/10.1007/978-94-024-1076-1_1

highly unified surgery. This technology has been gradually introduced to spinal surgery from its initial applications in neurosurgical, orthopedic, and ear-nose-throat procedures. Thus, a new field of computer-aided navigation surgery was created. The successful use of computer-assisted navigation in orthopedics also fully embodies the advanced nature of digital bone science, and its applications will only become more extensive [2].

In recent years, rapid prototyping and detection technology, such as spiral CT and magnetic resonance imaging (MRI) with three-dimensional image reconstruction functionality, have become more widely used in orthopedics, cardiovascular surgery, ear-nose-throat surgery, forensic medicine, tissue engineering, and oral surgery, among others. By combining rapid prototyping technology and reverse engineering science in bone applications, we can broaden the research scope in the field of bone science. Reverse engineering is used in mechanical engineering, biology, materials science, engineering, and various field of medicine; its applications will continue to expand with the development of biological materials science and medical imaging technology. At present, the medical applications of reverse engineering have been integrated with computer software, such as Geomagic, Imageware, and Rapidform. Its applications in digital orthopedics are mainly in the following areas: (1) design and production of implants; (2) design, teaching, and evaluation of complex surgical procedures; (3) creation and analysis of a three-dimensional model of human bone with body movement mechanics [3].

Through rapid prototyping technology and reverse engineering, we can build an orthopedic surgery planning system to design and evaluate orthopedic surgical procedures. This system can aid in the setup of internal fixation devices, the creation of a three-dimensional classification database for fractures, the three-dimensional simulation of the reconstruction and restoration of various fracture types, and the choice of internal fixators.

3 The Present Situation of Digital Orthopedics

Held in Beijing in 2001, the 174th Xiangshan Science Conference was attended by more than 40 scholars from different disciplines, who gathered to discuss the state of digital research in China. The theme of that meeting was Chinese digitized virtual human technology. In 2003, at the 208th Xiangshan Science Conference, with support from the national "863-Project" and the National Natural Science Foundation of China, the human body database with Chinese characteristics was presented. Early versions of virtual simulation software were also presented. This second conference theme was "digitized virtual human studies for

application and development in China." In 2007, the research emphasis on digital humans was transferred into the digital medicine sphere when a exploratory conference ("The First China Digital Medical Seminar") was held in Chongqing. To plan, communicate, and coordinate national academic activities, a Chinese digital medical research group was established in conjunction with national academic groups. In 2008, the Chinese Academy of Engineering's first "Digital Medical Conference" was held in Beijing. In May 2011, a digital medicine branch of the Chinese Medical Association was founded in Chongqing. Then, in November 2011, the Chinese Medical Association formally established a medical engineering branch of the digital orthopedic group in Xi'an.

4 The Development Trends in Digital Orthopedics

Orthopedic virtual simulation systems allow for image processing, virtual reality, electronic communications, and orthopedic surgery planning using rational, quantitative, and individualized interactive systems. The design, simulation, intervention, and evaluation of orthopedic surgery can be achieved using visual, auditory, touch, and other sensory experiences. The orthopedic surgeon can produce immersive interactive visual simulations, including computer graphics, image processing, and pattern recognition. The fields of intelligent technology, sensor technology, language processing, audio technology, network technology and many other sciences will contribute to the further development and application of digital medicine. Using a virtual simulation system, the orthopedic physician can effectively communicate with patients, inform patients on the basic procedures they will undergo, and thus reduce the number of patients experiencing stress about their surgeries.

Although digital technology and digital medicine provide a good theoretical basis for the realization of the concepts of digital bone science, many research institutions have obtained good results using the Visible Human Project dataset in their digital technology research and development. In digital anatomy, institutes have developed virtual simulations of adult males in a systemic model (Visible Photographic Man, VIP-Man); the Voxel-Man system (developed by the University of Hamburg, Germany); an ultrasound, CT, and MRI dataset to build individualized numbers (France); a computerized virtual human body system (jointly developed by the British PA consulting company with Orme Scientific); nerve function reconstruction of the brachial plexus (Fudan University); virtual human organs for study (China University of Science and Technology); and reconstructions of the uterus, liver, kidney, and bones (Southern Medical University, Third Military Medical University, Capital

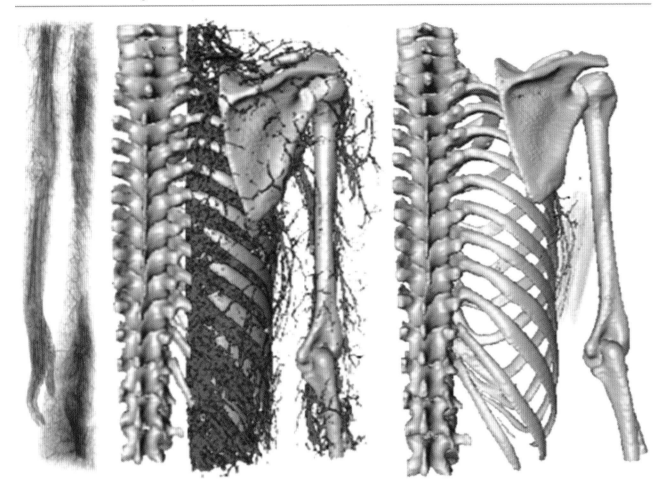

Fig. 1.1   Upper limb artery and three-dimensional reconstruction of the latissimus dorsi myocutaneous flap in digital bone anatomy

University of Medical Sciences). Other surgical procedure design and simulation research has been based on microcomputer technology, including a force feedback abdominal surgery simulator (C.S. Tseng), knee surgery training in a virtual environment (A.D. McCarthy), a force feedback endoscopic surgery simulator (C. Baur), and a complete atlas of the brain for surgical planning (Harvard University). In China, the design and implementation of virtual surgery has been successfully applied in bone, liver, neurosurgery and other areas, such as virtual vertebral spine bone resection (Southern Medical University) and functional simulation and clinical applications of the eye (Xiamen University). Digital technology is new to the field of orthopedics, however,.

Digital orthopedics has three aspects: digital bone anatomy, surgery, and virtual simulation systems. Three-dimensional digital bone anatomy is the basis of virtual teaching in orthopedics, allowing students to interactively browse a model of the human body. With digital bone anatomy, users can freely explore the body without causing any external disturbances to anatomical structures, learn about anatomy more quickly, and fully visualize individual anatomical characteristics (Fig. 1.1) [4, 5].

Digital bone surgery may apply a three-dimensional fracture or bone disease database model, intuitive analysis and observation of a fracture, fracture type classification using a database, and digital operation design and simulation to improve outcomes and enrich the database (Figs. 1.2 and 1.3) [6–8].

Digital bone surgery combines diagnosis tools, advanced equipment, and the surgeon in an organic union to ensure a patient's safety while providing accurate and minimally invasive surgery. This is a kind of human–computer interaction system, which reasonably and quantitatively uses multivariate data and navigation systems for surgical planning, intervention, and evaluation to promote the development of minimally invasive surgery. Virtual reality technology and virtual teaching are perhaps the most important applications of orthopedic simulation training. Use of the technology allows the physician to become immersed in the virtual scene, using several senses to learn about a surgical procedure.

Currently, multilayer spiral CT three-dimensional reconstructions provide good images, but the reconstruction results can only be displayed on a computer; they cannot be exported

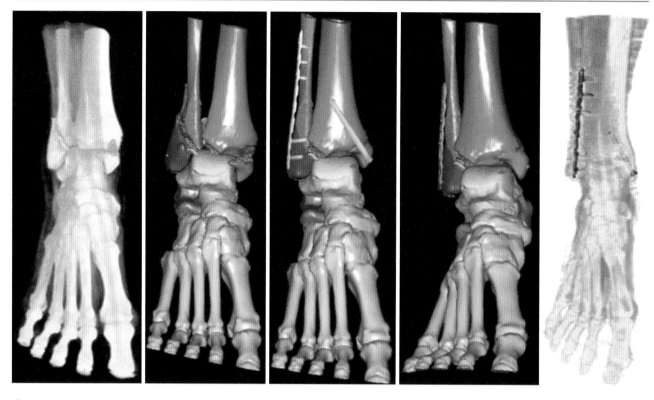

Fig. 1.2 Design and implementation of ankle fracture surgery in digital orthopedic surgery

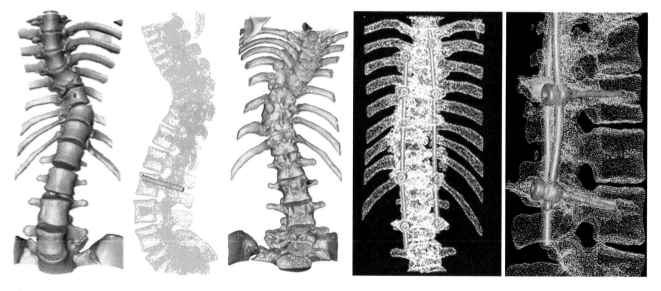

Fig. 1.3 Design and implementation of spinal corrective surgery in digital orthopedic surgery

to other interfaces. The use of three-dimensional reconstruction software in Initial Graphics Exchange Specification (IGS) and stereolithography (STL) formats allow the model to be created and then imported into other computer-aided design and reverse engineering software for further segmentation and manipulation to design a virtual surgery. Through the extraction of CT data, different digital operation models can be created, which in turn can provide a surgical model that has flexibility, a sense of tension, and authenticity (e.g., blood, sound). The simulation can provide a realistic surgical environment with multiple angles and a full view of the implant position, location of the injury, and adjacent anatomy, which can greatly improve the accuracy of the procedure and effectively avoid any complications (Fig. 1.4) [9].

Surgical simulation training can improve traditional teaching methods beyond the operating table. This type of

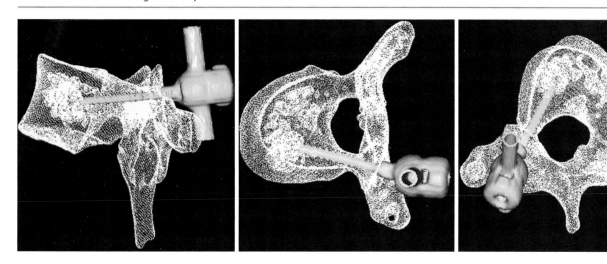

Fig. 1.4 Pedicle screw placement in an orthopedic virtual simulation

surgical training is beneficial to students. It also standardizes the training of surgeons, thus improving the quality of surgery and treatment outcomes.

A three-dimensional virtual simulation is a convenient, interactive teaching tool for young orthopedic surgeons. Fracture treatments can be viewed on an omnidirectional display using a virtual fracture model, according to the fracture location and information contained in the database. This allows the formulation of the surgical procedure and simulation of the operation and treatment results. An orthopedic virtual surgery simulation training system has low costs, zero risk, and repeatability. The advantages of automatic guidance have broad development and application prospects.

The emergence of digital orthopedics provides a new method for clinical training and teaching. The traditional teaching tools have become virtual, moving from two dimensions to three, from plane to solid, from static changes to dynamic. Digital orthopedics promises to implement systematization, standardization, and materialization in clinical orthopedics. Working in three dimensions, orthopedic surgeons can use the new model and technology platforms for simulation and training. As a new branch of orthopedics, digital orthopedics will greatly promote the development of the field as a whole.

References

1. Crowe JF, Mani VJ, Ranawat CS. Total hip replacement in congenital dislocation and dysplasia of the hip. J Bone Joint Surg (Am). 1979;61:15–23.
2. Harris WH. Traumatic arthritis of the hip after dislocation and acetabular fractures: treatment by mold arthroplasty. An end-result study using a new method of result evaluation. J Bone Joint Surg (Am). 1969;51:737–55.
3. Vedantam R, Capelli AM, Schoenecker PL. Pemberton osteotomy for the treatment of developmental dysplasia of the hip in older children. J Pediatr Orthop. 1998;18:254–8.
4. Zhang YZ, Li YB, Tang ML, et al. Application of digitalized technique in three-dimensional reconstructing of anterolateral thigh flap and arteria dorsalis pedis flap. Microsurgery. 2007;27:553–9.
5. Zhang YZ, Li YB, Jiang YH, et al. Three-dimensional reconstructive methods in the visualization of anterolateral thigh flap. Surg Radiol Anat. 2008;30:77–81.
6. Won YY, Cui WQ, Baek MH, et al. An additional reference axis for determining rotational alignment of the femoral component in total knee arthroplasty. J Arthroplasty. 2007;22:1049–53.
7. Lu S, Xu YQ, Lu WW, et al. A novel patient-specific navigational template for cervical pedicle screw placement. Spine. 2009;34:E959–64.
8. Sheng L, Xu YQ, Zhang YZ, et al. A novel computer-assisted drill guide template for placement of C2 laminar screws. Eur Spine J. 2009;18:1379–85.
9. Sheng L, Yong QX, Zhang YZ, et al. A novel computer-assisted drill guide template for lumbar pedicle screw placement: a cadaveric and clinical study. Int J Med Robot Comput Assist Surg. 2009;5:184–91.

2

Guoxian Pei and Su Xiuyun

1 Basic Equipment for Digital Medical Imaging

1.1 X-Ray

The digital image in common sense is the formation of image based on the reflected light of the 3D objects from the real world, and its 3D information can be understood through the fluoroscopy principle. However, x-ray imaging is a special kind of imaging formed by using a conical beam of light from a point source radiating through the body tissue on a photographic plate. The grayscale of images produced by x-ray reflects the different attenuation ratio of different human tissues. Due to the conical beam, the image will be more or less enlarged. At the edge of the image, the angles of the beam and photographic plate are a little large, which cause distortion of image to some extent. Thus, to measure the size of human body tissue based on an x-ray imaging accurately demands: on one hand, a reference is needed. According to some literature, a coin, the diameter of which has been known to us, can be used as a proportional scale during filming. Nowadays, clinical digital imaging all has its proportional scale. On the other hand, the tissues to be measured should be placed at the center of the image.

For bone tissue, compared with CT and MRI, x-ray imaging has the highest spatial resolution. Spatial resolution refers to the minimum distance distinguishing the adjacent two objects. The spatial resolution of the traditional x-ray film is 0.08 mm, digital radiography 0.17 mm, and the image of fluoroscopy 0.125 mm.

Because of easy access and moderate price, plain x-rays are widely used at clinical examination. But since x-ray imaging essentially is a projection of the 3D objects on the two-dimensional plane, more images from different angle will have to be filmed to get more information of the 3D structure. Meanwhile, it's difficult to convert x-ray imaging into 3D computer models.

1.2 CT

The progresses in medical imaging and information technology based on the progress of CT propel the birth and development of digital orthopedics. A CT scan, also called cross-sectional images, is in fact a tomography of a certain human part with a certain thickness. The space between the cross section of the early CT scan is normally 1 cm, way bigger than the spatial resolution of the cross-sectional images. However, at present, the spiral CT applied in clinic provides 3D volume data of human body, achieving 3D isotropy at spatial resolution.

Volume data refers to a set of discrete sampling of one or some kinds of physical property in a limited space, which can use regular sampling at the sampling point based on the rule of the same interval and layer space. Other sampling methods are also applicable. The value of sample at the sampling point can be single-valued or multi-valued. When it is single-valued, it is called scalar volume data; while it is multi-valued, it is called vector volume data. The value of sampling of spiral CT reflects the tissue's attenuation ratio to x-ray; thus it is a scalar volume data.

The imaging of CT applies principle that the different tissues have different attenuation ratio to x-ray. As a result, it has an advantage at imaging of bone. The spatial resolution of CT scan is 0.4 mm, lower than x-ray image, because it is discrete sampling of human body.

G. Pei
Orthopedic Hospital, Xijing Hospital Fourth Military Medical University, Xi An, China

S. Xiuyun (✉)
Department of Orthopaedics, Affiliated Hospital of the Academy of Military Medical Sciences, Beijing, China

© Springer Nature B.V. and People's Medical Publishing House 2018
G. Pei (ed.), *Digital Orthopedics*, https://doi.org/10.1007/978-94-024-1076-1_2

1.3 MRI

The principle of formation of MRI is to put human body in the magnetic field, then obtain electromagnetic signal by using the magnetic resonance of human tissue, and combine cross-sectional images through a computer. Every sampling point of MRI has three sample values, representing the proton density of tissue, T1 relaxation time, and T2 relaxation time, respectively, so it is a vector volume data. The imaging of MRI is based on the amount of protons of different tissues, the difference between T1 relaxation time and T2 relaxation time and other numerous parameters. Adopting different scanning sequences can better observe the lesion of bone, muscle, ligament, cartilage, and nervous tissues. MRI has a higher resolution than CT in imaging soft tissue. However, nowadays MR imaging still cannot be isotropic. The thickness of the section is generally 7 mm, so in the application of digital orthopedics, MRI is usually applied in combination with CT.

MR's spatial resolution of sections is 1 mm, while the thickness of the section is 7 mm [1].

2 Basis of Digital Image

2.1 Basic Concepts of Vision And Image

2.1.1 Visual Perception

The visible sense that the optical radiation stimulated the brain through the eyes is visual perception. It is the most important sensory organ for human beings. About 80% of external information people got come from eyes. Visual perception is synthetic reaction of a serial of physical, molecular biological, biochemical physiological, and psychological process. Under the light, the object would absorb a part of light and then reflect a part of light. The reflected light will enter into the eyes, hitting the refractive media, becoming focusing, and forming an image on the retinas. The signals of imaging will be "decoded" and recognized when they reach the occipital lobe cortex of the brain. Now the object is "seen" in consciousness, including its position, shape, size, color, surface texture, degree of transparence, and so on. Visual function can be decomposed into light perception, form perception, color vision, 3D perception, distance perception, and some other several aspects.

Form perception is the ability to distinguish the contour of the objects. Its quantitative criterion is called visual acuity, namely, the ability to discern tiny objects. When the eye balls look right ahead fixedly, the range of form perception they can perceive is called visual field. Color vision is the eye's ability to tell different colors due to the different visual reaction of optical wave with different wavelengths [2].

2.1.2 Image

Image is the entity that obtained by observing the world through various observing systems which directly or indi-

rectly work on the human eyes and produce visual perception. Visual perception is the main approach for human being getting information from nature. According to statistics, among the information people obtained, visual information accounts for 60%, auditory information about 20%, and the rest information only about 20%. This shows that visual information is very crucial for human beings. At the same time, image is the main way for people to get visual information and the most important, richest, and largest amount of information source that people can experience. Generally speaking, the object is three dimensional in space, but the image captured from the object is two dimensional. And the tomography cross-sectional images also can be considered as two dimensional in space.

Simulation Image

It includes optical image, camera image and television image, etc. For instance, the image people saw under a microscope is a simulation of optical image. The processing rate of simulation image is quick, but it has shortage in accuracy and flexibility, and it is hard to be found and judged.

Digital Image

Digital image is computer recognizable bitmap which is achieved through discretization of a continuous simulation image. Technically speaking, digital image is a two-dimensional function that goes through equidistance rectangular grid sampling and equal interval quantizing of amplitude. Thus, digital image in fact is a quantized two-dimensional array sampling. Grayscale image is one-dimensional matrix, while color image is 3D matrix.

Graphics

Graphics refers to the vector graphics constituted by the contour lines. Vector graphics, also named object-oriented image or graphic image, is defined mathematically a serial of dots connected by lines. That is to say, it includes the straight line, round, rectangular, curve, and chart drawn by computer. The graphic elements in vector file is called object. Each object is a self-contained entity with properties like color, shape, outline, size and screen position, etc. The object can be zoomed optional without distortion. Vector graphics are usually applied to geometric figure, engineering drawing, CAD, 3D modeling software, and so on.

2.2 Favorite Image Processing Software

Digital image processing is also called computer image processing, which refers to the course of transferring the image signal into digital signal and then processing them through computer. Early image processing is aimed to improve the quality of image by using people as objects in order to improve visual effect of people. During image processing, the image of low quality is inputted, and the improved image is outputted. Frequently used image processing methods are image enhancement, image restoration, image coding, image compression, and so on. There are a lot algorithms and software of image processing that can be easily understood and grasped by medical professionals. Here, two kinds of commercial software will be introduced: Adobe Photoshop and MATLAB. For medical researchers, these two have their own advantages and disadvantages that can compensate each other, which is a relatively better choice for medical image processing [3].

2.2.1 Adobe Photoshop

Photoshop is the world famous image processing and design software. Its functions can be divided into four parts: image editing, image composition, color correction and modulation, and special effects. Image editing can do amplifying, contracting, rotating, tilting, mirroring, changing perspective, and so on. It also can duplicate, remove speckles, repair and modify damaged image, etc. Image composition is to compound several images into an intact image conveyed a clear and definite meaning by applying layer operational tools. Color correction and modulation is to adjust the brightness and to correct color bias. They can also switch between different colors in order to meet the need of application of image in different fields. Special effects are mainly done through a synthetic application of filter, channel, layer, and other tools of Photoshop. Creative idea and words with special effect and some traditional painting techniques like oil painting, embossment, plaster oil painting, and sketch all can be made by it.

Photoshop has batch processing function and uses variables and event-based scripting, which makes it able to process repetitive tasks. It also integrates many mature algorithm of image processing, so it has advantages like great interactivity, fast operational speed, and easy to grasp. Now Photoshop is widely used in many aspects of scientific and medical image processing. However, due to its lack of accurate and flexible scientific computing ability, it is difficult to conduct image registration and segmentation.

2.2.2 MATLAB Image Processing

MATLAB is the abbreviation of Matrix Laboratory. It is a scientific computing commercial software using matrix form to process data and now is widely applied to analysis, simulation and design of scientific computation, control system, information processing, and other fields. With a specialized tool developed by the experts of each domain, our work would have a higher starting point. And MATLAB command is very close to the symbol and formula in mathematics, readable and easy to grasp.

MATLAB provides an intuitive and reliable integrated developmental tool for image processing engineers, scientists, and researchers. These tools are widely used in aerospace, remote sensing and measuring, biotechnology, medical imaging, scientific image processing, and other fields.

The image processing tools of MATLAB support many kinds of image data format, including DICOM format of medical image. At the same time, it offers a lot of functions to apply to image processing. By using these functions, people are able to analyze image data, obtain detailed information of image, design corresponding filtering algorithm, and filter the noise contained in the image data. Many functions of mathematical morphology are used to process grayscale image or binary image and realize quick edge detection, image denoising, skeleton extraction, watershed segmentation, and so on. And all of them can process multi-dimensional image data.

Image processing tools provide many high-level image processing functions, including operations like permutation, transformation, sharpening, etc. Also, image cutting and size changing can be achieved by employing these functions.

MATLAB itself is a powerful data visualization tool, which can present analyzed data through various forms, for example, gray level histogram, contour line, montage mixture, pixel analysis, layer transformation and texture mapping, etc. Using visualized image not only can assess the properties of graphic images but also can analyze the color distribution and other conditions of image.

3 Image Standard

3.1 Pixel, Resolution, and Pixel Size

Pixel is the most basic unit forming an image. It can be seen as an extremely tiny square color blocks. An image is usually made up by many pixels, which are arranged in rows and columns. When the user uses the scale tool to zoom in to a certain degree, he/she would see the result resembling mosaic and each block is a pixel. Pixel is an individual element of digital image matrix. Its position decides the objects' position in the image, and its size is the grayscale value of grayscale image and RGB value of color image.

The more pixels in a unit area will result in the higher resolution, so the effect of the image is better. The unit of image resolution is pixel/inch, namely, the amount of pixel in an inch. If the image's resolution is 72 pixel/in., it means each inch includes 72 pixels. The higher image resolution means there are more pixels in each inch, therefore more details and smoother color transition of image.

What is needed to be noted is that usually image resolution refers to the amount of pixels in a unit area of photographic paper after printing the image. And also the pixel size of the medical cross-sectional images is the proportion of raw distance between two dots on the image (whose unit is the number of pixel) and actual physical distance of an object (whose unit is cm). The references of these two distances are different: the previous one is printed photographic paper, and the latter is the actual object. Their applications are also different: raw distance is applied to photograph and photo printing industry, while the physical distance is used in medical imaging [4].

3.2   Color Depth

Color depth indicates the number of color in an image, namely, the binary digits storing matrix elements of digital image.

One binary number can only save 0 or 1 two numerical values, so it is also called binary image or logical image. Usually image segmentation is resulted in a single bit image. Meanwhile, the morphological operation of image is based on a single bit image. Sixteen bit is $2^{16} = 65,536$, which is able to save 65,536 grayscale value. It is the bit of storage of image of DICOM format. If these grayscales are all displayed in an image, then the human eyes cannot distinguish it. Thus, the DICOM format image displaying 16 bit can only choose a small scope (window width) of a certain position (window level) to display the grayscale. All the pixels lower than window width is shown as black, and the pixels higher than window width is shown as white.

3.3   Color Models of Image File

The frequently used color models are RGB, CMYK, and Lab.

RGB color model is also named RGB color space. It represents three colors: R for red, G for green, and B for blue. Red, green, and blue are known as three primary colors of light. Most visible spectrum in nature can be shown by mixing light of these three kinds of color with different proportions and intension.

CMYK color model is a subtractive color model, which is the fundamental difference between CMYK and RGB. We use this subtractive color model not only when we observe objects but also when it is applied to printing on the paper. CMYK refers to the four colors: C for cyan, M for magenta, Y for yellow, and K for key (black).

Lab color model is the color space of human vision. It based on the only principle of vision—the uniform color space that is the same amount of movement causing same sense of color changes to the eyes. Lab color space is device independent, producing colors matching with various devices like colors of display and printer. Lab color model makes up for the shortcomings of RGB and CMYK. Moreover, it can realize color change of various devices as intermediate color. In lab color model, L refers to lightness, a refers to the color changing from green to red, and b for the color changing from yellow to blue. L is definitely a positive value. When a or b is positive, it appears as red or yellow, respectively. When a or b is negative, it appears as green or blue, respectively.

3.4   Image Format

Bitmap, also called raster graphics, is the image displayed by pixel matrix. The color information of each pixel is presented by RGB combination or grayscale value.

BMP file is a method of data exchange and storage developed by Microsoft Company. Every version of Windows all supports files in BMP format. Windows provides a fast and convenient method to store and compress BMP file. The shortage of BMP format is that it would take up a relatively large storage space and the file size is too big.

TTFF (Tagged Image File Format) is a commonly used image format for desktop publishing system developed by Aldus and Microsoft Company. TIFF is a non-distorted compressed format (2–3 times compression ratio top). This compression is the compression of the file itself, namely, recording some repeated information in the file through a special method. The file can be completely restored maintaining the color and level of the original image. The strength of TIFF is the high quality of image, but it would occupy a larger space.

JPEG is the abbreviation of Joint Photographic Experts Group. It is the most common used image file format developed by a Federation of software development organizations. It is a lossy compression format that compresses the image into a very small storage space, so the repeated and unimportant materials will be lost. Thus it is easy to cause damage of image data. However, JPEG compression technique is advanced. It uses lossy compression to remove the redundant image data. As a result, it achieves an extremely high compression ratio and shows a vivid image at the same time. In another word, it can receive a relatively high image quality by using the least disk space. Besides, JPEG is a very flexible format which has the function to adjust the image quality, allowing compressing the file with different compression ratio and supporting multiple compression levels. The compression ratio is usually ranged from 10:1 to 40:1. The bigger the compression ratio is, the lower quality will be. Inversely, the lower the compression ratio means higher quality. JEPG mainly compresses information of high frequency which can better reserve the color information. It is suitable for application in the internet with advantages like saving transmission time and supporting 24-bit true colors. It is also commonly applied to continuous tone image.

3.5   DICOM Format

As of the early 1990s, with the rapid development of computer technology, communications technology, and network technology, image analysis, image processing, and PACS (Picture Archiving and Communication Systems) have been playing an increasingly important role in clinical diagnostics, telemedicine, and medical education. One of the technical problems to be solved in PACS is the standardization of image data formats of various digital imaging devices and data transmission. DICOM 3.0 (Digital Imaging and Communications in Medicine 3.0), an important network standard and communication protocol for PACS to become an open system, is a new standard of digital imaging and communications, in accordance with which the production of different types of digital imaging devices can be realized as one communicates with different manufacturers through PACS.

DICOM format image files are files stored in accordance with DICOM standard. A DICOM file generally consists of DICOM File Meta Information and DICOM data set.

DICOM File Meta Information contains information about the data set. It can be understood as recording all the useful information of a certain DICOM format image. For example, in a DICOM format CT image, the DICOM File Meta Information records the patient's name, image size, layer thickness, layer distance, pixel resolution, as well as other clinical and image-related information.

As for the description of the image, DICOM takes advantage of bitmaps, in which, as elaborated above, grayscale images are usually stored in 16-bit. DICOM allows three matrices to represent the three components, respectively, or one matrix for the representation of the entire image. The former can be used to store color images, such as the reconstructed three-dimensional color image we see in the PACS system and the latter to store 16-bit grayscale images.

4 Quality Control of Digital Human Images in China

4.1 Relationship Between Cutting Layer Space and Pixel

Thanks to the advancement of layer cutting machine and digital camera resolution, the layer distance of equally spaced digital human datasets has been substantially decreased. In America, the earlier male datasets of VHP was 1 mm, while the later female datasets distance reached 0.33 mm; the Korean datasets VKH and Chinese datasets CDH (of both gender, CDH-M1, CDH-F1) have an modified layer distance of 0.2 mm; Chinese Digital Human Famel-Child No. 1 (CDH C-F1) has an even smaller distance of 0.1 mm. But the key technology of achieving slice datasets with smaller spaces is not about layer distance, because with the help of CDH-VCH-FA00 gantry milling machine specially developed for DCH, the experimental layer distance can arrive at 0.02 mm, nor is that about camera resolution

which nowadays has reached more than 10 or even 20 mega pixels. Building a fine-pitch data layers are the key technologies and the resolution matches. The key technology to build datasets thin distance lies in the matching of layer distance with resolution.

CDH-M1 and CDH-F1, the two datasets of Chinese digital human have a cutting layer distance of 0.2 mm. And the resolution is 3024 × 2016, the cross-sectional area of the tomogram to be collected is 600 mm × 400 mm, and minimum side length of distinguishable pictures is 0.2 (mm). CDH C-F1 dataset has a cutting layer distance of 0.1 mm, the resolution of 4256 × 2848, the cross-sectional area of tomogram to be collected of 280 mm × 280 mm, and side length for the minimum unit of distinguishable pictures of 0.1 (mm).

4.2 Color Management

Color, the inherent properties of objects, is also susceptible to the environment. The image we get through digital camera or scanner should be revealed on the display and transmitted to the printer to be printed out. Different color modes lead to different color ranges; and different devices with the same color mode can bring out different color ranges. The way to ensure the faithfulness to the original color during shooting and transmission process and achieve accurate reproduction is called color management.

Color management, simply put, is the use of computer technology for orderly management of color system, namely, the color must be consistent through all the stages, from initially the image signal importing (such as shooting, scanning, etc.) to the middle stages (image processing with image editing software), and finally to the output (printing). The core of color management is ICC profile. ICC profile is a color description file of a digital device, which signifies the correspondence between the expression of this particular color device and standard CIE Lab color space. ICC profiles provide description files mainly for devices concerning the following three aspects: input (scanners, digital cameras), display (various displays), and output (printers or a variety of color output devices) and require a scientific and reasonable match among them to reach a correct color reproduction of the image.

Standard color card is the card printed with a number of standard colors. On the card are various gradient colors that all follow strict standards and have the color descriptions in the color card Text Description File (TDF). The more color on the card, the better the correction. The commonly used card is IT8 color cards. By synchronously shooting IT8 color or special CDH color on the tomogram and then testing color-coded images with colorimeter and spectrum analyzer, the color management profile of tomogram data for Chinese digital human datasets can be established for the completed property profile, thereby ensuring the tomographic image of Chinese digital human to be consistent in color throughout the subsequent processing.

4.3   Data Storage and Backup

Data backup is to store data in a suitable medium through a particular way for the purpose of ensuring that data will not be missing under any circumstances and will always be available. The core of data backup is to restore the data—a backup that cannot be restored makes no sense. Data backup of CDH is divided into two categories, namely, real-time backup while data collection and copy backup while data using. That involves data backup media, data backup hardware and data backup software.

Real-time backup data is also known as data synchronization backup. It is a means to prevent data loss during the collection process which might be caused by hardware failure or human errors. The real-time data backup of CDH, through dedicated real-time synchronization backup software, provides the backup machine with a synchronization tool with folder directories specified by the gathering machine of ready access. Thus the directory on the two computers can be synchronized and mirrored through a small local area network to achieve data backup purposes.

To prevent the dataset from falling short in the actual use and protect the established data set from failing which might be caused by system crashes, hardware failures, virus attacks, misuse, and natural damage, we need a backup copy of the data set, that is, the hardware backup. The backup CDH original data set currently uses hard disk as a storage medium for backup copy and conducts full backup regularly to achieve backup copies of the original data set. For safety reasons, promptly after a successful construction of CDH original data set, we produce two copies of the original data set and keep the two original sets and two copied ones in four different sites.

In addition, by depositing timely the CDH original data set on websites of partner organizations, such as the Institute of Computing Sciences of CSA (Chinese Academy of Sciences), the Shanghai Center for Biotechnology Information (CAS grid) Institute, Huazhong University of Science and Technology (Ministry of Education Grid), etc., whose network could backup the dataset, the function of automatic unattended backup, cross-platform data management, real-time subset backup, database management, disaster recovery, error alarm, and others can be realized. It is also an effective way to ensure the security, reliability, and efficiency of the entire data backup.

5   Image Registration

5.1   Basic Theory about Medical Image Registration

In the acquisition, transfer, and record keeping process of the image, due to various factors, such as the effects of atmospheric turbulence, diffraction of the optical system in the equipment, the nonlinearity of the sensor, aberration of the optical system, the relative motion between the imaging device and the object, the nonlinearity of photosensitive film, grain noise of the film, the nonlinearity of television camera scanning, and others, the image will inevitably result in distortion. Typically, the quality declining caused by these factors is called image degradation.

The typical examples of image degradation are blur, distortion and additional noise. Because of the degradation of the image, the image displayed in the receiving end is no longer the original image under transmission; thus the quality of the image drops dramatically. Therefore, to show better the image, it is a must to work on the degraded image and restore the original one. And such process is referred to as image restoration.

Image restoration technique is a very important technology in image processing. Similar to other basic image processing technology such as image enhancement, it also aims at the improvement of visual quality. But the difference is that image restoration process is an estimation process during which degraded images are restored according to the specified degradation model to get the original picture that has not been degraded. In short, image restoration is to improve the degraded image and to achieve amelioration in the visual image.

Since the image degradation can be caused by various factors, and the properties of each are not identical, there is currently no uniform method for restoration. Many researchers have worked out different restoration methods by studying the physical environment of application and thus employ different degradation models, processing techniques, and estimation criteria accordingly. Degradation and restoration are actually a pair of mutually positive and negative issues. Degradation is a well-posed problem, and restoration is an ill-posed problem. The estimation of degradation factors is the first step of image restoration.

Image distortion and registration is a special kind of degradation and restoration. In doing medical image analysis, several images of one patient are often analyzed together for comprehensive information about the patient, which contributes to the improvement of medical diagnosis and treatment. While doing quantitative analysis of several different images, we must firstly align the images strictly, and this is what we call the image registration.

Medical image registration refers to seeking a (or a series of) spatial transformation for a medical image so that it matches with the corresponding point of another piece of medical image. This correspondence means that the same anatomical points of the human body have the same spatial location on two matching images. Registration should make match all the anatomical points on the two images or at least all points essential to the diagnosis and those related to the surgery.

For two images I1 (x1, y1, z1) and I2 (x2, y2, z2) which are obtained at different times or under different conditions, to achieve registration is to find a mapping P: (x1, y1, z1) (x2, y2, z2), so that each point on I1 has a unique corresponding point on I2. And the two points should correspond to the same anatomical location. The mapping P takes on the form of a group of contiguous space transformations. The commonly used spatial geometric transformation is rigid body transformation, affine transformation, projective transformation, and nonlinear transformation.

5.2 Registration Method of Medical Image

Conventional medical registration is based on an important premise: the image of the same object filmed at the same time through different imaging modalities or the image of the same object filmed at different times through the same imaging modalities. The object shot here is assumed not to change or only partially changes. Such as an X-ray film in the same position before and after surgery of a patient and the different images formed by different spectrums under fluorescence microscopy.

5.2.1 Points
Points can be divided into internal points and external points. Internal points are obtained from images relevant to the patient, such as anatomical landmarks. Anatomical landmarks must be defined in three dimensions and can be seen in the images of two scanning modes. Typical anatomical landmarks can be a point-like anatomy. External points are screws embedded in the subjects' skulls, marks made on skin, and other additional markers in the two images that can be detected.

5.2.2 Moment and Spindle Method
Thanks to the concept of body mass distribution in classical mechanics, the pixel centroid and spindle of the two images can be calculated and then aligned by translation and rotation, so as to achieve registration [1]. This method is more susceptible to the lack of data, which requires that the body must appear entirely in the two images. In addition, this method proves to be of poor effect for some cases interesting to neurologist.

5.2.3 Correlation
For a sequence of images of the same object resulting from the differences in image acquisition conditions or small changes of the object itself, registration can be achieved by way of the principle of maximizing the similarity between images, namely, by optimizing the similarity criteria between two images to estimate the transformation parameters, mainly the translation and rotation of the rigid body. Photographic sequences, considering the prism system, should be given the necessary scaling. Intensity difference caused by different exposure time should also be amended. Intensity scaling should also be carried out in nuclear medicine images to diminish the impacts of the acquisition time, injection activity, background, and other factors. The similarity measure used can be varied, such as correlation function, correlation coefficient, sum of the squared difference or sum of absolute value of the difference, and so on. The similarity measure should be calculated for each possible value of the transformation parameters, so the amount of calculating becomes tremendously large. Some scholars have made efforts in this regard, such as using the Fourier phase correlation method to estimate the translational and rotational parameters, using genetic algorithms and simulated annealing to reduce search time and overcome local minima, and taking advantage of cross-correlation techniques of Fourier invariance and decomposition of logarithmic transformation. Correlation is largely limited to a single-mode image registration, especially for the comparison of a series of images so as to find the small changes caused by diseases.

5.3 Registration of Continuous Tomographic Image

Tomogram is an important way for people to understand the inside information of three-dimensional objects. In medicine and industry, people, in many cases, cannot know the internal three-dimensional information of some structures by conventional methods. As an alternative method of observation, tomograms of the three-dimensional structures help us infer internal information of the structure by observing the tomograms. The examples are tomograms of human body; continuous histopathology tomograms; tomographic data set obtained through CT, MRI, and other imaging equipment; and ultrafine cell tomographic information obtained through confocal microscope.

Continuous tomogram contains complete information about the internal structure of a three-dimensional object. Firstly, we can transect the object along the assumed Z-axis at equal intervals (d) to obtain a series of horizontal tomograms. Then take out randomly one tomogram and observe the piece corresponding to a certain internal part. Assume that the tomogram is placed in a three-dimensional coordinate system for the observation of the three-dimensional coordinates of *P*, a point on the contour of an unknown object. The coordinate values of P are X-axis and Y-axis (x, y), which can be determined by its location in the horizontal tomogram; *P* in the Z-axis has a coordinate value (z) that can be determined by the product of a cut distance (*d*) and tomogram order (*n*) ($z = d * n$). Therefore, the continuous tomogram point *P* contains accurate three-dimensional coordinate information that extends from the point to the surface and finally to the body. Thus it can be easily concluded: the three-dimensional structural information of an unknown object can be observed in a continuous tomogram.

It should be noted that the continuous tomographic image registration is a registration done in a special case where each of the tomographic image comes theoretically from different objects. If taking the conventional medical registration method, we will commit a serious mistake due to different premises. For example, the continuous tomographic images of a tilt cylinder prove to be an oval. If reconstructed three-dimensionally by the conventional registration method, the images will form an elliptical cylinder.

Accordingly, during the shooting and storage of tomographic images, because of different parameters of image forming devices, as well as varied relative positions and angles between the image forming device and tomogram, there is often a positional deviation between the image layers. So while embedding and shooting specimens, we need to add location marks to facilitate the registration of the original image, in order to ensure that each piece retains exactly the two-dimensional information of the original tomogram. Of course, the advanced quick-scanning image acquisition equipment of CT and MRI has made it unnecessary to consider the alignment between tomograms.

5.4   Registration of Continuous Tomographic Image of Chinese Digital Human

During the image acquisition process of Chinese Digital Human (CDH), the parameter setting of digital cameras remains unchanged. Since the shape of human tomograms change at different layers, factors of image degradation cannot be accurately estimated by the organ's changing shape presented in the tomograms. To facilitate the locational registration of photos collected, we have added four positioning rods while doing embedment. The positioning rods preset in the cutting specimens remain at the same spatial position on each actual layer, so changes of positioning rods in the continuous tomographic image may represent distortion of each image.

With respect to human tomogram plane, a digital camera can realize small pan and rotation in six degrees of freedom

in three-dimensional space (rotation of axis X, Y, Z and plane translation of X, Y, Z), causing tomographic translation, rotation, and scaling (square corresponds to square), shear (square corresponds to parallelogram), and tilt (square corresponds to arbitrary quadrilateral; straight line corresponds to straight line), which are collectively referred to as projective distortion. Thus registration of continuous tomographic images can be reduced to projective transformation based on coordinates of positioning rods.

Firstly, process the original tomographic images to get the images of the four positioning rods on every layer, calculate in MATLAB the centroid coordinate values of the four positioning rods which are used as the coordinate values of the positioning rods, and take the average of coordinate values of all the tomograms as the reference coordinates. Secondly, determine the dimensional projective transformation parameters based on the coordinate values of positioning rods on each layer, carry out projective transformations of tomographic images, and eliminate projective distortions. Then get images of the first positioning rod from corrected images reprocessed in Photoshop, calculate their coordinate values in MATLAB, and, based on the coordinate values of the positioning rod, cut the tomographic images into ones of the same size.

6   Image Segmentation

6.1   The Overview of Medical Image Segmentation

Victor Spitzer, the pioneer of the research of Digital Virtual Human, once said that there was just one challenge in the research, which is segmentation. Image segmentation is the foundation and the bottleneck of the succeeding image processing including 3D reconstruction. On the one hand, accurate image segmentation takes a lot of time and effort; on the other hand, the precision level of image segmentation will affect the results of the succeeding medical basic research and clinical application. Thus it is of particular significance to improve the efficiency and precision level of image segmentation.

Image segmentation is to differentiate areas of special implications from each other. Both the data sets of Chinese Digital Visual Human and those of clinical serial sections are volume data sets containing the 3D information of structure. The segmentation of volume data sets is similar to that of 2D images; namely, it's to segment voxels of special implications from volume data sets, which is like the process of carving a statue out of a huge stone. There are two ways to segment voxel data; one is to separately segment every 2D slice and the other is to directly segment 3D volume data sets. Thus, image segmentation can also be simply understood as a process of choice. For every pixel constituting 2D images and every voxel volume data sets, the result of choice is either removed or preserved. Thus the results of image segmentation can be preserved with binary image.

6.1.1 The Features of Medical Image Segmentation

One of the reasons why medical image segmentation is very challenging is that whatever imaging mode is adopted, the real information will to some degree be lost or distorted in the process of image acquisition, so that the results of section-image segmentation can only approximately but cannot completely reflect the real anatomical boundaries.

Medical researchers and surgeons hope that normal or pathological anatomical structures reconstructed by computer can truly represent the layer of structure shown in human anatomy and surgeries and even reproduce fine structures seen under a microscope. However, all imaging devices produce some noises, and each kind of imaging mode has some limitations in reflecting the real anatomical structures. For example, the optical photograph of the anatomical specimen of frozen section shows the reflectivity to visible light of different tissues. But it cannot clearly distinguish adipose tissue and nervous tissue that are similar in color as well as connective tissues like adjacent muscle compartments, periosteum, muscle tendons, and joint capsules. CT tomography reflects the attenuation rates to X-rays of different tissues, but it cannot clearly distinguish soft tissues that are similar in density. MRI tomography reflects the density of hydrogen protons contained in tissues and the time for relaxation of T1 and T2, but more often than not, the reflected pathological boundaries of the tissues are amplified compared with the real ranges.

The second reason is that whatever computer segmentation algorithm is resorted to, the accuracy of the computer automatic image segmentation can hardly be up to the anatomical level or the level of medical imaging experts' reading photographs when it comes to specific normal or pathological anatomical structures. In other words, the computerized algorithm cannot reach the level of visual thinking. For example, we see the changing clouds in the sky and imagine them sometimes as a flock of sheep and sometimes as running horses. The reason why out of the clouds we can see the images of sheep or horses is that the images are already in our mind. And this is the process of visual thinking. On the contrary, what the computer can recognize are just clouds. In medical image segmentation, there are two things needed to be done by the experts. One is to choose the computer automatic segmentation algorithm, and the other is to revise the results of the computer automatic segmentation. Thus, the process of medical image segmentation must involve the efforts of the medical experts, and the accuracy degree of the segmentation results is closely related to the experience of the operators, as the results it cannot be repetitive.

Thus, at the moment any single kind of section image cannot meet the precision demands of all the medical researches and clinical applications and any single kind of computer image segmentation algorithm is difficult to satisfactorily segment medical images. Although medical image segmentation is a hot research topic in the majority of computer graphics and it's continuously making progress, at the moment medical researchers cannot be replaced due to the reasons mentioned above. The purpose of medical image segmentation is to meet the precision demands to the maximum of the medical researches and clinical applications. Thus the author would like to give some suggestions to the process of segmenting the medical image data.

Firstly, raw data of high quality is to be prepared. As a saying goes, if you have no hand, you cannot make a fist. Therefore, to start, we should fully understand the research programs, as different research objectives require different precision degrees of segmentation. For example, anatomic teaching asks for segmenting adjacent tissues as much as possible, while the reconstruction precision degree of the brain visual operation project is higher than that of the orthopedics visual operation project. Then, we should fully understand the imaging features of all kinds of imaging devices, parameter conditions that affect imaging precision and how to choose suitable imaging mode according to the research objective, in order to go ahead with the succeeding image segmentation. For example, to perfuse the vessels of human body specimen in advance can make easy blood vessel segmentation; regular dyeing of tissue pathological slices or the immunohistochemical staining makes easy image segmentation of calibration structure; high scanning voltage of CT can improve the accuracy of the skeleton segmentation. Finally, we should frequently communicate with the section offices and researchers concerned in order to save resources and obtain the raw data of high quality.

Secondly, we should be familiar with the structure to be segmented. Reading slices based on the images require us to bear them in mind in advance. To start, before we segment anatomical structures, we need to review all the relating anatomical knowledge and literature, to learn their anatomical features and variations, to carefully observe anatomical specimen, and to conduct entity anatomy if possible. Then, by every means, we need to carefully observe the volume database to be segmented and to track the changes of anatomical structures layer by layer, in order to briefly segment the volume database in our mind before we start the work in practice. We should notice that the geometrical shapes of the anatomical structures are different, so that the fracture surfaces easily to be observed are different. For example, the cord-like cruciate ligaments of the knee joint are easier to be observed and segmented on the sagittal section than on the coronal plane and the cross section.

Thirdly, it is necessary to choose the suitable software or algorithm for medical image segmentation. As the old saying goes, good tools are prerequisite to the successful execution of a job. It is essential to consider how to choose segmentation algorithm or segmentation software for a particular task of segmentation when conducting medical image segmentation.

In brief, all the segmentation algorithms should be conducted by employing some features of the segmentation object, such as grayscale, color, texture, shape, and so on. Therefore, it is necessary to understand the principles of segmentation tools, to analyze the image's characteristics of the tissue to be segmented, and to select the appropriate tool for image segmentation.

Undoubtedly, it would get twofold results with half the effort if there was an appropriate automatic segmentation algorithm to accomplish segmentation. However, in many cases, it cannot meet the requirement of accuracy of segmentation by solely relying on the automatic segmentation methods. Hence, interactive segmentation method, in which users take part, has become a closely watched development direction. On one hand, ideal software for interactive medical image segmentation should provide the basic segmentation tools and flexible interactive platform; on the other hand, it should offer a variety of efficient segmentation tools available to be selected flexibly. Unfortunately, currently there are few softwares for interactive medical image segmentation available for medical researchers lacking engineering background to use, among which Mimics, with a friendly software interface, is easy to use and of good interactivity and can meet the general requirements for medical image segmentation, although the segmentation algorithm it provides is not exhaustive.

Finally, 3D segmentation methods should be applied to the segmentation of volume dataset. The objects of medical image segmentation are mostly volume dataset. There are two kinds of segmentation of volume dataset: one is conducting segmentation on every 2D image layer by layer, and the other is conducting 3D segmentation by using the correlation between layers. Making full use of the correlation between layers can accelerate the speed and improve the accuracy of segmentation.

6.1.2 Methods of Medical Image Segmentation

Technologies such as computer tomography (CT), magnetic resonance imaging (MRI), ultrasound imaging (UI), etc., have been widely applied to various medical links such as medical diagnosis, preoperative planning, treatment, postoperative monitoring, etc. It is the key point of medical image segmentation to separate the region of interest (ROI) from the image. Because of the complexity of human body's anatomic tissue, the irregularity of shapes of tissues and organs, and the differences among individuals, general methods of image segmentation do not provide satisfactory results for medical image segmentation.

Based on Hounsfield value, gray value, and RGB component value, many authors put forward a number of segmentation methods, mainly including threshold segmentation method, region growing method, and methods combining specific theoretical tools, such as pattern recognition method, artificial neural network method, method based on fuzzy segmentation, method of wavelet transform, evolutionary algorithm, and so on. Segmentation method of color image is an expansion of grayscale image segmentation method from one-dimensional matrix to three-dimensional matrix. In the following, it is a sketch of grayscale image segmentation method.

Threshold segmentation method is a method that transforms grayscale image into binary image so as to achieve the purpose of segmentation. It is a simple but quite effective method, especially when there is huge contrast of intensity between different objects or structures, it can receive a better effect. This method is usually interactive, and generally it can be employed as the first step of the procedure of a series of image processing. Its main limitation lies in which the simplest form of threshold value method can only produce a binary image to distinguish two different classes. Besides, it only takes into account the value of the pixel itself, and usually do not consider the spatial characteristics of the image; thus it is very sensitive to noise. For its shortcomings, many updated algorithms of the classic threshold value method have been proposed. Threshold segmentation does well for the effect of CT image, and it boasts easy algorithm and fast calculation. However, if selecting threshold value, the user needs to make a judgment based on his experience or adjust threshold value after several tentative segmentations until achieving a satisfactory result.

Region growing method is a method which, on the basis of predefined criteria, extracts connected region in images. These criteria can be information of grayscale, or the boundary of image, or the combination of the two. Just as threshold value method, region growing method is generally not used alone but used in a series of processing procedure, especially used to describe small and simple tissues such as tumors, wounds, and so on. Its main drawback is that each region needing to be extracted must be given an artificial seed point; thus corresponding number of seeds should be given to the multiple regions. This method is also very sensitive to noise, which can create a shape of aperture and even a discontinuous region. Instead, partial and numerous influences will connect the originally separated regions. To diminish these drawbacks, region growing method in a fuzzy classification and other methods emerge at the right moment.

Pattern recognition method can be further divided into classifier method and clustering method. Classifier method is a statistical pattern recognition method, which is used to distinguish characteristic space (e.g., grayscale histogram) that derives from the known marked image data. It is a kind of pattern recognition method with supervision. Compared to threshold value method, it has a higher computational efficiency in distinguishing multi-region images. Its disadvantage resides in the need to obtain the training data by human-computer interactive method. Moreover, if the same training sample is used to analyze a large number of biological images, it may lead to inaccurate results due to taking no consideration into anatomical and physical properties of different objects. The fundamental principles of clustering method are large identical with that of classifier method except that it does not require training data. It is a kind of pattern recognition method without supervision. In order to make up for the missing training data, clustering method repeatedly does two pieces of work: segmenting image and depicting the characteristics of each class, so as to achieve the goal of segmentation by using existing data to train themselves. Like classifier method, clustering method does not consider spatial modeling; hence it is rather sensitive to noise and nonhomogeneous grayscale. However, such a shorting speeds up the calculation. Because there exists the ambiguity in medical images by nature (e.g., the ambiguity of CT image with identical tissue's grayscale value, the ambiguity of edge and shape triggered by volume effect, and the image's uncertainty caused by motion artifacts), it is better to adopt fuzzy theory, which has a good ability to describe the uncertainty of image, when employing clustering method.

Artificial neural network (ANN) is a massively parallel continuously processing system. It possesses signal processing capabilities that simulate humans with analog of human, and it is adept at solving problems of pattern classification in the field of pattern recognition, while the problem of medical image segmentation is how to classify and mark each anatomical tissue in images. ANN is mainly featured by the ability to learn from examples and summarize what it has learned by using feed-forward networks, by the robustness for stochastic noise and by the fault-tolerant capabilities and capabilities of optimum search. Therefore, when performing image segmentation by using other methods, the adoption of ANN technology can solve problems such as noise, inhomogeneity of tissue, variability of biomorph, and so on. However, when using a neural network method, the spatial information can be easily contained in the process of classification due to numerous interactive connections in the network. Currently, a prominent feature of the application of ANN technology is its combination with fuzzy technology, which forms a fuzzy neural network system. Built on the basis of fuzzy set theory, fuzzy technology can better deal with inherent ambiguity of three-dimensional medical images, and it is not sensitive to noise. Fuzzy segmentation technologies principally include fuzzy threshold value, fuzzy clustering, and fuzzy edge detection. In recent years, fuzzy clustering technology, especially fuzzy C-means (FCM)

clustering technology, has achieved a wide range of applications. It is propitious to the solution of the uncertainty and fuzziness in medical images.

Wavelet transform with zooming characteristics at low- and high-frequency analysis has been widely used in medical image segmentation. The ideas of using wavelet to conduct medical image threshold segmentation are to use a binary wavelet transform to discompose histogram of image into wavelet coefficients at different levels and to select an appropriate numerical value of threshold according to the given segmentation criteria. The entire process progresses from coarsely to finely, which is strictly controlled by scale. If the segmentation is not desired, the wavelet coefficients of histogram in fine subspace will be employed to refine image segmentation step by step.

The fundamental idea of evolutionary algorithms is built on random, iteration, and evolution based on natural selection and the principles of population genetics. It adopts a strategy of non-ergodic optimization search, which is simple, suitable for parallel processing, of robustness, and of broad applicability. Evolutionary algorithms are good at global search, but in lack of capability of local search, thus they are often applied to medical image segmentation combined with other algorithms.

6.2 Image Segmentation Method in the Study of Digital Human

In terms of image segmentation, Chinese digital human color tomographic images are featured by complex adjacency, similar color, and discontinuous edge. On the same section, bone, periosteum, ligaments, muscles, nerves, and blood vessels are adjacent to each other; the color of the bone cortex is similar to that of the periosteum, ligaments, and muscle tendons, the color of muscle is similar to that of red marrow, and nerve's color is similar surrounding fibrous tissue's color. Colors are connected among different tissues; thus there is no color edge in a real sense, and it is necessary to rely on fiber orientation and change between the upper and lower layer when judging the edges. Such features lead to the fact that currently the result of computer automatic segmentation cannot reach the desired edge which anatomists perceive through eyes and with a combination of professional knowledge, and the result needs tremendous manual correction after segmentation.

With respect to Chinese Digital Human's data sets, Zhang Kun and other scholars proposed a segmentation method which combines a low-level segmentation method based on Regional Vector Confidence Connected Method and a high-level segmentation based on Boundary's Level Set. It maintains the smoothness of the boundary, while the semiautomatic segmentation method not only effectively integrates with medical background of medical experts but also improves the speed of segmentation processing. Song Tao put forward a three-dimensional segmentation method on the basis of the theory of fuzzy connectedness. In the intersection between tissue's edge and other tissue, the accuracy of segmentation is relatively low. Such a segmentation algorithm itself is an iterative process; hence the speed of segmentation is comparatively slow. Zheng Leibin employs an improved color structure code (CSC) segmentation algorithm to segment the color slices image of Chinese Virtual Human's (VCH) data set. It obtains a preferable segmentation of tissues that have consistent color or obvious boundaries, but it results in an over segmentation of tissues with a wider range of colors. Meanwhile, it should be pointed out that it is impossible to reach perfect segmentation without experts' guidance. In conclusion, these digital human's color tomographic image segmentation methods can be applied to segmentation experiments of individual tissue and organ, but they cannot be applied to the segmentation of all tissues on the same fault.

Su Xiuyun put forward a topical clustering segmentation method of Chinese digital human's continuous tomographic image. First of all, it uses knockout filter of Photoshop and the powerful function of masks to extract the target region interactively. Then, in MATLAB it uses the morphology to cope with functions and edge detection operators and extract smooth contour line accurately. Finally, it completes the segmentation and classification of bone, muscle, organs, large blood vessels, nerves, etc. With accurate location and relatively smoothness, the extracted contour line retains the precise details.

References

1. Birkfellner W. Applied medical image processing: a basic course. Boca Raton: CRC Press; 2015.
2. Xiuyun S, Liu S. Clinical mimics software tutorial. Bejing: People's Military Medical Press; 2011.
3. Xiuyun S, Guoxian P. A local clustering segmenting method for anatomical cross-sectional image of Chinese digital human. Acta Anat Sin. 2007;4:494–7.
4. Xiuyun S, Guoxian P, Bin Y, Yanling H, Jin L, Qian H, Xu L, Yuanzhi Z. Landmark-based automatic registration of serial cross-sectional images of Chinese digital human using Photoshop and Matlab software. J South Med Univ. 2007;27(12):1884–7.

Y. Z. Zhang

1 Three-Dimensional (3D) Reconstruction Technique Based on Sequence Images

1.1 Overview of a 3D Reconstruction Technology

3D reconstruction of medical image sequences is surface reconstruction and simplification of datum. In order to understand and study the internal structure and changes in the relevant part of the body or organism, people use the analysis and synthesis methods. The decomposition process is a cluster of equally spaced parallel planes, and the relevant part of the body was cut into thin slices, about slicing it down into a sequence. By observing every slice, one can understand its internal structure and change. Synthesis process is observed with each slice, which will result in superimposing together in order to form the original form of the relevant part of the structure of space, which is the original model from the slice sequence. Slice of the decomposition process can be physiological slice, or CT scanning images, and MR images.

Boundary extraction is an important means of data collection, and manifestations slice image is a very complicated structure. It is necessary to distinguish the different parts, the boundaries of the regions mapped out, that is to say, the image segmentation and edge detection to be made, can be used in image processing-related methods (such as threshold method, insect with law, etc.), but for the special nature of the medical image, the necessary human-computer interaction is essential. Image segmentation and edge detection purpose is to establish the boundary line in polygons for each area slice image or collect coordinate information from each vertex boundary line on the image. Sliced as hidden in the interior of the border acquisition and measurement provided for convenience, that is the necessary to prepare a 3D reconstruction.

Slice positioning required the images slice by slice relative position as overlapping them so that no deviation would occur. The method can be divided into hard slice location and soft location. The hard location uses slice image positioning coordinates of a reference point, when the two upper and lower images overlap as long as the reference point alignment can coincide; the soft location is in case of hard positioning element method to take into law. On the basis of integrity and continuity of biological tissue, adjacent sections of the biological structure should be consistent, when sliced thin, the adjacent sections of the image should be basically the same. The main method has characteristics of soft positioning point, regional overlap method, two-step positioning method, and flashing method.

Two-location method is to combine the feature point method and regional overlap method and methods used by the feature point method for coarse positioning, with regional overlap method for precise positioning, to improve the speed and positioning accuracy. Alternately flashing display method is performed by alternating adjacent image positioning method. The two adjacent slice images are alternately displayed on the computer screen. Wherein a still, another one can be used for translation, rotation changes, then produce a feeling of visual motion picture, take this motor and sensory relative position of the two images to achieve the most hours should be the selected location.

Flashing alternately display method is through the adjacent image for positioning method. One of the images is static, and another may change as translation, rotation, then visually produce a feeling of images in sports. The relative location should be selected as feeling the minimum movements of these two images.

Y. Z. Zhang
The Affiliated Hospital of Inner Mongolia Medical University,
Hohhot, China

1.2   Spiral CT Reconstruction Technique

Since the early 1970s, with the rapid development of micro-electronics and computer technology, CT equipment has also been developed and improved. Modern CT equipment is radiation diagnostics, clinical medicine, biomedical engineering, computer, and microelectric with a combination of many disciplines, such as learning. Both trends have advanced on the human body, i.e., slip ring scanning technology and high-resolution scanning technology. The slip ring scanning technology has triggered a rapid scan and spiral CT scanning technology. Spiral CT scanning has the speed, seamless, and makes it easy to carry out a variety of ways, such as image reconstruction from different angles and so on. In recent years, due to advances in technology, the use of computer software and fast arithmetic processing technology continues to develop, while many medical imaging are undertaking a comprehensive process. The situation can easily display the anatomy and other aspects. Spiral CT scanning is to rely on a combination of continuous operation and the continuous movement of the body axis of the X-ray tube, in a very short time to complete multi-data collection, resulting in a volume scanning resolution with good body axis direction. 3D images can be displayed through the "multi-phase scanning method," "volume perspective," "maximum intensity projection," etc., wherein the multiphase scanning is the surface shape of the object, a collection of 3D polygon display, because it to the surface of the object as the object does not have an internal structure of the data, it cannot be an internal perspective. Volume perspective due to the internal structure of the object can be displayed, it can be cut out or an internal perspective to observe any section of the line, but also to add false color, which can more accurately show the anatomy. Maximum intensity projection is a high-resolution method; while maintaining the original CT values, you can get a higher 3D image. However, the current reconstruction of CT images can be obtained, although a high-resolution display, but cannot export to some other interface formats such as IGS export and CAD design.

1.3   Amira Software

Amira is a 3D data visualization, analysis, and modeling system. It allows you to visualize scientific data sets from various application areas, e.g., medicine, biology, biochemistry, microscopy, biomed, and bioengineering. 3D data can be quickly explored, analyzed, compared, and quantified. 3D objects can be represented as image volumes or geometrical surfaces and grids suitable for numerical simulations, notably as triangular surface and volumetric tetrahedral grids. Amira provides methods to generate such grids from voxel data representing an image volume, and it includes a general-purpose interactive 3D viewer. Amira is a powerful, multi-faceted software platform for visualizing, manipulating, and understanding life science and biomedical data coming from all types of sources and modalities. Initially known and widely used as the 3D visualization tool of choice in microscopy and biomed research, Amira has become a more and more sophisticated product, delivering powerful visualization and analysis capabilities in all visualization and simulation fields in life science.

1.3.1   Overview

Amira is a modular and object-oriented software system. Its basic system components are modules and data objects. Modules are used to visualize data objects or to perform some computational operations on them. The components are represented by little icons in the Pool. Icons are connected by lines indicating processing dependencies between the components, i.e., of which modules are to be applied to data objects. Alternatively, modules and data objects can be displayed in a tree view Explorer. Modules from data objects of specific types are created automatically from file input data when reading or as output of module computations. Modules matching an existing data object are created as instances of particular module types via a context-sensitive popup menu. Networks can be created with a minimal amount of user interaction. Parameters of data objects and modules can be modified in Amira's interaction area. For some data objects such as surfaces or color maps, there are special-purpose interactive editors that allow the user to modify the objects. All Amira components can be controlled via a Tcl command interface. Commands can be read from a script file or issued manually in a separate console window. The biggest part of the screen is occupied by a 3D graphics window. Additional 3D views can be created if necessary. Amira is based on the latest release of Open Inventor from Mercury. In addition, several modules apply direct OpenGL rendering to achieve special rendering effects or to maximize performance. In total, there are more than 270 data object and module types. They allow the system to be used for a broad range of applications. Scripting can be used for customization and automation. User-defined extensions are facilitated by the Amira developer version.

1.3.2   Features Overview

Amira provides a large number of data and module types allowing you to visualize, analyze, and model various kinds of 3D data. The Amira framework is ideal to integrate the data from multiple sources into a single environment. This section summarizes the main features of Amira software suite. For more complete information, you may browse indexes for data types, file formats, and modules in the Reference Guide. This is accessible from the home page of the online help browser (Fig. 3.1).

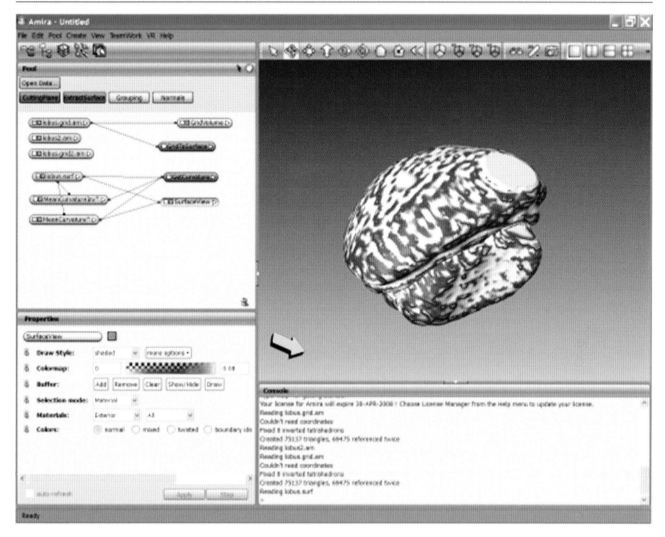

Fig. 3.1 Data objects and modules represented

Amira can load directly different types of data, including:

- 2D and 3D image and volume data
- Geometric models such as point sets, line sets, surfaces, grids
- Numerical simulation data
- Time series and animations

All visualization techniques can be arbitrarily combined to produce a single scene. Moreover, multiple data sets can be visualized simultaneously, either in several viewer windows or in a common one. Thus you can display single or multiple data sets in a single or multiple viewer windows and navigate freely around or through those objects. A built-in spatial transformation editor makes it easy to register data sets with respect to each other or to deal with different coordinate systems. Automatic registration of volume or geometric data is also possible. Direct interaction with the 3D scene allows you to quickly control regions of interest, slices,

probes, and more. Combinations of data sets, representation, and processing features can be defined with minimal user interaction for simple or complex tasks. You can quickly explore 3D images looking at single or multiple orthographic or oblique sections. Multiple data sets can be superimposed on slices, or displayed as height fields. You can cut away parts of your data to uncover hidden regions. Curved or cylinder slices are also available.

One of the most intuitive and most powerful techniques for visualizing 3D image data is direct volume rendering. Light emission and light absorption parameters are assigned to each point of the volume. Simulating the transmission of light through the volume makes it possible to display your data from any view direction without constructing intermediate polygonal models. By exploiting modern graphics hardware, Amira is able to perform direct volume rendering in real time, even on very large data when using the Very Large Data Option. Thus volume rendering can instantly highlight relevant features of your data. Volume-rendered images can be combined with any type of polygonal display. This improves the usefulness of this technique significantly. Moreover, multiple data sets can be volume rendered simultaneously—a unique feature of Amira. Transfer functions with different characteristics required for direct volume rendering can be either generated automatically or edited interactively using an intuitive colormap editor.

Isosurfaces are most commonly used for analyzing arbitrary scalar fields sampled on discrete grids. Applied to 3D images, the method provides a very quick, yet sometimes sufficient method for reconstructing polygonal surface models. Beside standard algorithms, Amira provides an improved method, which generates significantly fewer triangles with very little computational overhead. In this way, large 3D data sets can be displayed interactively even on smaller desktop graphics computers.

Image segmentation means assigning labels to image voxels that identify and separate objects in a 3D image. Amira offers a large set of segmentation tools, ranging from purely manual to fully automatic: brush (painting), lasso (contouring), magic wand (region growing), thresholding, intelligent scissors, contour fitting (snakes), contour interpolation and extrapolation, wrapping, smoothing and de-noising filters, morphological filters for erosion, dilation, opening and closing operations, connected component analysis, images correlation, objects separation and filtering, etc.

Surface generation is able to create a corresponding polygonal surface model. The surface may have non-manifold topology if there are locations where three or more regions join. Even in this case, the polygonal surface model is guaranteed to be topologically correct, i.e., free of self-intersections. Fractional weights that are automatically generated during segmentation allow the system to produce optionally smooth boundary interfaces. By this way, realistic high-quality models can be obtained, even if the underlying image data are of low resolution or contain severe noise artifacts. Making use of innovative acceleration techniques, surface reconstruction can be performed very quickly. Moreover, the algorithm is robust and fail-safe.

Surface simplification is another prominent feature of Amira. It can be used to reduce the number of triangles in an arbitrary surface model according to a user-defined value. Thus, models of finite-element grids, suitable for being processed on low-end machines, can be generated. The underlying simplification algorithm is one of the most elaborate ones available. It is able to preserve topological correctness, i.e., self-intersections commonly produced by other methods are avoided. In addition, the quality of the resulting mesh, according to measures common in finite element analysis, can be controlled. For example, triangles with long edges or triangles with bad aspect ratio can be suppressed.

Multiple data sets can be combined to compare images of different objects or images of an object recorded at different times or with different imaging modalities such as X-ray CT and MRI. In addition, fusion of multimodal data by arbitrary arithmetic operations can be performed to increase the amount of information and accuracy in the models. Amira allows manual registration through interactive manipulators, automatic rigid or nonrigid registration through landmarks, and automatic registration using iterative optimization algorithms.

1.3.3 Skeleton Option

All image data should be as stacks of numbered 2D images. The topmost slice should have the lowest number. File formats recognized by Amira can be found in the File Formats section of the user's guide. A good choice is TIFF because it provides lossless compression and is readable on many different systems. You should also know the position in 3D of the lower left front corner of the brick you're going to import and the voxel size.

Choose File/Open Data. A File Dialog pops up. You can now select all of the 2D images comprising the brick. After you press Load, another dialog pops up (Fig. 3.2).

Enter the position and the voxel size of your block. After you press OK, the files are loaded into one block. A new green icon will appear in the Pool. Select it and select File/Save Data As... to store it on disk. Name it 1ta.am. In this way you should proceed with all of your data.

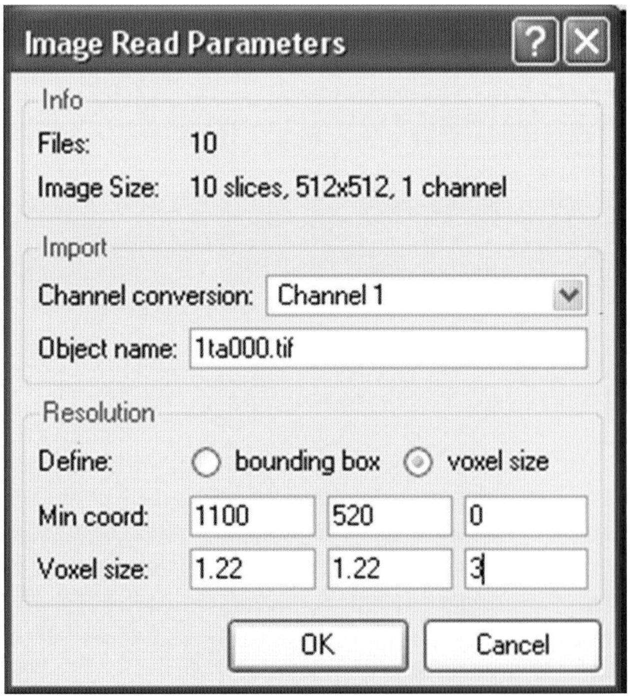

Fig. 3.2 Import your image data

After importing your data, you should copy the files to another directory where all the processing will be done. In this way the original data is not touched and you can revert back to it if something goes wrong.

Amira has a special data object to store links to files on disk and arrange them in 3D. It is called Mosaic.

- Create a Mosaic by selecting Mosaic from the Create/ Skeleton menu of the Amira main window.

A green icon appears. When you select it you see that it contains no bricks. The buttons below the info line are used to add data objects.

- Press the add files button.
- Select the files, e.g., 1ta.am, 1tb.am, 2ta.am, and 2tb.am, in the directory AMIRA ROOT/data/tutorials/skeleton. You can select multiple files at once by clicking on the first one and shift clicking on the last one.
- Press Load.

The selected files are added to the Mosaic. The Info port shows the overall number of the bricks added up to now. You can visualize the bricks with the DisplayMosaic module.

- Create a DisplayMosaic module by right clicking on the Mosaic and selecting Skeleton/DisplayMosaic from the context menu.
- Select the yellow DisplayMosaic icon and switch the highlighted brick by dragging the slider in the interaction area.
- Save the Mosaic.

1.4   Mimics Software

Mimics interfaces between scanner data (CT, MRI, technical scanner, etc.) and rapid prototyping, STL file format, CAD, and finite element analysis. The Mimics software is an image processing package with 3D visualization functions that interfaces with all common scanner formats. Additional modules provide the interface toward rapid prototyping using STL or direct layer formats with support. Alternatively, an interface to CAD (design of custom-made prosthesis and new product lines based on image data) or to finite element meshes is available. Materialise' interactive medical image control system (MIMICS) is an interactive tool for the visualization and segmentation of CT images as well as MR images and 3D rendering of objects. Therefore, in the medical field, Mimics can be used for diagnostic, operation planning, or rehearsal purposes. A very flexible interface to rapid

prototyping systems is included for building distinctive segmentation objects. The software enables the user to control and correct the segmentation of CT scans and MRI scans. For instance, image artifacts coming from metal implants can easily be removed. The object(s) to be visualized and/or produced can be defined exactly by medical staff. No technical knowledge is needed for creating on-screen 3D visualizations of medical objects (a cranium, pelvis, etc.) Separate software is available to define and calculate the necessary data to build the medical object(s) created within Mimics on all rapid prototyping systems. The interface created to process the images provides several segmentation and visualization tools (Fig. 3.3).

Mimics has a highly integrated and friendly interface of the 3D image editing and processing software, and it can quickly scan data into a complete 3D CAD, FEA (finite element analysis), the RP (rapid prototyping) data format, etc. Data input Mimics input 2D non-compressed package files such as CT and MRI scan data and also provide user-defined input module; input module reads the data on the disk or magnetic medium, conveys to Materialise-specific file format, retains all the information for further processing, has convenient operation, and guides customers to input operation. The software can merge multiple images in order to generate an object, the real-time images into different objects, and the choice of different images to generate objects (Fig. 3.4).

Display Mimics displays images in various ways, each a display method with relevant information and the window is divided into three views: the original axial views, coronal generated using slice data and sagittal views. Mimics has a variety of display functions such as contrast enhancement, drag, zoom, rotate, etc., and coloring can strengthen the details of soft tissue bone tissue showed in Mimics, a display image series or tracking image and display its position in the axis view.

3D 3D information Mimics provides a flexible interface, fast displaying a particular area of the 3D model, so you can set the resolution, the filtering, and the parameters, such as height, width, quantity, surface, etc., Mimics can be in any one window display 3D image, and the corresponding functions, such as real-time rotation, drag, amplification, and transparent processing, with OpenGL function can strengthen the reconstruction of the expressive force to provide high quality.

Slice Two heavy stratification tools are optional, double layer and output layer object tools online. Online stratification can show a local peace with image and display the user-defined

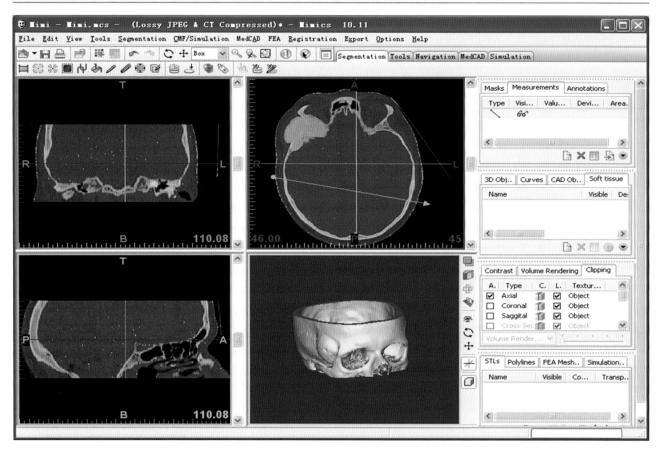

Fig. 3.3 Interface of Mimics

axis, and the user can custom a few line layer in the Mimics object. Output layer object tool is an easy-to-use interface, allowing output-layered Mimics object, any direction along the user to specify and view shows.

Measure Point to point can be done in the Mimics 3D or 2D view any point to point in the distance.

Contour and Gray Value Measurement Profile along the user-defined line shows the outline of strengthening line (based on gray level), four ways available accurate calculating gray scale, threshold method, four, four distance measurements, and the method is an ideal choice to CT technician.

Density Measurement Of ellipse and rectangle area density measurement, according to gray scale and density and the standard deviation, all the results are stored in the object file and listed in the object management.

Label Tag Label tag is used to add the information in the 3D model, the label can be placed in any direction, any view,

words and moving average, freedom, and only is the output with the a mask, only is restricted in a horizontal or vertical direction.

Output Report The report output enhances print function to print complete information of the object, 3D images, and all of the axial and heavy slice images can be printed in any view and stored as a BMP and JPEG format and also can output the BMP or JPEG1:1 format.

Project Management Project management function provides data file management, interface (such as partition mask, 3D reconstruction, contour, and so on), and their properties.

Segmentation Segmentation object function is used to highlight areas. Mimics can define and at the same time deal with multiple different partitions and mask. Setting up and modifying the mask need the following: (1) threshold segmentation, (2) the region growing, (3) the editor, (4, 5) dynamic regions which form adjustment, (6) Boolean operations, (7) volume filling, and (8) contour filling volume.

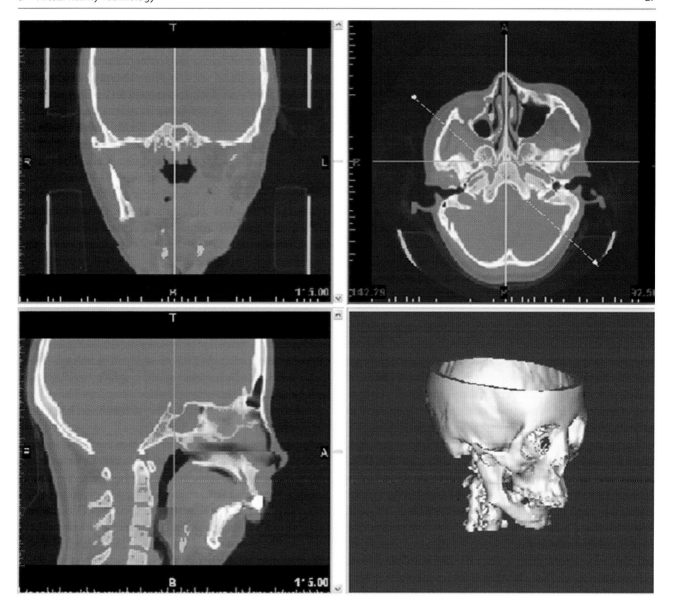

Fig. 3.4 Four view windows of Mimics

The basic modules are as follows (Fig. 3.5).

Mimics can input various types of CT, MRI scan data, 3D reconstruction, output, transformation, surface meshing, meshing and other processing, and output to the following modules (Figs. 3.6, 3.7, 3.8, and 3.9).

Finite Element Analysis Module One can scan image output to the appropriate file format after finite element analysis and the analysis of fluid dynamics. Users can be calculated according to the scanning images of 3D objects, also for finite element analysis for surface triangular mesh. The reconstruction of FEA module function could ensure the best input for FEA software pretreatment. In pretreatment, the conversion of surface triangular mesh body grid after the body of the grid can be input into the Mimics again. According to the scanning image of Hounsfield sets or project segmentation part, material can be assigned to the grid.

Rapid Prototyping Slice Module RP slice module provides an interface to rapid prototyping systems via sliced files with patented support structure generation. The perforated support structures are generated in no time and use less material. Supported formats are common layer interface files (*.cli), 3D systems layer interface files (*.sli), and 3D systems contour files (*.slc). To scan images of the model using high order interpolation (plane) within two elements, a linear

Fig. 3.5 Modules of Mimics

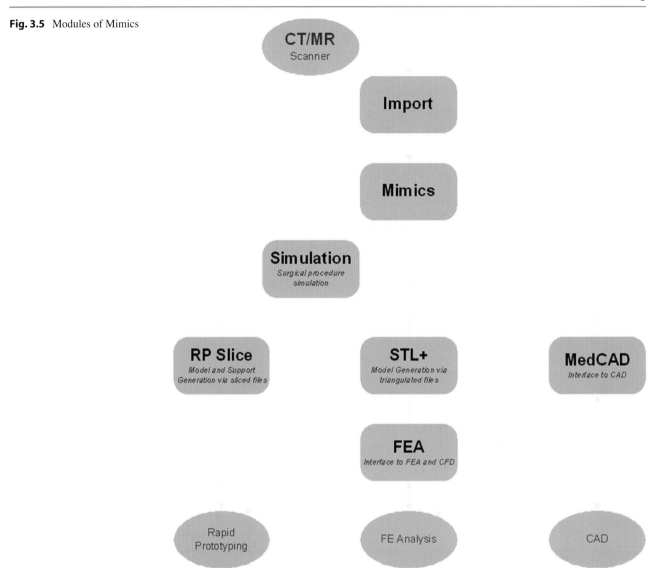

equation and algorithm can produce a perfect surface. Rapid prototyping slicing module supports color 3D laser rapid prototype manufacturing technology: as long as you give to the accuracy of the tumor, tooth and tooth root, neural network can be RP model of high-quality display. The patient's information users can use a fixed color labels show. This module allows the user to calculate contour file and from the contour to calculate generation support.

Surgical Simulation Module Surgical simulation module is a surgery simulation application platform, available anthropometric analysis template for details of data analysis. The osteotomy and separated operation and simulation, implanting or explaining the process of the implant, are very intuitive and simple.

STL + Module STL + module provide the triangle format of interface options: binary STL, ASCII STL, DXF, VRML 2.0, and the PLY. Using the STL+ module, on the surface of the object should be chosen to generate triangular mesh. The number of triangular mesh decides the quality of the refactoring: the more triangular mesh, the higher the quality. The disadvantage is that the more triangular mesh, the more need of memory. STL + module provide a powerful tool to reduce a lot of triangular mesh. STL + module through triangulation file format in Mimics and interaction between RP technology and the double linear and middle plane interpolation algorithm can guarantee the accuracy of rapid prototyping model finally.

Med-CAD Module Med-CAD Module is the bridge between medical image data and CAD, through two-way

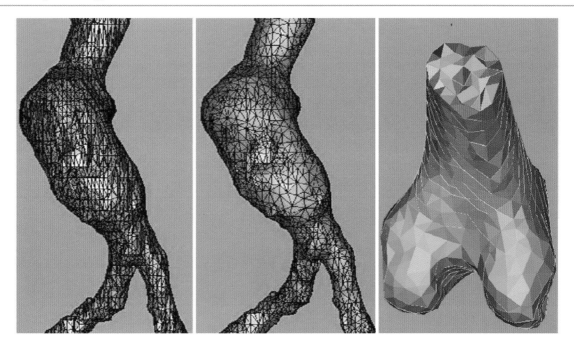

Fig. 3.6 Finite element analysis

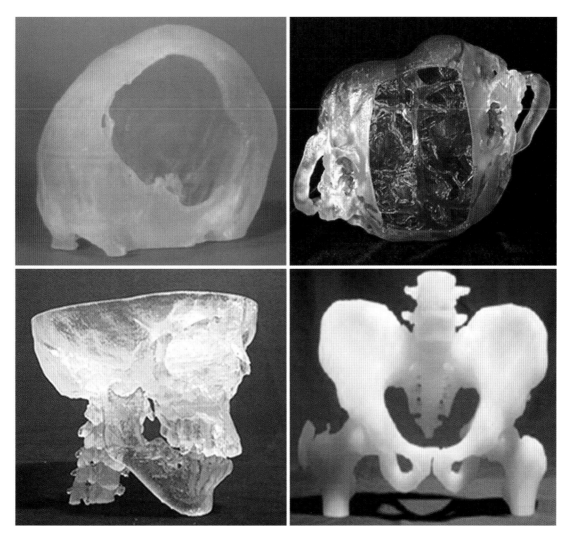

Fig. 3.7 Rapid prototyping models

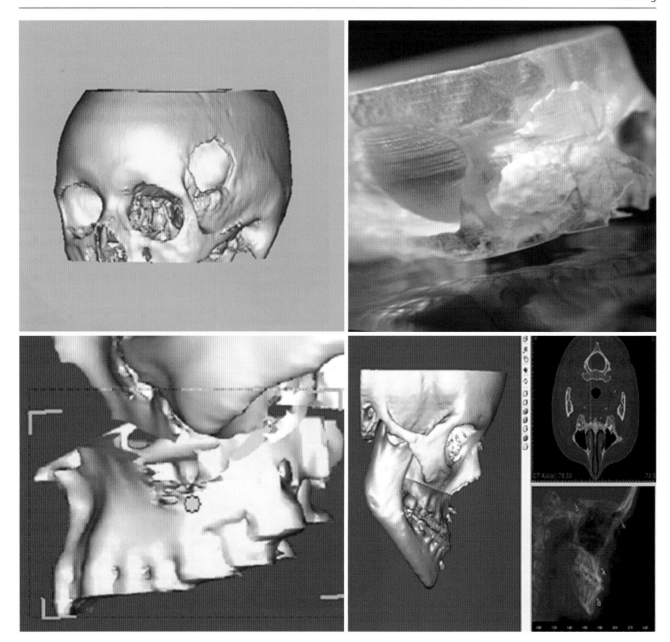

Fig. 3.8 Surgical cases (skull defect and mandibular simulation)

communication interaction pattern, which realizes the scan data and CAD data transformation.

Mimics FEA (Finite Element Analysis) This module can scan image output to the appropriate file format after finite element analysis and fluid dynamics analysis. Users can be calculated according to the scanning images of 3D objects, also for finite element analysis for surface triangular mesh. Reconstruction in the FEA module functions to ensure the best input for FEA software pretreatment.

1.5 3D Med Software

3D Med (3D Medical Image Processing and Analyzing System) is by the Department of Medical Imaging, Institute of Automation. Chinese academy of sciences based on MITK development of 3D Medical Image Processing and Analyzing System, due to the 3D Med purpose which is to form a scientific software, provides a more flexible framework, more powerful, easy-to-expand, and a friendly interface. 3D Med has the following characteristics: (1) supporting cross-platform, (2) strong scalability, and (3) easy to obtain (Fig. 3.10).

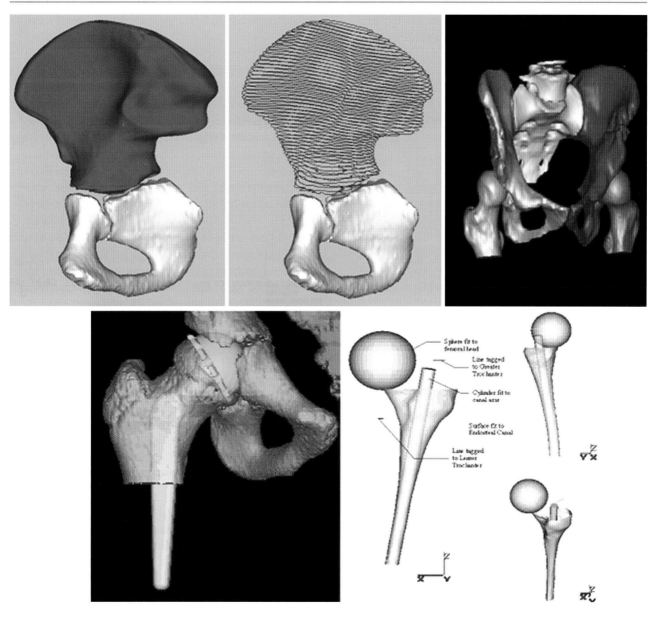

Fig. 3.9   3D reconstruction of skeleton

1.6   3D Slicer Software

3D Slicer software is produced by the Harvard Medical School Harvard Medical School affiliated with Brigham and Women's Hospital Surgical Planning Laboratory (Surgical Planning Lab) and Artificial Intelligence Laboratory at the Massachusetts Institute of Technology (determined by MIT Artificial Intelligence Lab). It is based on MRML (Medical Reality Modeling Language) language design; this is a description of the medical data sequence of various formats of 3D scene. 3D Slicer has the following functions: automatically importing the original data, semi-automatic image segmentation (extracted from the original data of interest structure), producing the integral structure of 3D surface model, 3D visualization and quantitative analysis, etc. (Fig. 3.11).

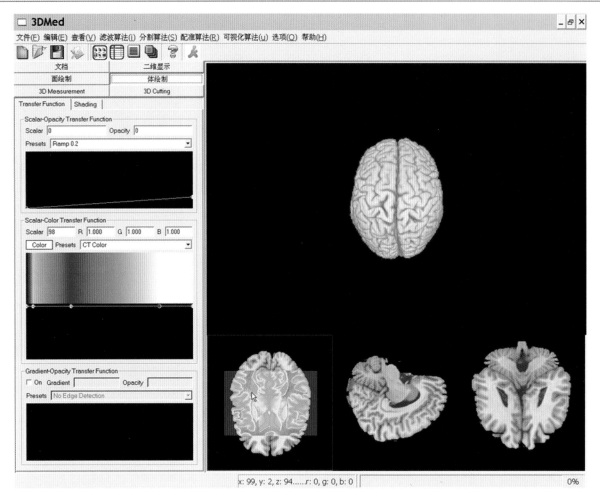

Fig. 3.10 The main interface of 3D Med

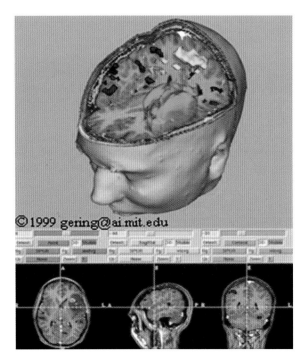

Fig. 3.11 The interface of 3D Slicer

2 Virtual Reality Modeling Language: VRML Profile

2.1 Overview

Virtual reality is a simulation of the real world; it can vividly describe the real environment and make people watching as immersive virtual environment interact with them. In the 1980s, many departments and organizations have been engaged in the research of virtual reality. NASA and the United States Department of Defense have organized a series of studies of virtual reality technology and obtained the encouraging results, which inspired people greater enthusiasm for virtual reality research as well as to the virtual reality technology. In 1984, NASA's Ames Research Center virtual planet detection laboratory organization developed for Mars, visual display of virtual environment, has been a success; the Mars rover back to input the data into the computer, for the ground researchers constructed 3D virtual environment on the surface of Mars. The research center in the subsequent virtual interactive environment workstation in the project has developed more than general sensing individual simulators and remote control equipment. As with many other disciplines, the development of related technologies of virtual reality plays a great role in promoting. The computer technology, the network technology, the rapid development of graphics technology, etc. make the virtual reality technology gain great progress. Into the 1990s, because of the development of 3D image technology, virtual reality has also made progress on the Internet, as the Internet 3D technology of VRML modeling language arises at the historic moment. VRML is a Virtual Reality Modeling Language and is a multimedia communication, and the Internet Virtual Reality is closely related to the new technology, which is used to describe a target object how to present on the Web. Like HTML, VRML can be explained by the browser. The VRML is not described as a page format, but as the layout of 3D environment and target. Its main features are 3D, interactive and dynamic, real time, etc. VRML is a term used to describe text information of 3D scene language, and it uses hierarchical modeling marshaling node, the basic element of VRML. The nodes include geometric modeling, lighting effects, viewpoint, the text, the basic dynamic effect, atomization, spatial modeling of material and material characteristics, etc. These nodes can be used to create a combination of 3D images, text, and voice of 3D objects page; this may be the basis of the virtual reality world online space in the future. The combination of VRML file by VRML nodes has layers complete scenario to describe the scene graph.

The characteristics of the objects in the scene graph mainly rely on the relationship between the structure and the node to the performance, its structure is a directed acyclic graph. Each node contains a series of attributes and types. By the diagram, one can see that VRML interaction and animation are driven by events. It can accept two event-driven: VRML scene from routing statements into the events and event directly by the external program interface written.

2.2 VRML Modeling

VRML provides a specification of virtual environment, combining the advantages of the existing 3D software scene description language. It has the basic elements, vertex, line, and plane definition, and coordinate transformation has scaling, rotation, and translation and has optimized data structure. The main function of VRML browser is read in VRML files and explain them into graphic images. VRML language has the basic objects: sphere, cone, cylinder, cube, and text, such as the basic object providing the convenience for creating a scene. VRML syntax is not complicated, but is more cumbersome, if you want to design the decoration of the

room, not only need to set up all kinds of equipment material but also need to set up the corresponding position, so the amount of code is considerable, and there are many to create VRML file model of the software, which can put the other 3D format file into VRML files, such as 3Ds Max, RAW, etc. But if using the software to complete 3D model is mapped in the various views by hand, time-consuming, laborious, truthful, and accurate enough, for those who need to use a large amount of data to accurately describe the structure, or a very irregular one, describing the object is difficult to precisely create by hand.

2.3 Virtual Reality Development Tools

VrmlPad is powerful and easy to use. VRML is a professional software, supporting VRML97 standard. Using VrmlPad to browse the VRML file editor, carry on the effective management of resource files, and provide a VRML file publishing wizard can help developers to write and publish their own VRML virtual reality. In addition, it provides plug-in functions and the VRML model can be easily created.

2.4 VRML Browser

VRML browser plug-in provides the interaction of the environment, which can carry on some simple 3D interactive control (such as translation, amplification, narrow, rotation, etc.). Due to lack of underlying control, VRML browsers usually can only provide 3D reconstruction, but cannot observe organs inside, which is not conducive to the doctor for a microscopic observation of the lesions and judgment. One can use VRML Script node, sensor node, combining with the JavaScript language, VRML 3D reconstruction of dynamic cutting, to enhance the VRML 3D reconstruction of dynamic control and interactivity.

References

1. Spitzer V, Ackerman MJ, Scherzinger AL, et al. The visible human male: a technical report. J Am Med Inform Assoc. 1996;3:118.
2. Ackerman MJ. The visible human project. J Biocommun. 1991;18:14.
3. Ackerman MJ, Spitzer VM, Scherzinger AL, et al. The visible human data set: an image resource for anatomical visualization. Medinfo. 1995;8:1195.
4. Chung MS, Kim SY. Three-dimesional image and virtual dissection program of the brain made of Korean cadaver. Yonsei Med J. 2000;41:299.

Finite Element Analysis (FEA) Technology

4

Yan Yabo

1 Introduction to Biomechanics

Biomechanics is a discipline to study the structure and function of biological systems including human, animals, plans, organs, and cells by means of applying mechanical methods. The terms "biomechanics" and "biomechanical" come from the ancient Greek words βίος and μηχανική, meaning life and mechanics, respectively. This word was created by Nikolai Bernstein. Biomechanics is a discipline to study the mechanical laws of biological tissues.

Biomechanics and engineering are closely related because the latter is always necessary to analyze biological systems in biomechanics. Some simple applications of Newton's laws and the material science are approximate to studies on mechanical laws in biological systems. Applied mechanics, including mechanics of continuous medium, mechanical analysis, structural analysis, dynamics, and kinematics analysis, play quite an important role in the study of biomechanics. However, biological systems are much more complex than artificial systems. Therefore, it is always necessary to introduce numerical methods of analysis in mechanical analysis of biological systems. In biomechanical analysis, we often need to use modeling, computational simulation, and mechanical testing.

The human skeleton system is comprised of single bones and connective tissues connecting the bones together so as to ensure that the body may make a variety of mechanical operations. Bone tissue is the most important part in the skeletal system and is biomechanically featured by high hardness. Bone tissue's features are dependent on its components which are mainly collagen matrix comprising minerals and collagen fibers as well as a variety of non-collagen proteins. The high hardness of bone tissue is applicable to the main functions it burdens: maintenance of the body's normal form; protection of intracranial, intrathoracic, and intrapelvic soft tissues; receiving bone marrow; and conduction of muscle contraction from the part of the body to another to complete motions. Bone tissue also serves as the body's ion storage warehouse, especially calcium ion; it also adjusts the composition of human extracellular fluid, especially the concentration of extracellular calcium ions. In addition, bone tissue is also a tissue capable of self-repair and reconstruction that may constantly reconstruct its shapes based on the burden of mechanical functions to ensure that human body may complete motions under optimal conditions.

Human skeleton mainly includes cortical bone and cancellous bone. Cortical bone is solid-cored tight structure and serves as part of the main cortical backbone and metaphysis shell. On histological level, cortical bone is mainly composed of bone cells (diameter 100–300 μm) and surrounding Haversian canal and simple straight bone. Cancellous bone is a hollow spongelike structure in which is filled with interconnected rodlike and platelike trabecular bones.

1.1 Application of FEA in Bone Biomechanics

FEM is a method to simulate, calculate, analyze, and predict a complicated entirety by decomposing it into finite elements. The main method of FEA is to divide a continuous object into finite simple elements and substitute and simulate a continuous elastic body with these idealized and simplified elements to calculate their displacement and stress distribution trends by mathematical methods for the purpose of obtaining their shapes and mechanical features; in short, it is to calculate the features of the entirety from simple elements by dividing the entirety into simple elements. Its basic process includes discrete the entirety, determining the element computation function, establishing the stiffness matrixes of elements and the entirety, solving and calculating the displacement and stress distribution, etc. As of today, FEA has been developed into the following basic steps: sample → 3D scanning → point cloud data → hook face establishment → shape optimization to 3D date modeling → model material assignment → simulation computation

Y. Yabo
Department of orthopaedics, Xijing Hospital, Airforce military medical university, Xi'an, China

and analysis; and the purpose of rapid prototyping and manufacturing may also be further obtained via reverse engineering technologies by means of computer-aided design (CAD).

1.1.1 Application of FEA in Spinal Researches

The establishment of finite element model (FEM) is the basis for FEA. With the development of imaging technology and computer technology, FEM established now is no longer just a re-rendering of structures, and it even includes related muscles. Jones et al. found that the FEMs assigned with properties of materials may also be used to simulate and compute the biomechanical properties of the whole spine [1]. Board et al. found, during spinal biomechanical simulation with FEM, that the impact of differences in ages on the spine morphology may also be taken into account in the impacts on the computation results [2]. Kallemeyn et al. established FEMs from C2 to C7 based on the specificity of each specimen, which may be used to calculate various biomechanical simulations of cervical spine [3]. Laville et al. established FEMs of lower cervical spine with experimental parameters reported in literatures and found that the torsion of lower cervical spine was closely related to the morphology [4]. As technology advances, spine FEM has been able to properly simulate and calculate biomechanical properties of the spine and provide valuable reference for clinical practice.

1.1.2 Application of FEA in Bone Joint Researches

With the development of artificial joint technology and application of FEA, FEA is also being applied to the design, optimization, and postoperative complication management of joint prostheses. Since some researchers firstly experimented to establish 3D FEM of proximal femur with CT-scanned data [5], a large number of 3D FEM-based analyses on the stress distribution of hip joint and characteristics of prosthesis have been reported in literatures. Brian et al. employed the 3D femoral FEMs prior to biological-type hip replacement to analyze and simulate changes in stress distribution and evaluate changes in bone-prosthesis interface in standing state, which showed well conformance to conventional mechanical experiment results [6]. Some researchers analyzed the impact of bone cements of different thicknesses on femoral stress distribution after replacement with FEA to explore the optimal consumption of bone cement in prosthesis replacement [7]. In recent years studies evaluating and optimizing hip prosthesis with FEA have been carried out one after another [8, 9]. Currently, FEA has become an essential means for design and application of prosthesis, prevention of complications, and many other similar studies.

1.1.3 Application of FEA in Design and Implantation of Prosthesis

By FEA, we may obtain a better understanding in terms of the properties of materials used for prosthesis and its design.

In the field of total hip replacement, Harrigan et al. [10] first reported stress analysis of cementless total hip replace-ment with 3D axisymmetric cylinder model. Reports show no significant changes occurred in surface longitudinal and medial distal end stress distributions of femur after cementless total hip displacement, the stresses at the internal point (i.e. contact of prosthesis shank and femur) and internal face of femur neck were significantly increased, and the proximal femur stresses reduced to 5–10% of the normal level. Proximal femur atrophy, thigh pain, stresses, etc. are conducted to distal femur directly via the prosthesis shank after cementless total hip replacement, resulting in significant reduction in proximal femur stresses, and they are related to uneven distribution of distal stress concentration. Experimental results show that the micro movement level of prosthesis-bone interface depends on the type of load rather than the prosthesis shape design and surface coating type. Micro movement of prosthesis-bone interface is more significant at torsion load than vertical load.

The individualized design of prosthesis is a trend in artificial joint replacement. A prosthesis designed based on the patient may change the irrational state that human body cannot be altered to accommodate the prosthesis. The high expense of 3D CT reconstruction limits its clinical application. However, its guidance significance to acetabular revision showed a good price-effective ratio. We need to combine FEM and 3D CT reconstruction technologies to make the proper judgment on whether an artificial hip replacement destroys the normal stress conduction and whether it obtains the best stress distribution after implantation of prosthesis. In addition, FEA is the priority method to establish objective indicators to guide doctors to choose the prosthesis fitting a patient the most. In short, since the introduction of FEA in biomechanics, it has obtained further improvement and development and there is a broader outlook in researches on artificial prosthesis.

2 Basic Concept and Method of FEA

3D-based digital models of all parts of the body are widely used, especially for the study of the biomechanical properties of the spine, some of which are difficult to study by mechanical experiments, for example, the study of internal force, stress, and strain of the vertebral body, in which the digital model has incomparable advantages upon physical models [11]. Results of digital simulation model of the spine can explain the inherent stress state of the spine, including the load distribution, reasons for injury, result of injury, and spinal aging behavior [12].

2.1 Development Process of FEA

In 1922, Richard Courant first proposed the method of FEA. However, due to limited computing capacity at that time, it is very laborious to solve a large number of linear equations unarmed, so this method is not widely used at the

Fig. 4.1 The principal of FEA is to break down complex problems into pieces

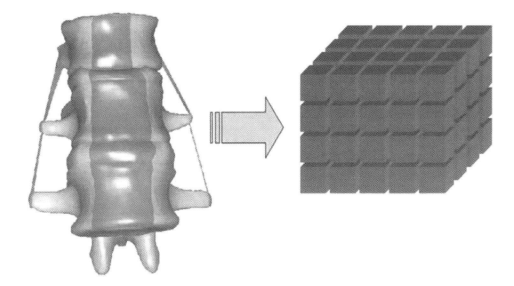

time. Until 1942, the advent of the computer starts the application and promotion of the method. In fact, in the early 1950s, John Argyris had used this method solving many problems, and published a series of papers, which laid the basis for the application of this method and recognized that computers play a very important role in the method. Although FEA had been widely used in engineering disciplines since the 1950s and 1960s, but until 1973, the method was first applied to the analysis of the human skeletal system. Then, FEA method gradually helps scientists to better understand the basic biomechanical properties of the human body. Up to now, several important reviews about the application of FEA method in orthopedics include Yoganandan et al. (1987) [13], Yoganandan et al. (1996) [14], Natarajan et al. (2004) [15], and Teo (2008) [16].

Like most of the numerical analysis methods, FEA method is to break down a very complex problem into hundred, thousand, or even million simple questions (as Fig. 4.1). Due to the significant improvement of computer speed and robustness and accuracy of modeling software, FEA method can solve extremely complex models. In 1965, one of the founders of Intel Corporation, Gordon Moore proposed the famous Moore's law, which is the computing capacities of computer that will double every 1–2 years, and halved its production costs (Fig. 4.2). In the past 40 years, Moore's law has been practiced all the time. For the enhancement of computing capacity of computer and the development of scientific computing software, FEM has become an important part of standard engineering analysis tool.

Finite element method, since the 1870s applied in thoracic, has become one of the key technologies in the field of computer-assisted applied orthopedic biomechanics [17]. This method is mainly used for the force analysis of simulation physiology, pathology, and implantation and fixation status of human body in the field of orthopedics [18, 19]. At present, most domestic and overseas scholars believe that FEA method is a reliable analysis method, which is an impor-

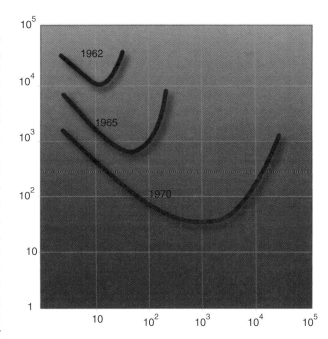

Fig. 4.2 Moore's law

tant tool in biomechanical research, and is valuable in the force analysis of simulation skeletal system [20]. Its application has been extended to reconstruction and simulation and biomechanical analysis of the spine, four limb bones and joints, and soft tissue and bone trabecular microstructure.

FEM application in orthopedic is focused on spinal research in the early stage, with the accumulation of FEM applications experience in orthopedic and the development of computer technology, now a 3D model has replaced the earlier 2D plane model, using nonhomogeneous anisotropic material simulation to replace the past homogeneous isotropic material simulation and developing from the simple stress analysis computing to simulation of bone tissue microstruc-

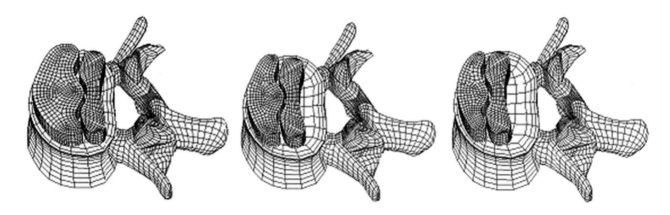

Fig. 4.3 Different finite element models with interbody fusion cages implanted into different positions

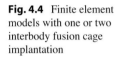

Fig. 4.4 Finite element models with one or two interbody fusion cage implantation

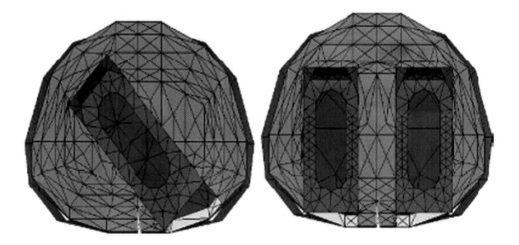

ture. Lee et al. [21] used the parametric method for evaluating the relationship between fusion cage implantation location and integration effect (Fig. 4.3). Changing the front and rear position of fusion cage, the change of axial stiffness, compressive stress, and endplate bulge of the model is not remarkable. The results suggest that in posterior lumbar interbody fusion, changing the position of fusion cage may not cause a significant impact on the biomechanics of the lumbar spine. Chiang et al. [22] studied the difference of using one or two fusion cages in the posterior lumbar interbody fusion of posterior lumbar interbody fusion (Fig. 4.4). The result showed that a fusion cage could achieve biomechanical stability and no earlier aging of near segments, but slight subsidence and slight increase of fixing screw stress occurred. According to this result, it is recommended to use single interbody fusion cage in the PLIF surgery combined with internal fixation in the clinical practice. Goel et al. [23] tested biomechanical impact of the surgical segment and the adjacent segment after implanted mobile artificial intervertebral disc (Charite artificial disc) with the model of L3-S1. Noailly et al. [24] designed compound equipment similar with the human lumbar intervertebral disc structure, of which compression, flexion, extension, and axial rotation force was applied to the model of L3-L5, evaluating the biomechanical properties, and found that the range of motion of the implanted model was poor compared with the normal model. Implanted internal fixation has an influence not only on the stress of surgical segment and adjacent segment but also on the stress distribution of adjacent segment, resulting in bone remodeling.

In bone tissue microstructure analysis, with the development of μCT technology, FEA is gradually applied in the prediction of intensity of bone tissue. In early stage, adopt geometric cellular structure to simulate and predict the intensity of bone tissue; however, due to the diversity of clinical diseases and the individualization of patients, a simple geometric structure model is clearly not efficient to assist μCT technology to make disease diagnosis and prognosis judgment in the clinical practice. In addition, with the development of computer technology, data processing capabilities of personal computers and workstations are improved significantly. The direct measurements of cancellous bone microstructure and mechanical features are more easily to implement. Liu et al. divided the trabecular bone into rod-shaped and platelike trabecular bones, according to the structural characteristics and space arrangement with the computer method, and proposed a series of structural parameters to evaluate the structural characteristics of cancellous bone [25]. They [15] believed that the relationship between volume fraction of vertical aligned trabecular bone and the intensity of bone is stronger than the total volume fraction ($r^2 = 0.83$ vs. 0.59, $p < 0.005$). Changes of trabecular bone microarchitecture are associated with many factors, although a large number of laboratory studies concluded that there was a correlation between the structural parameters and mechanical properties of cancellous bone. But a further study is required in how to apply 3D morphological indicators in the clinical diagnosis of osteoporosis.

For the 40 years of application of FEM, it has been considerably developed and widely applied in the field of orthopedic biomechanical simulation. With progress of the computer technology and numerical analysis method, we believe that, in the near future, with the continuous deep development in microstructure and constant expanding of macroscopic computing simulating capability of FEM method, the establishment and application of high-quality, multiple organizational large data model will unveil a new direction for orthopedic translational medicine.

2.2   Key Problems in FEA

Finite element simulation (FES) is a method to study the real-world physical principles by means of computer simulation methods; and FES is one of many simulation methods.

The main role of human motor system is to support the body's own load and skeletal-muscular coordinated motor so as to complete human motor functions. In stationary state, human motor system is to maintain body posture and mutually cooperate and antagonize with muscle tissues to form resultant forces; bone tissues bear the resultant forces of muscle tissues and gravity. In this state, it is static analysis to analyze the forces and stress distribution of muscle and bone tissues. In motor state, muscle tissues keep contract and relax to drive joint relative movement, maintaining the motor state, in which it is kinetic analysis to analyze the resultant forces of muscle and bone tissues as well as bone joint motor trajectories.

The increasing problems along with the wide application of FEM are misapplication. Attention must be paid to several key problems if you want a reasonable application.

2.2.1   Select Appropriate Solution Methods

Selection of solution methods is directly related to the mathematical equations used to solve specific problems, especially whether the problem involves large-size deformation. For single vertebral simulation computation with small strain, the appropriate choice may be linear solver [26–28]. For multi-segmental spinal simulation, due to the presence of the disc resulting in a large range of motors of the spine,

namely, large-size deformation, along with the presence of contact nonlinearity of the height of small joints, nonlinear solver applicable to large-size deformation is required [29–31]. Many important research problems may be solved by quasi-static analysis methods; however, the problems in connection with the inherent load of the spine also require dynamic simulation otherwise. Only dynamic simulation can solve some physiological viscoelastic problems [32–34].

2.2.2   Geometric Modeling

Bones and muscles have different geometric shapes and sizes in different individuals accompanied by, respectively, different densities and tissue structures. Furthermore, like the structure of other human body parts, the various parts of the spine do not exercise independent functions but mutually coordinate to maintain the body's physiological activities and stability. At present, it is difficult to establish a so-called appropriate model fitting each portion of the spine; and it is also difficult to determine which portion is required. Varied ligaments and skeletal muscles among different individuals also post a great challenge for geometric modeling. In addition to interindividual variations, it is also necessary to take into account in vivo changes in biological simulations. In a period of time, boundary conditions of the spine may also vary along with changes in respiration, circulation, gait, posture, and tissue water content. In the long run, material composition and geometry of the spine also change along with development, age, disease, and natural regeneration. For example, bone structure has been constantly changing based on collective external stimuli.

2.2.3   Proper Model Materials

Undoubtedly, all biological tissue materials are nonlinear [35, 36]. But it is necessary to hypothesize linearization in some specific problems. However, appropriate biomechanical experiments are required to substantiate the computation results of such hypotheses. For example, studies found that the linear model may effectively predict the origin of vertebral burst at the time of vertebral collapse [37, 38]. However, we may simulate the actual process of vertebral collapse if we can establish a nonlinear material model combined with corresponding fatigue criteria [39]. It is necessary to establish valid material model based on the macrostructure and microstructure, but few models may conform to the standards in both macrostructure and microstructure [40]. Most researchers studied mechanical properties of the disc [41–43] and the mechanical properties of the vertebral body [44, 45] with multiphase models. In addition, the prestress of ligaments on the spine may impose impacts on the biomechanics of the spine, yet the prestress of ligaments is considered in few models [46, 47]. Bone microstructure is anisotropic and nonhomogeneous [48, 36]; and in most of the models, the bone is assumed homogeneous and isotropic.

2.2.4 Boundary Conditions

It is extremely hard to determine the boundary conditions around a biological system. And many problems in engineering fields, such as bridge and automobile design, are relatively simple. The spine is a flexible structure that can not only bear the weight and load of upper body but also move within a certain range. It is necessary to consider physiological boundary conditions (connected with the skull, sacrum and rib, etc.), muscle traction force, and kinetic limitations in spine modeling. In addition, the process and speed of load application also requires attention. Currently, there remains a controversy with regard to the physiological load of spine. In particular, it is difficult to determine how much load and torque to be applied in mechanical experiments and numerical models.

2.3   Basic Steps of FEA

Basic steps of finite element modeling include data acquisition, geometric modeling, mesh generation, and providing material parameters. After completing these steps, the obtained model is a physical model. Then analysts add different loads according to purpose and requirements of the research to complete the appropriate analytical content.

2.3.1   Data Acquisition

Source data required in the establishment of 3D model:

1. Establish a 3D model directly from a CT scan file: CT and MRI is the process of fault scanning of the human body structure, after the scan is complete, virtual "cutting" the 3D human body to form a continuous series of 2D image, and different tissue density corresponds to different CT values in the picture, due to the density of bone tissue which is significantly higher than the surrounding soft tissue, and therefore, by setting the threshold, it is easy to extract the bone tissue from the CT image (Fig. 4.5). The 3D model of skeletal system based on CT scanning files has the following advantages: (1) fast speed, (2) high accuracy, and (3) CT values can provide density information to facilitate post-assigning operation of material value according to the density. Application scopes of this method include (1) systemic skeletal system modeling, which can be obtained by the CT scanning, and (2) soft tissue system modeling, such as the modeling of brain tissue, which can be obtained by MRI scanning. This method is not suitable for muscle, tendon tissue modeling.
2. Obtain the 3D model by surface scanning: 3D surface scanner is a common surface scanning tool. Establish the corresponding coordinate in a virtual coordinate system of the points on the surface of the 3D model, and then input these point cloud data into the computer software (the common software is the Geomagic software from Rapidrop Company) to conduct 3D reconstruction.

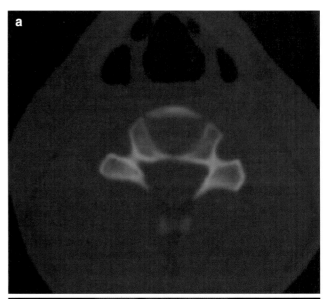

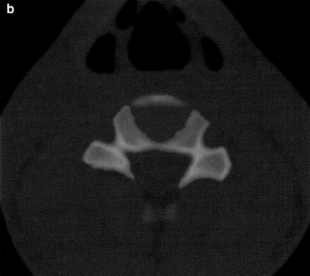

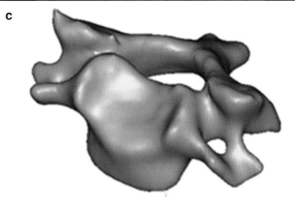

Fig. 4.5 3D model established by cross-sectional CT. (**a**) Cross-sectional CT. (**b**) Threshold extract. (**c**) 3D reconstruction

Skeletal system 3D model established by the surface scanning file has the following advantages: (1) fast speed, (2) no radiation, (3) good machine portability, and (4) the ability to complete a large-scale 3D reconstruction with

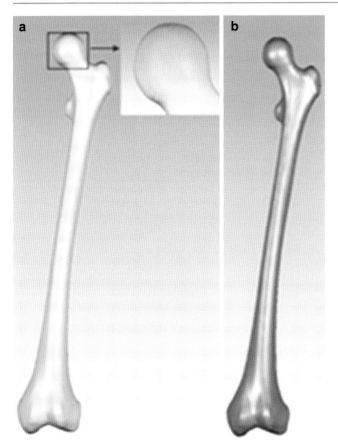

Fig. 4.6 Point cloud image 3D reconstruction. (**a**) Point cloud image.
(**b**) 3D model

small amount of data. The main disadvantage of this method is that only the surface information of model can be collected, and the internal structure of the model cannot be obtained. For the long tubal bone, the method cannot obtain information about the medullary canal. This method is also unable to obtain density information of the model, but the method has the advantage for the model with uniform material density.

3. Establish a 3D model by the anatomical structure. In the early stage of 3D modeling, since the 3D reconstruction algorithms and software are not well developed, no accurate complex 3D structure of bone tissue can be obtained, and therefore, researchers simplified the model according to the engineering theory, such as the vertebral model. The vertebral body can be simplified into cylindroid, and the processus transversus can be simplified into a rectangular, only extracting the feature size of the model to conduct modeling. Conducting modeling with the method has the following advantages: (1) extracting feature size to conduct modeling, from the bottom to the top, and the workload is relatively small, and (2) using the feature size to conduct modeling, feature size can easily be parameterized, enabling parametric modeling, which is important for the simulation of the variation of human tissue. The disad-

vantages of this method are (1) if the researchers lack understanding of the feature size, ignoring the important feature size of bone tissue, the results could lead to a larger deviation. (2) Due to the curved surface of human bone structure which is very complex and some locations which are difficult to simulate by simple feature sizes, only reasonable simplification is applicable, which leads to certain deviation of the results. Application scope of this method includes (1) model requiring parametric study, such as the study of the influence of human physiological curvature of cervical vertebra to the external load, to control the relative position between the intervertebral disc and vertebral body to change the physiological curvature of the cervical model and thus to complete the cervical corresponding research under different physiological curvature. (2) Suitable for the structure with a relatively simple anatomy, such as long bone and vertebral bone; the bone tissue with complex structure, such as the iliac and skull, since the structure is irregular, is difficult to extract the feature size, so it is difficult to establish the parameterized model (Fig. 4.6).

2.3.2   Mesh Generation

After completing the 3D reconstruction of model, finite element mesh generation is required to conduct for the model. There are two methods of mesh generation for the FEM:

1. Automatic generation by the computer: Due to the development of computer and the progress of algorithm, most common finite element analysis software has the function of automatic meshing generation. However, due to the complexity of the geometry of human bone tissue, the meshing function of common finite element analysis software often may not work. In years' study of our group, the commonly used automatic meshing software is the Altair Company's Hypermesh software and Ansys Company's ICEM software. The basic principle of these two automatic meshing software are as follows: firstly, divide the surface mesh of geometric model, and then the surface mesh works as a "boundary bag," in which there are tetrahedral, hexahedral, or prismatic blocks, thereby forming a volume mesh. Advantages of this method: (1) the speed is fast, due to the well-developed algorithm generating tetrahedron model from the triangle mesh, so the tetrahedron model can be easily obtained. (2) Not many human intervention is required. Disadvantages of this method: (1) Data used to form the tetrahedral model is large, since the number of tetrahedral model is large, so the number of node and element is large, which means the late calculation process requires more time. (2) If you want to reduce the number of units requested, taking post-computing costs into account, oversimplification of the geometric model may occur, leading to a larger error of results. Therefore, when using this method, you need to master the balance between quantity and quality of the unit (Fig. 4.8).

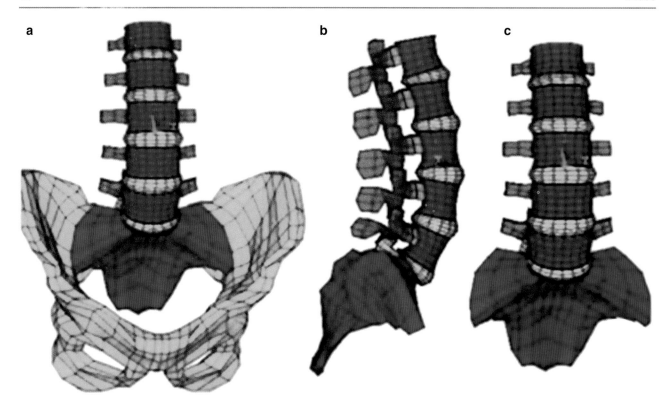

Fig. 4.7 FEM. (**a**) L-spine—model of pelvis. (**b**) Side view of lumbar sacral model. (**c**) Front view of lumbar sacral model

2. Manual mesh generation: Despite the rapid development of computers and algorithms, however, good algorithm cannot be comparable to the human brain. Especially for the mesh generation of structure of the human body, the researchers need to "guide" computer software to conduct rational division of high-quality mesh. Currently, there are two main methods of manual meshing. The central idea of the first method is "hexahedral segmentation," dividing an irregular object into hexahedral block manually. In accordance with the principle of "any hexahedron, it is made up of smaller hexahedron." Ultimately high-quality hexahedral meshing can be achieved. The central idea of the second method is "hexahedral mesh approximation." Inside the skeleton model, establish hexahedral block manually, and then project the fixed point on the surface of the skeleton model, and the computer will automatically generate high-quality hexahedral model in accordance with the corresponding points. Advantages of this method: (1) the unit quality is high, split irregular geometry into relatively regular hexahedron by the large amount of manpower, and therefore, the unit generated by the computer has a high quality. (2) Model computational efficiency is high, due to the high quality of unit, and the number of hexahedral units of a model is often less than the number of corresponding tetrahedral units, so the model computational efficiency is high. Disadvantages of this method: (1) it takes a long time for modeling, because the manual segmentation is required for irregular object, which will take a lot of time,

resulting in a long time for meshing. (2) It is necessary to master a large number of geometric segmentation techniques; for a same model, some people may soon be able to segment high-quality hexahedral meshes, while some others may not. It comes down to personal experience and his/her understanding of geometric shapes (Fig. 4.7).

2.3.3 Material Selection

The FEM shall be preliminarily established upon mesh generation of geometric model; subsequently, we will give life to the preliminary model, which is the assignment of materials. Assignment of materials is of great importance to the model, which depends on the purpose of analysis and determines whether the results of analysis make sense.

Generally, the choice of material properties depends on the complexity of the problem to be solved. For example, to study the spine dynamics in general, it may be possible to assume that the vertebral body is rigid, which can greatly reduce the complexity of the model and save computing time. But it is necessary to study mechanics of the femur in standing load with the isotropous materials and set the tissues as viscoelastic materials to study creep effects of bone tissues. Homogeneous and isotropic materials are mostly used for bone materials. Under normal circumstances, the internal cancellous bone and surrounding cortical bone may have different properties of material.

Different tissues are featured by different materials. In a motor system model, the common tissues include cortical bone, cancellous bone, cartilage, ligament, and muscle; special

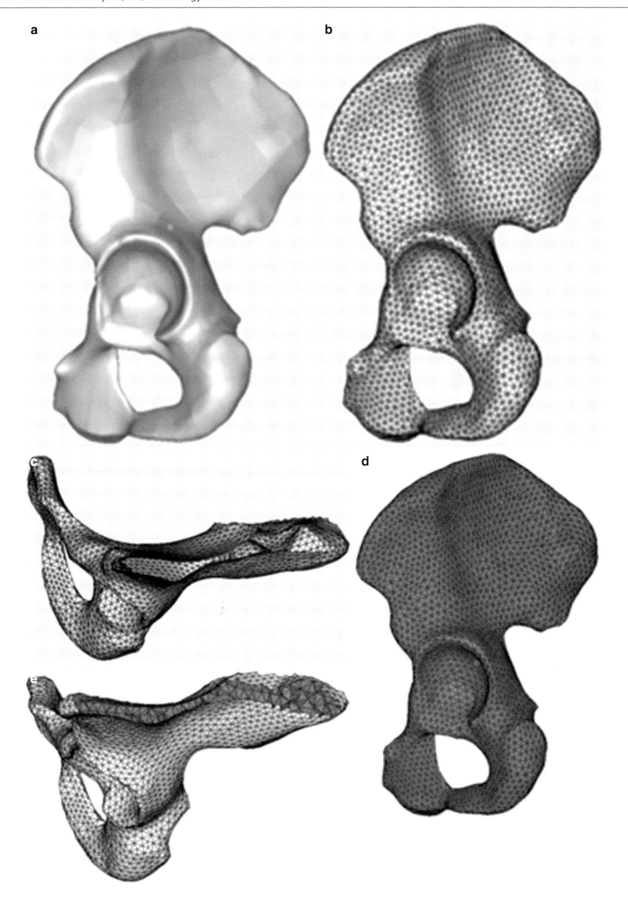

Fig. 4.8 Meshing process of volume mesh. (**a**) Ilium-ischium-pubis 3D model. (**b**) Surface mesh. (**c**) Split observation of the surface mesh. (**d**) Volume mesh. (**e**) Split observation of the surface mesh and volume mesh

tissues include meniscus, front and rear cruciate ligaments, and intervertebral disc. These tissues are featured by different material properties of their, respectively, different biological structures and functions.

2.4   Model Test

There may be a variety of factors leading to errors in the numerical model. The test process is to eliminate as many such factors as possible. Some of these factors are common causes, which may exist in various models. Some others may exist in spine models only. Although FEA method has been widely accepted and applied, it remains frequently misapplied. Therefore, the test process is critical. The comment made by Cook, Malkus, and Plesha is still applied today: "This powerful computing tool must be applied after training. If the operator does not understand the internal work processes and basic theory, the results may be of no credibility. In no way may computation errors caused by misunderstanding be corrected by refining the mesh or employment of a computer of better performances. Despite the fact that FEA method can make a good engineer more excellent, it may also make a poor engineer very terrible."

Linear FEA method is more fledged than nonlinear FEA method provided that the former's applicable scope and significance of computation results must be specified. The main criteria for testing a linear model are:

Is it a linear model? Linear FEM is applicable to elastic materials with small strain and small deformation only. However, the linearity hypothesis is generally not available for spine model.

Is the meshing sufficient? Are the results of the intensive meshing for the stress/strain regions improvable? General experiences are that after a twofold refinement of the meshing, the changes in maximum stress are not more than 5%.

Are the boundary conditions loaded to the model correct? In general, you should avoid point loading because this may cause stress intensification, while no such condition exists in actual physiological situation. Similarly, rigidly fixed boundary conditions may also lead to local stress intensification. For example, to the compression load of single vertebral body, general loading method is to apply a uniform pressure on the upper vertebral surface with rigidly fixed lower surface. However, under physiological conditions, the pressure load is not evenly distributed over the end plate on the upper surface, while the lower end plate is always not in a rigidly fixed state due to its contact with the elastic disc and the posterior arch support. Undoubtedly, different boundary conditions may lead to different computation results.

There may be more problems caused by the application of nonlinear FEA method. There are many solving options in nonlinear computation and most of such options significantly affect the results. Although solving options are greatly varied in different packages, almost all solving methods are included in every package. In addition to the said criteria for testing linear models, criteria for testing nonlinear models are as follows:

Is the solution process stable and convergent? Although sometimes a proposed nonlinear problem appears to be reasonable, the reality is not the case. Certainly, the solution results will not conform to the real physical results if the problem proposed is unreasonable. In addition to this problem, the most common cause of non-convergence computation result is that the researcher may take a so-called shortcut in order to save computing time for nonlinear problems.

Is the choice of elements reasonable? In the computation of 3D nonlinear strain, it is well accepted that hexahedral elements are reasonable. But programs that can generate hexahedrons are not yet available. In a large nonlinear model, it generally takes up most of the experimental time for hexahedral meshing of the model (50–90%). Given the fact that meshing is time and energy consuming, many researchers prefer to use the automatically generated tetrahedral meshes or hexahedral/tetrahedral mixed meshes. Generally good computation results may be obtained out of these elements, but it is necessary to examine carefully the convergence. Using higher-order elements may improve computation efficiency more than increasing number of meshes.

Is the material applicable to the simulation model of large deformation and large strain? As described above, all of biological materials are nonlinear and, under physiological conditions, act in a nonlinear way. In addition, the physiological load (such as flexion, extension, lateral bending, and rotation) is not qualified as a small deformation or a small strain. Nevertheless, many of the FEMs of the spine isotropic linear elastic materials are used to simulate the spine.

2.5   Validity Check (VC) of Model

In simple terms, the VC of model refers to the conformance between the computation results of the model and previously observed experimental results. There are many ways to check whether a spine model is valid, but not all have the same effect. The predicted parameters of a model, namely, parameters that are of concern in a study, are the most important parameters requiring a VC. For example, if a model is used to predict the kinematics of the spine only, the VC of cortical bone strain seems unnecessary and, it is not enough to make only such a VC. In the study of ligament strain model, dynamics and strain of ligaments must be verified [49].

In the VC of model, the most important problem to be considered is individual properties of biological models. Due to changes in the geometry and material, individualized experimental VC is autonomous without the necessity of the statistic results conforming to a large number of experimental studies [50]. Of course, it has to be established on the basis of correct modeling methods and rigorous tests and checks. Although individualized experimental studies are featured with such autonomy, it remains hard to carry out individualized VC; and most VCs of models are verified in the way of comparing with published experimental data [51]. Because of large interindividual differences, the standard error of this kind of studies is generally high.

Another necessary consideration for a VC is that FEA method provides the mechanical changes in a discrete area. For example, people may insert a probe manometer into the nucleus pulposus to measure disc pressure. If comparing with the simulation results of FES, they should be the average stresses of the positions at the corresponding levels rather than the maximum or minimum overall stresses.

2.6 Model Prediction

The ultimate goal of numerical modeling is not only to describe the biomechanical behaviors to be verified but also to accurately predict the biomechanical behaviors that have never been measured before. It is the common goal of all FEMs; however, in no way shall the goal be achieved once there is one model without rigorous simulation verification. Prediction modeling allows us to explore those mechanical experiments, which are hard or impossible to implement, by means of simulation processes.

For example, researchers establish a large number of spine models to study the biomechanics under high-speed blast injuries caused by car accidents. Other models allow us to learn about the biomechanical performances of the spine with new surgical fixation techniques. FEM may help us understand in vivo biomechanical properties of surgical internal fixation as well as the body's biomechanical responses to internal fixation and provide reference for improvement of such internal fixation. US FDA has acknowledged the effectiveness of FEM simulation performed in preclinical trials. The American National Standards Institution is considering the development of specifications and guidelines for orthopedic internal fixation FEA.

References

1. Jones AC, Wilcox RK. Finite element analysis of the spine: towards a framework of verification, validation and sensitivity analysis. Med Eng Phys. 2008;30:1287–304.
2. Board D, Stemper BD, Yoganandan N, et al. Biomechanics of the aging spine. Biomed Sci Instrum. 2006;42:1–6.
3. Kallemeyn N, Gandhi A, Kode S, et al. Validation of a C2-C7 cervical spine finite element model using specimen-specific flexibility data. Med Eng Phys. 2010;32:482–9.
4. Laville A, Laporte S, Skalli W. Parametric and subject-specific finite element modelling of the lower cervical spine. Influence of geometrical parameters on the motion patterns. J Biomech. 2009;42:1409–15.
5. Harrigan TP, Kareh JA, O'Connor DO, et al. A finite element study of the initiation of failure of fixation in cemented femoral total hip components. J Orthop Res. 1992;10:134–44.
6. McNamara BP, Cristofolini L, Toni A, et al. Relationship between bone-prosthesis bonding and load transfer in total hip reconstruction. J Biomech. 1997;30:621–30.
7. Vichnin HH, Batterman SC. Stress analysis and failure prediction in the proximal femur before and after total hip replacement. J Biomech Eng. 1986;108:33–41.
8. Scifert CF, Brown TD, Lipman JD. Finite element analysis of a novel design approach to resisting total hip dislocation. Clin Biomech (Bristol, Avon). 1999;14:697–703.
9. Messick KJ, Miller MA, Damron LA, et al. Vacuum-mixing cement does not decrease overall porosity in cemented femoral stems: an in vitro laboratory investigation. J Bone Joint Surg Br. 2007;89:1115–21.
10. Harrigan TP, Harris WH. A finite element study of the effect of diametral interface gaps on the contact areas and pressures in uncemented cylindrical femoral total hip components. J Biomech. 1991;24:87–91.
11. Panjabi MM, Ito S, Ivancic PC, et al. Evaluation of the intervertebral neck injury criterion using simulated rear impacts. J Biomech. 2005;38:1694–701.
12. Yoganandan N, Kumaresan SC, Voo L, et al. Finite element modeling of the C4-C6 cervical spine unit. Med Eng Phys. 1996;18:569–74.
13. Yoganandan N, Myklebust JB, Ray G, et al. Mathematical and finite element analysis of spine injuries. Crit Rev Biomed Eng. 1987;15:29–93.
14. Yoganandan N, Kumaresan S, Voo L, et al. Finite element applications in human cervical spine modeling. Spine. 1996;21:1824–34.
15. Natarajan RN, Williams JR, Andersson GB. Recent advances in analytical modeling of lumbar disc degeneration. Spine. 2004;29:2733–41.
16. Zhang QH, Teo EC. Finite element application in implant research for treatment of lumbar degenerative disc disease. Med Eng Phys. 2008;30:1246–56.
17. Natarajan RN, Williams JR, Lavender SA, et al. Relationship between disc injury and manual lifting: a poroelastic finite element model study. Proc Inst Mech Eng H. 2008;222:195–207.
18. Lu S, Xu YQ, Zhang MC, et al. Biomechanical effect of vertebroplasty on the adjacent intervertebral levels using a three-dimensional finite element analysis. Chin J Traumatol. 2007;10:120–4.
19. Little JP, Adam CJ, Evans JH, et al. Nonlinear finite element analysis of anular lesions in the L4/5 intervertebral disc. J Biomech. 2007;40:2744–51.
20. Teo EC, Zhang QH, Huang RC. Finite element analysis of head-neck kinematics during motor vehicle accidents: analysis in multiple planes. Med Eng Phys. 2007;29:54–60.
21. Lee KK, Teo EC, Fuss FK, et al. Finite-element analysis for lumbar interbody fusion under axial loading. IEEE Trans Biomed Eng. 2004;51:393–400.
22. Chiang MF, Zhong ZC, Chen CS, et al. Biomechanical comparison of instrumented posterior lumbar interbody fusion with one or two cages by finite element analysis. Spine. 2006;31:E682–9.
23. Goel VK, Grauer JN, Patel T, et al. Effects of charite artificial disc on the implanted and adjacent spinal segments mechanics using a hybrid testing protocol. Spine. 2005;30:2755–64.
24. Noailly J, Lacroix D, Planell JA. Finite element study of a novel intervertebral disc substitute. Spine. 2005;30:2257–64.
25. Liu XS, Sajda P, Saha PK, et al. Complete volumetric decomposition of individual trabecular plates and rods and its morphological

correlations with anisotropic elastic moduli in human trabecular bone. J Bone Miner Res. 2008;23:223–35.

26. Langrana NA, Harten RR, Lin DC, et al. Acute thoracolumbar burst fractures: a new view of loading mechanisms. Spine. 2002;27:498–508.

27. Teo EC, Ng HW. First cervical vertebra (atlas) fracture mechanism studies using finite element method. J Biomech. 2001;34:13–21.

28. Ng HW, Teo EC. Nonlinear finite-element analysis of the lower cervical spine (C4-C6) under axial loading. J Spinal Disord. 2001;14:201–10.

29. Zhang QH, Tan SH, Teo EC. A numerical study of the effect of axial acceleration on the responses of the cervical spine during low-speed rear-end impact. Proc Inst Mech Eng H. 2008;222: 1167–74.

30. Pearson AM, Panjabi MM, Ivancic PC, et al. Frontal impact causes ligamentous cervical spine injury. Spine. 2005;30:1852–8.

31. Panjabi MM, Ivancic PC, Maak TG, Tominaga Y, Rubin W. Multiplanar cervical spine injury due to head-turned rear impact. Spine. 2006;31:420–9.

32. Tropiano P, Thollon L, Arnoux PJ, et al. Using a finite element model to evaluate human injuries application to the HUMOS model in whiplash situation. Spine. 2004;29:1709–16.

33. Tschirhart CE, Nagpurkar A, Whyne CM. Effects of tumor location, shape and surface serration on burst fracture risk in the metastatic spine. J Biomech. 2004;37:653–60.

34. Wilcox RK. The biomechanics of vertebroplasty: a review. Proc Inst Mech Eng H. 2004;218:1–10.

35. Panjabi MM, Maak TG, Ivancic PC, et al. Dynamic intervertebral foramen narrowing during simulated rear impact. Spine. 2006;31:E128–34.

36. Morgan EF, Bayraktar HH, Keaveny TM. Trabecular bone modulus-density relationships depend on anatomic site. J Biomech. 2003;36:897–904.

37. Crawford RP, Cann CE, Keaveny TM. Finite element models predict in vitro vertebral body compressive strength better than quantitative computed tomography. Bone. 2003;33:744–50.

38. Crawford RP, Rosenberg WS, Keaveny TM. Quantitative computed tomography-based finite element models of the human lumbar vertebral body: effect of element size on stiffness, damage, and fracture strength predictions. J Biomech Eng. 2003;125:434–8.

39. Anderson IA, Bowden M, Wyatt TP. Stress analysis of hemispherical ceramic hip prosthesis bearings. Med Eng Phys. 2005;27:115–22.

40. Yeni YN, Hou FJ, Ciarelli T, et al. Trabecular shear stresses predict in vivo linear microcrack density but not diffuse damage in human vertebral cancellous bone. Ann Biomed Eng. 2003;31:726–32.

41. Ito S, Ivancic PC, Pearson AM, et al. Cervical intervertebral disc injury during simulated frontal impact. Eur Spine J. 2005;14:356–65.

42. Panjabi MM, Ito S, Pearson AM, et al. Injury mechanisms of the cervical intervertebral disc during simulated whiplash. Spine. 2004;29:1217–25.

43. Qiu TX, Teo EC, Zhang QH. Comparison of kinematics between thoracolumbar T11-t12 and T12-L1 functional spinal units. Proc Inst Mech Eng H. 2006;220:493–504.

44. Qiu TX, Tan KW, Lee VS, et al. Investigation of thoracolumbar T12-L1 burst fracture mechanism using finite element method. Med Eng Phys. 2006;28:656–64.

45. Ivancic PC, Coe MP, Ndu AB, et al. Dynamic mechanical properties of intact human cervical spine ligaments. Spine J. 2007;7:659–65.

46. Weiss JA, Gardiner JC. Computational modeling of ligament mechanics. Crit Rev Biomed Eng. 2001;29:303–71.

47. Hou FJ, Lang SM, Hoshaw SJ, et al. Human vertebral body apparent and hard tissue stiffness. J Biomech. 1998;31:1009–15.

48. Villarraga ML, Bellezza AJ, Harrigan TP, et al. The biomechanical effects of kyphoplasty on treated and adjacent nontreated vertebral bodies. J Spinal Disord Tech. 2005;18:84–91.

49. Nie WZ, Ye M, Liu ZD, et al. The patient-specific brace design and biomechanical analysis of adolescent idiopathic scoliosis. J Biomech Eng. 2009;131:041007.

50. Wagnac EL, Aubin CE, Dansereau J. A new method to generate a patient-specific finite element model of the human buttocks. IEEE Trans Biomed Eng. 2008;55:774–83.

51. Guo LX, Teo EC. Influence prediction of injury and vibration on adjacent components of spine using finite element methods. J Spinal Disord Tech. 2006;19:118–24.

Computer-Aided Design and Manufacturing for Digital Orthopedics

Xiaojun Chen

1 Introduction

Over the past decades, the surgical guides or templates as the high-precision technologic tools have been applied for various surgeries such as the oral implantology, oncology, nasal prosthesis implant placement, cervical or lumbar pedicle screw placement, total hip arthroplasty (THA), treatment of sacroiliac joint fracture, total knee arthroplasty (TKA), etc. The surgical template is a guide aiming at directing the drilling, osteotomy, or tumor resection, providing an accurate placement of the implant or prosthesis, etc. Therefore, with the use of it, the preoperative planning can be transferred to the actual surgical site, and the precision and safety and reliability of the surgery can be improved. The general workflow of the template design and manufacturing (shown in Fig. 5.1) is described as follows: on the basis of the original medical image data (computed tomography (CT), cone beam computed tomography (CBCT), magnetic resonance imaging (MRI), etc.), image processing (including segmentation and registration) is conducted through the preoperative planning software. Then, modeling of the critical anatomical structures is realized for 3D visualization. Based on the series of 2D images (coronal, sagittal, and axial) and the 3D-reconstructed models, preoperative planning is performed, including 2D/3D geometrical measurements, the optimization design of the position and orientation of surgical trajectory, the simulation of implant placement, etc. According to the result of preoperative planning, the surgical template can be designed using key technologies of reverse engineering, point cloud, and surface reconstruction. Then, it can be fabricated through numerical control machining, additive manufacturing (3D printing) technologies, etc., and the clinical application can be finally conducted.

Compared with the surgical navigation system, the advantages of surgical template applications are convenience and ease of use. Furthermore, the surgical procedures can be optimized and executed in a shorter time, with less time spent in the operating room, thus enabling significant cost savings to hospitals and fewer risks to the patient.

The early production of the surgical template is mainly dependent on manual design and fabricating methods, which are not standardized and efficient. Pesun et al. described a technique fabricating a guide with gutta-percha to be used for oral implant placement. Then, with the development of computer technologies, the computer-aided design (CAD) and the computer-aided manufacturing (CAM) have been widely used for producing the customized surgical guides in the field of digital orthopedics. Furthermore, the rapid prototyping (RP) or 3D printing has now become the mainstream fabricating method over the past years due to the great enhancement of production efficiency and accuracy. For example, Zhang et al. designed a patient-specific drill template through the CAD software (Imageware, Siemens PLM Software, Germany) and produced using the stereolithography rapid prototyping technique for total hip arthroplasty. The key technologies involved in this method are image processing, preoperative planning, template design, and fabrication, which are discussed as follows.

X. Chen
Institute of Biomedical Manufacturing and Life Quality Engineering, School of Mechanical Engineering, Shanghai Jiao Tong University, Shanghai, China

© Springer Nature B.V. and People's Medical Publishing House 2018
G. Pei (ed.), *Digital Orthopedics*, https://doi.org/10.1007/978-94-024-1076-1_5

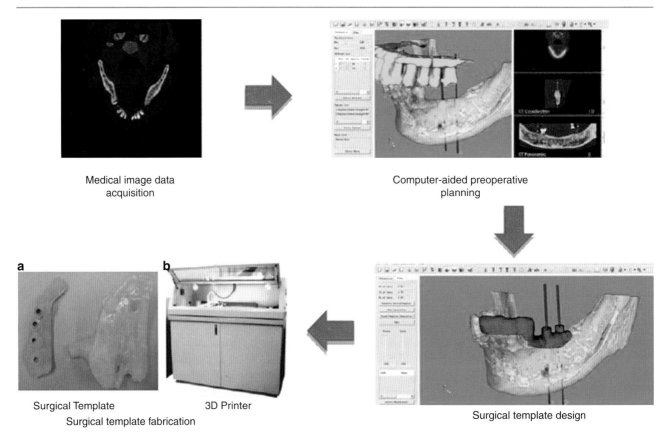

Medical image data acquisition

Computer-aided preoperative planning

Surgical Template   3D Printer
Surgical template fabrication

Surgical template design

Fig. 5.1 The general workflow of the template design and manufacturing

2   Image Processing

Medical image processing is the core and prerequisite of the preoperative planning. With the aid of image processing, the important information such as focus, hard and soft tissues, blood vessels, and nerves can be extracted for the clinical diagnosis and treatment.

2.1   Image Segmentation

Image segmentation is the key procedure of image processing, and its main purpose is to divide the image into different regions with special signification and make the results approximate to the anatomical structures.

Manual segmentation of medical images (CT, MR, PET, etc.) is time-consuming and can hardly deal with some complex situations when the difference in features between the targets and the surrounding tissues cannot be identified. Nowadays, researchers are focusing on the development of automatic image segmentation algorithm. Although some novel algorithm have been proposed, a related limitation is that the accuracy of the segmented result for some cases may not be sufficient to meet the clinical requirements. For exam-

ple, some tumors are detected as structures within or on the edge of the liver, and can be missed if some slices at the top or at the bottom of the liver are not segmented. So far, the major segmentation algorithms include region growing method, watershed algorithm, the deformable biomechanical model method, level set method, Markov random fields algorithm, Voronoi-diagram algorithm, fuzzy connectedness algorithm, etc. In addition, there are some methods based on special theories, for example, the artificial neural network algorithm, the methods based on wavelet transform, statistics, fractal theory, mathematical morphology, etc.

2.2   Image Registration

Medical images acquired from different sensors can provide more complete information to gain more complex and detailed scene representation for the treatment verification. For example, MRI records the anatomical body structures, and ultrasound or CT monitors functional and metabolic body activities. Therefore, multimodality image registration is a crucial procedure in all image analysis tasks which is the process of bringing two or more images into spatial alignment.

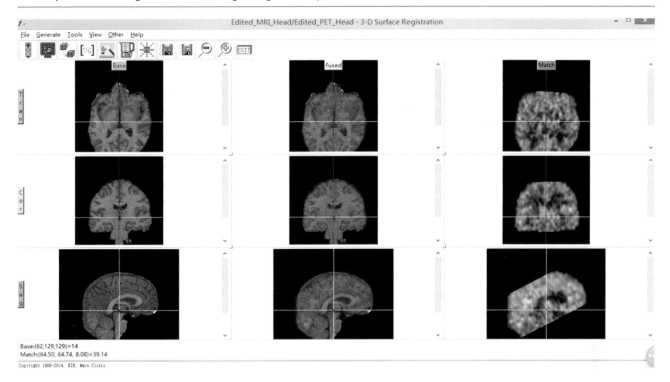

Fig. 5.2   3D surface registration between MRI head and PET head performed through the software of Analyze

Currently, the major registration methods are divided into two categories: the feature-based algorithms (e.g., iterative closest point) and intensity-based algorithms (e.g., maximization of mutual information). Nowadays, more advanced methods are presented for image registration, for example, iterative principal axes method, maximum likelihood approach, fast Fourier transform-based method, local frequency representations algorithm, etc. In addition, some softwares have been developed for image registration using various approaches based on the abovementioned methods. For example, the functions of 2D registration, 2D nonrigid registration, 3D surface registration, and 3D voxel registration are provided in the software of Analyze (Fig. 5.2 shows the result of 3D surface registration between MRI head and PET head).

However, the semiautomatic approach, still a great challenge since registration of images with complex nonlinear and local distortions, multimodal registration, and registration of N-D image (where $N > 2$), belongs to the most difficult tasks in this field.

Because of the deformations caused by the movements of the soft tissue or surgical manipulations, the current approach, the so-called rigid registration, is not accurate. Recently, numerous nonrigid, patient-specific, and fully automatic registration algorithms have been proposed for real-time enhancement of intraoperative images and "prediction" of the amount of deformations. For example, Rivaz et al. presented an algorithm for nonrigid registration of ultrasound images that modeled the deformation with free-form cubic B-splines.

2.3   Three-Dimensional Visualization

The purpose of visualization is to provide a 3D (and even 4D) image so that the surgeon no longer needs to refer to 2D images from multiple modalities (radiograph or CT/MRI image). Today, the 3D reconstruction algorithm can be categorized into two classifications: surface rendering and volume rendering.

Surface rendering is the method of extracting surfaces from the structures in the images and displaying groups of polygonal surfaces, and the surface is basically constructed through the cuberille method, marching cube method, or dividing cube method. The marching cube method is the most widely used one, for example, Fig. 5.3 shows a 3D surface mesh pelvis model reconstructed through the vector-based surface rendering command in 3D-DOCTOR.

Volume rendering is the technology of computing rays through the volumes to produce a projection image. Since it does not suffer from data misclassification as part of the segmentation stage and all the original data in the rendered image can be retained, volume rendering is generally considered to be the most appropriate volume visualization technique (Fig. 5.4 shows the volume rendering in Mimics). The methods of volume rendering have been developed such as ray-casting algorithm, splatting algorithm, or shear-warp algorithm.

However, even though computers are continually getting faster, the presented volume visualization algorithms still remain as challenges to improve the rendering speed of large

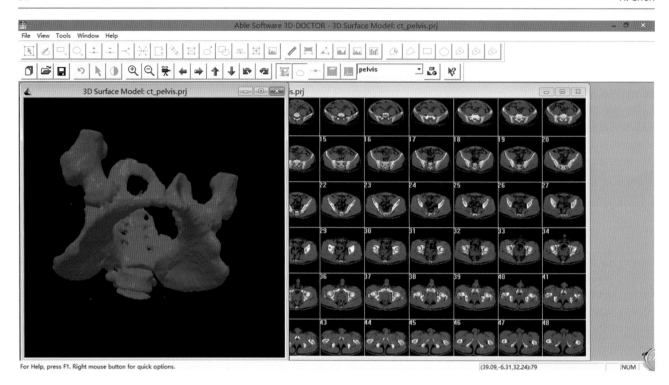

Fig. 5.3 The surface rendering of pelvis processed through the software of 3D-DOCTOR

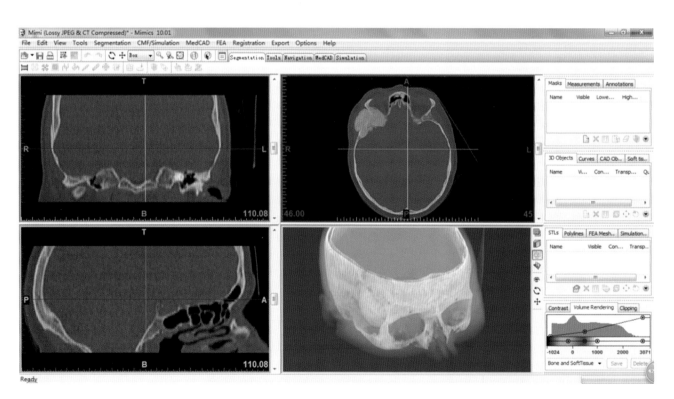

Fig. 5.4 The volume rendering method in the software of Mimics

datasets and the quality of their reconstructed images. Since the graphics processing unit (GPU) can deliver giant computational raw power compared to the central processing unit (CPU) on a per-dollar basis, the GPU-based volume rendering systems have been developed to produce clearer images and effectively convey visual information over the recent years. For example, Pelt et al. proposed an interactive GPU-based illustrative volume rendering framework to achieve real-time interaction and prompt parametrization of the illustrative styles. Schlegel et al. presented a novel approach in direct volume rendering based on GPU ray-casting for obtaining fast, plausible volume illumination and shading effects. Nelson et al. described a new GPU-based volume rendering method using the properties of spectral/hp finite element fields with the goal of producing accurate and interactive images. Liu et al. (2013) presented a novel approach for GPU-based high-quality volume rendering of large out-of-core volume data.

3   Preoperative Planning

The computer-aided preoperative planning has been a hot topic and the basis for the following template design and manufacturing. It is regarded to be the process of using computer technologies to design, simulate, and optimize the surgical scheme (3D geometrical measurement, virtual surgical trajectory of tumor resection, simulation of implant or prosthesis placement, etc.) according to both 2D and 3D data. Nowadays, some commercial computer-aided preoperative planning softwares have been developed and widely used, for example, Analyze, 3D-DOCTOR, Mimics, etc. In addition, there are also some open-source softwares such as CamiTK, 3D Slicer, GIMIAS, etc.

In the following, the details of self-developed software called Computer-Assisted Preoperative Planning for Oral Implant Surgery (CAPPOIS) are described. It is divided into five following modules:

1. The module for image importing and 3D reconstruction: Original CT image data in DICOM (Digital Imaging and Communications in Medicine) file format can be imported. The image grayscale and contrast can be adjusted; the bone can be segmented from its neighboring areas including soft tissue, water, adipose, etc.; and then a 3D cranio-maxillofacial model can be reconstructed and rendered.
2. The module for multi-planar reconstruction: A panoramic curve following the curvature of the jaw bone on one of the imported axial CT image slices can be drawn manually, and then on the basis of this panoramic curve, the

series of panoramic images and cross-sectional images can be reconstructed. With respect to a plan of the mandible type, several points of inferior alveolar nerves can be labeled according to the series of panoramic images, and then these nerves can be reconstructed and highlighted in the 3D view.
3. The module for basic operations in 2D/3D views: Translation, rotation, and zooming in and out of the 2D/3D views can be done interactively. 3D cranio-maxillofacial models can be rendered and the transparency of the models can be adjusted. In addition, geometrical measurement can also be realized in the 2D/3D views, e.g., after selecting the required anatomical landmarks on the cranio-maxillofacial model, the distance between any two points and the angle among any three points can be calculated.
4. The module for implant design and adjustment: A certain type of virtual implants can be selected from an implant system library, including Branemark, ITI, FRIALIT, AVANA, Replace, CAMLOG, etc., and placed into the ideal areas in a 2D/3D view. The position and orientation of the implant can be adjusted by taking into account prosthetic requirements and available local bone. If the information of an implant is changed on a 2D/3D view, its information in all the other views will be updated simultaneously. Distance between an implant and alveolar nerves can be calculated, and collision detection among implants and bone density analysis around an implant can be done as well. In addition, relevant abutments and dentures can be designed.
5. The module for graphical user interfaces (GUI): Export/import, redo/undo, storage, retrieval, and deletion of the preoperative planning data can be realized. The preoperative planning information can be saved and exported in a special file format, so that it can be used in the subsequent software for the design of surgical templates.

After comprehensively analyzing the abovementioned functions, we designed the architecture of the software. The key technology of the software involved some algorithms in the field of medical image processing and computer graphics. The major algorithms included DICOM file parsing, image segmentation and 3D visualization, spline curve generation, multi-planar reconstruction, spatial search and 3D distance computing, cutting, volume measurement, etc. For each algorithm, we developed a set of dynamic-link libraries (DLL) using Microsoft Visual C++, as well as the Visualization Toolkit (VTK, an open-source, freely available software system for 3D computer graphics, image processing, visualization etc., http://www.vtk.org/) and Insight Toolkit (ITK, an open-source software toolkit for

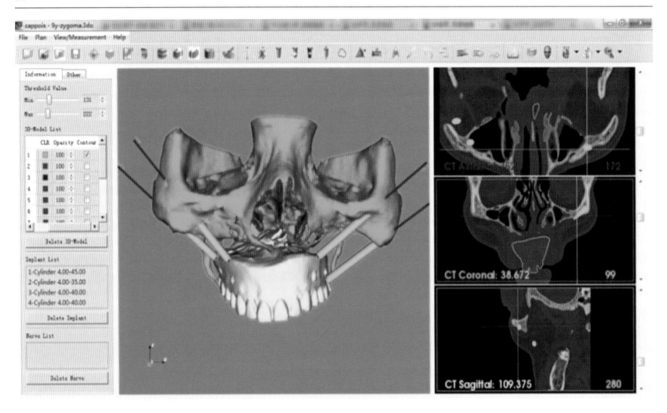

Fig. 5.5 The user interface of a self-developed preoperative planning software of CAPPOIS

performing registration and segmentation, http://www.itk.org/) via object-oriented programming methodology; therefore, a three-layer modular software model was developed. This basis can be extended by virtually any new approach or algorithm, which then becomes seamlessly integrated into the method set of the preoperative planning software framework. The aim is to provide well-defined levels of abstraction (the hiding of implementation details) from the individual components, so that new technology can be incorporated into the system without a complete software rewrite. We choose Qt (a free, open-source, and cross-platform application development framework widely used for the development of GUI programs, http://qt.nokia.com/products) for its powerful cross-platform support features. The main interface of the software is shown in Fig. 5.5.

The user interface and functions of CAPPOIS parallels Simplant (Materialise, Belgium), which is already commercially available; however, since the visualization and image processing algorithms involved in our software are developed by using VTK and ITK, a plug-in evolutive software architecture is established, allowing for expandability, accessibility, and maintainability in our system. In addition, aiming to make the software simply accessible and fulfill the research requirements in academia, our future work is to make CAPPOIS a free, open-source, and cross-platform

(Windows, Linux, and Mac OS X operating systems) software for preoperative planning in oral implantology.

4 Computer-Aided Design for Surgical Templates

On the basis of the preoperative planning result, the patient-specific template can be designed for improving the surgical accuracy and reliability. Currently, the major template designing approaches can be divided into two groups: (1) utilization of commercial softwares and (2) comprehensive applications of traditional CAD softwares.

4.1 Utilization of Commercial Softwares

Some commercial preoperative planning systems have been available for the design of surgical guides, including two approaches: (1) The software suppliers provide the service of designing a customized template according to the preoperative planning results such as NobelGuide® (Nobel Biocare, Kloten, Switzerland), SurgiGuide® (Materialise Dental, Leuven, Belgium), etc. (2) Some softwares also supply the specific modules of template design for local design such as 3Shape Dental System® (3Shape A/S, Copenhagen, Denmark), coDiagnostiX™ (IVS Solutions AG, Chemnitz, Germany), Signature® Personalized Patient Care (SPPC) (Biomet Inc., Warsaw, IN), etc.

For example, Vasak et al. performed the preoperative planning through NobelGuide®, and the result was then sent to a certified manufacturing facility (Nobel Biocare) for template design and fabrication. Since the designing process is often completed in the companies without the surgeon's participation, the final product may deviate from the expected object, and it is hard to correct or optimize. Particularly for larger surgical guides, this technology is associated with high cost and production time. Boonen et al. designed a drilling and cutting template through Signature® Personalized Patient Care for total knee arthroplasty (TKA). Kuhl et al. utilized the coDiagnostiX™ to design a surgical template for guided implant surgery.

In addition, some research groups also developed their own template designing software and presented in the literature. For example, Yang et al. developed a semiautomatic computer-aided software which enables surgeons to design and optimize the template individually for various surgeries, including oral implantology, cervical pedicle screw insertion, iliosacral screw insertion, and osteotomy.

Since most commercial softwares provide the solutions of template design for specified kinds of surgery (oral implantology and orthopedics), as for other surgeries such as nasal prosthesis implantation, cervical or lumbar pedicle screw placement, treatment of sacroiliac joint fracture, etc., the template design mainly depends on traditional CAD software.

4.2 Comprehensive Applications of Traditional CAD Softwares

Some CAD softwares and third-party 3D modeling software such as UG Imageware, Rhino 3.0 (Robert McNeel & Associates, Seattle, USA), and Magics RP (Materialise, Leuven, Belgium) are now utilized to design the template. Among them, UG Imageware is most widely used for total hip arthroplasty, iliosacral screw insertions, and C2 translaminar screw insertion. And, Ciocca et al. designed a template through Rhino 3.0 to guide the insertion of craniofacial implants for nasal prosthesis retention. Hirao et al. utilized Magics RP to design a custom-made drilling guide for malunited pronation deformity after first metatarsophalangeal (MTP-1) joint arthrodesis.

As the existing CAD software often consists of well-established system and powerful function modules, the engineer can design template according to almost any kind of preoperative planning result theoretically. However, the

design work is quite complicated and requires for high precision; the process may be with high cost and low efficiency.

5 Computer-Aided Manufacturing for Surgical Templates

Once the designing procedure is accomplished, the surgical template can be fabricated through special mechanical positioning devices or various types of CAD-CAM technology. With the tremendous development of manufacturing techniques over the past decades, additive manufacturing (AM) technology (also called rapid prototyping or 3D printing) has brought revolution for the surgical guide production. Rapid prototyping is the process of using the materials of ceramic powder, plastic, or metal powder to print any object layer by layer based on the virtual three-dimensional computer designed model. Compared with the traditional CAD-CAM technologies, rapid prototyping allows the creation of very complex geometries and has the advantages of humanization design, low cost and carbon, high production efficiency, etc. For example, it may take several days to produce a template for iliosacral screw insertion through the centralized facility, while the whole process may only need 6–20 h through the RP technology.

In addition, with the appearance of the metal fabrication strategies, the metallic biomaterials such as pure titanium and its alloys have been most frequently used for medical applications over the past years. Titanium is a particularly suitable material for work in the medical field due to its high mechanical strength and fracture toughness, low specific weight, nonmagnetic, and good biocompatibility properties, and the compact protective film of titanium oxide (TiO_2) on the metal surface provides high corrosion resistance.

In 2006, Electron Beam Melting (EBM) was one of the first metal additive manufacturing technologies used for producing a cranial implant by the Swedish company Arcam. Besides EBM, the technologies of direct metal laser sintering (DMLS) and selective laser melting (SLM) have been developed recently for manufacturing high-quality metallic components. For example, Mazzoni et al. fabricated a customized mandible cutting guide through the DMLS to precisely reproduce the site and orientation of the osteotomies for tumor ablation from the virtual plan into the surgical environment. Table 5.1 shows the detailed classifications of additive manufacturing (rapid prototyping or 3D printing) technology using different materials: stereolithography (SLA), selective laser sintering (SLS), fused deposition modeling (FDM), laminated object manufacturing (LOM), etc. Among these methods, the SLA can achieve the highest level of precision and the STL is the most common way for

Table 5.1 The types of additive manufacturing

Type	Material	Method	Systems for instance	Accuracy
Stereolithography (SLA)	Photopolymers	Curing by UV laser	3D Systems, Rock Hill, SC, USA	+++
Selective laser sintering (SLS)	Small particles of thermoplastic, metal, ceramic or glass powders	Fusing by a high power laser	EOS GmbH, Munich, Germany	++
Fused deposition modeling (FDM)	Fused thermoplastic materials or eutectic metals	Extruding	Stratasys Inc., Eden Prairie, MN, USA	++
Laminated object manufacturing (LOM)	Layers of paper or plastic films	Gluing together and shaping by a laser cutter	Cubic Technologies, Torrance, CA, USA	+
Melt 3D printing	Powdered pure titanium and its alloys	Electron Beam Melting (EBM), direct metal laser sintering (DMLS), selective laser melting (SLM)	EOS GmbH, Germany / Arcam, Sweden	++

fabricating surgical templates. Figure 5.6 shows various 3D-printed surgical templates and the adjacent tissue models using SLA technology.

6 Clinical Applications of Computer-Aided Design and Manufacturing of Surgical Templates

After all the preoperative work is accomplished, the surgeon can perform the surgery with the use of surgical template. The main clinical applications are in the subjects of nasal, oral, spine, hip, knee, metatarsophalangeal joint, etc., and the accuracy evaluations can be obtained through the comparison between the postoperative images and the preoperative planning images based on the image registration technique and statistical analysis.

As for the oral implantology, the accuracy has been improving since the early application of surgical template in 1990s due to the developing fabrication techniques. Usually, the global (apical and coronal), angular, depth, and lateral deviations are considered as the main parameters for the surgical assessment, and the depth deviation has been proven to be the extremely significant impact on the accuracy and clinical results. Cassetta et al. performed 112 cases of oral implant surgery using stereolithographic guides, and 111 implants were available for a comparison of accuracy [depth deviation]. The results showed that 45 were placed deeper to the planned implants with a mean deviation of −0.70 mm and a maximum deviation of −1.70 mm, and 66 were placed more superficially to the planned implant with a mean value of 0.78 mm and a maximum deviation of 2.29 mm. Scherer et al. recently conducted a total of 180 drilling actions of dental implants, and the mean position and angular deviations were $0.31° \pm 0.17°$ mm and $0.53° \pm 0.24°$. We intro-

duced a novel bone-tooth-combined-supported surgical template (shown in Fig. 5.7), which is designed utilizing CAPPOIS and fabricated via SLA technique using both laser scanning and CT imaging. The results show that the fixation was more stable than tooth-supported templates because laser scanning technology obtained detailed dentition information, which brought about the unique topography between the match surface of the templates and the adjacent teeth. The average distance deviations at the coronal and apical point of the implant were 0.66 mm (range 0.3–1.2) and 0.86 mm (range 0.4–1.2), and the average angle deviation was 1.84° (range 0.6–2.8°). In summary, the template-guided drilling procedure can improve accuracy on a very significant level in comparison with non-guided drilling surgery.

As for the nasal prosthesis retention surgery, surgical template can be used for craniofacial implant positioning. Ciocca et al. (2011) performed an accuracy evaluation between the planned and the placed final position of each implant, while the surgery was accomplished using a 3D printing template. The deviation values at the apex of the implants with respect to the planned position were 1.17 mm for the implant in the glabella and 2.81 and 3.39 mm, respectively, for those implanted in the maxilla, which means it has a more accurate positioning of craniofacial implants than unguided surgery.

As for the total hip arthroplasty (THA), Zhang et al. (2011) compared the accuracy between the conventional THA (control group, $n = 11$) and navigation template implantation (NT group, $n = 11$). After 1 year follow-up, the NT group showed significantly smaller differences ($1.6° \pm 0.4°$, $1.9° \pm 1.1°$) from the predetermined angles (abduction angle 45° and anteversion angle 18°) than those in the control group ($5.8° \pm 2.9°$, $3.9° \pm 2.5°$) ($P < 0.05$).

In the field of spine surgery, Hu et al. evaluated the accuracy of patient-specific CT-based rapid prototyping drill

Fig. 5.6 (**a1–d1**) The 3D-printed surgical templates and the adjacent tissue models (**a1**, mandibular phantom; **b1**, part of cervical vertebrae phantom; **c1**, part of cervical vertebrae phantom; **d1**, part of bone phantom); (**a2–d2**) matching of the surgical template with the adjacent tissue models

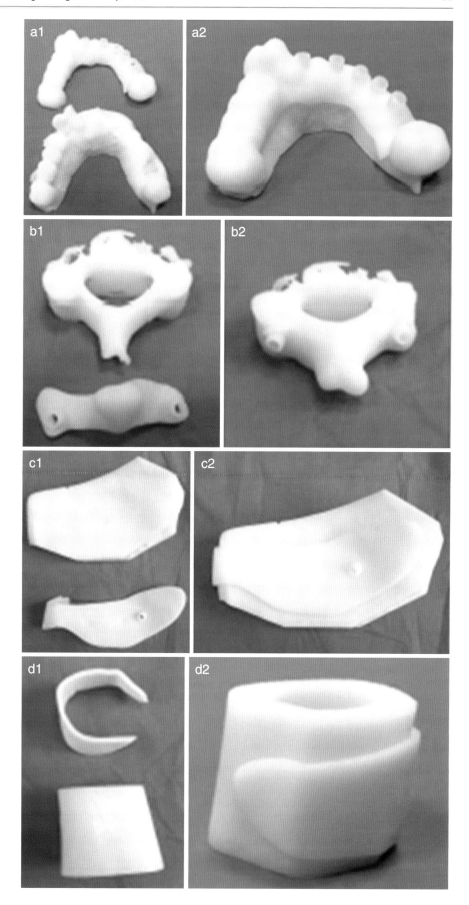

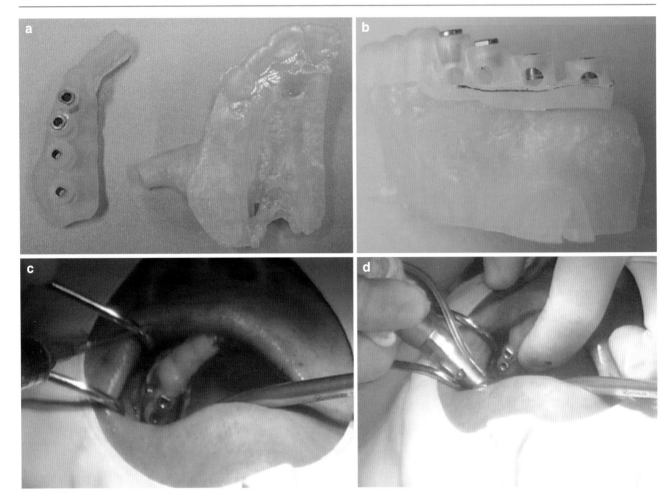

Fig. 5.7 (**a–d**) A novel bone-tooth-combined-supported surgical template and its clinical application, (**a**) The stereolithographic surgical template and maxillary phantom. (**b**) Matching of the surgical template with the maxillary phantom. (**c**) The template rested on the alveolar bone as well as the adjacent teeth. (**d**) The application of the template during the surgery

templates for C2 translaminar screw insertion. The results proved this technology can improve the safety profile of the fixation technique. In addition, Boonen et al. conducted 40 cases of total knee arthroplasty (TKA) using patient-specific guides. Compared with the conventional intramedullary alignment technique, the new method improved accuracy of alignment and a small reduction in blood loss and operating time.

In general, the accuracy of the surgical template applications depends on various factors such as the supporting ways of the template, the designing and fabricating methods, etc. As for the template-guided oral implantology, since the position of the implant has to be compatible with the intended final surgical restoration, there are three main types of template including bone supported, mucosa supported, and tooth supported. The oral surgery with the use of the template gets

a relative highest accuracy due to several reasons as follows: (1) Template is usually placed on the tooth, which is more stable than mucosa supported in other anatomy regions (spine, nasal, etc.). (2) Many commercial or open-source preoperative planning software and template design software are available. (3) The exposed region of oral presents is larger than other regions of anatomy so that the template can achieve the optimum position.

Nevertheless, some problems and complications may exist during the period of postoperative observation, due to that the template may have the problems of supporting or assembly. Therefore, the surgeons also need to check the CT images, the manufacturing progress of the template, the fixation of the template, the substantial allowance of drill in tubes, sharpness of the drill, entry points of the drilling performance, etc.

Additive Manufacturing Technology

6

Qin Lian, Wu Xiangquan, and Li Dichen

Additive manufacturing (AM) technology, also known as rapid prototyping (RP), is a set of technologies which are capable of fabricating 3D models and objects directly from CAD data by using the method of adding material in layers. The materials of different states, such as powder, liquid, and sheet, can be used by different AM technologies to fabricate 3D objects.

1 Basic Principle of Additive Manufacturing

AM is based on adding materials layer by layer, and each AM technology has its unique way of processing different materials to layers and bonding layers together (Figs. 6.1 and 6.2).

Basic AM process sequence is as follows:

1.1 Creation of CAD Model

The original model of AM part is created in the CAD software (like Pro/E, UG, CATIA, SolidWorks, Solid Edge, CAXA, AutoCAD, etc.), as shown in Fig. 6.3 [1].

1.2 Tessellation of CAD Model

Almost all AM machines accept STL files which are used as the basis of layering the model. STL is a simple way of describing the shape of the model by approximating the model surface with triangular facets. Most CAD software can convert the model to STL format, and the minimum size of the triangle can be set. Taking Pro/E software as example,

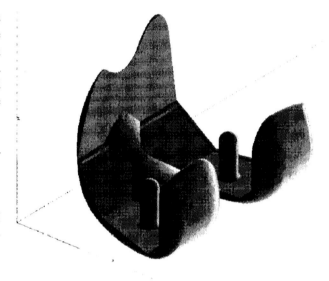

Fig. 6.1 CAD model

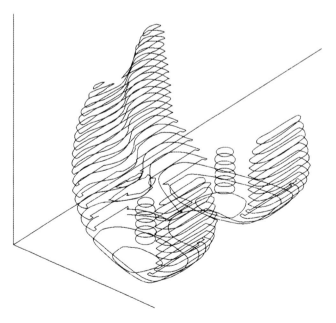

Fig. 6.2 Sliced model

Q. Lian • W. Xiangquan • L. Dichen (✉)
State Key Laboratory for Manufacturing Systems Engineering,
Xi'an Jiaotong University, 710054, Xi'an, Shaanxi, China
e-mail: dcli@mail.xjtu.edu.cn

© Springer Nature B.V. and People's Medical Publishing House 2018
G. Pei (ed.), *Digital Orthopedics*, https://doi.org/10.1007/978-94-024-1076-1_6

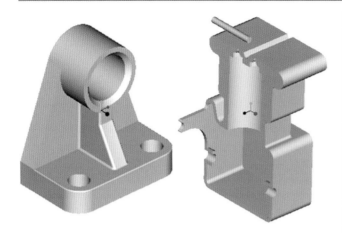

Fig. 6.3 Pro/E CAD model

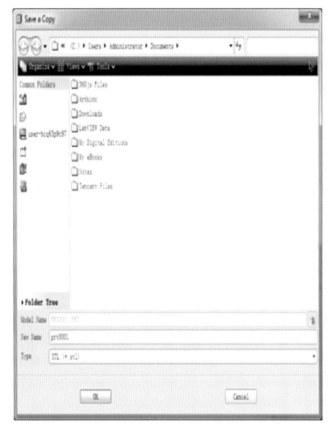

Fig. 6.4 Save as dialog box

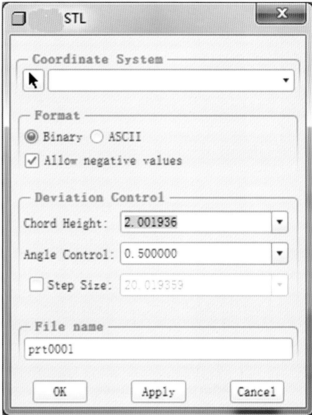

Fig. 6.5 STL output dialog box

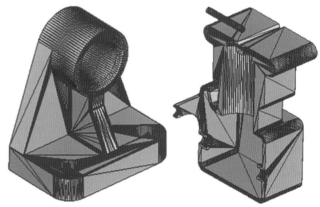

Fig. 6.6 STL format model

after finishing the CAD model, the user can save the model as STL format (Fig. 6.4) with different chord heights and angles (Fig. 6.5) which can control the accuracy of the tessellated model and the size of its file. The small chord height and angle are recommended for obtaining accurate and smooth tessellated model surface.

An example is shown in Fig. 6.6.

1.3   Slicing Process

Slicing refers to intersecting a STL format CAD model with a series of parallel planes in order to get the intersecting line to determine the 2D cross section. The distance between two parallel planes is the layer thickness of the building part. Since STL model is an approximation of the original CAD model and the sliced model is an approximation of the STL model, the slicing process will cause dimension and shape error of the original CAD model, and the error will be larger if thicker layer thickness is used. So the thinner layer thickness should be used in terms of increasing parts' dimensional accuracy [1].

1.4 Formation and Bonding of Layer Cross Section

There are several ways to form a cross section. Some AM machines use computer-controlled scan head (laser scanner, nozzle, cutting knife, etc.) to scan lines in order to form layer cross section (through curing resin, sintering powder, binding powder, cutting paper, etc.). Figure 6.7 shows a FDM nozzle's working path forming a single cross section. The newly formed layer will be bonded to the previous one until the whole part is finished.

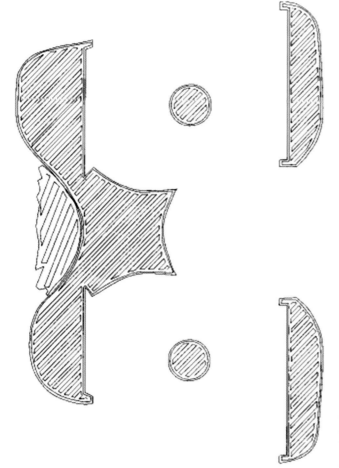

Fig. 6.7 FDM nozzle's working path

1.5 Post-process

Post-processing refers to the stages of finishing the parts for application purposes. This may involve abrasive finishing, like polishing and sandpapering, or application of coatings. In some specific cases, the part may also need high-temperature sintering in order to increasing its strength [1].

2 Process Techniques of AM

Since the AM techniques have developed, a dozen of process techniques emerged. The classification of AM process techniques is shown in Fig. 6.8. This present paper will only introduce those commonly used in industrial field, as shown below:

1. Stereolithography (SL)
2. Fused deposition modeling (FDM)
3. Selective laser sintering (SLS)
4. Laminated object manufacturing (LOM)
5. Laser direct metal rapid prototyping and manufacturing (LDMRPM)

2.1 Stereolithography (SL)

Stereolithography is the most wildly used AM process technique nowadays. The photosensitized monomer resin or solution which is used in stereolithography can be converted into solid parts through exposure to light of certain wavelengths. Monomers at the irradiated areas are polymerized upon their exposure to light, which can form a single-layer cross section.

As shown in Fig. 6.9, before the formation of the first layer, the vat surface is one layer thickness higher than the build platform. The computer uses the sliced model information to control the dynamic mirrors, which direct the laser beam over the vat surface, scanning the cross section of one layer of the part. After scanning a layer, the platform dips into the polymer vat, leaving a thin film from which the next layer will be formed. The next layer is drawn after a wait period to recoat the surface of the previous layer. Newly formed layer can cure strongly to the previous one. The resin which is not cured in the whole process can be used for next build process, so this kind of process technique can achieve the goal of being waste-free. For overhanging features of the part, synthetic supports are designed to ensure the correct formation. After finishing the whole part, the synthetic supports can be easily removed because of its network structure.

Fig. 6.8 Three-dimensional printing processes

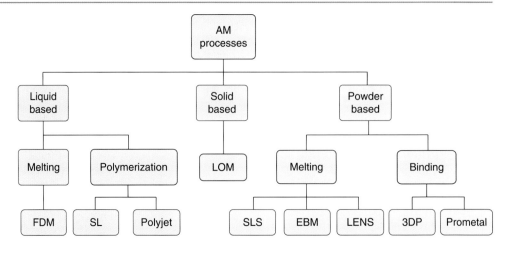

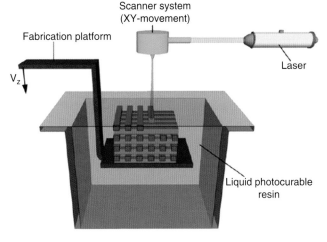

Fig. 6.9 A schematic of stereolithography [2]

Stereolithography is the first commercialized AM technology, and almost 70% of AM machines sold around the world are SL machines. Stereolithography can form highly sophisticated, fine part and meanwhile maintains the dimension accuracy of it (generally of ±0.1 mm) [1]. SL technology also achieves nearly waste-free raw material.

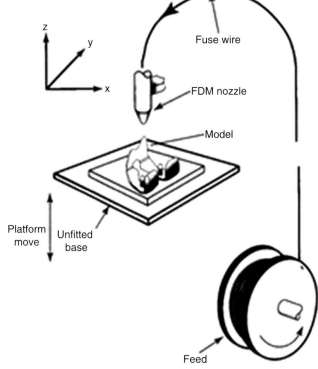

Fig. 6.10 Fused deposition modeling [1]

2.2 Fused Deposition Modeling (FDM)

A schematic diagram of fused deposition modeling is shown in Fig. 6.10. The nozzle that mounted on the gantry can move along the two main axes, and the platform can move upward and downward [1].

The nozzle can plot according to a predefined path and in a controlled manner, and meanwhile the thermoplastic plastics or wax fuse will be heated to semisolid state and extruded out at a constant speed. The first layer is formed on foam substrate, and the platform will move downward when the first layer is finished. The key of FDM process technique is maintaining the temperature of the semisolid material higher than its melting point (generally 1 °C higher).

The synthetic supports are needed since the overhanging structure (as shown in Fig. 6.11) can't be formed by FDM without supports. The supports can be formed firstly using other low-density or low-strength material which can be easily removed after finishing the whole part.

The thickness of each layer is determined by the diameter of the extruded material (generally 0.15–0.25 mm), and the thickness also represents the tolerance range of the vertical direction. In x–y direction, the dimension accuracy can reach to 0.025 mm [1].

There are several advantages of FDM, such as cheap, clean, easy to operate, and small impact to the environment, while its disadvantages, such as low accuracy, unable to form sophisticated or large part, poor surface quality, and low efficiency, limit its use. Based on its feature, FDM is used for forming conceptual model or prototype and can be used for shape and function test. The raw materials of FDM have good quality of toughness, and one of them, methacrylic acid (ABS), has good chemical stability and can be sterilized by gamma ray, making it fit for medical use [1].

2.3   Selective Laser Sintering (SLS)

Selective laser sintering is a process that nonmetal (nylon, synthetic rubber, etc.) or metal particles mixed with bonding agent are selectively fused by laser beam in a powder bed. A schematic diagram of SLS is shown in Fig. 6.12.

There are feed cartridges and build platform in the build chamber. Powder in the cartridge can be pushed out and spread across the build platform using a counterrotating powder leveling roller. The piston at the bottom of build platform can be lowered by the amount of one layer thickness each time and leave space for filling new powder.

The first layer of powder (0.1–0.2 mm) is selectively fused by computer-controlled laser beam according to the sliced model data. Then the counterrotating powder leveling roller will spread a new layer of powder to the lowered build platform. The unfused powder remains loose and serves as supports for subsequent layers, thus eliminating the need of

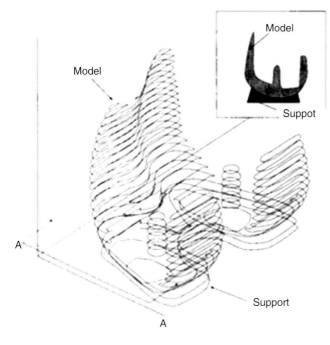

Fig. 6.11 Support [1]

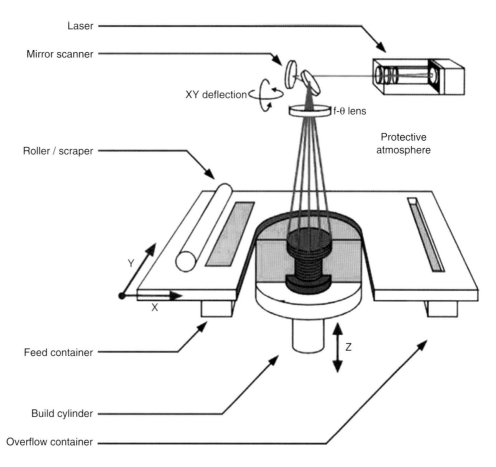

Fig. 6.12 A schematic of selective laser sintering [3]

synthetic supports. After the formation of the whole part, it is necessary to clean or do further process (grinding, drying, etc.) of the part.

There are many advantages of SLS, such as the high strength and mechanical property of the formed parts, no need for synthetic supports, lots of available raw material (functional plastics, durable synthetic rubber, ceramic and metal, etc.), utilization of raw materials close to 100%, large production capacity, high product quality and dimensional stability, short manufacturing cycle, etc. The disadvantages are low roughness of part surface, hard to form fine structures, loose and porous structure of the part which needs high energy cost post-process. The whole build chamber needs to be filled with nitrogen gas to minimize oxidation. The powder in the build platform needs preheating and the formed part needs 5–10 h for cooling, thereby causes low efficiency. During the process, sintering will produce toxic gases harmful to environment. SLS can be used for fabricating function test component. Since SLS can use different metal powder as raw material and the formed part can obtain the similar mechanical property similar to the metal component after post-process such as copperizing, it can be used for producing metal mold. SLS also can sinter wax powder to produce melt mold for producing small quantities of relatively complex and small components [1].

2.4   Three-Dimensional Printing (3DP)

A schematic diagram of 3DP is shown in Fig. 6.13. This process uses ink-jet technology to print binder into powder bed to form a part. The whole build process is similar to SLS. Post-process is also needed, like cleaning and sintering which can improve mechanical property.

2.5   Laser Direct Metal Rapid Prototyping and Manufacturing (LDMRPM)

Laser direct metal rapid prototyping and manufacturing is a technology combining both AM and laser cladding technologies. A schematic diagram of LDMRPM is shown in Fig. 6.14.

This process enables the creation of parts by melting and deposition of material from powder or wire feedstock. Unlike SLS, LDMRPM is not used to melt a material that is pre-laid in a powder bed but are used to melt materials as they are being deposited [5].

LDMRPM develops rapidly in recent years and it changes that AM can only make prototype of component using limited kinds of material (photosensitive resin, plastic, paper, wax and polymer, coated metal powder, etc.). The component made by LDMRPM has the property of high-density, high-strength, low-surface roughness, high-dimension accuracy and can be used directly as fully functional component with none or simple post-process. So this technology has broad market demand and application prospects in aerospace, energy, electrical engineering, instrumentation, military equipment, and medical field [5].

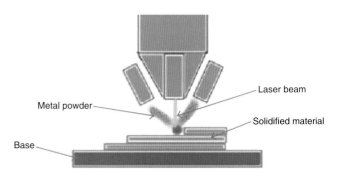

Fig. 6.14 A schematic of laser direct metal rapid prototyping and manufacturing [4]

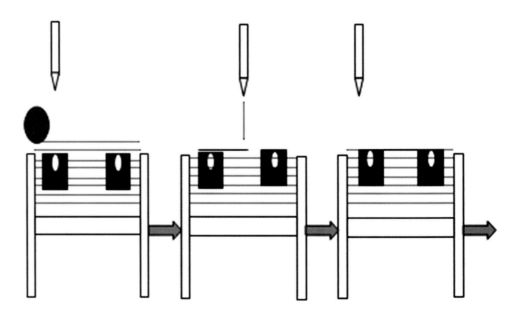

Fig. 6.13 A schematic of 3DP

3   The Development of AM Technology

Charles Hull created the world's first stereolithography equipment in 1986. He created the 3D System Company to market SL machines in the next year. Since then, a wide variety of AM technologies have been developed. A lot of fast-growing companies become famous and go public, such as Stratasys, Objet, etc. The direct revenue (sailing AM systems, producing prototypes, and downstream processing) of AM industry reached 1 billion dollars till 1998 [1]. In 2011, it was a $3.5 billion market of sailing AM machines and its material [6].

At present, major industrial countries pay much attention to AM and spend large amount of money in research and development. In United States, Obama proposed revitalization of manufacturing program and National Network for Manufacturing Innovation (NNMI) to congress, aiming to retake the leadership of manufacturing field and achieve 'design in America', 'manufacture in America'. In this way, more Americans will have job opportunities and American economy will become more sustainable. NNMI is led by Department of Defense and joined by manufacturing companies, universities, and nonprofit organizations. Its initial government investment was $30 million and company investment was $40 million. NNMI aims to make America the world center of AM and bridge the basic research with product development. The American government views supporting AM as a primary strategy for the development of manufacturing industry [6]. In 2003, Obama emphasized the importance of 3D printing again at the State of the Union address and viewed 3D printing as the symbol of the manufacturing industry renaissance.

In the early 1990s of the twentieth century, under the support of Ministry of Science and Technology, Xi'an Jiaotong University, Huazhong University of Science and Technology, Tsinghua University, Beijing Longyuan Company, etc. made great progress in research and industrialization of AM equipment, software, material, etc. Subsequently, many domestic universities and research institutions (such as Northwestern Polytechnical University, Beijing University of Aeronautics and Astronautics, South China University of Technology, Nanjing University of Aeronautics and Astronautics, Shanghai Jiao Tong University, Dalian University of Technology, North University of China, China Engineering Physics Research Institute, etc.) also conducted relevant research [6]. Nowadays, China has developed many kinds of AM machines and the quality of them is close to overseas products. Figure 6.15 shows the SPS SL machine developed by Xi'an Jiaotong University [7]. Figure 6.16 shows the medical use ceramic scaffold made by Xi'an Jiaotong University using SL technology [8].

Some technologies of Chinese AM machines are at the same level with overseas products, but China lags behind

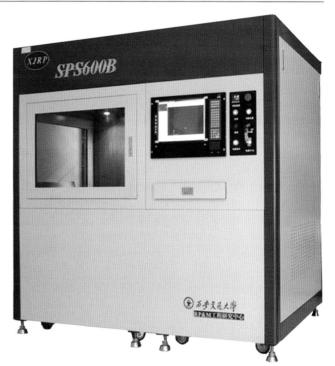

Fig. 6.15 SPS SL machine

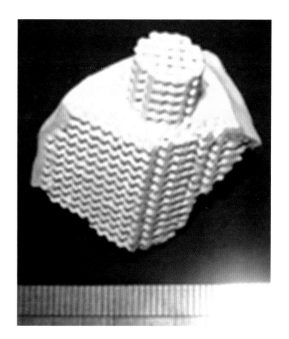

Fig. 6.16 Ceramic scaffold

overseas advanced level in key components, raw material, intelligent control, and application field. In China, AM is mainly used for manufacturing prototype other than directly producing components. In terms of basic theory and microforming mechanism, foreign countries have done lots of basic, deep, and system research work, but China only focuses on some specific problems. Advanced countries develop process technology based on theory mostly other than trial, and there is a huge gap between China and advanced countries with basic material research, material preparing technology, and material industrialization. The intelligence level of Chinese AM machines needs to be improved compared with overseas products. Chinese AM machines still need imported core components.

4   Application of Additive Manufacturing Technologies

AM technologies are able to quickly make sample parts for assessment, identification, and optimization, thereby avoiding faults and defects as much as possible. Using AM-made

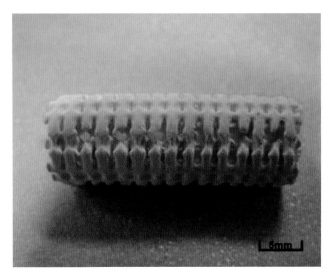

Fig. 6.17   AM application in various industries

sample parts, the designer can shorten the manufacturing cycle and increase the test items so that the finial component and product can be designed faster than before. As a result, AM technologies are widely used in designing new concept product, production feasibility study, product design approving, component engineer test, the overall coordination and evaluation of components, product function test and structure analysis, marketing promotion, etc. In rapid tooling area, AM can also provide parent parts of silicone mold and metal spraying mold. AM can be found in home appliances, automotive, aerospace, ship, industrial design, medical, and building areas, and it will have broader uses in the future.

Wohlers Associates Inc., specializing in additive manufacturing advisory service, analyzed AM application in various industries at its 2011 annual report. Figure 6.17 shows the situation of AM application in different areas. Consumer products and electronic field still hold a leading post, reducing the proportion from 23.7% to 20.6%. The motor vehicle proportion dropped from 17.9 to 9.1%. The proportion of research agency was 7.9%, and medical and dental field proportion increased from 13.6% to 15.9%. Industrial equipment field and aerospace field are 12.9% and 9.9%, respectively. During the past few years, medical and dental field has been the third largest field using AM [9].

Figure 6.18 shows the proportion of AM function applications. The functions include visual exhibition (using for communication between engineers, designers, toolmakers, architects, medical experts, and their customers), geographic information system model, functional model, assemble model, prototype (such as silicon rubber mold), metal casting model, mold parts, customized parts, substitute parts, etc.

Many countries are developing or using AM, and the amount of AM systems in a country responds to its economic

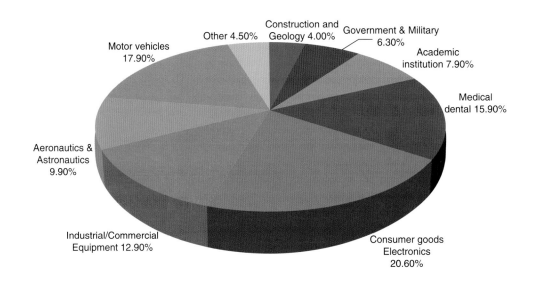

Fig. 6.18   Proportion of AM function applications

Fig. 6.19 The amount of AM systems in major countries

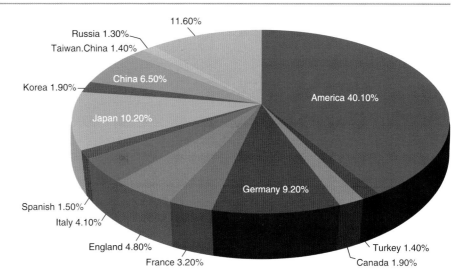

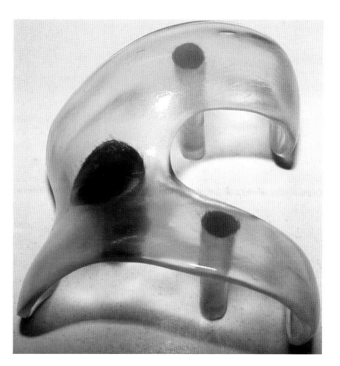

Fig. 6.20 Resin model of distal femur knee joint prosthesis [10]

vitality and creativity in certain degree. Figure 6.19 shows the amount of AM systems in major countries from 1988 to 2010. The United States, Japan, Germany, and China have most of the AM systems [9].

Currently, the major applications of AM are as follows:

4.1 Evaluation of Product Design and Function Test

Using prototype quickly made by AM, the designer can do assessment and verification of products and get feedback information from customer rapidly. Prototype can also enhance the manufactures' understanding of products so that they could determine the production principle and process flow reasonably. The new type of photosensitive resin material applied in AM can be used for making prototype good enough to do heat transfer and fluid mechanics test. Compared with the traditional way of model manufacturing, AM technologies are not only quick and precise but also can be changed or revalidated by CAD at any time so that makes the design more perfect. AM prototype maybe is the best thing for communicating between manufacturer and customer. For instance, the doctors will more likely want to see the physical prototype when they cooperate with engineers. Figure 6.20 shows the resin model of distal femur knee joint prosthesis made by stereolithography.

4.2 Rapid Tooling

With the technologies of precision casting, powder sintering, electrode grind, mold core, and die sleeve made by AM can be manufactured to function mold or equipment needed by enterprises. The manufacturing cycle of this method is 1/10–1/5 of traditional numerical control cutting, 1/5–1/3 of its cost. This kind of reduce will become larger when geometric complexity of mold is higher. Xi'an Jiaotong University made joint prosthesis (Fig. 6.21) by using investment casting to cast SL-made resin mold (Fig. 6.20).

4.3 Metal Parts Manufacture

As the LDMRPM matured, many metal components can be produced by AM with high production efficiency. Figure 6.22 shows the titanium alloy artificial joint sample parts.

4.4 Biomedical Engineering

In the 1990s of the twentieth century, Xi'an Jiaotong University Mechanical Engineering School proposed solving biomedical engineering problems by engineer method and applied AM in biomedical engineering research [11]. They have made progress on customized artificial prosthesis, bioactive artificial bone and joint, liver tissue engineering, etc [12]. Figure 6.23 shows the titanium mandibular implant made by Xi'an Jiaotong University using AM, and the implants have been used for clinical application [13].

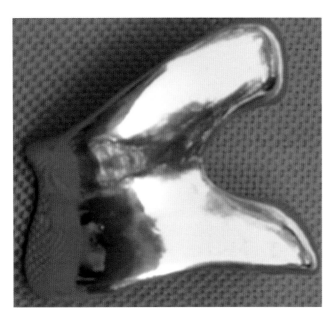

Fig. 6.21 Joint prosthesis [10]

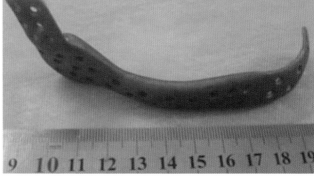

Fig. 6.23 Titanium mandibular implant

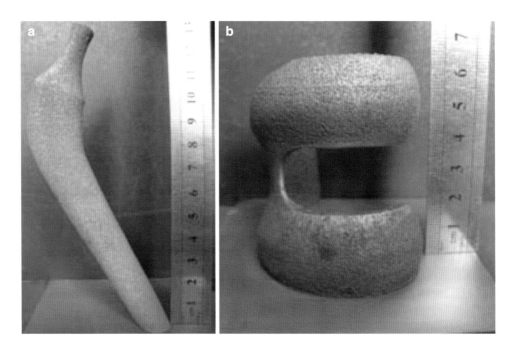

Fig. 6.22 Titanium alloy artificial joint sample parts. (**a**) Artificial hip joint. (**b**) Artificial knee joint

References

1. China Institute of Mechanical Engineering. 3D print: print the future. Beijing: Popular Science Publishing House; 2008.
2. Billiet T, Vandenhaute M, Schelfhout J, et al. A review of trends and limitations in hydrogel-rapid prototyping for tissue engineering. Biomaterials. 2012;33(26):6020–41.
3. Shahzad K, Deckers J, Zhang Z, et al. Additive manufacturing of zirconia parts by indirect selective laser sintering. J Eur Ceram Soc. 2014;34(1):81–9.
4. Wilkes J, et al. Additive manufacturing of ZrO_2-Al_2O_3 ceramic components by selective laser melting. Rapid Prototype J. 2013;19(1):51–7.
5. Anfeng Z, Dichen L, Bingheng L. Research progress of laser direct metal rapid prototyping technology. Ordnance Mater Sci Eng. 2007;30(5):68–73.
6. Bingheng L, Dichen L. Development of additive manufacturing (3D printing) technology. J Mach Manuf Autom. 2013;42(4):1–4.
7. Dichen L, He J, Xiaoyong T, et al. Additive manufacturing: the realization of macro-microstructure integration manufacturing. J Mech Eng. 2013;49(6):129–35.
8. Linzhong Z. Biomimetic interface design and fabrication technique of the hydrogel/ceramic composite joint scaffold. Xi'an: Xi'an Jiaotong University; 2012.
9. Dichen L, Xiaoyong T, Yongxin W, et al. The development of additive manufacturing technology. Elect Process Mold. 2012;(A01):20–2.
10. Hu Z, Dichen L, et al. Desert and rapid fabrication of custom-made unilateral knee joint prosthesis. Beijing Biomed Eng. 2003;22(4):266–9.
11. Qin L, Yaxiong L, Jiankang H, et al. The development of biofabrication technology. China Eng Sci. 2013;15(1):45–50.
12. Qin L, Dichen L, Cheng C, et al. Tissue-engineered soft tissue oriented manufacturing technologies and additive manufacturing. China J Tissue Eng. 2014;18(8):1263–9.
13. Mian Q, Yaxiong L, Jiankang H, et al. Application of digital design and three-dimensional printing technique on individualized medical treatment. China J Reconstr Surg. 2014;3:009.

Reverse Engineering Technology

Xie Le

1 The Basic Theory of Reverse Engineering

1.1 The Concept of Reverse Engineering

Reverse engineering [1–4], is based on modern design theory, method, and technology, to dissect, analyze, and recreate the existing products. Compared with the forward engineering, the differences are that it carries out some testing analysis for the existing product model and obtains the 3D contour data of the object. And then it deals with these data and proceeds 3D reconstruction and sets up the CAD data model. Engineering designers work on the CAD model for improvement or redesign, then they output the standard data file to rapid prototyping (RP) system or generate NC code to CNC machining system directly to generate realistic product or its mold. Finally, they will put it into production after the verification of experiment and finalizing the design product. Thus, reverse engineering technology is an effective way to shorten the development period of product, especially for the objects with complex shape or consisted by free surface, such as streamlined products, works of art, biological organs, mold, etc.

1.2 The Main Process of Reverse Engineering

Reverse engineering can be generally divided into four stages (Fig. 7.1):

1. Digitization of model: use digital means such as three coordinate measuring machine (CMM) or measuring devices such as laser scanning, to obtain the three-dimensional coordinate values of the point on the surface of the base model.

2. Extraction of geometrical characteristics of the parts' prototype from measured data: split measured data according to the geometrical properties of the measured data and adopt the method of geometric feature matching and recognition to obtain the design and machining features of parts' prototype.

3. The reconstruction of CAD model of parts' prototype: fitting of surface model in CAD system is carried out, respectively, with the 3D data after splitting, and the CAD model of the parts' prototype on the surface can be obtained through the intersection and joint of each surface piece.

4. The inspection and correction of the reconstructed CAD model: use the method of remeasuring the processed samples compared with the attained CAD model to test whether the reconstructed CAD model can meet the requirements of precision or other test performance indicators. As for those failing to meet the requirements, the above processes should be repeated until they meet the design requirements of parts.

1.3 The Application Fields of Reverse Engineering

Reverse engineering has a very wide demand in practical application. In summary, reverse engineering can play an important role in the following ways:

1. Transfer physical model to 3D CAD model through reverse engineering. At present, many shape designs are difficult to make some objects' three-dimensional geometric design yet by using the computer directly, such as complex artistic modeling, the body and other animals and plants' shape, etc., and more clay, wood, or plastic foam are inclined to be used to design the initial shape and then to design models.

2. Reverse engineering plays an irreplaceable role in modified design. Due to the reasons such as technology, beauty,

X. Le
Department of Plasticity Forming Engineering, Shanghai Jiao Tong University, Shanghai, China
e-mail: lexie@sina.com.cn

Fig. 7.1 Flow chart of
reverse engineering

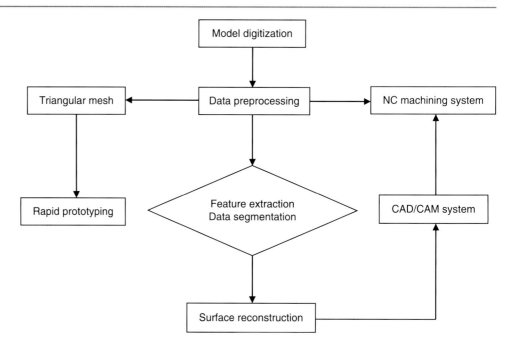

usage, etc., people often do some local modifications of existing component. In the occasion of original design without 3D CAD model, if physical component can generate CAD models according to the fact by data measuring and processing, it will significantly improve the production efficiency after processing the modified CAD model.

3. Some large equipment, such as aircraft engine, steam turbine unit, etc., often stop running because of certain part's damage. By means of reverse engineering, the replacement of the part can be produced quickly, so as to improve the efficiency and service life of equipment.

4. With the aid of industrial computed tomography (CT) technology, reverse engineering can not only generate the shape of the object but also can quickly find, measure, and position the internal defect of the object, so that it becomes the important means of nondestructive detection of industrial products.

2 Data Collection Methods

2.1 The Introduction of Several Digital Methods

Currently, with the development of sensor technology, control technology, image processing, computer vision, and some relevant technologies, a variety of solid surface geometric data acquisition methods appear; in terms of gauge head structure principle, it can be divided into contact and non-contact type.

2.1.1 Contact Measurement Method

Coordinate Measuring Machine (CMM)
The CMM, a kind of large precise three coordinate measuring instrument, which can measure the space dimension of workpiece with complex shape, is also commonly used. The CMM generally adopted touch-trigger probe, and one sampling can only obtain three-dimensional coordinates of one point. Main advantages of the CMM are high measurement precision and strong adaptability.

Chromatography
Chromatography is a kind of reverse engineering technology developed in the recent years. After filling the researched prototype parts, it adopts the method of combination of milling step by step and light scanning step by step to get the prototype parts inside and outside contour data of different section position and combines them to obtain the parts' three-dimensional data. The advantage of chromatography is measurement of inner and outer contour of arbitrary shape and arbitrary structure parts, but the measurement method is destructive.

2.1.2 Non-Contact Measurement Method
According to different measuring principle, non-contact measurement approximately includes optical measurement, ultrasonic measurement, electromagnetic measurement, etc. The most commonly used and relatively mature optical measurement method in reverse engineering will be introduced here.

Moire Fringe Method Based on the Phase-Shift Measurement Principle

This measure projects grating stripe onto the surface of tested object; grating stripe is modulated by object surface shape; the phase relationship of stripes will get change; and digital image processing method resolves the phase variation of the grating stripe images to obtain 3D information on the surface of the tested object.

Tomography Image Method Based on Industrial CT

This measurement method is to scan the fault section of tested object, based on the X-ray attenuation coefficient, and by processing the fault section reconstruction image, the object's 3D information can be established according to the fault images of different location. The method can be carried out to nondestructively measure the internal structure and shape of tested object. The method is of high cost and low spatial resolution of the measuring system, acquisition time of data is long, and the equipment volume is big. The high resolution of ICT system measuring accuracy is 0.01 mm developed by the LLNL laboratory.

The Stereo Vision Measurement Method

The stereo vision measurement is based on the parallax of the two (multiple) camera images of same three-dimensional space point in the different space position, and the location of space geometry relationship among the cameras to get the 3D coordinates of the point. Stereo vision measurement method can measure target feature points which are at two (multiple) cameras' common vision, without scanning device such as servomechanism. The biggest difficulty for stereo vision measurement is extraction and matching precision and accuracy of space feature points in many of the digital images. Recently a measure that structured light with the feature of spatial encoding projects onto the surface of tested object to make the measurement characteristics occurs to solve the problem of measurement feature's extraction and matching effectively, but it still needs to be improved in the measurement accuracy and the number of measurement point.

The Laser Scanning Method Based on Optical Triangle Principle

The principle and application of three-dimensional laser scanning, triangulation measurement principle, is one of the most widely used optical measurement, and one of the most mature methods in technology currently. Firstly surveying source (generally be laser point source or linear laser source) sent out by light source generator detects the surface of tested workpiece to be tested and projects to the position of linear CCD or array CCD through the optical system. As the datum for the calibration system, the projection position is point, so through the triangle, the height of the workpiece can be calculated from the length of CCD. All shape size of workpiece can be obtained by the movement of the measuring system

(that is, the scanning movement). Light source of 3D laser scanner adopts the semiconductor laser, and it has a long service life, low consumption and narrow laser scalpel and a series of advantages. Imaging system adopts the matrix CCD camera with imported resolution and high precision. Test platform of measuring system, which uses linear motion of three coordinates and four coordinate plan of one dimensional rotation movement, can scan and measure three-dimensional topography of 360° of objects. Schematic diagram of 3D laser scanning system is shown in the figure below. Linear laser projects the items placed on the worktable, and by taking use of one or two CCD camera to capture the image of the laser. When the relative position between the laser source and the CCD camera is known, the triangle method or other method may be used to convert the spot on the CCD image to spot position of items' three-dimensional coordinates X, Y, Z.

2.2 Comparison of Two Kinds of the Most Common Way of Data Acquisition Method (Table 7.1)

It can be seen from the table above that each of two kinds of common way has its advantages and disadvantages; the point is to choose the most appropriate method for the measured object.

3 Reconstructing CAD Model by Utilizing Reverse Engineering Technology

3.1 Method of Surface Reconstruction

The surface of the model may be divided into two parts. One kind is formed by elementary analytic surfaces such as plane surface, sphere, cylinder, cone, torus, ellipsoid, and so on; the other kind does not consist of elementary analytic surfaces and is formed by the freedom of surfaces that can change freely in a complex way, namely, the so-called freedom of surfaces.

1. For the first kind of shape regular surface, which consists of basic analytic surface, its identification and fitting is one of the key issues in computer vision and reverse engineering research. Especially, the algebraic surfaces of the two types have been studied extensively. The key technology is the segmentation of measurement data. So far, the main algorithms can be classified into two categories:
   (a) The method based on edge: This kind of method studies on the original surface of the features of the infinitesimal geometry and thus finds the sharp boundary. The surface

Table 7.1 Comparison between the advantages and disadvantages of the 3D laser scanner and the three coordinate measuring machine

Category	3D laser scanner	Three coordinate measuring machine
Unreached areas	1. Optical shadow	Probe radius limits the internal measure of workpiece
	2. Where the optical focal length changes	
Tolerance	With the change of surface	Partial distortion
Advantages	1. Fast, easy to get surface data	1. High precision
	2. Not necessary to do the probe radius correction	2. Specific geometric features of workpiece can be measured directly
	3. Can measure soft, fragile, untouchable, thin, fur, small deformation workpiece, and so on	3. Widely used, mature technology
	4. No contact force, won't destroy the precision surface	
Disadvantages	1. Unable to distinguish specific geometric features	1. Need to measure point by point, slow speed
		2. Radius correction should be done before measurement
		3. Size of contact force will affect the measurement value
		4. The contact force will cause the wear of the workpiece and the surface of the probe and affect the smoothness
		5. The method of radius correction is not easy to measure the inclined plane, and accuracy is also a problem
	2. Steep surface is not easy to measure, it cannot be measured where laser cannot be irradiated	6. For the internal measure of workpiece, the measurement value will be affected by the shape and size
	3. The surface of the workpiece surface is not perpendicular to the probe surface	
	4. The light and shade degree of workpiece surface will affect the accuracy of the measurement	

data is collected by discrete sampling, often represented in the difference format to estimate the derivative value everywhere, for example, the edge detection algorithm in image processing, such as analysis of gradient operator, Sobel operator.

(b) The method based on surface: This is a segmentation method combining the curved surface fitting. First, assign a surface expression to the point set in one region; then scale out from the near to the distant; meanwhile, check the fitting degree of the surface, it will not stop until the error exceeds the predetermined requirement. Because of considering the measurement information in the whole process, so this method is more stable than the former; the accuracy is also higher. But when the scale of the point cloud data to be processed is large, it takes a long time to complete the process. In addition, the method is not very effective for the segmentation problem of free surface. Curved surface fitting can be made after data segmentation. Segmentation and fitting are two processing steps that cannot be separated; especially for the segmentation method based on surface, segmentation and fitting are often closely connected. It often boils down to solve least squares problem for the problem of quadric surface fitting.

2. For the second type of free surface, it should be emphasized on developing automatic subregion and subarea of the point cloud data and then singly divided into point clouds surfaces by CAD operators using mathematical surface NURBS or Bezier to approach approximately.

The curved surface fitting is through all the data points with interpolation method, usually used for the measurement of precision point.

With the approximation method, surface fitting does not have to pass all the data points, but it expresses the overall optimal approximation degree of data points. It is usually used to handle a large number of data points, or in the condition when it needs to average the measurement error and noise. In most cases, if the surface of measured object is free curved surface model, it can be used directly to control vertex method to establish its geometric model. Thus the constructed surface can easily meet required mathematical properties to ensure the continuity of the higher order derivative which is over the first or second order derivative in the surface joint.

When we build free-form surface modeling, we first need to reverse surface control point through arbitrary distribution type points. After the surface control points is calculated, the existing free surface modeling technology can be used to establish corresponding geometrical model. For some objects, we can fit through a set of parallel section or translate a section. Rotation operation is to establish the three-dimensional geometric model. Skinning, sweeping, or swing technology can be used to construct geometric model in the form of non-uniform rational B-spline (NURBS) surface. The skinning method is mainly used for object with cross section of uniform variation, and the discrete point data of all parallel sections can be measured first, correspondingly fitting out NURBS curve of each closed section. Then use skinning technology to construct three-dimensional geometric model. The more cross section, the more precise the model structure is. Sweeping and swing method is mainly used for constant across section and rotary object; it needs to measure discrete data line of the section contour and then combine these two methods to construct the corresponding geometrical model. When the contour line is closed, it builds an entity model; otherwise, it builds a surface model. Free curved surface fitting is much more difficult; it is the key to construct CAD modeling for the reverse engineering.

Fig. 7.2 Surface reconstruction flow

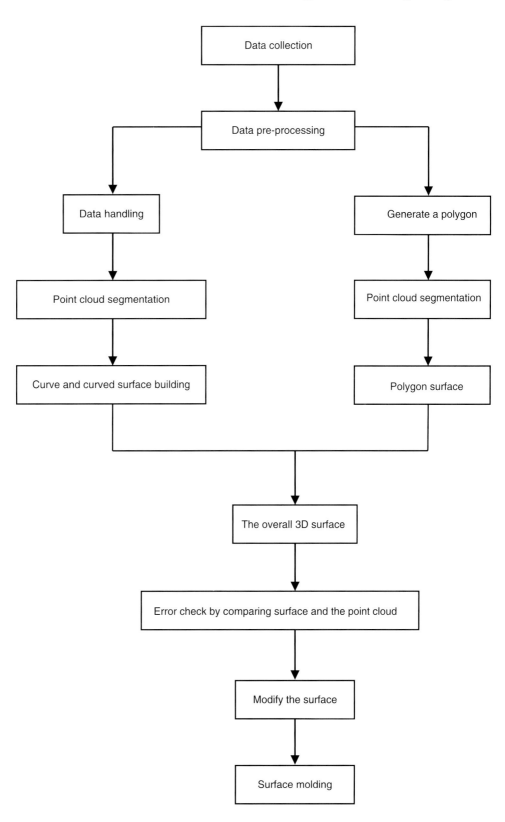

3.2 The Process of Model Reconstruction
(Fig. 7.2)

3.3 Introduction and Comparison of Several Kinds of Reverse Engineering CAD Software

The implementation of the reverse engineering needs the support of reverse engineering CAD software. The main function of reverse engineering CAD software is to receive product data from measuring equipment, good quality of curve or surface model is obtained by a series of edit operation, and through the standard data format. These data of curves and surface will transfer to the existing CAD/CAM system, and a final modeling in these systems will be completed.

With further studies of the theory of reverse engineering modeling, a number of commercial reverse engineering CAD software have emerged, very commonly used software include EDS's Imageware, ParaForm's ParaForm, DELCAM's CopyCAD, CISIGRAPH's STRIM100, ICEM company' ICEM Surf, etc. A few of the commonly used reverse engineering CAD software will be compared as follows.

3.3.1 EDS' Imageware Software (Formerly Surfacer)
Imageware software mainly has four aspects functions:

1. The function constructing the surface model, quickly and accurately constructing NURBS surface models according to the measuring data.
2. The analysis function of surface model's precision and quality.
3. The surface modification function, curves, and surfaces can be real-time modified interactive shape.
4. The analysis processing function of the measurement point can accept all kinds of different sources of data, such as CMM, Laser sensors, Mouse sensors, Ultrasound, and so on.

3.3.2 ParaForm Software
ParaForm software has been widely used; its main function includes:

1. Receive the ASCII and IGES format of measurement data and implement fast triangulation.
2. Based on the analysis of curvature characteristic, the characteristic curve is extracted for data blocking.
3. NURBS surface fitting in a given accuracy and under the restriction of cross-border continuity.
4. By editing curve network and global linkage function, implement surface deformation.

3.3.3 DELCAM's CopyCAD Software
CopyCAD software mainly has the following functions:

1. Input and transform process of various measuring data, and according to the given tolerance triangles, construct model.
2. According to the triangle patch model, interact or automatically extract characteristic curves.
3. The analysis of surface model's precision and quality.
4. Use the characteristic curves to construct NURBS surface patch and achieve smooth joining of surface patch according to the continuity requirement.

3.3.4 CISIGRAPH's STRIM 100 Software
Curved surface reconstruction mainly has the following several processes with STRIM 100 software:

1. Read the measurement point, and collect noise data.
2. Interactively define model's characteristic curve, and set up the wire frame model.
3. Define the continuity constraint between the surface patch, and construct NURBS surface patch on the wire frame model.
4. Finally check the surface model.

3.4 The Key Steps in the Process of Model Reconstruction

3.4.1 Advance Planning in Model Reconstruction
Before reconstruction, it is very crucial to plan the decomposed method and the range of the entire surface in advance. Various measurement tools in Imageware were mainly relied on observing the point cloud curvature distribution, continuity, and the extracted features. For example, direct point cloud fitting method, UV grid fitting method, curve rotating method, scanning method, lofting curve surface construction, etc. It is important to identify the basic characteristics of the point cloud block, choose the most suitable and high-precision method, and take into account the continuity of it with the surrounding surface.

3.4.2 The Process to Create Curve
First it is necessary to judge and decide which type of curve to generate. The curve can be exactly through the lattice, or can be very smooth (Capturing the main shape of a curve represented by a dot matrix), or between the two.

In the process of creating curves, the author will create curves to meet the need for lofting surface construction and the UV grid method fitting, and the more curve the structure is, the more accurate the resulting surface will be. Thus, in the place where the surface curvature is big, the authors will usually construct more cross-sections. The same principle applies to curve control points, the curve can be adjusted by changing the number of control points. When control points increase, the shape is well agreed, otherwise, the curve is relatively fairing.

The step to diagnose and modify curves is also very important. The smoothness of curves can be judged by the curvature of curves. For important curves, you can check them with the agreement of point cloud; you can also change the continuity of curve with other curves (connection, tangent, and curvature continuity). This step has great impact on the quality of surface to be created subsequently.

3.4.3 Process of Creating Surface

We first need to decide to generate what kind of surface. As with curves, we can consider to generate more accurate surface or need more smooth surface, such as class 1 surface, but continuous surface of G1 already has a smooth surface. It depends on the need of the parts' design and accuracy that can be achieved in the process.

In the process of creating surface, as mentioned above, there are lot of methods to create surfaces. Lattice can be used directly to generate surface; curve surface can also be created by skin, scanning, four methods of boundary surface, and so on; of course, surface can be generated by combination with lattice and the information of curves; there are also other ways such as rounded corners, composite, bridge to generate surface. But these ways were limited by the purpose and surface shapes of point cloud characteristics, curve, and the constructed object; the authors usually choose low error and point cloud good inosculation as a selection criteria.

Surface diagnosis and modification are also the necessary steps. Although compared with the curve, it is more difficult to modify the surface by means of the control points. But by tools provided by Imageware, we can compare the adjacent degree between surface and lattice, check surface fairing and other surface continuity, and revise at the same time. For example, we can make the surface and lattice alignment, adjust the surface control points to make the surface more smooth, or reconstruct the surface and so on. It takes a skilled and experienced software operating personnel. Therefore, the authors usually try their best in the first two steps, but do not easily modify the surface by manual adjustment of the surface control points. But this function is quite useful for the product designers; they can adjust the control point to change surface to meet their requirements and inspire their imagination.

3.4.4 Piece of Surface

As mentioned in the error analysis, errors are usually larger in the process of curved surface fitting than directly constructed surface.

References

1. Yu Z, Yu F, Xuefeng C. Reverse engineering technology principle and its key technology. Kunming University of Science and Technology. 2001;24.
2. Guangzao F. Reverse engineering technology and applications. Taipei: Gau-Lih Book. 2003.
3. Zhiqing X, Changku S. 3D reverse engineering technology. Beijing: China Metrology. 2002.
4. Yuanqing J. UG/Imageware reverse engineering training tutorial. Beijing: Tsinghua University Press. 2003.

Digital Technology Used in Orthopedics

8

Lin Yanping and Le Xie

1 Digital Technology Used in Orthopedics

1.1 Digital Technology Used in Orthopedic Surgery

Toward precise, minimally invasive, customized, and remote surgery is the four directions of clinical surgery in twenty-first century, and the trend exacerbates the need of digital technology. Orthopedic surgery is the fastest-growing application of digital technology and a complete digital system has been formed. This system mainly consists of these following parts:

1. Computer-assisted preoperative planning, including medical image processing, 3D modeling and editing, operative scheme design, and database interface.
2. Digital design and manufacture of surgical template and customized implant, including the design of the template and implant, 3D printing technology, and digital manufacturing.
3. Image-guided surgery, including the registration and real-time tracking of the instruments. The 3D models are registered to the patient during the operation in order to provide spatial navigation and guidance. The registration is achieved using a rigid body transformation.
4. Robot surgical system, including surgical extenders and auxiliary surgical supports, to assist in the accurate execution of the planned interventions.
5. Integrated operating room, including the information integration of visual information and data from multiple sources, to provide maximum visual information and data to the surgeon in real time.
6. Computer-aided rehabilitation, including the measurement and analysis of the postoperative condition to assess the effect of operation, to make scientific rehabilitation planning.
7. Virtual surgical simulator, including virtual reality and haptic feedback, to provide a realistic, cost-effective, safe, and repeatable alternative to traditional surgical training methods.

With the development of digital technology, the structure and composition of this system will be continuously developed.

1.1.1 Computer-Assisted Preoperative Planning

Through image processing such as image fusion and image segmentation, the 3D virtual model of the patient is constructed, in which surgeons can observe, measure, and compare directly to design the operation planning. The major work includes:

(a) Acquiring the medical image CT/MRI from the PACS/HIS system
(b) Medical image processing and 3D model reconstruction using professional software, to establish 3D model of the patient
(c) Observing and editing the 3D model by rotating, translating, zooming, mirroring, measuring, analyzing, cutting, or repositioning
(d) Getting more intuitive information by 3D printing and preoperative operating on it when necessary
(e) Designing the individualized implant for special case with preoperative planning
(f) Database supporting, in which the surgeon can acquire all sorts of implants, and the related case information

Computer-assisted planning software is the necessary tool for surgeons to design the operative planning. The planning software usually contains the following modules: image processing module, 3D reconstructing module, 3D editing module, database module, and design module of the individualized implant. At present, the famous preoperative planning

L. Yanping (✉) · L. Xie
The National Center of Digitizational Manufacture Technique, Shanghai Jiaotong University, Shanghai, China
e-mail: yanping_lin@sjtu.edu.cn

software includes Mimics, Simplant, SurgiCase of Materialise, 3D Slicer of Harvard University, Amira of ZIB company, Voxel-Man Dental, TempoSurg, SinuSurg of the University of Hamburg, and iPlan of BrainLab. The trend of the software development is more specialized, for adapting the professional needs of orthopedic surgery.

1.1.2 Surgical Template and Customized Implant

According to the different clinical applications, surgical guide can be classified into two kinds. One is the basic template with definite shape and structure, such as dental implant template and pedicle screw implant template. This template has the definite structure and the design is relatively simple

and mature. The other one is customized implant, which structure is completely dependent on the surgical region and the operation scheme.

(a) Basic template with definite structure. Take the pedicle screw implant; for example, the insertion point, orientation, and depth of screw channel are determined by surgical planning on the 3D model (Fig. 8.1a). The structure of the template has basic shape and even can be generated automatically (Fig. 8.1b).

(b) Customized guide. Take the pelvic tumor excision; for example, the shape and structure of the surgical guide are dependent on the tumor and the operation scheme, which is completely customized (Fig. 8.2).

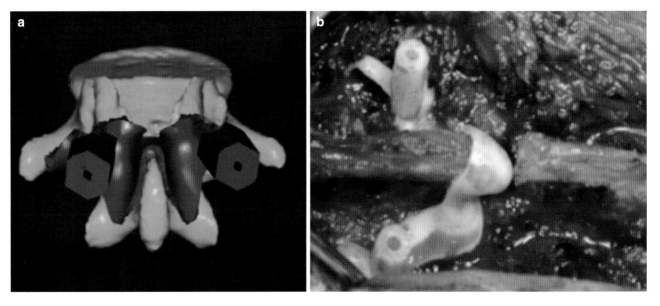

Fig. 8.1 Template for pedicle screw implant. (**a**) 3D design of the template. (**b**) 3D printing model

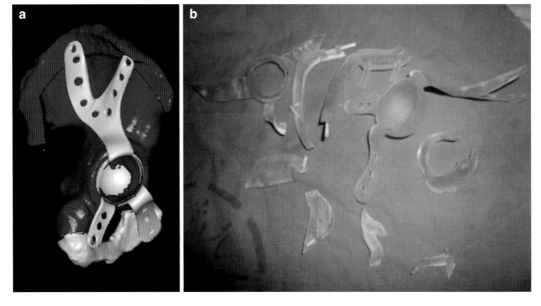

Fig. 8.2 Customized guide for pelvic tumor excision. (**a**) 3D design of the guide. (**b**) 3D printing model

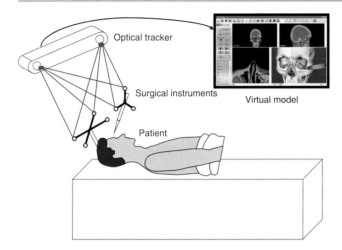

Fig. 8.3 Image-guided surgery

Individual guide can guarantee the operation accuracy, but its application is limited by various factors. The guide design and application should meet the following requirements:

(a) Design. The guide is designed based on 3D model and operation scheme to determine the cutting path, drilling point, direction, and depth.
(b) Locating. The hard tissue matched to surgical guide should have relative complex geometry, and the soft tissue should be stripped to locate the guide correctly.
(c) Manufacturing accuracy. Suitable 3D printing method and materials of surgical guide should be selected in order to guarantee the manufacturing accuracy.
(d) Stiffness. The guide should have sufficient stiffness and have no deformation to credibly guide the instruments.

1.1.3   Image-Guided Surgery

Image-guided surgical navigation is the import method to operate accurately with minimal invasion. Using a rigid transformation, the 3D reconstructed model is registered to the corresponding surgical anatomy. The instruments and patient are tracked in real time by positioning tracker. Surgeons can operate guided by the images on the screen (Fig. 8.3).

The advantages of image-guided navigation technology are as follows:

(a) The virtual 3D model can be easily manipulated by the surgeon to provide views from any angle and at any depth within the volume. The operation scheme can be planned and simulated virtually before actual surgery takes place. This way, the surgeon can easily assess most of the surgical risks and difficulties and has the confidence about how to optimize the surgical approach and decrease surgical morbidity.
(b) During the operation, the surgeon can locate the tracked instrument in relation to the patient's anatomy on images

using the navigation system. The system provides the accurate location of the instrument where the surgeon cannot actually see the tip of the instrument. This way, the surgical accuracy is improved, and the risk of surgical error is decreased.
(c) Assisted by the image-guided navigation, the surgeries can be carried out with minimal invasion and less time.

At present, many famous medical companies from the USA, Germany, Japan, and other countries, such as BrainLab from Germany, have developed a variety of navigation systems. Surgical navigation system is used in standard surgical procedures in many surgeries, such as computer-assisted neurosurgery, computer-assisted oral and maxillofacial surgery, guided implantology, computer-assisted ENT surgery, computer-assisted orthopedic surgery, and so on.

1.1.4   Robotic Surgery

The classification of surgical robotic systems depends on the actual point of view one takes. There are multiple classifications of robotic systems applied in medicine. Robotic surgery can be divided into three subcategories depending on the degree of surgeon interaction during the procedure: supervisory controlled, tele-surgical, and shared control. For surgical assistant systems, the surgical robot systems are further divided into two classes: surgical extenders and auxiliary surgical supports.

The RoboDoc developed by the Integrated Surgical Systems in the 1980s was the first commercial surgical robot system used in orthopedic surgery. It is currently used in hospitals in Europe. It is first used in total hip replacements, and its use is now extended to revision hip replacement and total knee replacement.

At present, there are many companies focused on surgical robots for orthopedic surgery. Acrobot from the Imperial College London is designed for total knee replacement. CASPAR from the German company OrtoMaquet is mainly used for knee surgeries. SpineAssist from Mazor Surgical Technologies is the first commercially available mechanical guidance system for spine surgery, which was approved by the FDA in 2004. The SpineAssist is a semi-active robotic system that is employed by a surgeon to perform a surgical procedure, compared with a fully automatic robotic system that performs the procedure autonomously (Fig. 8.4).

Surgical robot can access the body much easily through the small incisions than a surgeon can. It can integrate large amounts of data and images to access areas deep within the body with precision. And though they cannot process qualitative information to make judgments during the surgery, they are still able to filter out hand tremors and scale the surgeon's large movements into smaller ones in the patient. Robots do

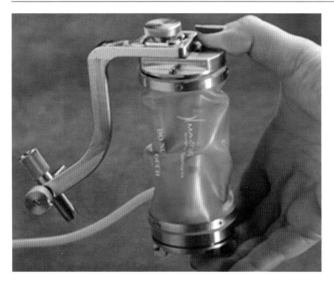

Fig. 8.4 SpineAssist from Mazor Surgical Technologies

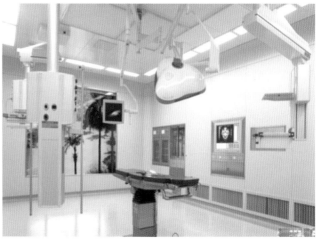

Fig. 8.5 Integrated operating room of the Jiuxin Mediclean Company

not actually replace surgeons but rather improve their ability to operate through the small incisions.

1.1.5 Integrated Operating room

The development and growth of minimally invasive surgery claim higher requirements to the doctor and spur the creation of integrated operating room. Integrated technologies augment surgeons' skills and help the surgical team work more efficiently. They can:

(a) Get the patients' information with PACS, HIS, and pre-operative planning at any time.
(b) Communicate with the experts, students, or patients' dependents through audio and video information.
(c) Control all medical equipment more effectively and safely.
(d) All technology can be manipulated from a central command console by one operator with friendly user interface.

Generally, the immediate availability of the data and information from multiple sources allows surgeons to operate more efficiently and safely. The integrated control system can provide maximum visual information and data to the surgeon in real time. The sophisticated, intuitive, and user-friendly interface allows the operating room staff to provide this support for the surgeon without distracting from their focus on the patient.

Many famous companies have launched digital integrated operating room successfully, and some domestic enterprises are also developing similar products. In cooperation with the Shanghai Jiao Tong University, the Jiuxin Mediclean Company has developed the integrated operating room (Fig. 8.5) and has achieved good sales performance.

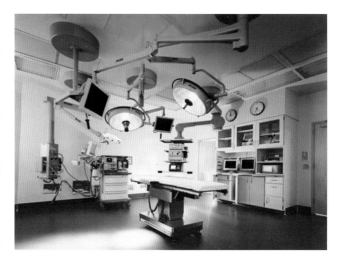

Fig. 8.6 Digital operating room from Stryker, Inc.

The further developments of the integrated operating room are the following:

• Integrating the navigation and robot system. Figure 8.6 is the digital operating room with navigation system, which is integrated into the control system. This system is applied in many hospitals of China for the orthopedic surgery.
• Integrating the intraoperative CT/MRI. Figure 8.7 is the digital operating room with the intraoperative CT system, which can scan and reconstruct the patient's model during operation.

1.1.6 Computer-Aided Rehabilitation

Computer-aided technology is more and more widely applied in the field of medical rehabilitation, to evaluate the effect of operation through professional software, to determine the

Fig. 8.7 Digital operating room from Medtronic, Inc.

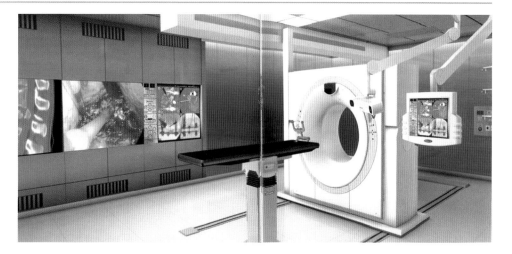

recovery degree of the postoperative function based on the biomechanics theory, to design the rehabilitation training program using rehabilitation robot, and to quantitatively detect the results of rehabilitation treatment for effective rehabilitation.

In the application of biomechanical methods, the scientific rehabilitation training program can be designed according to the data of motion measurement and analysis of further biomechanical rehabilitation.

- By comparing the measurement results of the joint motion to normal motion data, the joint and the movement which are not in the right place can be found.
- By comparing the postoperative motion data with the preoperative data, the quantitative evaluation of operation effect can be determined and the rehabilitation program can be planned.
- By human dynamic analysis such as motion measurement, plantar force measurement, EMG signal measurement, and so on, the factors that led to motion instability can be determined by the analysis of joint force and muscle force data. The customized rehabilitation training program is conducted with the help of rehabilitation training robot.
- By comparing the data of regular measurements, the effect of rehabilitation treatment can be evaluated.

Rehabilitation robot has been researched for quite a long time, such as the first rehabilitation robot CASE in the early 1960s, the MASTER of CEA company in France, the DeVAR system of Tolfa Corporation in the USA, the RAID system of the Oxford Intelligent Machines in England, the MELDOG system researched by Professor S. Tachi, and the MOVAID system of the Scuola Superiore S. Anna lab.

1.1.7   Virtual Surgical Simulator

Virtual surgical simulators with both visual and haptic feedback have been rapidly developed in recent years. The

surgical simulator can provide a cost-effective, realistic, and repeatable alternative to traditional surgical training methods and can play an increasing role in surgical education and training. With these simulators, novice surgeons can practice surgical operations safely, and they are allowed to make mistakes without serious consequences. Virtual surgical simulator is the important part of the digital technology.

Recently, many researchers have undertaken studies to improve the surgical skills in many minimally invasive surgeries, such laparoscopic, gastroscopic, bronchoscopic, and arthroscopic surgery. In virtual surgical simulator, virtual reality system is used to create virtual environments for simulating real-world scenarios, and haptic device is employed to assist in surgical training through virtual simulations of surgical procedures with haptic feedback. The simulator should have the following functions:

- Construction of virtual environment and virtual patients. By rendering the virtual models through 3D stereoscopic display, the users can experience the operative scene realistically.
- Haptic device. By employing the haptic device, the users can operate the virtual instrument with force feedback.
- Real-time virtual and haptic interaction. By utilizing collision detection technology, the real-time simulation of the deformation and force feedback is realized.
- Other sensory simulations. The system should simulate more interactions during operation such as sound and smell for more realistic feeling in the future.

For orthopedic surgery, virtual surgical training simulator has broad prospects. In the future, the individual and difficult cases are expected to be operated in virtual simulator to optimize the surgical results.

1.2 Biomechanical Simulation and Application of Musculoskeletal System

The biomechanics of human movement describes, analyzes, and assesses human movement including the gait of the physically handicapped, the lifting of a load by a factory worker, the performance of a superior athlete, the opening of space hatch by an astronaut, and so on [1]. The physical and biological principles applied are the same in all cases. The orthopedic surgeons, athletic coaches, rehabilitation engineers, therapists, kinesiologists, prosthetists, psychiatrists, orthotists, sports equipment designers, astronaut coaches, and so on are all interested in applied aspects of human movement. The application of analytical, numerical, and experimental characterization methods allows us to model, analyze, and understand the behavior and biological structures, which can make it possible to know the speed and acceleration of the mass center of each human bone segment, the joint force and torque, the muscle force, and the distributions of deformation and stress/strain in the bone [2]. Theory algorithm and numerical simulation of bone remodeling can explain how the mechanical environment influences bone remodeling and predict the changes of bone amount and structure.

In this part, the development of a biomechanical musculoskeletal model of human movement based on kinematic and dynamic analysis theory, theoretical calculations of muscle force, and on bone remodeling theory [1, 2] was described. The musculoskeletal geometric modeling, kinematic modeling (including development of a joint coordinate system, collection of experimental data, transformation of muscle model coordinates, and model scaling and matching), calculation of multi-rigid kinematics, estimation of muscle force, and simulation of bone remodeling were separately discussed. Additionally, a biomechanical simulation analysis software to predict BMD and muscle performance and to assess how these factors affect risks such as bone fracture or prosthesis loosening was introduced.

1.2.1 Musculoskeletal Biomechanical Model

The overall biomechanical model of a human musculoskeletal system includes a geometric model of the musculoskeletal system, a kinematic analysis model, a kinetic analysis model, a muscle force prediction model, and a bone remodeling model. The geometric model of the musculoskeletal system was developed to visualize human movement using powerful software. The kinematic parameters were calculated using the kinematic analysis model, while joint forces and joint torques were determined using kinetic analysis model. The muscle force model calculated muscle force. The bone remodeling simulated changes in bone density utilizing a bone remodeling control equation, which mathematically describes the relationship between density changes and mechanical loads.

Constructing the Musculoskeletal Model

Color images of human cadaver cryosections, computed tomography (CT) images, or magnetic resonance images are commonly used for musculoskeletal modeling. We constructed a musculoskeletal model using the CT data from a volunteer so that detailed BMD information contained in CT images could be incorporated. An integrated three-dimensional (3D) musculoskeletal model was reconstructed through image processing, including skeleton profile extraction, skeleton surface modeling, and muscle modeling (Fig. 8.8a, b). There are two types of muscle modeling approaches: a straight-line model, which uses a straight line to connect the origin and insertion attachment points of the muscles, and the muscle-path-plane (MPP) method [3, 4], which uses a physiologically relevant curved path to connect the origin and insertion attachment points.

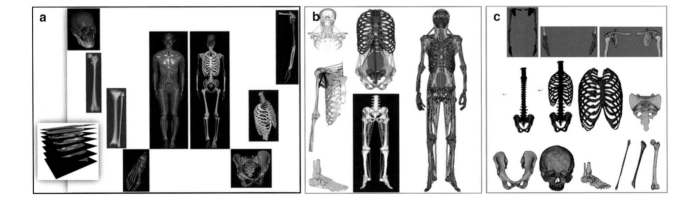

Fig. 8.8 Biomechanical models of the human musculoskeletal system. (**a**) Geometric model, (**b**) visualization model, (**c**) FE model

Establishing a Joint Coordinate System

Defining a standard joint coordinate system (JCS) of the entire human body is the key for determining the kinematic and dynamic parameters of astronaut movement. We used the same standard to define a JCS for both of our musculo-skeletal models (straight line and MPP) as well as for the actual subjects. This facilitated our ability to determine the relative position of each body segment during a subject's movement and to reproduce the movements with a model. In addition, changes in the muscle's length can be instantly observed using this analysis. In a 2009 study, we proposed a method for defining a local coordinate system for the entire body, which can be applied to the analysis of the kinematics and dynamics of normal human body movement [5]. The ter-minologies we used for the anatomical landmarks of the body came from anatomical related literature resources; therefore, each anatomical landmark could be easily identi-fied on both the musculoskeletal model and the subject.

Gathering Experimental Data

Experimental data is needed in order to calculate kinematics and dynamics or to estimate muscle force. For example, electromyography (EMG) measurements are required for making estimations of muscle force, while ground reaction force or other contact reaction forces are needed in order to use the static optimization method for estimating muscle force. Additionally, motion capture systems are required for recording movement and translating those movements into a digitized model [6].

EMG measurements were generally obtained, while sub-jects performed an operation or maximum voluntary contrac-tion (MVC) tests. MVC tests involved an experimenter manually applying increasing loads on the limbs of the sub-ject, while surface EMG information was simultaneously being collected. The peaks of the EMG signals, indicating maximum contraction, were used to estimate muscle force. Standard terminologies for anatomical landmarks were used, and the positions of the anatomical landmarks were obtained using a motion capture system while the subject was moving. To reduce the chance errors when determining the anatomical landmark positions, rigid plates with four markers for each segment of the subject were used to indirectly calculate the positions of virtual markers in JCS.

Transforming Muscle Model Coordinates

To obtain the spatial location of the muscle attachment points (MAPs) during joint movements, we had to transform the coordinates of the MAPs from the world coordinate system (WCS) A (the standard human body coordinate system of the musculoskeletal system often used for 3D musculoskeletal system reconstruction of space-related operations) to our JCS. If it is assumed that the JCS of the musculoskeletal model is identical to the JCS of the subject, then the MAPs can be easily transformed from the JCS to world coordinate system B (WCS B, the coordinate system defined by the motion capture system of the subject) at any time during movement [7]. We hypothesized that during a subject's movement, their bones and segments would be rigid bodies; therefore, the relative spatial coordinates of the MAPs for bones remained unchanged. We could then explore the dynamic properties of the muscles (such as changes in mus-cle length and muscle contraction speed) by analyzing the changes in the MAP locations [8]

Scaling and Matching Models

Scaling and matching a model representation to a human subject is necessary for studies of the musculoskeletal model. Since there may be many obvious differences between the musculoskeletal model and the subjects, the model has to be scaled to match the anthropometry of the subject. Maintaining consistency for the kinematic parameters between the mod-els and the subjects is also very important. In our study, the heights of the subjects were considered to be the major factor impacting the calculation of kinematic parameters. Therefore, the dimensions for each body segment in the model were scaled based on relative distances between the two joint cen-ters obtained from anatomical landmarks of the subject. Muscle fiber lengths and tendon slack lengths were scaled according to the relative location of MAPs. This process allowed all the features of the subject to be reproduced in the model [8].

Calculating Multi-Rigid Kinematics

Kinematic parameters, such as linear and angular accelera-tion for each segment of a subject's body, play an important role in the calculation of dynamic parameters such as joint force, joint torque, and muscle force during movement. After defining the JCS of each body segment based on the ana-tomical landmarks, we calculated the kinematic parameters by analyzing the relative position of the JCS to WCS at spe-cific time points and exploring the relationship between each JCS at different moments [7].

Calculating Multi-Rigid Dynamics and Estimating Muscle Force

Following the determination of the multi-rigid kinematic parameters, we were able to calculate the multi-rigid dynamics, space force system equilibrium equation estab-lishment, and static optimization value. For the multi-rigid dynamic calculation, an inverse dynamic algorithm was used. Thus, when calculating the joint torque or force of the elbow, we started with the hand before moving up to ana-lyze the forearm. Similarly, when calculating the joint torque or force of the knee, we started with the foot and then analyzed the lower limb, followed by the thigh. We could obtain the raw EMG data by taking EMG measurements along with the MVC tests. The raw EMG data was then imported to the software we developed for signal analysis and processing. Finally, the processed data could be used to calculate the muscle activation function in order to estimate muscle force.

Simulating Bone Remodeling

Bone remodeling is a complicated biological activity, which must be represented in models by nonlinear characteristics due to the anisotropic properties of the bone and the complex load conditions imposed on bones. To generate a simulation algorithm for bone remodeling, we coupled the bone remodeling control equation with a finite element model for the bone (Fig. 8.8c). The initial densities and elastic modulus were defined according to the gray value of bone CT images, determined by the degree of X-ray attenuation during imaging. New densities and elastic modulus were calculated from the initial bone densities using specific simulation criteria, which were taken into consideration in building this simulation model. The final solution of the remodeling process generated by the algorithm following an iterative computational process represented the final density distribution of the bone. The bone remodeling simulation allowed analysis of bone turnover, loss, and adaptation [9].

Developing Simulation Software

We are currently developing biomechanical simulation and analysis software using C++ programming language and biomechanical model described above. The software includes a kinematic analysis module, a kinetic analysis module, a muscle force prediction module, and a bone remodeling module. The four software modules can be applied to a wide range of applications, such as comparing different exercises designed to counteract the physical effects of weightlessness in order to optimize their effectiveness. Moreover, it can be used to analyze task requirements as well as record the state of an astronaut's strength and endurance at a particular time during a mission.

1.2.2   Application in Clinic

The musculoskeletal biomechanical model has been widely used in clinic. Geometric model of the musculoskeletal model was mainly used for visualization during kinematic and dynamic analysis (shown as Fig. 8.9). The kinematic and dynamic calculation models were applied to analyze the data measured from kinematic and dynamic experiments of motion of the normal persons and patients. The muscle force and joint force, the position and speed, and the acceleration of the mass center of every bone segment can be obtained by kinematic and dynamic calculation.

The FE model of musculoskeletal system was used to calculate the stress or strain in the bone to evaluate the stress level or changes in the bone under special load or after fracture fixation. All these analysis results can help the surgeon to select better schemes for fracture fixation, skeletal deformity correction, and bone defect reconstruction (Figs. 8.10, 8.11 and 8.12).

1.2.3   Parametric Investigation of Bone Remodeling Simulation

The bone is a living tissue that is capable of modifying its structure in response to environmental changes, known as adaptive bone remodeling. For instance, immobilization and weightless spaceflights cause bone density and size reductions, and bone density and mass are increased by mechanical loads resulting in bone growth. Several different bone remodeling models have been proposed to explain how the mechanical environment influences bone remodeling and to be able to predict changes in bone density and structure [13, 14]. The results of numerical simulations are strongly dependent upon a set of parameters that are based on remodeling equations. We studied the effect of mechanical stimuli on the numerical simulation of bone remodeling to elucidate how the bone density distribution is affected by the different parameters that govern the remodeling process.

A finite element (FE) model of a proximal femur was constructed and imposed the forces at different phases of the gait cycle as the load conditions to simulate the bone's daily loading history [13]. Bone remodeling predictions were assessed

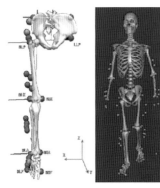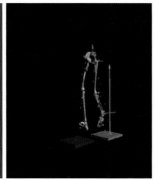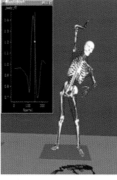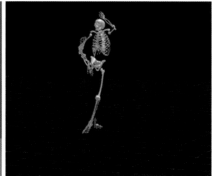

Fig. 8.9 Geometric model of the musculoskeletal model displayed in kinematic and dynamic analysis

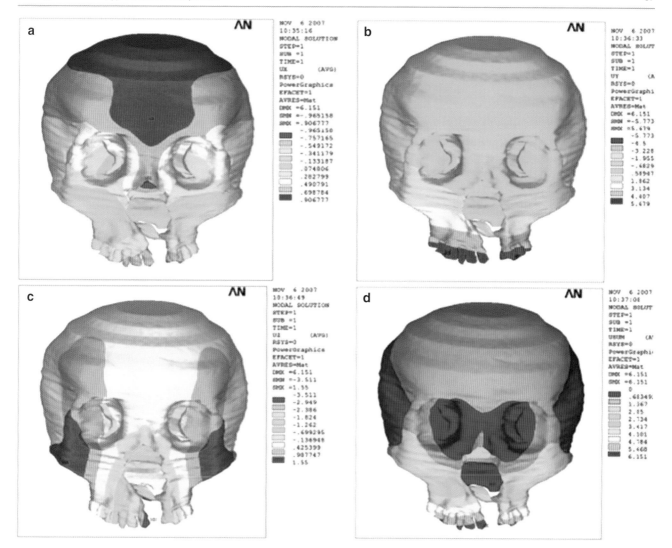

Fig. 8.10 Displacement distribution (mm) in the craniofacial complex during 5-mm expansions [10]. (**a**) the sagittal (X) displacement, (**b**) the transversal (Y) displacement, (**c**) the vertical (Z) displacement and (**d**) the total displacement.

using three different mechanical stimuli: strain energy density, equivalent stress, and equivalent strain. Then for each stimulus, several remodeling predictions were also made using different sets of parameters, such as varying width of the dead zone, reference stimulus values, and remodeling coefficients. The simulation results were compared quantitatively with calculating results obtained from CT images.

Remodeling takes place based on maintaining a homeostatic equilibrium between a strain-induced stress state and the bone density distribution. Any local perturbation in the mechanical state would stimulate local changes in bone density [15].

As shown in Fig. 8.13, the rate of this change for the apparent bone density at a particular location $d\rho/dt$, with $\rho = \rho(x, y, z)$, can be described as an objective function that depends upon a particular stimulus at the location (x, y, z). Whether bone formulation or resorption occurs depends on the stimulus, S. If S is greater or less than the reference stimulus by only a small amount, then bone remodeling will not occur; this is called the dead zone.

All the simulation results (Fig. 8.14) showed the characteristic form of the proximal femoral structure (A, cortical bone; B, intramedullary canal; C, Ward's triangle; D, typical cancellous density patterns).

The density values of proximal femur at different positions were shown in Fig. 8.15. It was shown that bone density distributions from all simulated results agreed well with those in the real structure of proximal femur. The predicted bone density distribution of the model using equivalent stress as the mechanical stimuli was the most consistent result. It was further indicated that the equivalent stress played a leading role in the mechano-regulation algorithms of bone remodeling. All these results provide a significant theoretical basis for the selection of stimulus parameters during bone remodeling simulation, which makes it possible to accurately predict bone remodeling process when stress level in the bone is changed because of weightlessness, prosthesis replacement, or orthopedic treatment.

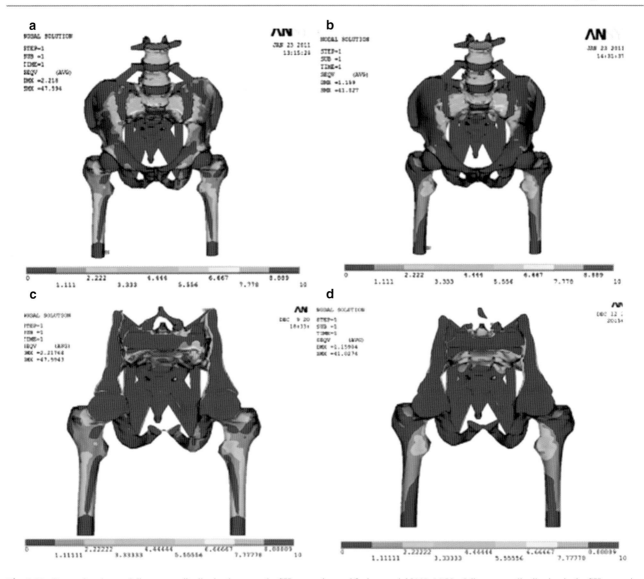

Fig. 8.11 Comparing the von Mises stress distribution between the SIJ contacting and fusing model [11]. (**a**) Von Mises stress distribution in the SIJcontacting model; (**b**) Von Mises stress distribution in the SIJ fusing model; (**c**) cross-section view of the Von Mises stress distribution from the SI joints to the hip joints inthe SIJ contacting model; (**d**) cross-section view of the Von Mises stress distribution from the SI joints to the hip joints in the SIJ fusing model

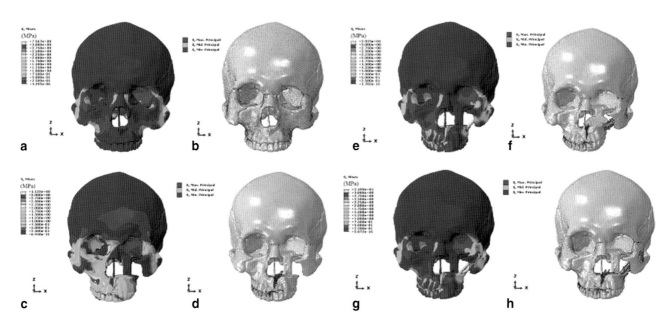

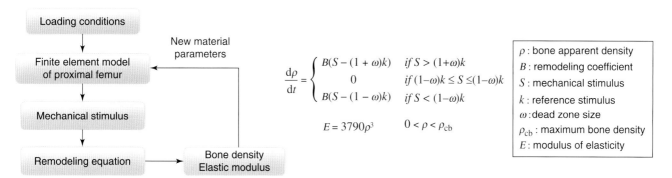

Fig. 8.13 Algorithm of bone remodeling simulation

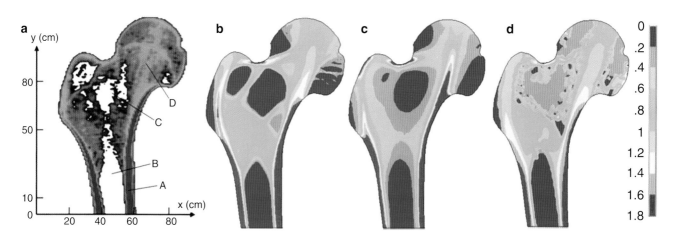

Fig. 8.14 CT scan image and predicted density distribution of proximal femur. (**a**) CT image, (**b**) strain energy density as stimuli, (**c**) equivalent stress as stimuli, (**d**) equivalent strain as stimuli

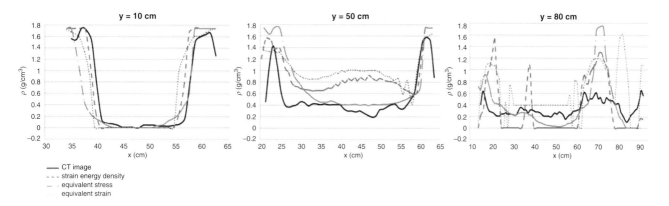

Fig. 8.15 Density of proximal femur in different positions

Fig. 8.12 Von Mises stress and principal stress vector distribution in normal craniofacial complex model and reconstructed model with unilateral maxillary defect [12]. (**a**) Normal model with Von Mises stress distribution; (**b**) Normal model with Principal stress vector distribution; (**c**) Reconstruction model 1 with Von Mises stress distribution; (**d**) Reconstruction model 1 with Principal stress vector distribution; (**e**) Reconstruction model 2 with Von Mises stress distribution; (**f**) Reconstruction model 2 with Principal stress vector distribution; (**g**) Reconstruction model 3 with Von Mises stress distribution; (**h**) Reconstruction model 3 with Principal stress vector distribution

1.2.4 Summary

The musculoskeletal biomechanical model and dynamic simulation have a great potential not only for clinical biomechanics research but also for enhancing spaceflight research, including for predicting musculoskeletal system performance, assessing spaceflight risks, and developing techniques to counteract the predicted effects of microgravity.

2 Virtual Reality Technology and Its Applications

2.1 Overview of Virtual Reality Technology

2.1.1 The Basic Concept of Virtual Reality

Virtual reality [16–20], also called spiritual environment, is a comprehensive technology in the computer field, combined with computer graphics technology, multimedia technology, sensor technology, technology of parallel real-time multidisciplinary technical computing, artificial intelligence, and simulation technology.

In 1965, Ivan Sutherland, the founder of computer graphics, gave us the classical concept of virtual reality which is popular today. (1) Computer generates the world which looks, sounds, and touches like real virtual world (also known as the model world). The model world also provides the involved people with a variety of sensory stimulation like visual, auditory, and tactile stimulations. (2) The virtual world that computer generates should give a sense of immersion immersive. (3) People interacted with objects in the virtual world in a natural way. That is to say, people use gestures, body language, human languages, and other natural ways instead of regular input devices like keyboard and mouse. We can get the concept of virtual reality model, just like that in Fig. 8.16.

2.1.2 The Basic Features of Virtual Reality Technology

We can use three Is to represent the basic features [21, 22] of virtual reality technology – immersion, interaction, and imagination. The triangle of virtual reality technology which is short for I^3 is shown in Fig. 8.17.

Immersion refers to the operator that works as the man-machine-environment leader, existing in a virtual environment. Interactive means the interactive ability that the operator has encountered with the objects in the virtual world.

It is a key factor in the harmonious relationship between people and machines, reflecting the various sensory stimulation signals the virtual environment provides and the different response actions people make to the virtual world. Interactivity includes objects' operational level, the natural level that users get feedback from the natural environment, and the extent of physics movement that objects perform according to physics movement laws in the virtual environment. With the combination of virtual reality and qualitative and quantitative binding of comprehensive integration environment, imagination guides people to deepen the concept and germination of new ideas, further developing people's creativity. So virtual reality is not only a connector between the users with the terminals but also allows users to immerse in this environment to acquire new knowledge, thus improving emotional and rational knowledge and resulting in new ideas. When the results are input into the system, the state of the system will handle the real-time display or feedback to the user by the sensing device. This is the process of learning-creating-relearning-recreating process.

2.2 Virtual Reality Research Status

2.2.1 The Status of Foreign Virtual Reality Research

The USA is the birthplace of virtual reality. In the early 1940s, the flight simulator as a predecessor of virtual reality was invented in the USA. In 1966, with the auspices of the Office of Naval Research, the US MIT Lincoln Laboratory developed the first helmet-mounted display (HMD), and

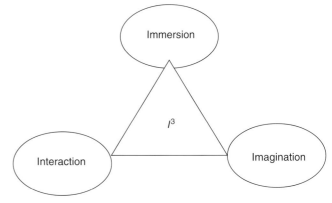

Fig. 8.17 Virtual reality technology feature

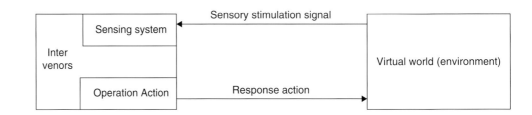

Fig. 8.16 The concept of virtual reality model

then the analog force and tactile feedback device were added to the system. In 1970, the first HMD system with more complete features was developed. Since the late 1980s, the US VPL companies have developed a more practical helmet-style three-dimensional display, which could provide six degrees of freedom of data gloves, stereo headphones, and a corresponding computer hardware and software system. In the early 1980s, the US Defense Advanced Research Projects Agency (DARPA) developed a practical system of virtual battlefield called SIMNET for the formation of combat training tank. In addition, the US NASA actively applied VR technology to the research programs such as the space activities outside the space vehicle, free to manipulate space station research and research on the Hubble Space repair projects, leading to important results.

Britain didn't show any weakness in the research and development of the virtual reality technology. In some aspects of VR development, especially in the fields of distributed parallel processing, ancillary equipment (including haptic feedback) design, and applied research in Europe, the UK is ahead of other countries. Some other developed European countries such as France, Germany, Sweden, and Spain also actively pursue the development and application of VR. Japan is one of the leading countries in the field of current virtual reality technology research and development, whose focus is on the establishment of large-scale VR knowledge base. It has also done a lot of work in the field of virtual reality games. Japanese universities are working on applying virtual reality technology to industry and business that also have achieved fruitful results.

2.2.2 The Status of Domestic Virtual Reality Research

The research on the VR technology in our country started in the early 1990s and it has achieved preliminary till now. Some domestic research institutes, such as the key laboratory of spot induction technology of the Beijing University of Aeronautics and Astronautics and Tsinghua University, the key laboratory of computer simulation of the National Defense University, Shanghai Jiao Tong University and Zhejiang University, China Civil Aviation College, Air Force Aviation College, and Air Force Engineering College, all have made great achievements in the research of virtual reality, and the PLA Information Engineering University has achieved important results. In some aspects of the research, they even have been close to the international advanced level.

2.3 The Application Fields of Virtual Reality

The application prospect of virtual reality technology is very broad, starting from the demands in the military field, now to the fields of education, industry, commerce, engineering, entertainment, education, medical and visualization, and many other fields.

2.3.1 Military Applications

It was first used in military simulation and the initial simulation was used to train pilots. When the pilot is in the simulator, he would just feel like he was in a real plane. All equipment would perform like the real ones, but it would never hurt pilots nor the simulator, which is considered as the ideal training method. Currently, virtual reality technology has been used in the large-scale combat exercises in realistic combat environment of land, sea, and air forces.

2.3.2 Manufacturing Industry Applications

Virtual reality technology has great potential in the manufacturing industry, from initial market research to processed products as well as after-sales service. In recent years, many countries have undertaken actions in the field of virtual manufacturing research and application, including the shape virtual design, virtual design layout, motion and dynamic simulation, thermal processing simulation, process simulation, assembly simulation, virtual prototype and product performance evaluation, advertising and roaming, production process simulation and optimization, virtual corporation's cooperation optimizer, and so on.

2.3.3 Medical Applications

The main applications [23, 24] are as follows: virtual dissection training systems, surgical simulation systems, remote operation, and so on. With virtual reality technology to simulate training, it can not only save expenses of entity material but also allow students to repeat operations on an issue, so as to achieve purposes of effective training.

2.4 Virtual Surgery System

2.4.1 Virtual Surgery Background

Since the concept of virtual reality (VR) proposed in the 1980s, it is booming as a new discipline in recent years. Meantime, it is more and more widely applied in the fields of engineering, military, construction, aerospace, medicine, and so on. As one major application of virtual reality technology, virtual training system is now becoming a hot topic of research institutions at home and abroad. Many countries, especially developed countries, have paid great attention on the virtual medical training system in the medical field and have put much effort into the research.

2.4.2 Virtual Surgery Meaning

Virtual medical surgery simulation training is an application with great technical difficulties. Conventional surgery is generally performed by on-site observation and animal experiments. All these methods have some shortcomings, such as non-repeating, some damage caused to the operation targets, and so on. Virtual reality technology can provide surgeries in a virtual environment and can also be used in surgical procedures for teaching, training, and surgical planning. At the same time, the virtual training system can significantly shorten training time of training a professional doctor for an operation. The success of the operation is closely related to the patient's life. Therefore, in general, before primary doctors have obtained the ability of a certain operation, they need to watch the operation procedure with experienced doctors' guidance. Then they would experiment on animal or human specimen and finally to clinical operations. Because of this, it takes a long time to develop a qualified surgeon. With the increasingly sophisticated and complex surgical procedures, it needs new ways to train doctors. And as the VR technology-based virtual training systems have been introduced, it is of great practical significance to train surgeons.

In the virtual training environment, trainees are immersed in the virtual scene. They would roam and observe three-dimensional structure of the training content, experience, and learn how to cope with the reality of the practical problems that may be encountered in operation. They can also learn all kinds of practical technical movements through eyes, ears, and feelings. It greatly saves training costs and time, so that the risk of non-skilled personnel to operate is greatly reduced. It is of important significance to improve the efficiency and quality of training with surgical experience and examples of experts training for beginners.

The National Digital Manufacturing Technology Center of Shanghai Jiao Tong University and the Eye and ENT Hospital of Fudan University have a long-time cooperation on the research of microsurgical anatomy of the ear and ear microsurgery (refer to Fig. 8.18).

2.4.3   Virtual Surgery Research Status

Conditions of Virtual Surgery Implementation

The four conditions to carry out the virtual surgery are as follows:

Constructing virtual scene in surgery of human organ or individual three-dimensional model from one or more of the medical examination equipment such as CT, MRI, and other patient image data

Displaying three-dimensional virtual human body and organs vividly and real time

Providing a virtual force feedback function with surgical instruments for surgical operation virtual contact

Providing more real human and physical characteristics of the organ and feeling the interaction and feedback of the models' deformation real time

Demand of Virtual Surgical Instrument Library

Medical electronic devices developed from the development of virtual surgery techniques are now growing at 10% per annual growth rate. However, the hardware of virtual surgery is to solve the input and output signals; virtual surgery software is the key, which can easily change, increase and decrease, and improve function and size of the system. Studies of virtual reality systems in the software include:

1. Geometric modeling and simulation based on computer graphic virtual environment
2. Based on the physical characteristics of complex objects' kinematic and dynamic simulation modeling and visualization

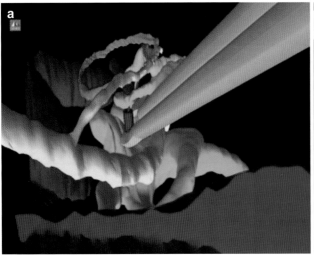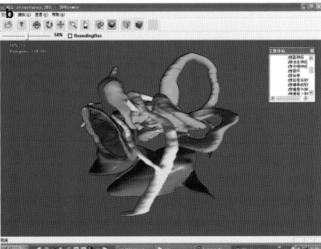

Fig. 8.18 (**a**, **b**) are the different angles of view about virtual ear microsurgery

3. Sensing information description and simulation based on human senses
4. Scientific visualization based on virtual reality technology
5. Intelligence and naturalization of man-machine interface

In conditions of virtual surgery, it is very important to provide surgical instruments with a virtual force feedback function. We could say that virtual operating room is built on a virtual environment based on computer graphic geometric modeling and simulation. Virtual surgical instruments provide platform and tools for the implementation of virtual surgery, which is a prerequisite for virtual surgery. Once the standard surgical instrument libraries are established, they can be ported to multiple virtual surgery system. It can share statics with many doctors through the Internet, avoid repeated work, decrease the workload, and save the resources. Therefore, it is necessary to develop a virtual library of surgical instruments used in surgery, to create a virtual environment for virtual surgery and to provide technical support for the subsequent development of the early virtual surgery.

2.5   Establishment of Knee Knowledge Systems and Motion Simulation

Human knee is the body's most important and most complex joint, also the site of multiple lesions. Due to its significance and value in all areas of clinical treatment, medical research, biomechanical design, application, and research, it has long been a widespread concern.

2.5.1   Data Acquisition and Processing

Data Collecting [25]
The data of this chapter are through two ways:

Data of the Southern Medical University are from virtual digital Chinese people, by adding each layer's image data to the obtained Mimics reconstruction.

The data of the Shanghai Ninth People's Hospital is through this way of CT scanning men's fresh body through the knee at 0, 45, 90, and 120° in four different positions. In order to obtain data ligament, before scanning the ligament was labeled with a metal wire. Then CT data were reconstructed and obtained in the Mimics.

Data Processing and Outputting
Belgium Materialise's [26] interactive medical image control system (MIMICS) is the interface of data scanning and rapid prototyping, STL file format, CAD, and finite element. Mimics software is an image processing software with three-dimensional visualization function and could support all common scanning file format. In addition, as a CAD or finite element, mesh interface is also available. Also, the software enables the user to adjust and revise division section of CT scans and MRI scans for later restoration model. Additional modules use Mimics STL file format or file format directly cut layer to provide the interface for the rapid prototyping and can be applied to all rapid prototyping system. It can also be used in other software to describe and calculate must-data which are intended to create medical objects.

Standard 3D file output formats include ASCII STL, Binary STL, DXF, VRML 2.0, and PointClouds.

2.5.2   Knee Motion Modeling [27]

Data Integration on Java3D Platform
From 3D max conversion output data to its display on the Java3D platform, several stages need to be added like importing obj. files, arranging the scene, adding simple features, and so on.

Importing Obj. Files
In obj. file import interface written in Java3D application, you need to write a three-dimensional shape or other contents such as background, lighting, and other branches, namely, a content branch.

Fig. 8.19 is the effect after the initial setting.

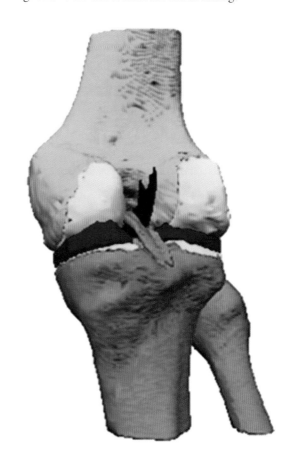

Fig. 8.19 The effect after the initial setting

Material and Transparency Settings
Material obj. format has its own file format mtl. in the material library, and modifications can be accessed in the program.

The movement of the knee ligament changes is needed in medical research. So the bone parts need transparent process

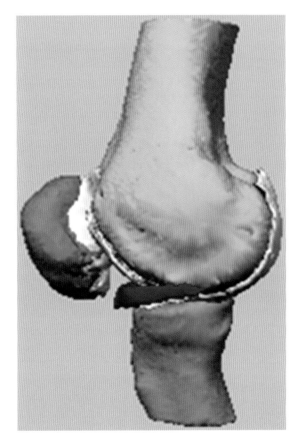

Fig. 8.20 The effect of materials of each component after the operation

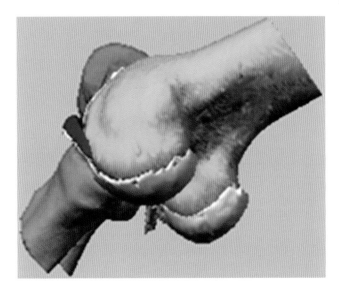

Fig. 8.21 The effect pictures after mouse functions

and you need to access obj. material library file. Figure 8.20 is the effect of materials of each component after the operation.

Add Simple Functions to the Established Platform
Define mouse functions: mouse to drag the rotation, the middle mouse button to enlarge, and drag the mouse. Figure 8.21 is the effect pictures after mouse functions are added.

Java3D Animation Realization
The key and difficulty of 3D animation realization is the body's movement. There are two different ways of Java3D to deal with the physical simulation of real-time animation. Interpolator is used in this section. By using position PathInterpolator object, you can make the body at the specified path shift, and the use of objects can make the body Rot Position PathInterpolator achieve translational motion of the shaft at the same time special about the rotation specified manner.

Scanning Data Interpolation Animation
CT scans knees' four-location data. On the basis of the data, we can interpolate knee motion animation. As the four sets of data's location in the collection are not precisely positioned, it influences the animation's positions to some extent. Meanwhile, as the derived data are composed of the triangle and can't be characterized and operated in UG and SolidWorks, it somewhat restricts to the animation software. However, with the doctor's explanation, knees vary by people. What femoral and neck bone animations show are mainly the trend movement, so it does not need to be accurate and complete with the collected data.

Simulation in Java3D The position of the neck bone at 0, 45, 90, and 120° is added to different position of timeline.

Simulation in 3dmax Steps of 3dmax animation are as follows. The main advantages of CT animation: imported knee information at four positions can be moved randomly in the same scene, so it brings much convenience to the animation data collection at different positions. Please refer to Fig. 8.22.

That is, after setting a certain angle as the key point, you can coincide the data with the knee information in the animation (Fig. 8.23).

Analysis and Optimization of Animations
1. As animation made by Java3D is imported into the Java platform, with the different knee coordinate systems and modeling, there are some mistakes of the animation data at the certain position. To solve this problem, we need to convert the data at the four positions into the same absolute coordinate system. However, we can't select the certain feature points and determine bone position and angle

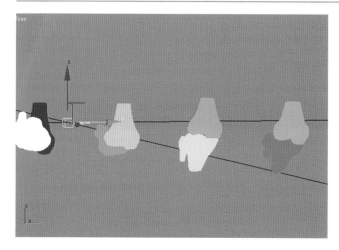

Fig. 8.22 The effect of four position data

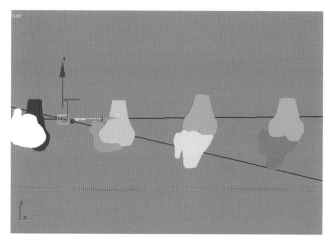

Fig. 8.23 Key point setting

data only by manual movement and alignment, which can't assure the accuracy. At the same time, Java3D's interactive performance is limited, so the workload of the whole process is relatively large. But on simple motion simulation for the trend, Java3D can quickly simulate a trend bones' basic movement path and movement, as a rough guide. In terms of simple motion simulation for the trend, Java3D can quickly simulate a trend of bones' basic movement path and movement for a rough reference.

2. 3dmax animation is the animation of CT data. As it is a professional flash software and easy to operate, it could assure the flash accuracy under the same workload. First of all, the data of the four key positions are relatively accurate. Although we can't choose the feature point in 3dmax, imported components' rotary and translation are very convenient, which is of great help to add the position data at the important time. Secondly, analog intermediate interpolation curve can be freely chosen. Animation of

interpolation curve during the simulation at the key points in this passage is selected by Shanghai Ninth People's Hospital orthopedic surgeon. Because knee motion varies, the key is to meet the medical requirements. In addition, in order to make it convenient for doctors to observe the knee movements, all animation is modified by bone doctors of SNPH that are more in line with human motion laws.

2.5.3   Establishment of Knee Knowledge Platform

Knowledge Platform Architecture

Architecture is the carefully chosen software architecture after analysis of needs and system module. It directly determines the software development tools, material, etc., types of support systems, and the quality of the system structure selection. It greatly influences on modifiability, scalability, maintainability, and development pace of the software.

System implementation structure can be divided into the following three forms:

1. It is called the material integrated systems implementation structure by using production tools like Dreamweaver and FrontPage and the output material integrated development approach like HTML, XML, and so on.
2. It is called the dynamic relationship between the data structure of the interactive system implementation by using databases like SQL Server and MySQL to manipulate objects and using PHP, ASP, and JSP as the dynamic development of output.
3. It is called dynamic and interactive multimedia integration system implementation structure by using multimedia database to manipulate object on the basis of development platforms like Author2ware and Director.

This system mainly uses the second system architecture design. We can build a three-dimensional presentation of the network platform with the full use of 3D function of Java.

Achievement of Acknowledge System

1. Realization of Two-Dimensional Animation
   The most popular graphic image processing software include Photoshop, CorelDraw, Photostyle, Fireworks, etc., among which Flash is the commonly used animation software. Flash can not only import graphics, images, sound, video, 3D animation, and other media, which itself is a powerful animation software, but also has a sound object-oriented program design, implementation, and various types of multimedia courseware interactive features.

   To achieve interact function through film clips, such as the drag of objects, the reproduction of objects, the change of property (location, size, color, transparency and so on) of the object in the courseware, please refer to the codes shown above in Chap. 3.

2. Interactive Animation Operation in the Java3D Scene
   Interactive performance for knowledge systems is crucial and Java3D interactive applications have mainly three types of behavior. The first category is the use of Java event handling model. The second is the use of Java3D objects' utility package offer, and the third category is to define your own behavior objects. Based on the Java platform, using SQL Server, MySQL, and other databases as the back end database, with JDBC connection to the database, it saves lots of accessing time to the system.

   After exporting obj. file, you can use the complete API Java3D scene to go on interactive operations. In the realization of three-dimensional animation, the main application within Java3D is the generation of interpolator object called Interpolator. You can write various types of three-dimensional animation program by combining interpolation object with another alpha objects together. Interpolator is an abstract class of Java3D. And actually what you use are its subclasses or grandchildren classes, such as PositionInterpolator, RotationInterpolator, and PathInterpolator. They can make objects move, rotate, sport, and go on in the specific path. Alpha object is used to provide animated programming of time controlling.

Eclipse Applications

1. Introduction of Eclipse Software
   Eclipse was originally created by IDE product development group of OTI and IBM companies in April 1999. IBM provided the initial Eclipse code base, including the Platform, JDT, and PDE. Currently led by IBM, around the Eclipse project, it has been developed into a huge Eclipse Union with more than 150 software companies involved in the Eclipse project, including Borland, Rational Software, Red Hat and Sybase, and so on.

   Eclipse is an open-source project. It is actually an alternative for VisualAge for Java and its interface is almost the same. But because of its open source, anyone can get it for free and can develop their own plug-ins on this basis, which has been attracting more and more attention. Recently more and more large companies including Oracle have also joined in the project and claimed that Eclipse may become the IDE master for any language development. Users simply download plug-ins in various languages.

2. Addition and Optimization of Interactive Functions
   Overall interfaces after the addition of interactive functions are shown in Figs. 8.24 and 8.25.
   (a) The function of add button is to click to select the represented structure file. And meantime, the case color is changed and the structure introduction is displayed. Button functions have been achieved.

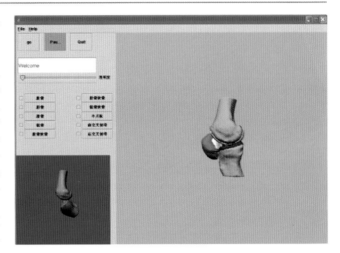

Fig. 8.24 Southern Medical University data platform

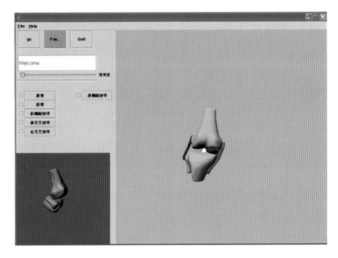

Fig. 8.25 Shanghai Ninth People's Hospital data platform

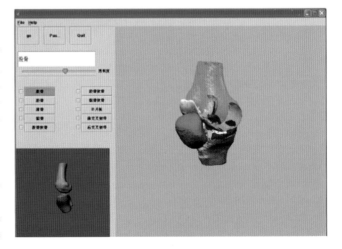

Fig. 8.26 Choose transparent display

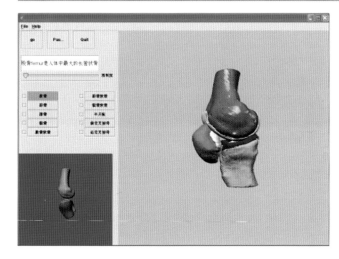

Fig. 8.27 Knowledge introduction

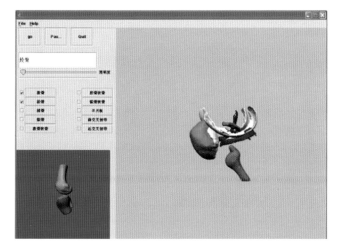

Fig. 8.28 Check blanking display

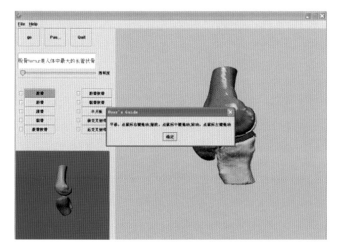

Fig. 8.29 Menu function introduction

(b) Add drag strip that can be selected to adjust the structure's transparency (Fig. 8.26).

(c) Add a text box to display the text. Figure 8.27 is the knowledge introduction.

(d) Add a check box, and then you can check the blanking and display the corresponding structure.

Figure 8.28 shows a check function. Add menu functions. Figure 8.29 displays a menu function.

References

1. Winter DA. Biomechanics and motor control of human movement. 4th ed. Hoboken: Wiley; 2009.
2. Öchsner A, Ahmed W. Biomechanics of hard tissues. Singapore: Wiley; 2010.
3. Tang G, Qian LW, Wei GF, et al. Development of software for human muscle force estimation. Comput Methods Biomech Biomed Engin. 2012;15(3):275–83.
4. Tang G, Wang CT. A muscle-path-plane method for representing muscle contraction during joint movement. Comput Methods Biomech Biomed Engin. 2010;13(6):723–9.
5. Tang G, Wei G, Nie W, et al. Simple method on definitions of coordinate systems for human lower limb. Biomed Eng. 2009;28(6):606–9.
6. Zhou H, Liu A, Wang D, Zeng X, Wei S, Wang C. Kinematics of lower limbs of healthy Chinese people sitting cross-legged. Prosthetics Orthot Int. 2013;37(5):369–74.
7. Tang G, Zhang XA, Zhang LL, et al. A technical method using musculoskeletal model to analyze dynamic properties of muscles during human movement. Comput Methods Biomech Biomed Engin. 2011;14(7):615–20.
8. Tang G, Ji W, Li Y, et al. JCS-based method on coordinate transformation of attachment points between muscle and bone. J Med Biomech. 2010;25(1):40–4.
9. Doblaré M, Garcı́a JM. Anisotropic bone remodelling model based on a continuum damage-repair theory. J Biomech. 2002;35(1):1–17.
10. Wang D, Cheng L, Wang C, Y Q, Pan X. Biomechanical analysis of rapid maxillary expansion in the UCLP patient. Med Eng Phys. 2009;31:409–17.
11. Wang M, Qu X, Cao M, Wang D, Zhang C. Biomechanical three-dimensional finite element analysis of prostheses retained with/without zygoma implants in maxillectomy patients. J Biomech. 2013;46:1155–61.
12. Shi D, Fang W, Wang D, Li X, Wang Q. 3-D finite element analysis of the influence of synovial condition in sacroiliac joint on the load transmission in human pelvic system. Med Eng Phys. 2014;36:745–53.
13. Mellal A, Wiskott HWA, Botsis J, et al. Stimulating effect of implant loading on surrounding bone. Clin Oral Implants Res. 2004;15(2):239–48.
14. Beaupré GS, Orr TE, Carter DR. An approach for time-dependent bone modeling and remodeling—theoretical development. J Orthop Res. 1990;8(5):651–61.
15. Mullender MG, Huiskes R, Weinans H. A physiological approach to the simulation of bone remodeling as a self-organizational control process. J Biomech. 1994;27(11):1389–94.
16. Min L. Virtual reality interactive multi-sensory information feedback technology research and implementation [Master's Degree Thesis]. Shanghai: Shanghai Jiaotong University; 2006.

17. Qiaojiao W. Research and development of virtual reality application software system [Master's Degree Thesis]. Shanghai: Shanghai Jiaotong University; 2006.
18. Bohan Z. The establishment of China-based digital human knee knowledge systems and motion simulation [Bachelor's Degree Thesis]. Shanghai: Shanghai Jiaotong University; 2007.
19. Ruixian Z. Preliminary study of human joint motion simulation and virtual surgery simulation of pedicle positioning [Bachelor's Degree Thesis]. Shanghai: Shanghai Jiaotong University; 2007.
20. Haipeng W, Ke R, Yanlin Z, You W, Le X. Establishment of dimensional finite element model around the knee ligament. Shanghai Jiaotong Univ Newsp (Med Sci). 2008;28(4):367–70.
21. Wang C, Gao W, Wang X. Spiritual environment (virtual reality) technology in theory, implementation and applications. Beijing: Tsinghua University Press; 1996.
22. Fenfang Z, editor. Virtual reality technology. Shanghai: Shanghai Jiaotong University Press; 1997.
23. Xie L, Shaoxiang Z, Wang Y, Lei T, Tianyu Z, Jiantie L, Tan L, Peidong D, Meichao Z, Yanbing L. Digital manufacturing technology applied in surgery. J Orthop Trauma. 2008; 10(2):109–10.
24. Le X, Bo X, Qiaojiao W, Min L. Applications of virtual reality technology in the surgeries. In: Symposium of Chinese Mechanical Engineering Society in 2005. Chongqing; 2015. p. 31.
25. Shizhen Z. Progress of problems and recommendations during human data acquisition. In: The 208th Xiangshan Science Conference Symposium. Beijing; 2003. p. 12–13.
26. Gao Y, Weidong Z, Yikai L, Wu Y, Xuemei J, Lin S, Shizhen Z. Interactive virtual reality technology and its application in the analysis of the stability of the knee. First Mil Med Univ Learn J. 2005;25(9):1145–8. www.materialise.com.cn
27. Tan G, Guo G, Wang Y, Wu P. Virtual reality technology applied in medical surgery simulation training. Med Train Coll Learn J. 2002;23(1):77–9.

Preliminary Study of Digital Technology on Orthopedics

Y. Z. Zhang, Sheng Lu, Yuanzhi Zhang, Yongqing Xu, Yanbing Li, Zijia Zhou, Shizheng Zhong, Zhijun Li, and Shaojie Zhang

1 Visualization of Digital Flap

1.1 Introduction

Anatomical and experimental studies of flaps have made a great leap forward, especially when the angiosome concept was introduced in 1987 by Taylor and Palmer, whereby the body was considered to be composed anatomically of multiple three-dimensional (3D) composite blocks of tissue supplied by particular source arteries. Since then, detailed studies of the forearm, leg, head, and neck have been carried out by Taylor and coworkers. The application of various flaps has resolved numerous problems in microsurgery. The traditional clinical training on flap anatomy, however, is conducted by means of textbooks, two-dimensional pictures, or cadavers. The rapid development of computer-based digitalization has made it possible to demonstrate flap anatomy in 3D, all-perspective, visualized, and vividly dynamic images, which will greatly enhance the understanding of the complex relationships between vessels, nerves, muscles, skin, and bones. It is expected that these possible images can be used in clinical anatomic training.

1.2 Application of Three-Dimensional Digitalized Reconstruction of Latissimus Dorsi Myocutaneous Flap

1.2.1 Section of the VCH-M III Dataset

Four VCH (Virtual Chinese Human) datasets, three males and one female (named VCH-M I, VCH-M II, VCH-M III, and VCH-F I), were reviewed to study the anatomic structures of thoracodorsal artery and latissimus . The VCH-M III dataset was chosen to be reconstructed for the LDM flap because it was finished recently with more distinct vessel illustration than other VCH datasets. The VCH-M III dataset consists of 8952 images, whose resolution is 302,462,016 pixels in TIF format. One thousand six hundred serially sectioned slices of VCH-M III, from the 1401st to the 3000th, were taken as the source for the 3D models. The cross-sectional images of the main structures of LDM, thoracodorsal artery, and its branches were analyzed on a section-by-section basis. From all the selected 1600 slices, one 2D section was chosen from every ten slices on an equidistant basis. The 160 sections chosen were directly digitized at a maximum resolution, and 160 color images were obtained, which were stored in JPEG format with middle-quality compression. The images were reframed, retouched, re-digitized, and restored in JPEG format without compression. The retouching was done by manual retouching with Adobe Photoshop 7.0 software.

1.2.2 CT Section of the Cadaver Specimen

Two adult fresh cadaver specimens, one male and one female, were subject to radiographic CT scanning before and after perfused with lead oxide–gelatine mixture, whose collimation is 0.625 mm (120 kV, 110 mA, pitch 2 mm, 5,126,512 matrix). By using Amira 3.1 (TGS) software, the 2D images in DICOM format were transformed into the 3D models of the entire region.

Y. Z. Zhang (✉) · Y. Zhang · Z. Zhou · S. Zhong · Z. Li · S. Zhang
The Affiliated Hospital of Inner Mongolia Medical University, Hohhot, China

S. Lu · Y. Xu
Department of Orthopedics, Kunming General Hospital of Chengdu Military Area Command, Kunming, China

Y. Li
Shanghai Jiao Tong University, Shanghai, China

Three-Dimensional Reconstruction

The skin, bone, subclavian artery, and thoracodorsal artery were used as marks for segmented areas in Amira software through a custom-written discrete snake procedure. The segmented structures of skin, bones, LDM, thoracodorsal artery, and its branches were displayed using toolbars of Brush, Lasso, and Magic wand. The 3D reconstruction consisted of (1) tracing the contours of the anatomical structures to be reconstructed, (2) adjusting the contours of stacked points by geometrical alignment, (3) modeling the surfaces by meshing the framework of the points transformed into polygons (wireframed object) and smoothing the contours of the object reconstructed from points (surface rendering), and (4) 3D-interactive visualization of the reconstructed structures. In order to demonstrate the LDM flap vividly, the images from pre-perfusion and post-perfusion reconstructed models were merged.

1.2.3   Sectional Observation

In the section images of VCH-M III dataset, the relationship of arteries and other tissues could be displayed clearly. We could trace the arteries from subclavian to the branches of thoracodorsal artery.

Three-Dimensional Reconstruction

The 3D images could display the main structures of LDM, thoracodorsal artery, and other adjacent structures. And the images could be transformed into movies with distinct and fluent frames by means of a moviemaker software.

1.2.4   Discussion

The latissimus dorsi muscle is the largest muscle in the body, up to 20 by 40 cm, allowing coverage of extremely large wounds. The latissimus dorsi flap is comprised of the skin paddle and underlying fat and muscle. It is the largest flap that can be harvested on a single pedicle and even can be combined with the serratus, scapular, or parascapular flaps, to create a flap complex that can cover massive wounds. The latissimus muscle is supplied by the subscapular artery, a branch of the axillary artery. The subscapular artery sends out the thoracodorsal artery, a circumflex scapular branch posteriorly, and then a serratus branch before it enters the substance of the muscle from its undersurface. The images of LDM flaps reconstructed from VCH can be displayed individually or continuously in different layers, directions, or tissues depending on the needs of the users, which directly exhibit the anatomical relationships of local tissues. One significant shortcoming of this technique, however, is that petty vessels and tiny nerves cannot be demonstrated. Therefore, we combined the above two different techniques in modern computers in order to reconstruct overall views of LDM flaps from cadavers. It shows that the vascular anatomy can be demonstrated digitally.

1.3   Three-Dimensional Reconstructive Methods in the Visualization of Anterolateral Thigh Flap

1.3.1   CT Angiography

Six healthy adult volunteers (five males, one female) underwent bilateral examination with a 64-row multi-slice spiral CT after median cubital vein injection with Ultravist (3.5 ml/s). Thin-layer image extents were from the abdominal aorta to toes. The date were tube tension 120 kV, tube current 100 mA, rapid 47.5 mm/circle, pitch 0.891, collimation 0.5 mm, and 512×512 matrix. Two-dimensional images in DICOM format were transformed into Amira 3.1 (TGS) software.

1.3.2   CT Section of the Cadaver Specimen

Two adult fresh cadaver specimens, one male and one female, were subject to radiographic CT scanning before and after perfused with lead oxide–gelatine mixture, whose collimation is 0.5 mm. Through Amira 3.1 (TGS) software, the 2D images in DICOM format were transformed into the 3D models of the entire region.

Three-Dimensional Reconstruction

The segmented areas of skin, bone, and ACFL structures were displayed in different colors using toolbars of Brush, Lasso, and Magic wand. Segmentation was performed through a custom-written discrete snake procedure. The 3D reconstruction via the Amira 4.1 (TGS) software consisted of tracing the contours of the anatomical structures to be reconstructed, adjustment by geometrical alignment of the contours of stacked points, modeling the surfaces by meshing the framework of the points transformed into polygons and smoothing the contours of the object reconstructed from points (surface rendering), and 3D-interactive visualization of the reconstructed structures. Then merging volume rendering with surface-rendered reconstruction from lead oxide–gelatine mixture perfused dataset. Three-dimensional models of these structures were saved as STL format, and then input Imageware 9.0 software to be retouched and re-divided.

1.3.3   Sectional Observation

In the section images of CT angiography from volunteer datasets, the relationship of arteries and other tissues could be displayed distinctly. The anatomy of ACFL could be traced from section to section in different layers. Perfusion with lead oxide–gelatine mixture angiography has the advantage of distinctly displaying the vessels and their perforation branches but incapable of demonstrating other tissues section by section.

Three-Dimensional Reconstruction

The 3D reconstructed visible models established from these datasets perfectly displayed the characteristic of ACFL and ALT flap anatomy, especially the blood supply of the flap. And the images also displayed the variation types of ACFL. The perforating branch of the lateral superior genicular artery and skin vasoganglion of the flap was also shown.

1.3.4 Discussion

The anterolateral thigh flap lies on the axis of the septum dividing the vastus lateralis and the rectus femoris muscles. Arterial inflow is supplied by the descending branch of the arteria circumflexa femoris lateralis and perforating branches of lateral superior genicular artery. The descending branch of ACFL arises from the profunda femoral trunk. The arteria circumflexa femoris lateralis distributes both ascending and descending branches, the latter supplying the perforators to the anterolateral thigh flap. This descending branch travels deep within the space between the rectus femoris muscle and the vastus lateralis muscle but on occasion within the substance of the rectus femoris muscle. In 80% of cases, the descending branch distributes musculocutaneous perforators to the flap. When it runs its entire course inferiorly in the substance of the rectus femoris muscle, flap dissection can be difficult. The skin paddle can be as large as 8 × 25 cm with primary closure attainable. Wider flaps can be harvested if the surgeon is prepared to skin graft the donor area. The flap has a large caliber pedicle, but the anatomy can be variable. There were three types of branches for arteria circumflexa femoris lateralis, the ascending, transverse, and descending branches, that came from the arteria circumflexa femoris lateralis and directly belonged to type I; in type II, the ascending, transverse, and descending branches were sent from the profunda femoris artery patterned with two shafts or from the femoral artery; the ascending, transverse, and descending branches originated from the profunda femoris artery that solely belonged to type III. Our study showed that merging volume rendering with surface-rendered reconstruction from lead oxide–gelatine mixture perfusion database is a more effective way of understanding the ACFL anatomy. This study established a foundation for observation on the state of skin flap blood supply stereoscopically implementing the development from plane anatomy to stereoscopic and digital anatomy. At present a detailed visualization of nerves in flap anatomy images is a problem that no one has currently resolved. So, we still have a long way to go before all the structures of the flap will be displayed in 3D models.

1.4 Three-Dimensional Digitalized Virtual Planning for Retrograde Sural Neurovascular Island Flaps: A Comparative Study

1.4.1 Introduction

Sural neurovascular flaps have advantages in treating ankle, foot, and leg defects, including proximity to the recipient site, easy excision, no injury to large blood vessels, good sensation recovery in the flap, and good skin quality. However, the clinical application of sural neurovascular flaps has been restricted by some complications such as postoperative swelling, congestion, and flap necrosis. It has been reported that an inappropriate-sized flap or an oversized flap without inadequate blood supply contribute to low survival rates of the flap. Traditionally, the preoperative design of the flap is to examine the blood vessels using two-dimensional imaging techniques such as Doppler ultrasonography and digital subtraction angiography. However, the caliber of the sural nerve nutritional blood vessel is very small and cannot be detected by Doppler ultrasonography and angiography. Therefore, the size and shape of the excised flap cannot be accurately designed before operation.

1.4.2 Materials and Methods

This study included 20 patients (13 males and seven females) with soft tissue defects of the ankle and foot who underwent soft tissue reconstruction. The average age of patients was 41.36 ± 5.65 years (range, 15–65 years). Inclusion criteria were (1) patient age between 15 and 65 years; (2) male or female patients; (3) deep wound defects in the distal one-third of the lower leg, ankle, or foot with exposure of larger blood vessels, nerves, tendons, and bones; and (4) shallow wound defects with exposure of unnamed smaller blood vessels, nerves, tendons, and bones or had a large soft tissue defect that was poorly repaired using a skin graft. Exclusion criteria were (1) severe cardiovascular, pulmonary, renal, hepatic, and gastrointestinal diseases; (2) extensive burn and frostbite injuries associated with inhalation injuries and shock; (3) severe injuries of the vital organs in the head, chest, and abdomen or multiple injuries associated with shock; and (4) osteomyelitis and intraarticular infection. Patients were examined using a 64 spiral CT scanner (GE, USA). The preoperative iodine allergy test was negative for all patients. Patients were injected with 90 ml of the nonionic contrast agent Ultravist 300 (Guangzhou Pharmaceuticals Corporation, Guangzhou, China) via the median cubital vein at a rate of 3 ml/s. The main CT scanning parameters were as follows: 120 kV, 200 mA, and slice thickness 2.5 cm (final reconstructed images were partitioned into 0.625 mm thick images). Serial data from the lateral malleolus to the tibial plateau regions in DICOM format were imported to a personal computer. Three-dimensional reconstruction was then performed using Amira 4.1 software. The 3D reconstruction consisted of (1) tracing the contours of the anatomical structures to be reconstructed, (2) adjusting the contours of stacked points by geometrical alignment, (3) modeling the surfaces by meshing the framework of the points transformed into polygons (wire-framed object) and smoothing the contours of the object reconstructed from points (surface rendering), and (4) 3D-interactive visualization of the reconstructed structures. The anatomical location of blood vessels, skin, and muscles was observed to determine the position of the flap. The 3D Lasso tool was used to select areas in the image based on the size and shape of the defects. The subcutaneous fat pixels were automatically measured and assigned to the skin, and the data were saved. The surface view in the Surface Gen module was used to visualize the sural neurovascular flap and the anatomical relationship of the flap with blood vessels and muscles. The source and pattern of blood supply as well as the number of perforating branches in the flap were recorded, and the length of the vascular pedicle and position of the perforating branches were measured using the Amira measurement tool.

For patients, the size and shape of the flap were designed according to the 3D digitalized reconstruction. The flap axis was marked between the midpoint of the popliteal fossa and the midpoint between the lateral malleolus and the Achilles tendon. The flap pivot point was located at the flap axis 5 cm above the tip of the lateral malleolus. An incision was made starting 0.5 cm bilateral to the flap pivot point longitudinally toward the proximal margin of the flap. A strip of skin (approximately 1 cm in width) was retained if the flap was transferred to the defect by opening the intervening skin. No skin was retained if the flap was transferred to the defect through a skin tunnel. The subdermal layer was dissected, and the deep fascia was longitudinally cut open 2 cm lateral to the flap axis to expose the sural nerve and its accompanying small saphenous vein. The pedicle of the flap was approximately 4 cm in width. The dissection was carried under the deep fascia until the perforating branches of the sural artery were found between the flexor hallucis longus and peroneus brevis muscles. The largest cutaneous branch was selected as the flap pivot point, and the design of the flap was adjusted according to the position of the flap pivot point. Dissection continued toward the proximal margin of the flap and deepened to include the deep fascia in the flap. Because the sural nerve was located in the deep part of the muscular layer in the middle of the leg, the nerve and some muscles were included in the flap. At the proximal margin of the flap, the sural nerve was severed, and the accompanying small saphenous vein was ligated. The flap was retrogradely transferred to the recipient site. Based on the tension of the distal pedicle of the flap, the flap was transferred by opening the intervening skin or through a skin tunnel. If the tension in the donor site was small, the flap was directly sutured. If the tension in the donor site was large, the defects were repaired with autologous thick pieces. The surgical method was the same for patients in both groups. The operation time, the surgical accuracy, and the survival rate of the flap were compared between the two groups. The surgical accuracy was determined using the following formula: surgical accuracy = (area of the flap area of the defects in the recipient site)/area of the flap.

1.4.3 Results

All flaps survived, and the recipient site primarily healed. During the 6–12 month follow-up period, the flaps provided a good quality of ski, and a satisfactory effect was achieved at the recipient site.

1.4.4 Discussion

Identification of the anatomy of the sural nerve and its blood supply is critical for surgical reconstruction of soft tissue defects in the ankle and foot. The medial sural cutaneous nerve originates from the tibial nerve of the sciatic nerve at the back of the mid-femur and descends to join with the anastomotic branch of the common peritoneal nerve to form the sural nerve at the popliteal fossa. The sural nerve passes between the medial and lateral head of the gastrocnemius and descends at the posterior-lateral side of the leg. The sural nerve pierces the deep fascia above the lateral malleolus and bifurcates into lateral cutaneous nerve and lateral dorsal cutaneous nerve, which supply the skin on the posterior and lateral surface of the foot. The peroneal artery has 3–5 intermuscular septum perforating branches and anastomoses with the vascular axis of the sural nerve. The most distal perforating branch of the peroneal artery is closest to the sural nerve and can be used as the vascular axis for the sural neurovascular island flaps. The sural artery supplies the retrograde sural fasciocutaneous island flap, and blood supply for the flap is segmental. The cutaneous branch of the sural artery provides blood supply to the sural nerve as the nutritional blood vessel, as well as to the adjacent skin. These nutritional blood vessels are anastomosed with the perforating branches of the peritoneal artery and the musculocutaneous branch of the posterior tibial artery. Anatomically, rich vascular networks exist above, below, and inside the deep fascia. These vascular networks are interconnected, and blood can flow bidirectionally among vascular networks.

In this study, we report that digitalization can be used to produce 3D images, which clearly demonstrate the stereoscopic anatomic structures of the sural neurovascular flap and the perforating branches of the sural artery toward the pedicle of the flap. The reconstructed 3D images can be used in the preoperative planning of the flap. Based on the preoperative measurements of the flap and blood vessels, we accurately located the position of the blood vessels, outlined the effective blood supply of the flap, designed the flap, and successfully reconstructed soft tissue defects. In addition, the distal perforating branch point of the peroneal artery in the pedicle was selected as the flap pivot point, which was marked preoperatively. In this way, the surgeon can pay attention to the flap rotation axis point, carefully avoid surgically damaging it, and reduce unnecessary surgical procedures to shorten operation time. The good condition of the flap pedicle guarantees the blood supply of the flap.

The growing demand for complex and minimally invasive surgical interventions is driving the search for ways to use computer-based digitalized technology in a wide range of medical applications, including disease diagnosis, treatment strategy, surgical simulation, clinical training, etc. One of the uses of 3D visualizations is to display and examine anatomical structures. Developments in the field of digital technology and 3D reconstruction from serial sections (CT or MRI) have allowed a precise description of morphology of tissues and organs and their relations. With the introduction of Visible Human Project (1989) and the development of Virtual Chinese Human (VCH) techniques, we could get more precise anatomic images. The graphics accelerator and digitalized visualization techniques make 3D visualization of some structures of the Chinese Visible Human dataset feasible, especially in the display of vessels. The improvement of the vascular injection technique has made more precise description of arteries possible. There are two methods for reconstructing the 3D volume from the 2D images: surface rendering and volume rendering. Surface rendering requires that the medical data be segmented and that a geometric surface representation of the structures of interest be extracted. The advantage of this technique lies in the relatively small amount of contour data, accelerating rendering speeds. Volume rendering, on the contrary, enables the visualization of 3D data without fitting geometric primitives to the data, but volume image datasets are characteristically large, taxing the computation abilities of volume-rendering techniques and the systems on which they are implemented. Of the methods available, shaded surface displays (SSD) have been the most commonly used 3D technique, because it requires a small amount of data and can be implemented in less powerful computers. This is why we chose SSD to display the outline of LDM flap. Our 3D reconstruction models displayed their anatomical characteristics. Correlation of cross-sectional images to 3D models is a more effective way of understanding the LDM anatomy. Perfusion with lead oxide–gelatine mixture has the advantage of distinctly and three-dimensionally displaying the vessels and their perforating branches which are reconstructed from a fresh cadaver specimen by direct visualization, while it also possesses the disadvantage of the incapability of demonstrating other tissues section by section, such as muscle structure. Manual efforts are needed to display a perfect anatomic structure diagram in case of oxide–gelatine perfusion.

2 The 3D Visualization of Perforator Flap

2.1 Related Concept and Principles of Clinical Application of Perforator Flap

Perforator flap [1] refers to the axial pattern skin flap with a blood supply through the skin perforating vessels (perforating arteries and perforating veins) which have fine calibers.

The clinical application of perforator flaps can be divided into two types: pedicled perforator flaps and free perforator flaps. Pedicled perforator flaps are mostly septocutaneous perforator flaps, which have a major donor site of upper and lower limbs and have been widely employed in repairing the sacral trauma [2]. Free perforator flaps are mostly musculocutaneous perforator flaps, which have a major donor site of the torso. The caliber of the cut perforating vessel is generally about 1 mm.

2.2 The Digital Construction of Perforator Flap

In perforator flap design, CTA becomes a reliable tool gradually, and it has been regarded as the golden standard in the detection of deep inferior epigastric perforating vessels. The surgery time would be considerably reduced by applying CTA in flap design [3].

After applying CTA scanning to the target area, the resulting data can be saved as DCM format. The software included in the machine can be used in three-dimensional reconstruction, observing and recording the amount and location of perforating arteries. These data can also be three-dimensionally reconstructed, assembled, and stained in Mimics software in order to extract the visualized anatomical image of the original artery and perforate vessels in any angle, which can be applied in the designing and operating of flap incision in the virtual environment.

2.2.1 The Digital Reconstruction of CT In-Built Software

Take DIEP as an example. Phillips et al. [4] offer a full description of the technical method and effect of the preoperating CTA examination of DIEP by 64 multi-detector helical CT and 16-slice spiral CT, summarized as follows. The patient takes consistent dorsal position as the position in the operation, preventing the natural abdominal contour being bounded or constricted by clothes, etc. Administer 100 mL highly concentrated low-osmolar (350–370 mg/L) nonionic contrast media and 50 mL physiological saline by intravenous injection using the dual channel syringe pump in the speed of 4 mL/s. The latter one is used to clean the blood vessels. When the CT value which is monitoring on the common femoral artery of pubic symphysis area is bigger than 100HU, the tail-to-head scanning will be launched automatically, which has a delay time of 4 s. Technical parameter: Tube voltage is 120 kV and current is 180–200 mA s. The auto-adjusting radiation dose quantity function is forbidden; the scanning layer is 0.6 mm thick, and it has a 0.9 mm pitch, 0.75 mm reconstructing layer. The space between layers is 0.4 mm. According to this setting, the balance (in the average

30 cm scanning area from the pubic symphysis to 3–4 cm above the navel, valid radiation dose is only 6 mSv) between radiation dose and image quality could be achieved.

The image reconstruction method and effect of the in-built software: maximum intensity projection (MIP) imaging – (1) the axial transverse scan is 5 cm thick, and it can be observed that the perforating branch arranges differently since its starting point to the tissue (Fig. 9.1) and (2) the coronal scan image requires employing image processing software to cut the front area of the skin and the back layer including the omentum, the mesenteric artery, and the volume of intestinal canal, to make a clear image of inferior epigastric artery and its branches and anatomic classification, which is similar with angiography. The image measurement is the most accurate when the caliber of the perforating branch is located at the axial transverse section.

2.2.2 The Digital Reconstruction of Mimics Software Platform

Take peroneal artery perforator flaps as an example. The CTA preoperative examination will be carried out for the patients. After preoperative vein patefaction, the patient will be asked to take the supine and feet-first position and keep the position during the examining process. The scanning area is from the lower segment of the abdominal aorta to the bilateral anterior and posterior tibial artery. The trigger points are the popliteal artery, which are all automatic. The delay time is 10–13 s. The contrast medium injecting speed

is 5 mL/s, and the total amount is 100–150 mL. The average amount is 120 ± 5 mL. The obtained data after scanning should be saved as DCM format and record on the CD-ROM, which can be three-dimensionally reconstructed by the in-built software and be used to observe and record the amount and location of peroneal artery perforating branches of each shin. Afterward, the patient's data can be three-dimensionally reconstructed, assembled, and stained in Mimics software in order to extract the visualized anatomical image of the peroneal artery perforating vessel in any angle, which can be applied in the designing and operating of flap incision in the virtual environment.

Operating steps:

1. Import the CTA data of the shin vessels into Mimics 10.01. After defining the direction of up, down, left, right, front, and back, Mimics 10.01 will show the two-dimensional image of the sagittal, coronal, and frontal position (Fig. 9.1).
2. Apply Thresholding on the lower limbs, set the parameter as 202, apply this Thresholding, and save as layer mask. Apply Region Growing to "YELLOW" mask in the shin bone part of the "GREEN" mask. Separate the tibia and fibula and the vessels from softer tissues. After the Region Growing, apply Edit Masks to the mask, scan the fault plane, and separate the tibia and fibula and the vessels. Apply Region Growing on the vessel area to "CYAN," and apply Thresholding -178 to the whole lower limbs and get "FUCHSIA." The three-dimensional model of the

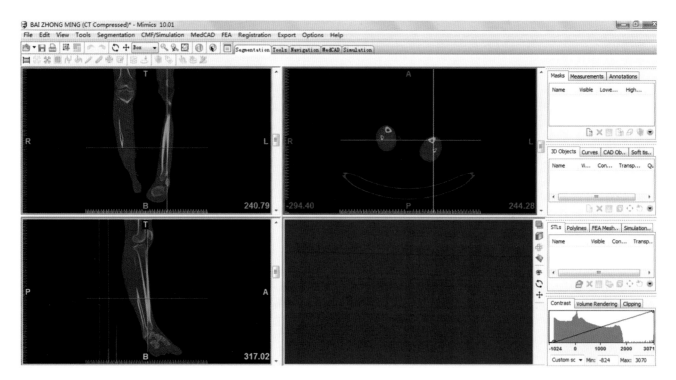

Fig. 9.1 Importing the CTA data into Mimics 10.01 software

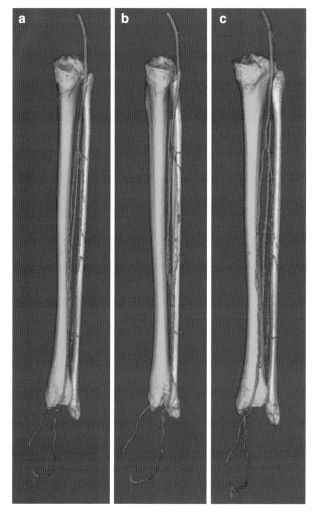

Fig. 9.2 After importing (**a–c**) CTA data into Mimics software, the reconstructed image can be observed in any angle, which offers the more accurate and complete information of peroneal artery perforator

patient's tibia and fibula, vessel, and soft tissue will be created by applying Calculate 3D. The peroneal artery can be separated from the vascular network by using cutting, separating, and Boolean calculation. The location and condition of each perforating branch is clear (see Fig. 9.2). And then design and simulate flap incision (Figs. 9.3, 9.4, 9.5, and 9.6).

2.3 The Clinical Application of the Digitalized Perforator Flap

Case 1: The patient was a 50-year-old male. The excision of the tumor in the left hypochondrium left a wound. Operate the ipsilateral inferior epigastric artery propeller flap by the first intention. (This case was provided by Professor Zhang Yixin from the ninth affiliated hospital of Shanghai Jiao Tong University.)

2.3.1 Using Preoperative CT Scanning and Three-Dimensional Reconstruction

1. Detection method: Using PHILIPS 64-slice spiral CT, the patient will be asked to take the supine position as in the surgery after setting up all the parameters (including tube current, voltage, moving speed of the CT-bed, pitch, thickness, etc.) Inject 90–100 mL (350 mg/mL ioversol injection) nonionic contrast media through dorsal hand vein by using the binocular high pressure. Apply the auto-track contrast system to trigger the scanning process. Set the CT value of descending part of aorta as 100HU and delay time in 5 s, which would make the perforating vessel develop clearly. Require the patient to hold his breath during the scanning process.

2. Establishing the coordinate: Send to original image to the image postprocessing workstation to reconstruct the two-dimensional and three-dimensional image of the vessel by using volume rendering and maximum intensity projection. Take the navel as the center of a circle, the medio-ventral line which crosses the navel as Y axis and the vertical which crosses the naval as X axis, establish a coordinate and mark the detected perforating branch, and move this coordinate and marked points to the body surface of the patient.

3. Choosing perforating branch: Choose the best perforating vessel as the pedicle to design the flap by analyzing the coronal section, vertical section, and axial section of the detected perforating branches.

Two musculocutaneous perforators P1 and P2 were found around the navel that originate from the left inferior epigastric artery. P1 and P2 have higher and better positions for propeller DIEP flaps. P1 perforating branch is larger than P2 and comparatively nearer to the edge of wound. So P1 perforating branch is chosen as the main perforating branch (Fig. 9.7).

2.3.2 Surgical Methods

The flap is separated on the surface of the sarcolemma of the rectus abdominis, cutting 21 × 7.5 cm DIEPF. The intraoperative anatomical exploration shows the position and caliber of P1 and P2 branches anastomose 100% with the CTA iconographic data. Adequately mobilize the surrounding tissue of the perforating branch. Repair the tumor excision wound after rotating the flap (Figs. 9.8, 9.9, 9.10, 9.11, and 9.12).

Case 2: The patient was a 19-year-old female. Traffic injury caused the compound and comminute fracture of the second and third metacarpal bone of the left hand, injury of extensor tendon of index finger, and soft tissue defect of the skin. Debridement, Kirschner wire, and VSD treatment were used as emergency treatment. After 16 days, the ultrathin peroneal artery perforator flaps were used to repair the wound. (This case was provided by Professor Chen Xuesong from the 59th Hospital of PLA.)

Fig. 9.3 (**a**) The three-dimensional reconstruction that only keeps the fibula, peroneal artery, and its perforating vessel. In figure (**b**, **c**) the flaps that nourishing by these perforating branches (pointed by the *black arrows*) which can be designed and cut in virtual environment

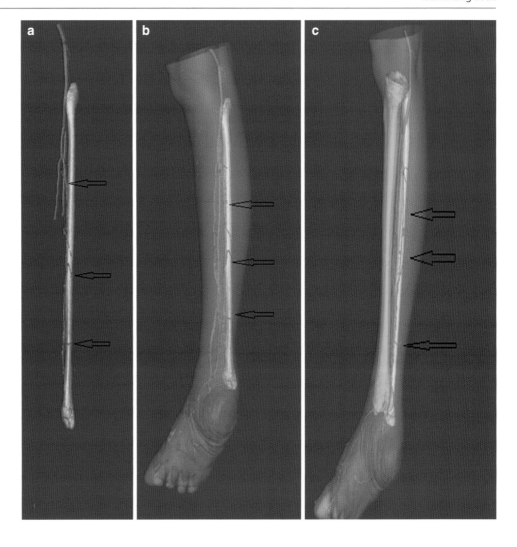

1. Using preoperative MDCT scanning and three-dimensional reconstruction.
2. According to CDFA and CTA detected data, a perforating vessel of the peroneal artery located above the lateral malleolus 16 cm of the right shin was chosen to be the supply vessel to design the ultrathin free flap to repair the wound. Import the CTA data into the Mimics software and reconstruct the three-dimensional image of the vessel, bone, and skin of the shin. In a virtual environment, the flap design can be completed in advance according to the wound shape, the location, and the vessel of the donor site.
3. Cut the flap during the operation. The pedicle has an external diameter of 1.44 mm, absolute length of 4.5 cm, and proportion of 10.0 cm × 7.0 cm; apply the ultrathin process after the incision. After the flap was moved to the recipient site, the circulation of the perforating arteries and veins and the dorsal carpal branch of radial artery was built, and the rest of the wound can be repaired after the donor site tightened. The flap survives after the operation and the suture is primary healing.

The postoperative reexamination shows that the flap is not bloated, and the finger function recovered well (Figs. 9.13, 9.14, 9.15, and 9.16).

3 Three-Dimensional Visualization of the Peripheral Nerve

Y. Z. Zhang

3.1 Introduction

Research on 3D reconstruction and visualization of the peripheral nerve can be divided into two aspects. One is the reconstruction of the external anatomical structure, and the other is the reconstruction of the internal anatomical structure (including the composition and distribution of the motor and sensory fiber). There is an external anatomical study on the traditional basis of fault specimen section 2D ultrasound and MRI images, 2D images, but these images have difficulty in reflecting the spatial position and, adjacent to the relationship between peripheral nerves, according to the two-dimensional image to imagine their spatial relationships, tend to be going through a difficult process of thought, and there is a big subjectivity. With the development of computer technology, computer-aided 3D reconstruction tech-

nology is widely applied in the medical field; its advantage that lies in the three-dimensional anatomic structure can be from any angle, at any direction. In the aspect of medical image, the Visible Human Project (1989) caused a big stir in the world. So far, only two countries have launched the plan, one in the United States and another in South Korea. In November 2001, the 174th Xiangshan science conference put "digitized virtual human body several key technology" listed in the national high technology research and development program "863" project, to start the research work of digitized virtual human body in our country, "virtual Chinese I number (male), II number (female)" of the human body section modeling research work has been launched in the first military medical university, the slicing accuracy of VHP, VKH increased 0.33 mm and 0.2 mm to 0.1 mm, and vascular perfusion in Virtual Chinese Human (VCH) No. 1, for building can represent the Chinese characteristics of digitized virtual human to lay a solid foundation. The visualization of virtual human research puts forward the possibility

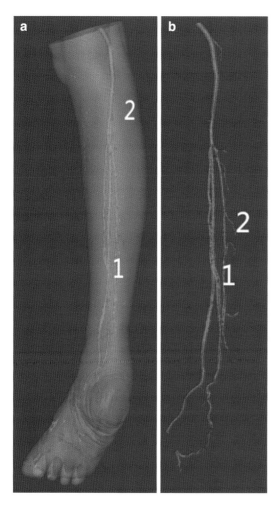

Fig. 9.4 (**a**) Shows the semitransparent skin and blood vessel; (**b**) Only shows the form of the blood vessel: 1, peroneal artery; 2, perforating vessel of peroneal artery

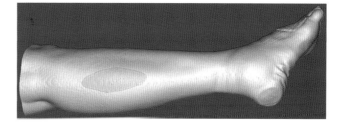

Fig. 9.5 The perforator flap designed in a virtual environment, according to the proportion, shape of the wound surface, and vessel positions of the recipient site

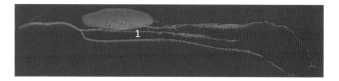

Fig. 9.6 The adjacent relations among flaps, perforating vessels, and original arteries

Fig. 9.7 Preoperative angiography and MDCT scanning

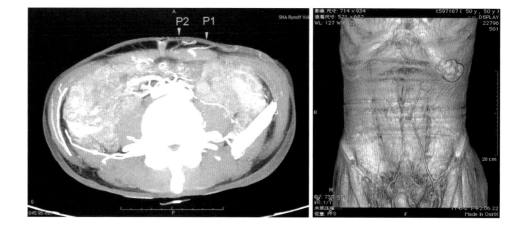

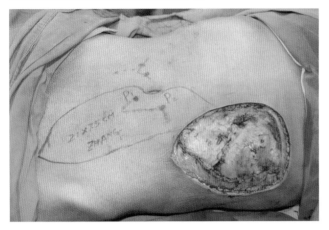

Fig. 9.8 The wound after the tumor excision and the flap design based on the preoperative CTA reconstruction of the vessel

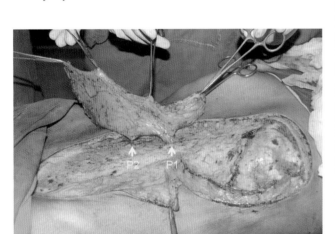

Fig. 9.9 Cut the flap. The perforating vessel of inferior epigastric arteries is pointed out by the *arrow*

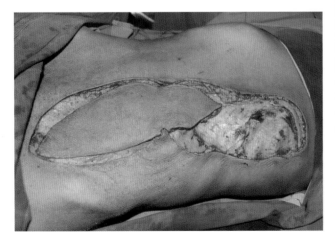

Fig. 9.10 The contour of the cut flap

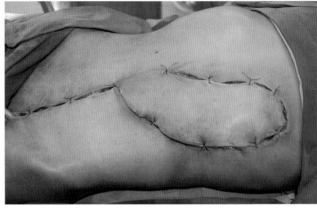

Fig. 9.11 Rotating approximately 180° to cover the wound surface

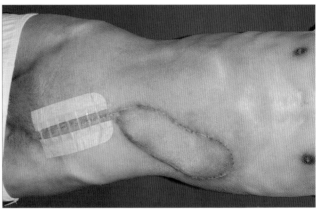

Fig. 9.12 Postoperative follow-up

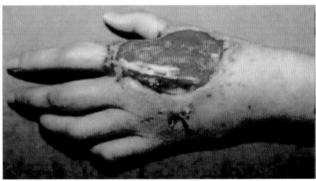

Fig. 9.13 Preoperative wound surface on the left hand

for visual nerves. How to display the nerve on virtual human is a worldwide problem, at present, can you find a can detect peripheral nervous system of the structure of the organization, chemical properties of chemical markers to differentiate between nerve images and the surrounding tissue, it can be for real samples of 3D reconstruction.

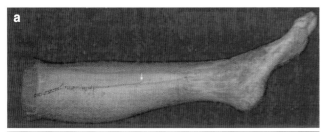
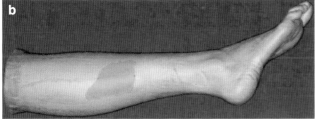

Fig. 9.14 According to the CTA data, a three-dimensional image can be reconstructed on the Mimics software platform. Selecting a peroneal artery from the patient's right shank as the nourishing vessel for the flap (pointed by the *yellow arrow*), the surgeon could design the free flap according to the proportion, the shape of the wound surface, and the vessel positions of the recipient site

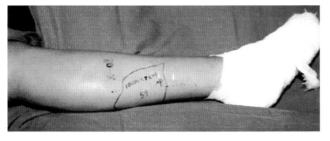

Fig. 9.15 According to the locating point on the surface (pointed by the *yellow arrow*), draw the flap contour as the preoperative virtual design on the posterolateral area of the right shin

Fig. 9.16 The shape of the cut flap is similar as the virtual design. The skin flap has been transplanted to the recipient site to repair the wound surface accurately

The cross-sectional images of VCH lack nerve information; in terms of the peripheral nerve showed, there are still no good countermeasures. Germany therefore in highly reality of VHP data set based on Voxel-Man body 3D reconstruction of blood vessels and nerves information had to be from outside to join (Fig. 9.17).

Unlike the peripheral nerve vascular system which has a pipeline space and uses infusion technology to display, the section of the peripheral nerve may no longer be dyed with other organizations; for the computer experts, further image registration and segmentation are difficult. But the peripheral nerve is a significant system in the medical science, and the project of VHP is put forward and competent people are struggling to find Dr. Ackerman group dyeing and broadspectrum method, in order to enhance the visibility of the nerve and its surrounding tissue and organ corresponding visual nerve branches. Peripheral nerve visualization technology of virtual human body, therefore, is one of topics in today's world and the difficulty, at present did not make a 3D virtual human with neural structures.

3.2   Three-Dimensional Reconstruction and Visualization of the Brachial Plexus

Neck dissection structure is complex, and the structure of brachial plexus injury adjacent to the relationship between the pathogenesis, clinical manifestation, diagnosis, and treat-

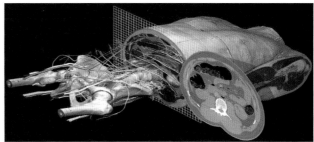

Fig. 9.17 Voxel-Man

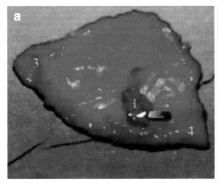
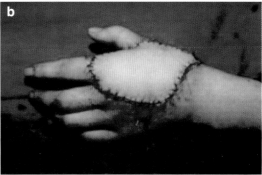

ment is of important guiding significance. At present a great deal of research about the anatomy of the brachial plexus based on fresh corpse neural anatomy and imaging anatomy (Fig. 9.18), or ultrasound (Fig. 9.19), for the neck section of

the continuous thin-layer section anatomy study is not very perfect. Conventional freezing fault technology can only provide 0.5 mm thickness; the neck structure of other relatively less in terms of brachial plexus is not good according to its structure. Using VCH I women dataset, the external structure of the brachial plexus was reconstructed. VCH dataset using frozen thin-layer milling technology, the neck of the milling spacing is 0.2 mm, this data set; a total of 8556 level continuous layer thickness is 0.2 mm, entire 149.7 GB of data sets. Every level image resolution is 6 096,384 (3024 × 2016 pixels), the file size is 17.5 M, uncompressed TIFF format, using Photoshop TIFF image format conversion into JPG format, image option for high quality, the parameters of eight, the converted each image size is 0.77 M. Extract edge from images on C_4 vertebral body plane to T_3 edge of vertebral body thin layer of frozen ct images in a row, a total of 527 layer, extract has the typical image, with Photoshop CS pruning the range image processing software, continuous observation (Fig. 9.20) and three-dimensional reconstruction, on the surface, on the basis of the static display of 3D reconstruction, to calculate the image

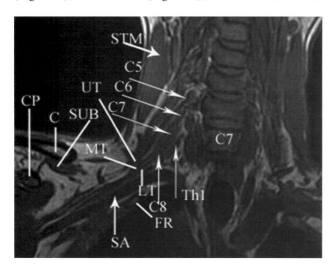

Fig. 9.18 MRI images of normal brachial plexus

Fig. 9.19 Cervical nerve exports in color Doppler ultrasonography. *Left*, the probe location. *Right*, display the root of C_5, C_6, C_7, and C_8 (1, 2, 3, 4)

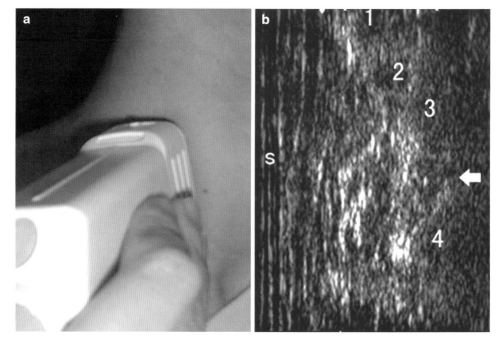

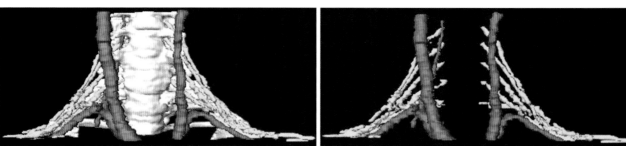

Fig. 9.20 3D surface reconstruction images of brachial plexus and vertebral artery

Fig. 9.21 Three-dimensional reconstruction of the lumbosacral plexus nerve and its surrounding structures of VCH-FI dataset (raw data and rendering)

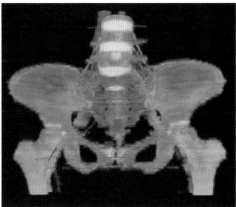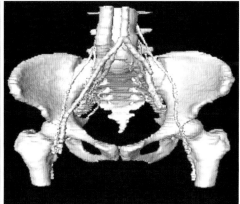

completely preserved, using film production program, its production for film, screen clear fluid, dynamic display.

Although small and less than the blood vessels and nerves of milling spacing structure it is difficult to identify, together with the nerve is soft and lack of support and sometimes appear in the process of milling around some tear, making it difficult to identify the main structure of brachial plexus and the surrounding muscle, ligament, cartilage, clearance and other large structures are clearly visible, which guarantee the data integrity of the structure, continuity and accuracy.

3.3 Three-Dimensional Reconstruction and Visualization of the Lumbosacral Plexus Nerve

Local anatomic relationship of Lumbosacral plexus nerve is complex, caused by pelvic fracture and dislocation after hip easily lumbosacral plexus injury, although the lumbosacral plexus nerve injury is a rare clinical, but its diagnosis and treatment is still a difficult problem, understanding the anatomy of the fault help explain the possible damage mechanism, at the same time provide damage after surgical exploration with good surgical approach to provide some information. Dataset of VCH I women were analyzed, and the exterior of the lumbosacral plexus nerve was also rebuilt. The original file size is 17.5 M, uncompressed TIFF format, using Photoshop TIFF image format conversion into JPG format, image option for high quality, the parameters of eight, the converted each image size is 0.77 M. Extract L_3 central vertebral body plane to femoral great trochanter thin layer of frozen ct images in a row, a total of 1491 layer, extract has the typical image, with Photoshop CS pruning the range image processing software, continuous observation on every level of the vertebral body, spinal cord and nerve root structure and L_4, L_5, lumbosacral dry, S_1–S_4 and femoral nerve walk line and its location; pay special attention to observe the nerve blood vessels around the composition and direction. In the progress of three-dimensional reconstruction, considering the perfor-

mance and the personal computer to display the gross anatomy structure, adopt the method of every ten take one from the whole data set, pitch extraction such as pictures, data extraction, reconstruction of the main structure and adjacent to the lumbosacral plexus nerve structure (Fig. 9.21).

On the basis of the static display of 3D reconstruction, to calculate the image completely preserved, partial reconstruction, and then use the software of Movie making process, the production for film, output, storage in AVI format. Three-dimensional image can fully display the lumbosacral plexus nerve and its main branches and the relationship between the major blood vessels and pelvis (Fig. 9.22), or so inclined a can be clear that the lumbosacral dry and S_1, S_2, S_3 merge sciatic nerve (Fig. 9.22), can also be shown separately nerve and the pelvis or the relationship between nerves and blood vessels (Fig. 9.22).

From the reconstruction of the image one could see behind the sciatic nerve is just located in the femoral head and acetabulum and femoral head dislocation or wall and posterior column after acetabulum fracture after large displacement of bone block is easy to cause the sciatic nerve injury, studies show that consolidation of sciatic nerve injury of nerve stretch, contusion or oppression, not broken, if the sciatic nerve by dislocation of femoral head or shifting bone block oppression for a long time, there will be a secondary ischemia of the nerve and the epineurium and bundles of scar tissue, causing irreversible neurological damage.

3.4 Clinical Anatomy and 3D Virtual Reconstruction of the Lumbar Plexus

Sheng Lu, Yuanzhi Zhang, and Yongqing Xu

Abstract The exposure of the anterior or lateral lumbar via the retroperitoneal approach easily causes the injuries of the lumbar plexus. The lumbar plexus injuries, which take place when exposing the spine and placing instruments therein, have been reported. To study the applied anatomy of the lum-

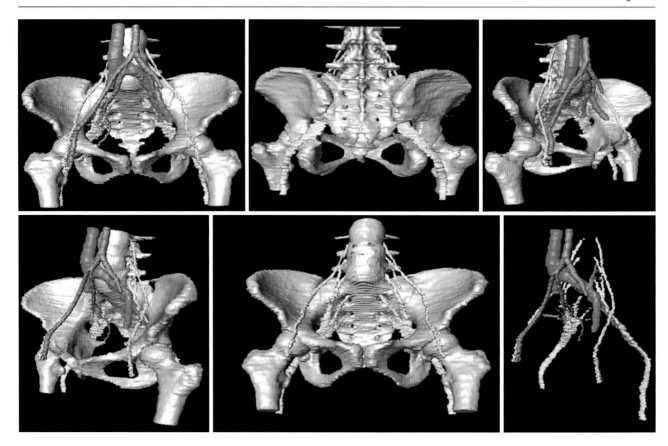

Fig. 9.22 Three-dimensional reconstruction of the lumbosacral plexus nerve and its surrounding structures

bar plexus by formaldehyde-preserved cadavers, two groups of sectional images of the lumbar segment and three series of the Virtual Chinese Human (VCH) dataset are established. Three-dimensional computerized reconstructions of the lumbar plexus and their adjacent structures were conducted from VCH Female I dataset. The order of the lumbar nerve is regular; from the anterior view, the lumbar plexus nerve arranges from medial to lateral from L_5 to L_2; from the lateral view, the lumbar nerve arranges from ventral to dorsal from L_2 to L_5. The angle of each nerve root exiting outward to the corresponding intervertebral foramen increases from L_1 to L_5. The lumbar plexus nerve was revealed to be in close contact with transverse process (TP). By sectional anatomy, all parts of the lumbar plexus nerve were located in the dorsal third of the psoas muscle; thus, the safety zone of the psoas major muscle to prevent nerve injuries is ventrally 2/3. The 3D reconstruction of the lumbar plexus based on the VCH data can clearly show the relationship between the lumbar plexus and blood vessel, vertebral body and kidney, and lumbar plexus and psoas muscle. Psoas muscle can be considered as a surgery landmark when exposing the lateral anterior of the lumbar by incising the psoas muscle, which prevents lumbar plexus injury by incising the psoas muscle ventral 2/3. The lumbar transverse process can be used as a marker, with which we can sure the position of lumbar plexus and as reference in

operation. The 3D reconstruction of the lumbar plexus based on the VCH data can provide a virtual morphological basis for anterior lumbar surgery.

3.4.1 Introduction

Exposing the anterior or lateral lumbar using the retroperitoneal approach assumes one of two methods: manipulating the major vessels inward or incising the lateral psoas muscle (transpsoas approach). The latter procedure is the less risky of the two, but it risks injuries to the lumbar plexus. Though the L_5 nerve is not part of the lumbar plexus, its intimate relationship with the lumbar plexus makes it natural to study along with the lumbar plexus nerve. Lumbar plexus injuries, which can occur when exposing the spine and placing instruments therein, have been reported. Potential complications of the lateral approach are mostly related to the psoas and the nerves of the lumbar plexus that lie within it. The nerves of the lumbar plexus and the genitofemoral nerve are at risk as the psoas is traversed. The real-time EMG monitoring during this critical stage of the procedure can reliably detect the proximity of neural structures and signal the surgeon to redirect. Still, postoperative groin or thigh dysesthesias may occur in some patients. In one recent series of patients with degenerative lumbar scoliosis, three of 12 patients experienced transient groin or thigh dysesthesias.

Though the possibility of injury to the lumbar plexus at the anterior approach to expose lumbar vertebras via the retroperitoneum has been emphasized, surgeons faced a dearth of anatomical knowledge on the lumbar plexus during this procedure. Once such knowledge became widely known, surgeons could either avoid nerve injury or determine the injury's location. However, applied anatomy of the lumbar plexus with respect to the anterior lumbar surgery has not been reported. Thus, we need more anatomical data concerning the lumbar plexus relative to clinical application, so as to prevent lumbar plexus injuries while increasing the safety of lumbar surgery.

3.4.2 The Gross Anatomy of the Lumbar Plexus

We collected 15 formaldehyde-preserved cadavers with integral lumbar plexus: nine were male and six were female. The mean age of the cadavers was 69 years, with a range of 56–87 years. Samples of 30 sides in total could be observed and studied. Clearing away all organs in front of the peritoneum to expose the posterior abdomen cavity, we left the psoas major muscle intact and in its original location as much as possible. We then dissected and exposed the lumbar plexus. We studied the anatomical relationship of the lumbar plexus nerve and the surgical landmark and took measurements of the plexus with a flexible surgical ruler.

3.4.3 Anatomic Observation of the Lumbar Nerve Roots

Lumbar nerve roots were situated in the posterior part of the psoas muscle. The majority traveled across the corresponding intervertebral foramens, under the surface of the lumbar pedicle, and across the transverse process (TP) ligament. The lumbar plexus was formed by tight loops, widening in the lower vertebra. There were anatomic rules of the lumbar plexus in the lateral vertebra: lumbar nerves arrange from medial to lateral, from L_5 to L_2, and from ventral to dorsal, from L_2 to L_5.

3.4.4 Angles of the Lumbar Plexus Nerve to the Intervertebral Foramen

The angle of each root exiting outward to the corresponding intervertebral foramen ranged 200–400 from L_1 to L_5; the largest angle was 32.90 at L_5.

3.4.5 Anatomic Relationship of Lumbar Plexus and Transverse Process

The lumbar plexus was located anterolateral to the lumbar vertebras. When exited from the intervertebral foramina, it was laid anterior to the transverse process for the duration. We used the transverse process as a landmark to protect the lumbar plexus during the operation. The distance between the upper level of the transverse process to its corresponding nerve trunk was 4.9–5.9 mm (3.6–7.9 mm); from L_2 to L_5, the distance between the lower level of the transverse process to its corresponding nerve trunk was 8.9 ± 1.0 mm (7.1–10.9 mm) at the level of L_2, 7.8 ± 1.1 mm (5.3–9.4 mm) at L_3, 6.8 ± 0.9 mm (4.9–8.4 mm) at L_4, and 6.2 ± 0.9 mm (4.8–8.4 mm) at L_5. We concluded that the distance between the anteromedial border of the transverse process and its corresponding nerve trunk decreased from the upper level to the lower level.

3.4.6 The Sectional Anatomy of the Lumbar Plexus

We applied five sets of Virtual Chinese Human (VCH) data from the Anatomic Department of South Medical University. Sectional photos displayed the lumbar plexus nerve. The sectional plane was divided into three average sections. The upper part was the superior margin of psoas major, and the lower was the intersection of the psoas major and lumborum muscles. We thus observed the relationship of the psoas major and the lumbar plexus nerve. In the 3D virtual reconstruction of the lumbar plexus nerve, the TIFF format of VCH Female 1 was translated to JPG format by software Photoshop CS. We selected a part from L_1 to the trochanteric of the femur. We had a total of 1491 pictures. The 3D virtual model of the lumbar plexus nerve was established using Amira 3.1 software to observe the 3D relationship of the lumbar plexus and vessel, vertebral body, kidney, and major psoas muscles.

Anatomical relationship between the lumbar plexus and the major psoas muscle.

During the operation, the major psoas muscles should be dissected to expose the vertebral body. According to both the anterior border of the major psoas muscle and the space between the major psoas muscle and lumbar quadrate muscle, the major psoas muscle could be fractionated to three equal parts that would be helpful in judging the location of the lumbar plexus. From our study, we found that the lumbar plexus is located always in the 1/3 posterior aspect of the major psoas muscle at different sections. Hence, injury can be avoided by incising the ventral 2/3 of the psoas major.

Moro et al. [5] studied the problem of the safety zone and the lumbar plexus via retroperitoneum by laparoscope; they concluded that the safety zone was L_2–L_3, as well as L_4–L_5, if we ignore injury to the genitofemoral nerve. At the L_5–S_1 level, the risk of injury to the iliac vessel is higher because it is just presented at the lateral surface. Going through the space between the major psoas muscle and the lumbar quadrate muscle and drawing the major psoas muscle forward to reach the lateral to lumbar vertebra presented another challenge. Here nerve roots of L_4 and L_5, femoral nerve and obturator nerve, presented and formed a dangerous area for this approach. Thus, sufficient exposure of the lumbar plexus was required. Entering the lumbar vertebras required pulling away or incising the major psoas muscle, but it was impossible to localize the exact point of the lumbar plexus during the operation. Hence, we considered the position of the lumbar plexus versus the major psoas muscle as critical. In our study, we found that entering the retroperitoneum revealed the anterior and posterior borders of the major psoas muscle. According to this finding, we believed the position of the lumbar plexus versus the anterior and posterior borders could serve as a landmark to incise the major psoas muscle and safely enter the lumbar vertebras or intervertebral disks. It is very important to choose the correct place to incise the major psoas muscle. The approach to such a place should avoid injury to the lumbar plexus during the process of dissecting or passing through the major psoas muscle. According to the sectional anatomy, with respect to the lumbar plexus and major psoas muscle, we found that the location of the lumbar plexus at the major psoas muscle was comparatively constant, which made it possible to separate the 2/3 ventral parts of the major psoas muscle to reach the safe area of the intervertebral space. We then drew the lumbar plexus backward. We suggest retaining 1/3 dorsal parts of the major psoas muscle to avoid injury to the nerve roots.

3.4.7   3D Reconstruction of the Lumbar Plexus

In the Chinese digital-visible database, from the level of lumbar vertebras to the level of the superior segment of the femur, all of the sectional images were clear so that we could the discern bone tissue, major psoas muscle, kidney, fibrous connective tissue, nerves, and vessel. The images of those tissues—nerve roots of L_1–L_5, the lumbosacral trunk (LST), the abdominal aorta and its branches, and the inferior vena cava and its branches—could be viewed clearly and consecutively. The static display of the 3D reconstruction images was entirely preserved and then reconstructed regionally. Benefits of the reconstructed images included (1) a clear display of the relationship between the lumbar plexus nerve or its main branches and important blood or vertebral body or kidney and (2) a clear display of the relationship between the lumbar plexus and the major psoas muscle, as well as the convergence of the lumbar plexus and the lumbosacral trunk.

Unfortunately, it is difficult to determine the location and adjacent space relation of the lumbar plexus from sectional images of the anatomical layers. If we wanted to visualize such space location from a 2D image, we would have to speculate carefully and precisely, but this method is problematical. Currently we take advantage of the 3D reconstruction technique to review anatomical structures of the lumbar plexus from any angle and thus understand the lumbar plexus and its surrounding tissues. We hope that this study's anatomical data will prove useful for anterior approach to the lumbar plexus and will help avoid injury during surgery.

4   The Digital Anatomic Study of Pedicle Screw Channel

Yanbing Li, Zijia Zhou, and Shizheng Zhong

1. The establishment of the digital analysis method of pedicle screw channel by the use of digital technology
2. The digital anatomic study of pedicle screw channel
3. The accurate positioning analysis of 3D relations of pedicle screw channel, screw entry point, and vertebra body boundary in thoracic vertebras
4. The accurate positioning analysis of 3D relations of pedicle screw channel, screw entry point, and vertebra body boundary in lumbar vertebras

4.1   Establish the Digital Analysis Method of Pedicle Screw Channel by the Use of Digital Technology

The pedicle is a bridge between the vertebral body and lamina, which is the only channel of pedicle posterior internal fixation techniques. As the implanted channel of screw, its 3D morphology structure should be fully considered. We established the digital analysis method of pedicle screw channel by the use of digital technology and conducted a 3D digital quantitative research of pedicle and its relationship of the overall structure, which is an important foundation for the development of digital spine surgery.

4.1.1   Materials and Methods

1. Design: A repeated measure design was conducted.
2. Object of study: CT scanning images of healthy adult physical examination were collected.
3. The experiment methods:
   (a) 3D reconstruction: We imported the CT images to Mimics and reconstructed the 3D model of vertebra, and then the model of the cervical spine, thoracic spine, and lumbar spine was saved, and database was established.
   (b) Analysis of pedicle screw channel in a 3D way: Firstly, we opened a 3D model in UG imageware and located 3D coordinate system. The horizontal plane was located in the middle of the pedicle, and the sagittal section was located in the median sagittal plane that passed through the vertebral body. The 3D rotation reference coordinate system was defined as the default coordinate system, and we conducted all the analyses according to this system. Then, we extracted the pedicle on the 3D model and reconstructed pedicle screw channel in any 3D direction. The cross section was located in the vertebra middle sagittal and the transverse direction. Secondly, lumbar pedicle channel was projected to the

plane along the vertical direction and obtained inscribed circle of each projection direction, respectively, as well as fitted excircle and inscribed circle of each inner borderline. The specific process is as follows: firstly, the vertical plane was defined by revolving model, then projected the pedicle to the plane along normal direction, and fitted the projection object interior boundary line, and 50 points were extracted from the line. And then in the inscribed circle, ellipse could be fitted. Some diameters like radius, ellipse long axis, and ellipse short axis should be noted, and the offset curve perpendicular to the ellipse could be obtained as well. Then projected the interior boundary line, the inscribed circle to centrum and lamina surface along the 3D direction, and replicated the center point. The point should be translated to the centrum and lamina surface along the 3D direction. By fitting curve on the vertebral plate surface projection point and line on the corresponding center point of the vertebral plate surface, we obtained the loft curved surface. Lofting curve surface between the interior boundary projection curve was the pedicle screw channel. Lofting curve surface between the inscribed circle projection curve was the biggest screw channel. Lofting curve surface between the fitting ellipse projection curve was the approximate pedicle screw channel. Lofting curve surface between offset curve projection curve was the approximate axes channel. The straight line between the translation inscribed circle center was the best axis in its 3D direction. The straight line between the translation ellipse center was the approximate axis in its 3D direction.

4.1.2 Results

Through this study, we got a precise definition of pedicle screw channel. Pedicle screw channel (PSC) was the channel between the interior boundary of the positive projection of pedicle 3D space corresponding on the centrum and lamina in the random orientation. In a certain scope, a 3D direction corresponded with a PSC, this PSC corresponded with the biggest screw channel, the channel corresponded with the best axis, and the entering screw point also corresponded with safe area and safe angle scope of a certain-size screw (Fig. 9.23).

Our study designed the pedicle screw trajectory accurately according to each centrum and the physical truth of each segment by the use of converse project technology and on the basis of 3D reconstruction digital model. And we could confirm the accurate diameter, length of the screw, and the location of direction axis. We could obtain the accurate screw insertion area on the vertebral plate surface and, therefore, provide an accurate reference to the preoperative plan. What's more, the principle of individualization and segmental variability could be fully reflected.

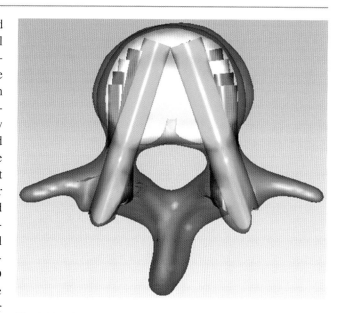

Fig. 9.23 The pedicle screw channel (raysum)

4.2 The Digital Anatomic Study of Pedicle Screw Channel

On the basis of the analysis methods mentioned above, we can make a 3D dynamic analysis of the changeable rule between each diameter and insertion channel by the use of a digital technique at a visible environment. At the same time, we can realize the relationship between the size, length, and direction of screw channel in different segments, make further analysis of their feature, and finally provide a theoretical foundation for the application.

4.2.1 Materials and Methods

1. Design: A repeated measure design was conducted.
2. Object of study: CT scanning images of healthy adult physical examination were collected.
3. The experiment methods:
   (a) Select the 3D digital anatomical models of cervical, thoracic, and lumbar vertebral from the database and then import into UG Imageware.
   (b) Locate 3D coordinate system. The cross section is located in the vertebra middle sagittal and the transverse direction.
   (c) The location analysis of insertion channel of the vertebral body in each segment.
1. Cervical vertebra: import the vertebral model of C_{3-7}, keep 0° SSA invariable, TSA from 0° to 45° is evenly separated by 5°, and study the changeable rule of PSC in different TSA, without considering SSA.
2. Thoracic vertebra: import the vertebral model of T_{2-12}, keep 0° SSA invariable, TSA from 0° to 40° is evenly

separated by 5°, and study the changeable rule of PSC in different TSA, without considering SSA.

3. Lumbar vertebra: import the vertebral model of L_{1-5}, keep 0° SSA invariable, TSA from 0° to 40° is evenly separated by 5°, and study the changeable rule of PSC in different TSA, without considering SSA.

4.2.2 Results

The Digital Anatomical Feature of Cervical Vertebra Pedicle Insertion Channel in Different TSA (Tables 9.1, 9.2, 9.3, and 9.4; Fig. 9.24)

The Digital Anatomical Feature of Thoracic Vertebra Pedicle Insertion Channel in Different TSA
Tables 9.5, 9.6, 9.7, and 9.8 and Fig. 9.25.

The Digital Anatomical Feature of Lumbar Vertebra Pedicle Insertion Channel in Different TSA
Tables 9.9, 9.10, 9.11, and 9.12 and Fig. 9.26.

4.3 The Accurate Positioning Analysis of 3D Relations of Pedicle Screw Channel, Screw Entry Point, and Vertebra Body Boundary in Lumbar Vertebras

The lumbar vertebra is the most centralized segment which transfers the gravity better in the spine; it is also the relatively flexible part of the spine. The development of pedicle internal fixation techniques in the lumbar segment is the earliest and the most mature one. With the development of digital technique, the use of spinal orthopedic navigation in

Table 9.1 The inscribed circle radius of the left and right pedicle channel from three to seven cervical vertebras (mm)

Segment	C_3	C_4	C_5	C_6	C_7	F	P
Left	2.3 ± 0.37	2.4 ± 0.48	2.0 ± 0.54	2.4 ± 0.40	2.6 ± 0.35	24.629	<0.000
Right	2.8 ± 0.37	2.6 ± 0.46	2.4 ± 0.57	2.7 ± 0.46	2.6 ± 0.44		
t	−57.712	−19.328	−37.881	−15.232	0.281	128.64	<0.000
P	0.000	0.000	0.000	0.000	0.785		

Table 9.2 The inscribed circle radius of the left and right pedicle channel from three to seven cervical vertebras in different TSA (mm) ($\bar{x} \pm s$) $n = 5$

Angle	0°	5°	10°	15°	20°	25°	30°	35°	40°	45°	F	P
Left	1.5 ± 0.28	1.8 ± 0.40	2.1 ± 0.36	2.3 ± 0.32	2.5 ± 0.27	2.6 ± 0.22	2.7 ± 0.19	2.7 ± 0.14	2.7 ± 0.13	2.6 ± 0.14	101.706	<0.000
Right	1.8 ± 0.25	2.0 ± 0.23	2.3 ± 0.19	2.5 ± 0.16	2.7 ± 0.14	2.9 ± 0.13	2.9 ± 0.10	3.0 ± 0.07	3.1 ± 0.05	3.0 ± 0.04	11.006	<0.029
t	−4.909	−1.041	−1.226	−1.618	−2.173	−2.855	−3.115	−5.943	−7.997	−6.407		
P	0.008	0.357	0.287	0.181	0.096	0.046	0.036	0.004	0.001	0.003		

Table 9.3 The size of the length of the left and right pedicle channel from three to seven cervical vertebras (mm) ($\bar{x} \pm s$)

Segment	C_3	C_4	C_5	C_6	C_7	F	P
Left	23.1 ± 2.99	20.6 ± 4.01	23.3 ± 5.17	22.7 ± 4.02	22.6 ± 6.26	20.092	<0.000
Right	20.4 ± 4.15	18.5 ± 4.16	22.1 ± 3.47	24.9 ± 4.71	23.4 ± 5.02		
t	3.449	4.505	1.740	−6.183	−1.623	13.011	<0.006
P	0.007	0.001	0.116	0.000	0.139		

Table 9.4 The size of the length of the left and right pedicle channel from three to seven cervical vertebras in different TSA (mm) ($\bar{x} \pm s$)

Angle	0°	5°	10°	15°	20°	25°	30°	35°	40°	45°	F	P
Left	17.8 ± 2.03	18.3 ± 1.26	18.6 ± 1.61	19.1 ± 1.29	20.5 ± 1.29	22.1 ± 1.40	24.2 ± 2.09	26.3 ± 2.61	28.3 ± 2.35	29.5 ± 2.99	69.991	<0.000
Right	17.9 ± 1.89	18.1 ± 1.66	18.4 ± 1.77	18.8 ± 2.32	19.4 ± 2.52	20.9 ± 3.22	23.2 ± 4.06	24.9 ± 3.48	27.6 ± 2.88	29.4 ± 2.26		
t	−0.084	0.213	0.182	0.431	0.982	0.853	0.619	1.030	0.631	0.120	0.472	>0.530
P	0.937	0.842	0.865	0.689	0.382	0.442	0.569	0.361	0.562	0.910		

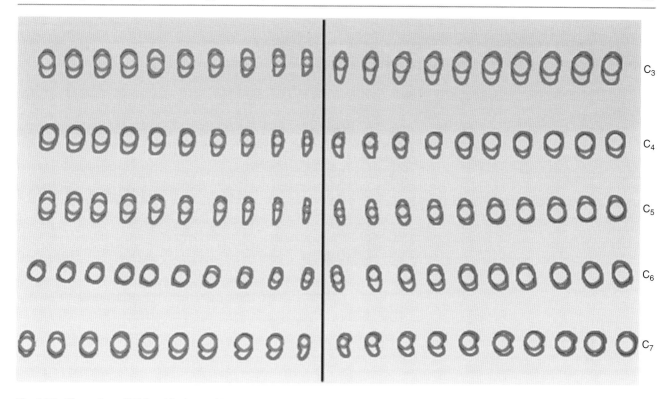

Fig. 9.24 The project of PSC and its internal boundary and inscribed circle from three to seven cervicals in different TSA

Table 9.5 The inscribed circle radius of the left and right pedicle channel from two to twelve thoracic vertebras (mm) ($\bar{x} \pm s$) $n = 9$

Segment	T_2	T_3	T_4	T_5	T_6	T_7	T_8	T_9	T_{10}	T_{11}	T_{12}	F	P
Left	3.8 ± 0.36	2.6 ± 0.25	2.5 ± 0.41	2.8 ± 0.35	2.7 ± 0.39	2.4 ± 0.51	2.6 ± 0.46	3.3 ± 0.33	4.1 ± 0.33	4.5 ± 0.62	4.2 ± 0.64	104.404	<0.000
Right	4.0 ± 0.21	3.1 ± 0.34	2.9 ± 0.51	2.3 ± 0.42	2.5 ± 0.58	2.3 ± 0.52	2.5 ± 0.33	3.0 ± 0.38	3.9 ± 0.35	3.9 ± 0.69	3.9 ± 0.77		
t	−1.277	−10.925	−9.346	8.588	3.204	10.581	2.073	14.803	8.183	19.327	5.856	10.528	<0.012
P	0.238	0.000	0.000	0.000	0.013	0.000	0.072	0.000	0.000	0.000	0.000		

Table 9.6 The inscribed circle radius of the left and right pedicle channel from two to twelve thoracic vertebras in different TSA (mm) ($\bar{x} \pm s$) $n = 11$

Angle	0°	5°	10°	15°	20°
Left	3.4 ± 0.91	3.5 ± 0.84	3.5 ± 0.79	3.5 ± 0.78	3.4 ± 0.78
Right	3.5 ± 0.77	3.5 ± 0.75	3.5 ± 0.69	3.4 ± 0.69	3.3 ± 0.70
t	−0.425	0.106	0.470	0.665	0.916
P	0.680	0.918	0.648	0.521	0.381

Table 9.7 The size of the length of the left and right pedicle channel from two to twelve thoracic vertebras (mm) ($\bar{x} \pm s$) $n = 9$

Segment	T_2	T_3	T_4	T_5	T_6	T_7	T_8	T_9	T_{10}	T_{11}	T_{12}	F	P
Left	26.9 ± 7.3	34.5 ± 13.5	36.3 ± 12.0	37.9 ± 11.0	39.7 ± 10.5	42.7 ± 9.4	44.3 ± 7.3	47.8 ± 13.9	42.0 ± 12.8	37.5 ± 10.1	37.0 ± 9.8	20.309	<0.000
Right	29.5 ± 6.6	34.3 ± 11.6	40.6 ± 11.9	43.5 ± 9.50	41.9 ± 10.6	43.7 ± 9.8	43.8 ± 7.3	45.2 ± 7.3	41.3 ± 12.6	40.7 ± 8.30	40.6 ± 10.7		
t	−4.540	0.166	−3.105	−5.391	−2.596	−1.189	1.343	2.026	0.777	−3.555	−3.980	22.683	<0.001
P	0.002	0.872	0.015	0.001	0.032	0.269	0.216	0.077	0.460	0.007	0.004		

Table 9.8 The size of the length of the left and right pedicle channel from two to twelve thoracic vertebras in different TSA (mm) ($\bar{x} \pm s$) $n = 11$

Angle	0°	5°	10°	15°	20°	25°	30°	35°	40°	F	P
Left	23.1 ± 5.09	26.8 ± 5.40	31.5 ± 5.48	36.0 ± 6.25	39.7 ± 6.05	42.9 ± 6.29	45.1 ± 7.76	51.2 ± 7.70	52.8 ± 8.00	99.396	<0.000
Right	24.8 ± 4.79	29.7 ± 4.36	34.7 ± 4.65	38.2 ± 4.50	41.6 ± 5.83	43.8 ± 5.32	46.6 ± 6.24	51.4 ± 6.96	53.2 ± 7.92	5.021	<0.049
t	−3.979	−3.462	−3.653	−2.295	−1.603	−0.776	−0.758	−0.173	−0.563		
P	0.003	0.006	0.004	0.045	0.140	0.456	0.466	0.866	0.586		

Fig. 9.25 The project of PSC and its internal boundary and inscribed circle from two to twelve thoracic vertebras in different TSA

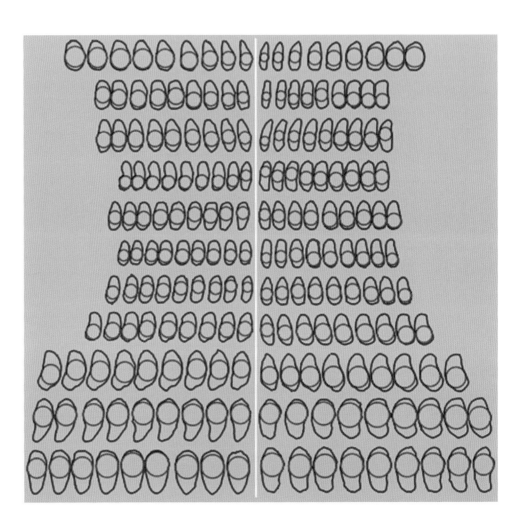

Table 9.9 The inscribed circle radius of the left and right pedicle channel from one to five lumbar vertebras (mm) ($\bar{x} \pm s$) $n = 9$

Segment	L_1	L_2	L_3	L_4	L_5	F	P
Left	2.6 ± 0.58	3.7 ± 0.35	4.0 ± 0.21	5.3 ± 0.33	5.7 ± 0.41	119.568	<0.000
Right	3.1 ± 0.41	4.0 ± 0.40	4.5 ± 0.23	5.3 ± 0.30	5.6 ± 0.39		
t	−7.765	−11.593	−8.891	−0.952	2.657	104.485	<0.000
P	0.000	0.000	0.000	0.369	0.029		

Table 9.10 The inscribed circle radius of the left and right pedicle channel from one to five lumbar vertebras in different TSA (mm) ($\bar{x} \pm s$) $n = 5$

Segment	0°	5°	10°	15°	20°	25°	30°	35°	40°	F	P
Left	4.1 ± 0.94	4.3 ± 0.97	4.4 ± 1.02	4.5 ± 1.16	4.5 ± 1.23	4.5 ± 1.36	4.3 ± 1.41	4.0 ± 1.66	3.8 ± 1.72	3.037	<0.012
Right	4.2 ± 0.71	4.5 ± 0.82	4.7 ± 0.79	4.7 ± 0.84	4.8 ± 0.95	4.7 ± 1.09	4.6 ± 1.14	4.4 ± 1.32	4.1 ± 1.39	4.136	>0.112
t	−1.414	−3.007	−2.535	−1.373	−1.775	−1.653	−1.872	−2.469	−1.717		
P	0.230	0.040	0.064	0.242	0.151	0.174	0.135	0.069	0.161		

Table 9.11 The size of the length of the left and right pedicle channel from one to five lumbar vertebras (mm) ($\bar{x} \pm s$) $n = 9$

Segment	L_1	L_2	L_3	L_4	L_5	F	P
Left	44.0 ± 7.1	43.1 ± 8.3	46.9 ± 6.80	39.9 ± 6.50	28.2 ± 5.1	46.975	<0.000
Right	44.9 ± 7.7	45.1 ± 7.4	40.3 ± 12.2	37.1 ± 11.4	29.6 ± 5.3		
t	−1.429	−3.622	3.377	1.445	−2.208	1.661	>0.233
P	0.191	0.007	0.010	0.186	0.058		

Table 9.12 The size of the length of the left and right pedicle channel from one to five lumbar vertebras in different TSA (mm) ($\bar{x} \pm s$) $n=5$

Angle	0°	5°	10°	15°	20°	25°	30°	35°	40°	F	P
Left	30.5 ± 4.48	32.2 ± 5.76	37.9 ± 5.91	39.1 ± 7.09	41.8 ± 8.28	41.3 ± 9.39	43.4 ± 10.52	47.4 ± 9.25	50.2 ± 6.60	32.614	<0.000
Right	24.8 ± 8.03	29.1 ± 6.58	35.0 ± 5.45	39.0 ± 6.47	40.7 ± 7.90	43.0 ± 9.39	44.8 ± 8.40	47.5 ± 8.47	50.5 ± 5.31		
t	1.325	0.829	1.646	0.037	0.927	−1.847	−1.226	−0.104	−0.316	0.411	0.557
P	0.256	0.454	0.175	0.972	0.407	0.139	0.287	0.922	0.768		

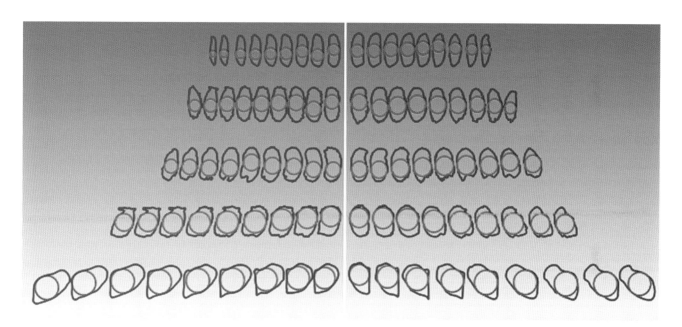

Fig. 9.26 The project of PSC and its internal boundary and inscribed circle from the first to fifth lumbar in different TSA

lumbar vertebras is becoming more and more extensive. Because the limited fundamental research of lumbar pedicle internal fixation, the study of lumbar vertebras adapts to the needs of the development of modern digital medicine.

4.3.1   Materials and Methods

1. Design: A repeated measure design was conducted.
2. Object of study: CT scanning images of healthy adult physical examination were collected.
3. The experiment methods: Select the 3D digital anatomical models of cervical, thoracic, and lumbar vertebral from the database and then import into UG Imageware 12.0.
   (a) Locate 3D coordinate system. The cross section was located in the vertebra middle sagittal and the transverse direction.
   (b) The location analysis of each segment in lumbar vertebras.

The centrum was divided into ten equal parts from front to back. Those ten equal parts were the present standard of borderline depth. From the front to the back, ten equal-part mark lines on the centrum were 100%, 90%, 80%, 70%, 60%, 50%, 40%, 30%, 20%, 10%, and 0% of borderline depth.

The pedicle profile was acquired from an anatomical model of the vertebral body, so we got the pedicle surface boundary. The internal 3D space of the pedicle and its projection boundary could be arbitrarily rotated and observed. Locate the 3D coordinate system of the objective and observe the overlap portion of the lateral margin of pedicle projection border and ten equal-part mark lines on the centrum in the condition of vertical axis rotation. Taking the lateral margin of pedicle projection border tangent to mark lines on the centrum as a standard, we defined this rotation angle as the slant angle in its depth. In the basis of this angle, we could locate the internal boundary of orthographic projection of the pedicle's 3D structure and its inscribed circle. Then the pedicle insertion channel and the biggest screw channel could be established. The center of the inscribed circle could be translated to the surface of the vertebral plate, the corresponding point on the vertebral plate was the best insertion point in its angle, and the translation distance was the length of the channel, so inscribed circle radius was the biggest radius of

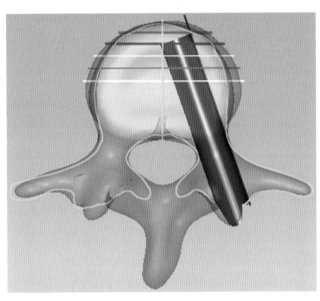

Fig. 9.27 The tangent plane of the outer boundary of the right pedicle projection and 80% boundary depth mark line

screw. By this method, we confirmed the radius, the TSA, and the length of PSC in 50–90% borderline depth. Then measure the perpendicularity distance from the best entering point in five different borderline depths to the middle horizontal plane through the pedicle and to the pedicle projection lateral borderline in 0°TSA of L_{1-5} (Fig. 9.27).

4.3.2 Results

The 3D Analysis of Pedicle Insertion Channel from One to Five Lumbar Vertebra in Different Boundaries
Tables 9.13, 9.14, and 9.15.

The 3D Analysis of the Best Entry Point from One to Five Lumbar Vertebras in Different Boundaries
Tables 9.16 and 9.17.

4.3.3 Discussion

Perpendicularity distances from the best screw point in 50–90% borderline depth to pedicle projection lateral borderline in 0° TSA of L_{1-5} were following: left and right of L_1 were −0.6 mm–4.1 mm and −1.0 mm–3.5 mm. Left and right of L_2 were −0.6 mm–3.9 mm and 0.3 mm–4.7 mm. Left and right of L_3 were −0.3 mm–4.5 mm and −1.4 mm–3.8 mm. Left and right of L_4 were −2.2 mm–1.6 mm and −1.6 mm–2.1 mm. Left and right of L_5 were −4.2 mm to −5.8 mm and −4.6 mm to −6.00 mm. The mean difference value of perpendicularity distance of L_{1-4} between the interior and the lateral screw point in 50–90% different boundary depth was (3.7 ± 1.70) mm to (5.4 ± 0.97) mm and of L_5 was (1.5 ± 2.74) mm to (1.7 ± 1.40) mm. The difference between

Table 9.13 The inscribed circle radius of the pedicle channel from one to five lumbar vertebras in different boundaries (mm) ($\bar{x} \pm s$)

Boundary depth	Segment				
	L_1	L_2	L_3	L_4	L_5
50%					
Left	3.4 ± 0.61	4.0 ± 0.52	4.8 ± 0.83	5.8 ± 0.53	6.1 ± 0.45
Right	3.6 ± 0.45	4.1 ± 0.35	4.7 ± 0.67	5.6 ± 0.68	6.1 ± 0.89
60%					
Left	3.6 ± 0.55	4.1 ± 0.62	4.9 ± 0.83	5.8 ± 0.54	6.1 ± 0.45
Right	3.7 ± 0.47	4.3 ± 0.40	4.9 ± 0.62	5.7 ± 0.65	6.1 ± 0.89
70%					
Left	3.7 ± 0.53	4.2 ± 0.58	5.1 ± 0.85	5.8 ± 0.57	6.1 ± 0.45
Right	3.8 ± 0.48	4.4 ± 0.34	5.0 ± 0.67	5.7 ± 0.70	6.1 ± 0.89
80%					
Left	3.8 ± 0.53	4.3 ± 0.55	5.1 ± 0.87	5.8 ± 0.52	6.1 ± 0.44
Right	3.8 ± 0.45	4.4 ± 0.35	5.1 ± 0.65	5.8 ± 0.73	6.2 ± 0.95
90%					
Left	3.6 ± 0.50	4.3 ± 0.53	5.1 ± 0.78	5.8 ± 0.56	6.1 ± 0.45
Right	3.8 ± 0.41	4.4 ± 0.22	5.1 ± 0.57	5.7 ± 0.80	6.0 ± 0.87
Difference					
Left	0.3 ± 1.03	0.3 ± 0.16	0.3 ± 0.11	0.0 ± 0.17	0.1 ± 0.08
Right	0.2 ± 0.61	0.3 ± 0.14	0.4 ± 0.13	0.1 ± 0.38	0.2 ± 0.07

Table 9.14 The size of the length of the pedicle channel from one to five lumbar vertebras in different boundaries (mm) ($\bar{x} \pm s$)

Boundary depth	Segment				
	L_1	L_2	L_3	L_4	L_5
50%					
Left	35.4 ± 1.77	36.6 ± 2.63	36.9 ± 2.31	36.0 ± 3.73	38.9 ± 3.91
Right	36.7 ± 2.57	36.6 ± 2.89	36.8 ± 2.48	35.7 ± 4.87	36.0 ± 6.84
60%					
Left	38.8 ± 2.44	39.9 ± 3.27	40.1 ± 2.22	39.4 ± 4.07	38.9 ± 3.91
Right	40.6 ± 2.54	39.9 ± 3.34	40.6 ± 2.26	39.2 ± 4.66	36.0 ± 6.84
70%					
Left	43.1 ± 2.99	43.4 ± 3.62	43.9 ± 2.48	42.7 ± 3.47	38.9 ± 3.91
Right	43.8 ± 3.90	43.0 ± 3.59	43.9 ± 2.57	42.6 ± 5.07	36.0 ± 6.84
80%					
Left	46.9 ± 3.78	46.7 ± 3.73	47.3 ± 2.89	45.4 ± 3.33	39.2 ± 3.80
Right	47.2 ± 3.73	46.2 ± 3.57	47.0 ± 2.92	45.7 ± 4.80	40.0 ± 5.85
90%					
Left	49.3 ± 3.90	48.8 ± 3.37	51.7 ± 1.87	48.6 ± 3.53	43.6 ± 3.46
Right	50.5 ± 4.22	47.9 ± 2.71	50.7 ± 3.18	47.8 ± 3.94	44.5 ± 4.93
Difference					
Left	13.9 ± 2.60	12.2 ± 1.64	14.2 ± 2.18	12.6 ± 3.12	17.0 ± 3.77
Right	13.8 ± 1.76	11.3 ± 2.46	13.9 ± 0.84	12.1 ± 3.28	16.6 ± 2.70

Table 9.15 The entry angle of the pedicle channel from one to five lumbar vertebras in different boundaries ($\bar{x} \pm s$) (degree)

Boundary depth	Segment				
	L_1	L_2	L_3	L_4	L_5
50%					
Left	−1.5 ± 3.36	0.0 ± 4.81	1.2 ± 2.75	10.3 ± 1.88	35.2 ± 6.47
Right	−2.1 ± 2.09	−1.5 ± 1.52	1.8 ± 4.79	9.7 ± 5.93	36.2 ± 4.49
60%					
Left	1.8 ± 2.66	3.3 ± 4.10	4.3 ± 2.23	12.0 ± 3.11	35.2 ± 6.47
Right	0.1 ± 1.27	1.5 ± 1.65	5.0 ± 5.32	11.80 ± 6.19	36.2 ± 4.49
70%					
Left	4.5 ± 1.80	5.9 ± 3.16	7.4 ± 2.04	14.2 ± 2.01	35.2 ± 6.47
Right	3.4 ± 1.55	4.5 ± 1.33	7.5 ± 3.67	14.18 ± 5.75	36.2 ± 4.49
80%					
Left	9.0 ± 1.46	9.4 ± 1.93	11.7 ± 2.03	17.1 ± 1.71	36.2 ± 5.37
Right	7.5 ± 1.45	8.2 ± 1.25	11.8 ± 3.14	17.3 ± 5.67	36.7 ± 3.41
90%					
Left	15.7 ± 2.48	14.8 ± 1.47	18.3 ± 1.87	22.6 ± 2.09	39.8 ± 5.69
Right	13.6 ± 1.63	13.9 ± 2.06	18.8 ± 2.80	22.8 ± 3.95	39.0 ± 4.18
Difference					
Left	17.2 ± 4.14	14.8 ± 4.32	17.1 ± 2.41	12.3 ± 2.19	4.6 ± 1.65
Right	15.7 ± 2.10	15.4 ± 2.44	17.0 ± 2.78	13.0 ± 2.45	2.8 ± 1.65

one to four lumbar vertebras was bigger than five lumbar vertebras and indicated that the entry point in 50–90% borderline depth of one to four lumbars had a large range of movement on the vertebral plate. Although the inscribed circle radius of the pedicle insertion channel of L_5 was bigger than L_{1-4}, the scope of entry point was smaller, which was closely related to their 3D space characteristics.

We concluded that with the increase of boundary depth and slant angle, the location of the entry point corresponded to the pedicle channel that moved from the inside to outside.

The biggest boundary depth we set was 90%, and the lumbar pedicle channel didn't break the center of the vertebral body. The size of inscribed circle radius in this depth was almost at the peak of the maximum radius. When the boundary depth was in 80% and 90%, the best entry point from one to four lumbar vertebras was located in the vertical distance of 1mm away from the outer boundary of the pedicle, and the vertical distance to the central level of the pedicle was also about 2 mm; the vertical distance to the central level of the pedicle of L_5 was the same as L_{1-4}, but the verti-

Table 9.16 The vertical distance from the best entry point to the central level of the pedicle from one to five lumbar vertebras in different boundaries (mm) ($\bar{x} \pm s$)

Boundary depth	Segment L_1	L_2	L_3	L_4	L_5
50%					
Left	0.5 ± 2.27	0.8 ± 2.43	0.5 ± 1.82	0.4 ± 0.58	0.2 ± 0.82
Right	0.5 ± 2.36	0.4 ± 2.67	0.4 ± 1.69	0.1 ± 1.19	-0.3 ± 0.60
60%					
Left	1.2 ± 1.33	0.0 ± 2.27	-0.3 ± 1.57	0.3 ± 0.52	0.2 ± 0.82
Right	1.1 ± 1.79	2.1 ± 1.05	0.8 ± 1.97	-0.1 ± 1.41	-0.3 ± 0.60
70%					
Left	1.4 ± 1.40	1.2 ± 1.59	-0.1 ± 1.69	0.2 ± 0.52	0.2 ± 0.82
Right	-0.3 ± 2.41	0.9 ± 1.75	0.8 ± 1.97	-0.3 ± 1.30	-0.3 ± 0.60
80%					
Left	0.1 ± 1.77	0.7 ± 1.73	0.1 ± 1.52	0.2 ± 0.52	0.2 ± 0.82
Right	-0.1 ± 1.83	0.9 ± 1.47	0.6 ± 2.08	-0.6 ± 0.95	-0.3 ± 0.51
90%					
Left	0.3 ± 1.81	0.5 ± 1.44	0.2 ± 1.12	-0.3 ± 0.46	0.1 ± 0.79
Right	0.0 ± 1.79	-0.1 ± 1.39	0.4 ± 1.63	-0.4 ± 1.26	-0.2 ± 0.41

Table 9.17 The vertical distance from the best entry point to the outer boundary of the pedicle from one to five lumbar vertebras in different boundaries (mm) ($\bar{x} \pm s$)

Boundary depth	Segment L_1	L_2	L_3	L_4	L_5
50%					
Left	3.5 ± 1.41	3.9 ± 1.94	4.5 ± 1.07	1.6 ± 0.97	-4.2 ± 2.11
Right	4.1 ± 1.37	4.7 ± 0.83	3.8 ± 1.84	2.1 ± 2.53	-4.6 ± 2.44
60%					
Left	2.9 ± 1.20	2.7 ± 1.44	3.5 ± 1.14	0.9 ± 1.16	-4.2 ± 2.11
Right	3.5 ± 1.10	4.0 ± 0.98	2.8 ± 2.02	1.4 ± 2.69	-4.6 ± 2.44
70%					
Left	2.0 ± 1.15	2.0 ± 1.01	2.5 ± 0.89	-0.2 ± 0.73	-4.2 ± 2.11
Right	2.7 ± 0.82	2.8 ± 1.12	1.8 ± 1.69	0.6 ± 2.11	-4.6 ± 2.44
80%					
Left	0.7 ± 0.95	0.8 ± 0.75	1.0 ± 0.68	-0.7 ± 0.45	-4.6 ± 2.22
Right	1.2 ± 0.71	1.7 ± 0.89	0.5 ± 1.49	0.1 ± 1.90	-4.9 ± 2.44
90%					
Left	-1.0 ± 0.81	-0.6 ± 0.72	-0.9 ± 1.10	-2.2 ± 0.82	-5.8 ± 2.66
Right	-0.6 ± 0.53	0.3 ± 1.08	-1.4 ± 1.21	-1.6 ± 1.25	-6.0 ± 2.85
Difference					
Left	4.5 ± 1.40	4.5 ± 2.11	5.4 ± 0.97	3.8 ± 0.38	1.7 ± 1.40
Right	4.7 ± 1.34	4.4 ± 0.95	5.1 ± 0.77	3.7 ± 1.70	1.5 ± 2.74

cal distance to the outer boundary of the pedicle of L_5 was about 5–6 mm on the outside. Just set the outer projection boundary line as the entry point; the depth of the insertion channel from one to four lumbar vertebras was between the depth of 80% and 90%. The depth of 80% and 90% could be used to analyze the insertion angle scope; the results were the following: left and right of L_1 were 9.0–15.7° and 7.5–13.6°. Left and right of L_2 were 9.4–14.8° and 8.2–13.9°. Left and right of L_3 were 11.7–18.3° and 11.8–18.8°. Left and right of L_4 were 17.1–22.6° and 17.3–22.7°. Left and right of L_5 were 36.2–39.8° and 36.7–39.0°. Among the results, the angle scope of L_5 was the smallest change, which could be associated with its big pedicle and small change of

boundary curve of the vertebral body. In our studies, we found out that when the slant angle reached to a certain degree, the mark lines of L_5 in 50%, 60%, 70%, and 80% depth were almost in the same level, which are different from another lumbar vertebra. Therefore, we should make a distinction between L_5 and other lumbar vertebras; for its small angle, it's easy to break the boundary.

Finally, it is easy to get to a conclusion by method of anatomical landmark: Lots of former studies took the intersections of the vertical line of zygapophysial joint space, center of zygapophysial, outer edge of zygapophysial and mastoid concave, and transverse process bisector as the positioning reference points, the location of these points on the vertebral plate changed from medial to lateral. And we concluded that the entry point in 50–90% boundary depth moved from medial to lateral, which was consistent with former studies. And we found that the inscribed circle radius in a different insertion depth was almost the same, the length of the channel in 50–60% depth from one to four lumbar vertebras was less than 40 mm, and the length in 70–90% depth was more than 40 mm. The length of the channel in 50–80% depth of L_5 was less than 40 mm, and the length in 90% depth was more than 40 mm. In consequence, we asserted that the entry point on the outside was better than on the inside; of course the insertion angle on the outside should increase.

4.4   The Accurate Positioning Analysis of 3D Relations of Pedicle Screw Channel, Screw Entry Point, and Vertebra Body Boundary in Thoracic Vertebras

4.4.1   Materials and Methods
1. Design: A repeated measure design was conducted.
2. Object of study: CT scanning images of healthy adult physical examination were collected.
3. The experiment methods:
   (a) Select the 3D digital anatomical models of cervical, thoracic, and lumbar vertebral from the database and then import into UG Imageware 12.0.
   (b) Locate 3D coordinate system. The cross section was located in the vertebra middle sagittal and the transverse direction.
   (c) The location analysis of each segment in thoracic vertebras.

The centrum was divided into ten equal parts from front to back. Those ten equal parts were the present standard of borderline depth. From front to back, ten equal-part mark lines on the centrum were 100%, 90%, 80%, 70%, 60%, 50%, 40%, 30%, 20%, 10%, and 0% of borderline depth.

The pedicle profile was acquired from the anatomical model of the vertebral body, so we got the pedicle surface boundary. The internal 3D space of the pedicle and its projection boundary could be arbitrarily rotated and observed. Locate the 3D coordinate system of the objective, and observe the overlap portion of the lateral margin of the pedicle projection border and ten equal-part mark lines on the centrum in the condition of vertical axis rotation. Taking the lateral margin of the pedicle projection border tangent to mark lines on the centrum as a standard, we defined this rotation angle as the slant angle in its depth. In the basis of this angle, we could locate the internal boundary of orthographic projection of the pedicle's 3D structure and its inscribed circle. Then the pedicle insertion channel and the biggest screw

channel could be established. The center of the inscribed circle could be translated to the surface of vertebral plate, then the corresponding point on the vertebral plate was the best insertion point in its angle, and the translation distance was the length of the channel, so the inscribed circle radius was the biggest radius of screw. In this method, we confirmed the radius, the TSA, and the length of PSC in 50–90% borderline depth. Then measure, respectively, the perpendicularity distance from the best entering point in five different borderline depths to the middle horizontal plane through the pedicle and to the pedicle projection lateral borderline in 0°TSA of T_{1-12}.

By the method mentioned above, we could, respectively, confirm the fitting ellipse of the pedicle projection boundary and its center point in 90% boundary depth and then translate the center point to the surface of vertebral plate, and the corresponding point on the vertebral plate could be defined as the reference point of the best entry point in different boundary depths, and then measure, respectively, the perpendicularity distance from pedicle projection lateral borderline to mark lines on the surface of vertebral body in 0° TSA (Fig. 9.28).

4.4.2   Results

The 3D Analysis of the Pedicle Insertion Channel from One to Five Lumbar Vertebras in Different Boundaries
Tables 9.18, 9.19, and 9.20.

The 3D Analysis of the Best Entry Point from One to Five Lumbar Vertebras in Different Boundaries
Tables 9.21 and 9.22.

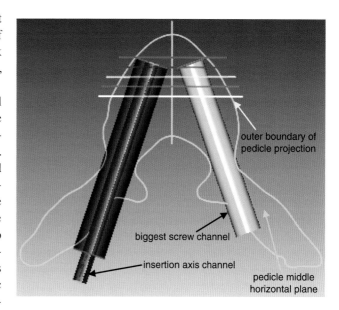

Fig. 9.28   3D analysis of PSC of thoracic vertebra

Table 9.18 The inscribed circle radius of the pedicle channel from three to twelve thoracic vertebras in different boundary depths (mm) ($\bar{x} \pm s$)

Segment	Boundary depth					Difference
	50%	60%	70%	80%	90%	
T_3						
Left	2.9 ± 0.41	2.9 ± 0.46	2.9 ± 0.49	2.9 ± 0.50	2.9 ± 0.51	0.0 ± 0.14
Right	3.0 ± 0.37	3.0 ± 0.40	3.0 ± 0.39	3.0 ± 0.34	3.0 ± 0.36	0.1 ± 0.09
T_4						
Left	2.7 ± 0.50	2.8 ± 0.50	2.9 ± 0.53	2.7 ± 0.57	2.7 ± 0.56	0.1 ± 0.17
Right	2.6 ± 0.41	2.6 ± 0.42	2.7 ± 0.37	2.6 ± 0.37	2.6 ± 0.41	0.0 ± 0.10
T_5						
Left	2.5 ± 0.60	2.6 ± 0.58	2.6 ± 0.58	2.6 ± 0.57	2.5 ± 0.46	0.1 ± 0.19
Right	2.6 ± 0.55	2.7 ± 0.54	2.7 ± 0.57	2.7 ± 0.50	2.6 ± 0.43	0.1 ± 1.66
T_6						
Left	2.7 ± 0.65	2.7 ± 0.61	2.7 ± 0.62	2.7 ± 0.56	2.6 ± 0.55	0.1 ± 0.06
Right	2.7 ± 0.64	2.7 ± 0.58	2.7 ± 0.60	2.8 ± 0.52	2.7 ± 0.49	0.1 ± 0.26
T_7						
Left	2.7 ± 0.67	2.7 ± 0.71	2.7 ± 0.69	2.7 ± 0.70	2.7 ± 0.64	0.0 ± 0.17
Right	2.9 ± 0.57	3.0 ± 0.54	3.0 ± 0.54	2.9 ± 0.52	2.9 ± 0.47	0.1 ± 0.11
T_8						
Left	2.8 ± 0.63	2.8 ± 0.56	2.9 ± 0.64	2.8 ± 0.61	2.8 ± 0.58	0.1 ± 0.37
Right	2.8 ± 0.63	2.9 ± 0.61	2.9 ± 0.57	2.9 ± 0.53	2.9 ± 0.57	0.1 ± 0.43
T_9						
Left	3.1 ± 0.52	3.1 ± 0.58	3.1 ± 0.55	3.1 ± 0.55	2.9 ± 0.55	0.0 ± 0.12
Right	3.2 ± 0.69	3.1 ± 0.62	3.2 ± 0.67	3.2 ± 0.64	3.1 ± 0.64	0.2 ± 0.29
T_{10}						
Left	3.7 ± 0.68	3.8 ± 0.69	3.7 ± 0.63	3.6 ± 0.66	3.5 ± 0.76	0.2 ± 0.15
Right	3.8 ± 0.60	3.8 ± 0.59	3.8 ± 0.58	3.7 ± 0.64	3.6 ± 0.70	0.2 ± 0.14
T_{11}						
Left	4.6 ± 0.40	4.5 ± 0.39	4.4 ± 0.42	4.3 ± 0.56	4.1 ± 0.48	0.5 ± 0.21
Right	4.4 ± 0.59	4.4 ± 0.56	4.4 ± 0.53	4.3 ± 0.49	4.1 ± 0.57	0.3 ± 0.20
T_{12}						
Left	4.9 ± 0.78	4.9 ± 0.79	4.8 ± 0.74	4.6 ± 0.76	4.4 ± 0.80	0.5 ± 0.19
Right	4.7 ± 0.82	4.7 ± 0.82	4.6 ± 0.82	4.6 ± 0.81	4.3 ± 0.81	0.5 ± 0.13

Table 9.19 The size of the length of the pedicle channel from three to twelve thoracic vertebras in different boundaries (mm) ($\bar{x} \pm s$)

Segment	Boundary depth					Difference
	50%	60%	70%	80%	90%	
T_3						
Left	24.2 ± 3.26	26.5 ± 2.62	28.9 ± 3.09	31.1 ± 2.97	33.5 ± 2.22	9.1 ± 2.21
Right	25.7 ± 1.81	27.7 ± 0.91	30.5 ± 1.61	33.5 ± 1.53	37.3 ± 2.31	11.3 ± 3.39
T_4						
Left	26.6 ± 2.33	29.3 ± 2.51	31.9 ± 2.33	34.0 ± 1.71	36.5 ± 1.54	9.9 ± 1.01
Right	27.2 ± 2.45	29.3 ± 2.79	31.9 ± 2.34	33.5 ± 3.10	37.3 ± 3.32	10.0 ± 2.29
T_5						
Left	28.2 ± 2.14	30.6 ± 2.30	32.9 ± 2.00	34.8 ± 1.76	38.2 ± 0.82	10.0 ± 2.42
Right	28.9 ± 2.74	31.3 ± 2.68	33.7 ± 3.05	36.4 ± 3.37	40.0 ± 4.20	9.6 ± 1.82
T_6						
Left	30.4 ± 2.59	33.1 ± 2.84	35.8 ± 3.38	38.7 ± 3.95	42.1 ± 4.37	11.7 ± 1.94
Right	30.5 ± 2.33	32.7 ± 2.49	35.5 ± 2.69	38.5 ± 2.87	41.7 ± 3.21	11.2 ± 1.87
T_7						
Left	29.8 ± 1.03	33.0 ± 1.16	36.3 ± 2.02	39.3 ± 2.89	41.9 ± 4.26	12.1 ± 3.38
Right	31.1 ± 1.93	33.8 ± 2.05	36.6 ± 2.32	39.8 ± 2.95	42.3 ± 3.76	11.2 ± 1.95

continued

Table 9.19 (cont.)

Segment	Boundary depth					
	50%	60%	70%	80%	90%	Difference
T_8						
Left	30.8 ± 1.69	33.1 ± 1.52	36.5 ± 1.16	40.4 ± 2.01	45.6 ± 2.85	14.9 ± 3.36
Right	30.4 ± 1.00	33.4 ± 0.71	36.0 ± 0.61	39.0 ± 0.84	42.9 ± 0.83	12.6 ± 1.97
T_9						
Left	30.5 ± 2.21	33.9 ± 2.20	36.6 ± 1.30	39.9 ± 1.67	44.1 ± 1.00	13.6 ± 2.23
Right	30.6 ± 1.79	32.5 ± 1.38	34.9 ± 1.24	39.4 ± 2.44	43.6 ± 3.45	13.0 ± 1.85
T_{10}						
Left	30.1 ± 1.75	32.5 ± 1.47	35.3 ± 1.51	38.0 ± 2.23	41.9 ± 2.28	11.8 ± 0.95
Right	30.1 ± 0.75	33.3 ± 1.34	35.3 ± 1.00	38.6 ± 1.12	42.9 ± 2.31	12.8 ± 1.69
T_{11}						
Left	31.8 ± 5.04	32.9 ± 1.73	37.2 ± 2.54	44.2 ± 6.95	46.7 ± 5.81	14.9 ± 3.78
Right	29.6 ± 1.85	32.6 ± 1.74	35.5 ± 1.36	39.2 ± 2.47	42.6 ± 2.42	13.0 ± 1.02
T_{12}						
Left	39.7 ± 3.07	42.9 ± 2.62	45.5 ± 2.16	48.9 ± 1.68	51.3 ± 1.96	11.6 ± 4.09
Right	40.5 ± 3.26	43.4 ± 3.19	46.1 ± 3.19	48.7 ± 3.16	51.5 ± 3.01	11.0 ± 0.62

Table 9.20 The entry angle of the pedicle channel from three to twelve thoracic vertebras in different boundaries ($\bar{x} \pm s$) (degree)

Segment	Boundary depth					
	50%	60%	70%	80%	90%	Difference
T_3						
Left	6.4 ± 3.78	9.3 ± 3.20	12.1 ± 3.14	15.0 ± 3.21	18.8 ± 1.62	12.1 ± 2.21
Right	9.0 ± 3.12	10.7 ± 2.75	13.3 ± 1.99	16.6 ± 2.70	20.7 ± 1.98	12.0 ± 3.44
T_4						
Left	4.0 ± 4.95	6.8 ± 5.07	9.3 ± 4.99	11.7 ± 4.53	14.1 ± 4.60	10.1 ± 1.97
Right	5.6 ± 4.05	8.3 ± 4.08	11.3 ± 3.97	14.2 ± 3.30	16.9 ± 3.24	11.3 ± 3.11
T_5						
Left	4.4 ± 3.73	6.6 ± 3.59	8.9 ± 3.66	11.3 ± 3.14	13.7 ± 3.17	8.4 ± 1.66
Right	2.7 ± 2.95	5.1 ± 3.70	7.4 ± 3.96	10.1 ± 4.31	13.6 ± 4.56	9.9 ± 3.08
T_6						
Left	3.8 ± 3.17	6.6 ± 3.50	9.2 ± 2.93	11.5 ± 3.09	15.0 ± 2.79	10.7 ± 2.02
Right	2.4 ± 3.79	4.6 ± 3.38	7.1 ± 3.46	9.9 ± 3.30	13.4 ± 2.79	11.0 ± 3.00
T_7						
Left	3.6 ± 4.72	5.7 ± 4.96	7.6 ± 5.63	10.4 ± 4.70	13.3 ± 4.56	9.7 ± 2.73
Right	1.30 ± 4.41	3.4 ± 4.33	5.0 ± 4.45	7.5 ± 4.04	10.7 ± 4.03	9.4 ± 1.83
T_8						
Left	1.7 ± 4.58	4.0 ± 4.75	6.8 ± 4.36	10.0 ± 4.03	14.2 ± 3.55	12.5 ± 1.97
Right	−3.2 ± 5.50	2.1 ± 5.12	4.4 ± 4.13	7.3 ± 4.56	11.4 ± 3.75	11.7 ± 2.73
T_9						
Left	3.1 ± 3.82	3.9 ± 3.38	6.8 ± 2.86	9.9 ± 2.48	14.5 ± 2.13	11.4 ± 2.02
Right	−0.2 ± 3.76	1.4 ± 3.62	3.8 ± 3.18	6.7 ± 3.14	11.0 ± 2.87	11.2 ± 1.79
T_{10}						
Left	3.7 ± 4.79	6.1 ± 4.57	8.0 ± 3.53	10.8 ± 3.44	15.1 ± 3.04	11.4 ± 2.80
Right	1.1 ± 3.43	2.7 ± 2.54	4.7 ± 2.18	7.4 ± 2.28	11.1 ± 2.31	10.0 ± 2.51
T_{11}						
Left	6.0 ± 2.97	7.3 ± 2.89	9.6 ± 2.80	12.7 ± 2.23	16.9 ± 2.32	10.9 ± 2.63
Right	5.3 ± 1.32	6.6 ± 1.03	7.9 ± 0.98	10.4 ± 0.99	14.0 ± 1.20	8.7 ± 2.38
T_{12}						
Left	8.9 ± 3.57	9.9 ± 3.30	11.9 ± 3.67	14.0 ± 2.76	18.0 ± 2.91	9.1 ± 1.47
Right	7.1 ± 3.83	8.0 ± 3.09	9.4 ± 2.92	11.8 ± 2.64	15.0 ± 2.02	7.9 ± 1.87

Table 9.21 The vertical distance from the best entry point to the central level of the pedicle from three to twelve thoracic vertebras in different boundaries (mm) ($\bar{x} \pm s$)

Segment	Depth				
	50%	60%	70%	80%	90%
T_3					
Left	−0.5 ± 0.56	0.4 ± 1.95	0.1 ± 1.98	0.7 ± 1.97	0.4 ± 2.27
Right	−0.1 ± 1.95	0.0 ± 1.92	0.8 ± 2.08	0.4 ± 2.20	0.1 ± 1.88
T_4					
Left	1.0 ± 1.46	0.46 ± 1.98	0.2 ± 1.73	0.7 ± 1.55	0.4 ± 1.45
Right	−0.2 ± 1.68	0.10 ± 1.92	0.26 ± 2.14	0.9 ± 1.95	0.2 ± 2.07
T_5					
Left	0.6 ± 1.47	0.9 ± 2.06	0.5 ± 1.68	0.8 ± 1.61	0.2 ± 2.25
Right	0.1 ± 0.79	−0.1 ± 1.29	0.7 ± 1.10	0.8 ± 1.89	0.2 ± 1.35
T_6					
Left	1.3 ± 1.20	0.9 ± 1.52	1.9 ± 0.96	1.6 ± 0.89	1.8 ± 1.26
Right	−0.2 ± 1.30	0.8 ± 1.61	0.6 ± 2.01	0.3 ± 1.87	0.2 ± 1.76
T_7					
Left	1.5 ± 1.66	1.4 ± 2.16	0.6 ± 2.38	1.4 ± 2.16	1.5 ± 2.18
Right	0.3 ± 1.79	0.7 ± 1.64	0.8 ± 1.55	0.1 ± 1.88	0.2 ± 1.15
T_8					
Left	1.4 ± 0.85	1.50 ± 1.73	1.2 ± 1.31	1.4 ± 1.16	0.9 ± 2.17
Right	1.8 ± 1.10	0.9 ± 1.88	1.3 ± 1.70	1.2 ± 2.39	0.3 ± 2.54
T_9					
Left	1.1 ± 1.14	0.3 ± 2.08	0.6 ± 1.47	0.7 ± 1.35	0.4 ± 2.04
Right	1.2 ± 1.63	1.7 ± 0.76	1.3 ± 1.56	0.8 ± 1.89	0.8 ± 2.25
T_{10}					
Left	0.9 ± 1.42	2.0 ± 1.97	1.7 ± 1.44	1.7 ± 1.66	1.6 ± 0.96
Right	1.2 ± 2.08	1.2 ± 1.97	0.7 ± 1.84	1.1 ± 2.19	0.4 ± 2.04
T_{11}					
Left	3.3 ± 0.85	2.7 ± 0.90	2.5 ± 1.35	2.2 ± 1.75	2.9 ± 1.23
Right	3.0 ± 1.54	3.0 ± 1.54	3.0 ± 1.54	3.0 ± 1.62	2.9 ± 1.67
T_{12}					
Left	1.7 ± 0.81	1.6 ± 0.75	1.1 ± 1.16	1.3 ± 1.04	1.3 ± 1.15
Right	0.6 ± 0.82	0.5 ± 1.02	0.4 ± 1.01	0.2 ± 0.57	0.4 ± 1.38

Table 9.22 The vertical distance from the best entry point to the outer boundary of the pedicle from three to twelve thoracic vertebras in different boundaries (mm) ($\bar{x} \pm s$)

Segment	Boundary depth					Difference
	50%	60%	70%	80%	90%	
T_3						
Left	1.3 ± 0.57	0.8 ± 0.27	0.0 ± 0.09	−0.2 ± 0.27	−1.0 ± 0.67	2.3 ± 1.02
Right	0.8 ± 0.76	0.3 ± 0.45	−0.3 ± 0.27	−1.5 ± 1.16	−2.9 ± 1.32	3.7 ± 1.69
T_4						
Left	1.7 ± 0.88	0.9 ± 1.22	0.3 ± 1.20	−0.1 ± 1.01	−0.6 ± 1.20	2.3 ± 0.45
Right	0.9 ± 1.02	0.5 ± 1.06	−0.5 ± 1.12	−0.6 ± 0.69	−1.6 ± 1.51	2.5 ± 0.73
T_5						
Left	1.5 ± 1.12	1.0 ± 0.73	0.7 ± 0.71	0.5 ± 0.79	0.0 ± 1.46	1.5 ± 1.66
Right	1.6 ± 1.25	1.3 ± 0.79	1.0 ± 0.61	0.4 ± 0.65	−0.4 ± 0.89	2.0 ± 0.94
T_6						
Left	1.7 ± 0.84	0.9 ± 1.08	0.6 ± 1.43	−0.3 ± 1.64	−1.0 ± 2.06	2.7 ± 1.79
Right	2.1 ± 0.69	1.7 ± 0.45	0.8 ± 0.32	0.3 ± 0.57	−0.9 ± 0.96	3.0 ± 1.31
T_7						
Left	2.2 ± 0.76	1.3 ± 0.57	0.8 ± 1.04	0.0 ± 1.17	−0.6 ± 1.67	2.8 ± 1.64
Right	2.8 ± 1.35	2.4 ± 1.43	1.8 ± 1.15	1.4 ± 1.17	0.4 ± 0.89	2.4 ± 0.65

continued

Table 9.22 (cont.)

Segment	Boundary depth					
	50%	60%	70%	80%	90%	Difference
T_8						
Left	2.5 ± 0.79	2.0 ± 0.71	1.3 ± 1.20	0.8 ± 1.26	−0.1 ± 2.19	2.6 ± 2.53
Right	3.0 ± 0.89	2.2 ± 0.84	2.0 ± 0.61	1.3 ± 0.83	0.1 ± 0.74	2.9 ± 0.47
T_9						
Left	2.4 ± 0.97	2.5 ± 1.23	1.8 ± 1.04	1.2 ± 1.32	0.1 ± 1.56	2.8 ± 0.87
Right	3.3 ± 0.75	3.2 ± 0.76	2.4 ± 0.72	1.6 ± 0.96	0.5 ± 1.41	2.8 ± 1.02
T_{10}						
Left	3.4 ± 0.65	3.0 ± 0.67	2.7 ± 0.61	2.1 ± 0.55	1.20 ± 0.76	2.2 ± 0.14
Right	3.7 ± 0.42	3.1 ± 0.70	2.7 ± 0.67	2.3 ± 0.48	0.90 ± 1.29	2.8 ± 1.36
T_{11}						
Left	4.1 ± 0.56	3.5 ± 0.46	3.0 ± 0.72	1.2 ± 1.44	0.4 ± 1.52	3.7 ± 1.51
Right	3.9 ± 0.89	3.6 ± 0.71	3.2 ± 0.81	2.6 ± 0.92	1.9 ± 1.08	2.0 ± 0.79
T_{12}						
Left	1.7 ± 1.32	1.5 ± 1.16	0.8 ± 1.04	0.3 ± 0.45	−0.7 ± 0.43	2.5 ± 1.72
Right	2.6 ± 0.50	2.1 ± 0.47	1.7 ± 0.34	1.2 ± 0.57	0.1 ± 0.96	2.5 ± 1.01

4.4.3 The Characteristic of the Digital Pedicle Channel of the Thoracic Vertebra

The inscribed circle radius of the pedicle channel from three to twelve thoracic vertebras decreased at the start and then increased gradually. The radius of T_5, T_6, and T_7 was at about the minimum peak, and the T_{12} was the maximum value. The scopes of T_{3-12} inscribed circle radius in 50–90% different boundary depths, respectively, were the following: left and right of T_3 were 2.9–2.9 mm and 3.0–3.0 mm. Left and right of T_4 were 2.7–2.8 mm and 2.6–2.7 mm. Left and right of T_5 were 2.5–2.6 mm and 2.6–2.7 mm. Left and right of T_6 were 2.6–2.7 mm and 2.7–2.8 mm. Left and right of T_7 were 2.7–2.7 mm and 2.9–3.0 mm. Left and right of T_8 were 2.8–2.9 mm and 2.8–2.9 mm. Left and right of T_9 were 2.9–3.1 mm and 3.1–3.2 mm. Left and right of T_{10} were 3.5–3.7 mm and 3.6–3.8 mm. Left and right of T_{11} were 4.1–4.6 mm and 4.1–4.4 mm. Left and right of T_{12} were 4.4–4.9 mm and 4.3–4.7 mm. The greatest depth and the smallest depth mean difference value was 0.0 ± 0.19 mm and 0.5 ± 0.19 mm. The T_{12} difference value was the biggest, about 0.5 mm, and other sections mostly were between 0 mm and 0.2 mm; it explained that with the change of depth, the size of the inscribed circle radius of the pedicle channel from three to twelve thoracic vertebras was in a stable scope. According to the *t*-test results analysis of the inscribed circle radius of the pedicle channel between the left and right in different boundary depths in each segment, there was a significant difference of T_7 in 50% depth and T_8 in 90% depth; others revealed no significant difference.

The length of PSC from three to twelve thoracic vertebras showed a consistent change rule: they increased gradually, and the PSC in 90% boundary depth didn't break the central vertebra body. The scopes of T_{3-12} PSC length, respectively, were the following: left and right of T_3 were 24.2–33.5 mm and 25.7–37.3 mm. Left and right of T_4 were 26.2–36.5 mm and 27.2–37.3 mm. Left and right of T_5 were 28.2–38.2 mm and 28.9–40.0 mm. Left and right of T_6 were 30.4–42.1 m and 30.5–41.7 mm. Left and right of T_7 were 29.8–41.9 mm and 31.1–42.3 mm. Left and right of T_8 were 30.8–45.6 mm and 30.4–42.9 mm. Left and right of T_9 were 30.5–44.1 mm and 30.6–43.6 mm. Left and right of T_{10} were 30.1–41.9 mm and 30.1–42.9 mm. Left and right of T_{11} were 31.8–46.7 mm and 29.6–42.6 mm. Left and right of T_{12} were 39.7–51.3 mm and 40.5–51.5 mm. The mean different value of the biggest and the smallest PSC length of T_{3-12} in 50~90% boundary depth was 9.1 ± 2.21 mm to 14.9 ± 3.36 mm. From 50–90% boundary depth different value was consistent, and maximum value was 14.9 mm, mostly concentrated between 10 and 12 mm. Various segments in 90% boundary depth, the PSC length scope was the following. T_3 was 33.5–37.3 mm. T_4 was 36.5–37.3 mm. T_5 was 38.2–40.0 mm. T_6 was 41.7–42.1 mm. T_7 was 41.9–42.3 mm. T_8 was 42.9–45.6 mm. T_9 was 43.6–44.1 mm. T_{10} was 41.9–42.9 mm. $T_{11}$was 42.6–46.7 mm. T_{12} was 51.3–51.5 mm.

The scope of T_{3-12} PSC slant angle in 50–90% boundary depth showed a consistent rule: they increased gradually. The scopes of T_{3-12} PSC slant angle, respectively, were the following: left and right of T_3 were 6.4–18.8° and 9.0–20.7°. Left and right of T_4 were 4.0–14.1° and 5.6–16.9°. Left and right of T_5 were 4.4–13.7° and 2.7–13.6°. Left and right of T_6 were 3.8–15.0° and 2.4–13.4°. Left and right of T_7 were 3.6–13.3° and 1.3–10.7°. Left and right of T_8 were 1.7–14.2°and −3.2° to 11.4°. Left and right of T_9 were 3.1–14.5° and −0.2° to 11.0°. Left and right of T_{10} were 3.7–15.1° and 1.1–11.1°. Left and right of T_{11} were 6.0–17.0° and 5.3–14.0°. Left and right of T_{12} were 8.9–18.0° and 7.1–15.0°. The mean different values of the biggest and the smallest PSC slant angle of T_{3-12} were 7.9 ± 1.87° to 12.5 ± 1.97°. The different values of angle in 50–90% boundary depth maintained consistently and changed between 9° and 11°.

80–90% boundary depth angle scopes were the following: the left and right of T_3 were 15.0–18.8° and 16.6–20.7°. Left and right of T_4 were 11.7–14.1° and 14.2–16.9°. Left and right of T_5 were 11.3–13.7° and 10.1–13.6°. Left and right of T_6 were 11.5–15.0° and 9.9–13.4°. Left and right of T_7 were 10.4–13.3° and 7.5–10.7°. Left and right of T_8 were 10.0–14.2° and 7.3–11.4°. Left and right of T_9 were 9.9–14.5° and 6.7–11.0°. Left and right of T_{10} were 10.8–15.1° and 7.4–11.1°. Left and right of T_{11} were 12.7–17.0° and 10.4–14.0°. Left and right of T_{12} were 14.0–18.0° and 11.8–15.0°.

The SSA of T_{3--12}, respectively, was −14.94°, −14.64°, −16.52°, −10.18°, −13.2°, −6.76°, −3.2°, −5.46°, 0°, 0°, 0°.

We used the same mark lines like the lumbar vertebra and defined the vertical distance between PSC best entry point and pedicle central level in boundary depth as the horizontal vertical distance and the vertical distance of the lateral line of projection boundary corresponded on the surface of vertebral body in 0° declination as the vertical distance of pedicle boundary. Then these relevant parameter indexes could be used to analyze the relationship between PSC best entry point, insertion direction, and PSC depth from three to twelve thoracic vertebras in different boundaries.

The mean different value of T_{3-12} between the interior and the lateral screw point in 50–90% boundary depth was (1.5 ± 1.66) mm to (3.7 ± 1.51) mm. With increasing depth, the entering screw point position moves outside. Motion scope was 2–4 mm.

Perpendicularity distances from best screw points in 80% and 90% boundary depth to pedicle boundary, respectively, were the following: left and right of T_3 were −0.2, −1.0 mm, −1.5 mm, and −2.9 mm. Left and right of T_4 were −0.1, −0.6 mm, −0.6, and −1.6 mm. Left and right of T_5 were 0.5 mm, 0.0 mm, 0.4 mm, and −0.4 mm. Left and right of T_6 were −0.3 mm, −1.0mm, 0.3 mm, and −0.9 mm. Left and right of T_7 were −0.0 mm, −0.6 mm, 1.4 mm, and 0.4 mm. Left and right of T_8 were 0.8 mm, −0.1 mm, 1.3 mm, and 0.1 mm. Left and right of T_9 were 1.2 mm, 0.1 mm, 1.6 mm, and 0.5 mm. Left and right of T_{10} were 2.1 mm, 1.2 mm, 2.3 mm, and 0.9 mm. Left and right of T_{11} were 1.2 mm, 0.4 mm, 2.6 mm, and 1.9 mm. Left and right of T_{12} were 0.3 mm, −0.7 mm, 1.2 mm, and 0.1 mm. Just set the lateral border of pedicle projection boundary as the reference line of entry point in different boundaries; we obtained the minimum boundary depth corresponding to the entry point on the lateral border of line from three to twelve thoracic vertebras. Left and right of T_3 were 70% and 70%. Left and right of T_4 were −80% and 70%. Left and right of T_5 were 90% and

80%. Left and right of T_6 were 80% and 80%. Left and right of T_7 were 80% and 90%. Left and right of T_8 were 80% and 90%. Left and right of T_9 were 90% and 90%. Left and right of T_{10} were 90% and 90%. Left and right of T_{11} were 90% and 90%. Left and right of T_{12} were 80% and 90%. The boundary depth of T_3 was relatively small, and depth of T_{9-11} was relatively bigger, so to take the measured value into consideration, the entry point of T_3 should move outside 1–2 mm, T_{9-11} should move inside 1–2 mm, and other segments could choose the point on the lateral border of pedicle projection as the entry point.

Perpendicularity distances from best screw points in 50–90% borderline depth to pedicle central level of T_{3-12}, respectively, was the following: left and right of T_3 were −0.5–0.7 mm and −0.1–0.8 mm. Left and right of T_4 were 0.2–1.0 mm and 0.20–0.9 mm. Left and right of T_5 were 0.2–0.9 mm and −0.1–0.8 mm. Left and right of T_6 were 0.9–1.9 mm and −0.2–0.8 mm. Left and right of T_7 were 0.6–1.5 mm and 0.1–0.8 mm. Left and right of T_8 were 0.9–1.5 mm and 0.3–1.8 mm. Left and right of T_9 were 0.3–1.1 mm and 0.8–1.7 mm. Left and right of T_{10} were 0.9–2.0 mm and 0.4–1.2 mm. Left and right of T_{11} were 2.2–3.3 mm and 2.9–3.0 mm. Left and right of T_{12} were 1.1–1.7 mm and 0.2–0.6 mm.

Perpendicularity distances from best screw points in 80% and 90% borderline depth to pedicle central level of T_{3-12}, respectively, were the following: left and right of T_3 were 0.7 mm, 0.4 mm, 0.4 mm, and −0.1 mm. Left and right of T_4 were 0.7 mm, 0.4 mm, 0.9 mm, and 0.2 mm. Left and right of T_5 were 0.8 mm, 0.2 mm, 0.8 mm, and 0.2 mm. Left and right of T_6 were 1.6 mm, 1.8 mm, 0.3 mm, and 0.2 mm. Left and right of T_7 were 1.4 mm, 1.5 mm, 0.1 mm, and 0.2 mm. Left and right of T_8 were 1.4 mm, 0.9 mm, 1.2 mm, and 0.3 mm. Left and right of T_9 were 0.7 mm, 0.4 mm, 0.8 mm, and 0.8 mm. Left and right of T_{10} were 1.7 mm, 1.6 mm, 1.1 mm, and 0.4 mm. Left and right of T_{11} were 2.2 mm, 2.9 mm, 3.0 mm, and 2.9 mm. Left and right of T_{12} were 1.3 mm, 1.3 mm, 0.2 mm, and 0.4 mm.

In this study, we made an approximate analysis of PSC in 90% boundary depth and entry point, and the perpendicularity distance from best screw point to pedicle central level of T_{3-12} was all positive, 0.10–0.90 mm above the pedicle central level, and was in close proximity to it.

5   Study on the Application of Digital Technology in Cervical Pedicle Screw Internal Fixation in Children

Zhijun Li and Shaojie Zhang

The cervical pedicle screw internal fixation technology has been developed rapidly in recent years. It has been widely used in internal fixation of spinal injury in adults due to its features such as three-point fixation, biomechanical rationality, stability, and fastness. Scholars at home and abroad have applied the technology in internal fixation of spinal injuries in children. Ruf et al. reported that hemivertebrectomy combined with vertebral pedicle screw internal fixation in 28 patients with congenital scoliosis aged 1–6 achieved very satisfactory effects; 19 patients aged 1–2 who underwent pedicle screw internal fixation at thoracic and lumbar vertebras also showed that the method was safe and feasible. Li Jing et al. successfully performed ten patients of pedicle screw internal fixation at lower thoracic vertebras and lumbar vertebras in children aged 1–3, Chen Liyan et al. successfully performed 19 patients of pedicle screw internal fixation at thoracic vertebras and lumbar vertebras in children under ten (6.5 averagely), and Lin Bin et al. successfully performed pedicle screw internal fixation at upper cervical vertebras. They all concluded that pedicle screw internal fixation was safe and feasible based on rigorous preoperative plan, selection of pedicle screw of appropriate diameter, and exquisite surgical technology.

Most spinal injuries in children occur in cervical vertebras. Cervical vertebra of a child is in a stage of persistent growth and development with morphological characteristics largely different from those of adults. The pedicles of vertebral arches of children are thin and small and those of cervical vertebras are thinner and smaller with largely variable anatomy structures and complex correlation with adjacent tissues. The form of the pedicle of vertebral arch is varied significantly with age and segment. The application of pedicle screw insertion based on adult data in children in the stage of growth and development has very high risk. Improvement of screw fixation accuracy and reduction of error rate become the key points for in-depth development of cervical pedicle internal in children. Therefore, applying the concept of digital and individualized screw insertion in pedicle screw fixation in children is extremely important.

5.1 Preliminary Discussion on the Application of Digital Technology in the Morphology of Children Atlantoaxial Pedicle and the Screw Insertion Mode

Most spinal injuries in children occur in cervical spines, especially in upper cervical spines. Tan Ming-Sheng and Desai et al. have applied the atlantoaxial pedicle screw internal fixation technology in children and achieved very satisfactory effects. However, since children are in a stage of growth and development and their atlantoaxial pedicles are thin and vari-able with complex correlation with adjacent tissues, screw insertion in this segment has higher risk. To reduce the surgical risk, atlantoaxial pedicle screw internal fixation in children should lay more emphasis on individualization and digitalization and take advantages of digital orthopedics, thereby improving the accuracy of screw insertion.

5.1.1 Materials and Methods

Imaging data of atlantoaxial vertebra of children who underwent MSCT scan (for GE Light QX/I 64-slice spiral CT, layer thickness and interval are both 0.625 mm, Fov 30 cm × 30 cm, the matrix 512 dip × 512 dip) were collected. After children with cervical injuries and malformations as well as obvious neurological symptoms and signs that were excluded, a total of 60 patients aged 4–12 were selected and divided into three groups at an interval of 3 years of age, namely, group for 4–7 (group A), group for 7–10 (group B), and group for 10–12 (group C), with 20 patients included in each group.

Measurement method: import the original DICOM format scanning data into Materialise Mimics Innovation Suite 16.0 software (Materialise Company, Belgium), select appropriate HU threshold value for 3D reconstruction, select and adjust corresponding central axis of atlantoaxial vertebra pedicle on the reconstruction model and three axial views, and mark their cross points with the cortex of the anterior edge and the cortex of posterior edge of the vertebral lamina (A, A′ and B, B′ respectively). Use a 3D measurement tool of the software to measure the pedicle width (PW) and pedicle height (PH) as well as the intervals of AB (POCL) and BB′ on the reconstruction of 3D model. Use cross section of the pedicle axis to measure E angle and use the sagittal plane of the pedicle axis to measure F angle. At last, observe the anatomic location of point B on the atlantoaxial vertebra to direct the insertion point.

Measurement content (Figs. 9.29, 9.30, 9.31, 9.32, 9.33, and 9.34):

1. Pedicle width (PW): PW of C_1 is the shortest distance between the exterior margins of the medial and lateral cortex of the groove for the vertebral artery; PW of C_2 is the shortest distance between the exterior margins of the medial and lateral cortex of the pedicle isthmus.
2. Pedicle height (PH): PH of C_1 is the shortest distance between exterior margins of the upper and lower cortex of the groove for the vertebral artery; PH of C_2 is the shortest distance between the exterior margins of the upper and lower cortex of the pedicle isthmus.
3. The entire length of the pedicle osseous channel (POCL): the shortest distance from the cortex of the posterior edge of the vertebral lamina to the cortex of anterior edge along the pedicle axis, namely, the distance between A and B.

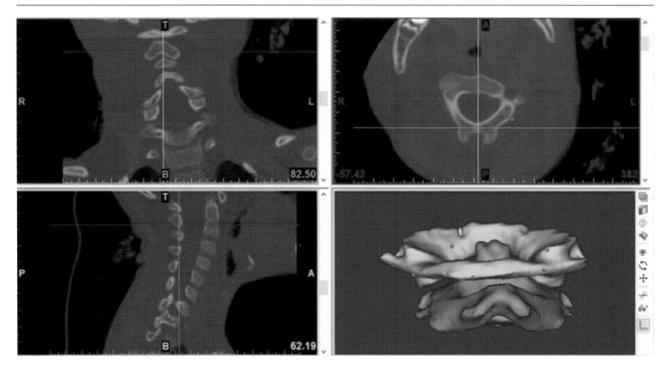

Fig. 9.29 Atlantoaxial reconstruction and definition of the pedicle axis

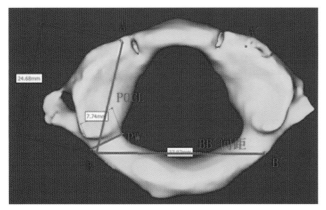

Fig. 9.30 Measurements of POCL, PW, and BB′ distances by using 3D measurement tools

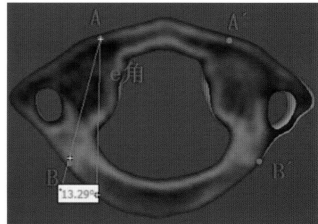

Fig. 9.32 Measurements of *E* angle on cross sections of atlas

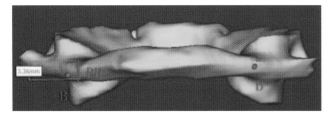

Fig. 9.31 Measurements of atlas PH by using 3D measurement tools

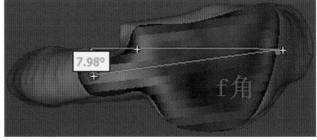

Fig. 9.33 *F* angle on cross sections of atlas pedicle axis

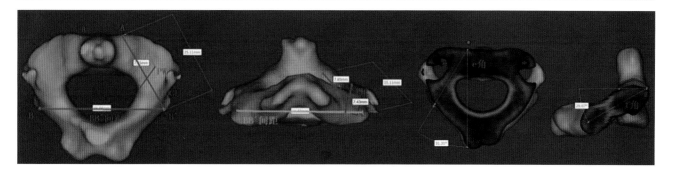

Fig. 9.34 Measurements of POCL, PW, PH, E angle, F angle, and BB′ distance of axis by using 3D measurement tools

Table 9.23 Measured results of PW, PH, I value, POCL, and BB′ distance of atlas in various age groups ($\bar{x} \pm s$, mm)

Group	PW	PH	I value	POCL	BB′ distance
Group A	6.10 ± 1.19	4.18 ± 0.74	1.46 ± 0.17	23.05 ± 2.67	35.04 ± 2.97
Group B	7.33 ± 0.73#	4.72 ± 0.78	1.58 ± 0.23	25.68 ± 1.93#	39.06 ± 2.70#
Group C	8.04 ± 0.99#	4.98 ± 0.67#	1.65 ± 0.34	26.51 ± 1.88#	42.41 ± 2.90#&

Note: #$P < 0.05$ vs. group A; &$P < 0.05$ vs. group B

Table 9.24 Measured results of PW, PH, I value, POCL, and BB′ distance of axis in various age groups ($\bar{x} \pm s$, mm)

Group	PW	PH	I value	POCL	BB′ distance
Group A	4.23 ± 0.63	5.15 ± 0.69	0.83 ± 0.14	25.27 ± 2.85	31.72 ± 2.76
Group B	4.62 ± 0.30	5.99 ± 0.44#	0.77 ± 0.07	26.57 ± 1.41#	35.25 ± 2.32#
Group C	5.95 ± 1.04#&	6.88 ± 0.92#&	0.86 ± 0.10	26.68 ± 1.98#	36.15 ± 2.71#

Note: #$P < 0.05$ vs. group A; &$p < 0.05$ vs. group B

Table 9.25 Measured results of E angle and F angle of atlantoaxial vertebra in various age groups ($\bar{x} \pm s$, degree)

| Groups | Atlas | | Axis | |
	E angle	F angle	E angle	F angle
Group A	10.80 ± 3.31	5.06 ± 3.12	29.92 ± 7.56	29.06 ± 4.69
Group B	12.16 ± 3.80	7.33 ± 4.48	31.29 ± 4.24	32.05 ± 2.75
Group C	12.15 ± 3.79	8.51 ± 2.67#	33.92 ± 5.43	31.64 ± 2.77

Note: #$p < 0.05$ vs. group A

4. E angle: the angle between the pedicle axis and the sagittal plane of the corresponding vertebra, namely, transverse screw angle.
5. F angle: the angle between the pedicle axis and the horizontal plane of the corresponding vertebra at the caudal side, namely, caudal screw angle.
6. BB′ distance is the distance between the screw insertion points of right and left sides of the atlantoaxial vertebra.

Statistical analysis: the data was imported into Excel and SPSS 13.0 for summarization, and statistical analysis and the data were presented as $\bar{x} \pm s$. Changes of the same indicator in different age groups were analyzed by multiple comparisons of sample means using one-way ANOVA. A comparison between any two means was performed by using SNK method. The significant level was that $\alpha = 0.05$; $P < 0.05$ indicated a statistically significant difference.

5.1.2   Results

Measurement Results of Parameter Related with Atlas in Different Age Groups (Tables 9.23 and 9.25)

In general, PW, PH, and POCL of atlas showed an increasing trend with age. PW of group A was statistically different from those of group B and group C ($P < 0.05$), while there was no significant difference in group B and group C ($P > 0.05$). PH of group A was statistically different from that of group C ($P < 0.05$). POCL of group A was statistically different from those of group B and group C ($P < 0.05$). F angles of group A were statistically different from those of group C ($P < 0.05$). E angles and I values had no statistical difference between the groups ($P > 0.05$), and I values in all age groups that were above 1.0. BB′ distances in three groups were not statistically different from each other ($P < 0.05$).

Measurement Results Of Parameter Related with Axis in Different Age Groups (Tables 9.24 and 9.25)

In general, PW, PH, and POCL of axis showed an increasing trend with age. PW of group C was statistically different from those of group A and B, while there was no statistical difference in group A and B. PH of group C was statistically different from that of group A and B ($P < 0.05$). POCL of group A was statistically different from that of group B and C ($P < 0.05$). E angles, F angles, and I values of all age groups were not statistically different from each other ($P > 0.05$). I values in all age groups were less than 1.0. BB′ distance of group A which was statistically different from those of group B and group C ($P < 0.05$), while there was no significant difference in group B and group C ($P > 0.05$).

Positioning of Pedicle Screw Insertion Point and Simulation of Screw Insertion in Various Age Groups

In adults, the anatomic relationship between inferior articular process of axis and axial pedicle is relatively constant; therefore, it can act as an anatomic maker for insertion of axial pedicle screw. In the experiments, the authors observed that children and adults were similar in these anatomic locations, suggesting that inferior articular process of axis could be used as a reference marker for pedicle screw insertion. It was observed that, in group A, the pedicle axis was mainly projected around the central point of the inferior articular process of the axis; in group B, the pedicle axis was mainly projected slightly above and medial to the central point of the inferior articular process of the axis; in group C, the pedicle axis was mainly projected around the cross point of the vertical line from the central point of the inferior articular process of the axis and the horizontal line from the point between the middle one-third and upper one-third of the inferior articular process of the axis.

Data of one patient was randomly selected from group A, B, and C and then imported into Mimics 16.0 software for 3D reconstruction; the Med CAD module of the software was used to construct a cylinder (parameter of radius was 1.75 mm) for simulation of pedicle screw insertion: in group A, the central point of the inferior articular process was selected as the screw insertion point and the screw insertion was performed with a transverse screw angle of 30° and downward angle of 29° (Fig. 9.35); in group B, screw insertion was performed at the point slightly above and medial to the central point of the inferior articular process with a transverse screw angle of 31° and downward angle of 30° (Fig. 9.36); in group C, screw insertion was performed at the cross point of the vertical line of the medial margin of the inferior articular process and the horizontal line from the point between the middle one-third and upper one-third of the inferior articular process with a transverse screw angle of 33° and downward angle of 32° (Fig. 9.37). The screw insertion points of three patients were visually observed, and the

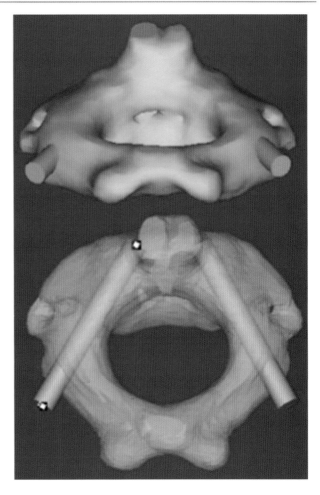

Fig. 9.35 Simulation of pedicle screws insertion in children axis for group A

results showed that screw insertion in each group was successfully performed in satisfactory points.

5.1.3 Discussions

This part will discuss the definition of children atlas pedicle and the insertion mode of pedicle screw. Atlas is a special cervical vertebra; its "pedicle" is not at the connection of the vertebral body and vertebral arch. Domestic and overseas scholars have proposed that the connection part of the massa lateralis atlantis and posterior arch is structurally and mechanically similar with the pedicle of the vertebral arch of other vertebras and thus being called "atlas pedicle." Atlas pedicle screw fixation is also called as atlas screw fixation via posterior arch and lateral mass, wherein the screw is fixed into the lateral mass of the atlas via the posterior arch of the atlas, the groove for vertebral artery, and isthmus of the posterior arch of the atlas. Of which, the groove for vertebral artery is the key part for screw insertion. In this study, related parameters of this "pedicle" were measured. Both width and height of atlas pedicle of child increase with age, but I value is always greater than 1.0, namely, width is

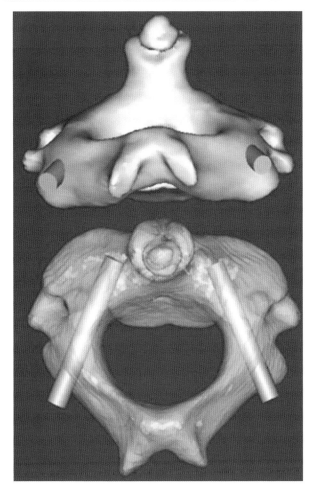

Fig. 9.36 Simulation of pedicle screws insertion in children axis for group B

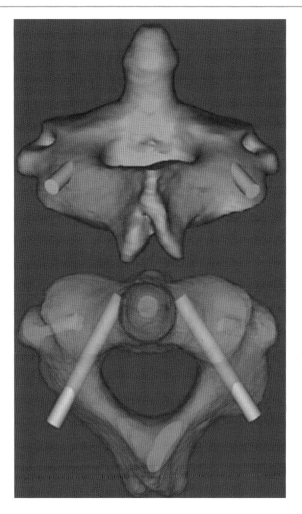

Fig. 9.37 Simulation of pedicle screws insertion in children axis for group C

higher than height; therefore, the screw diameter depends on the PH of the atlas. Ma Xiangyang et al. believed that when the atlas pedicle height was less than 4.0 mm, a screw with a diameter of 3.5 mm should not be recommended. In this study, the average PH of group A (4–7 years old) was 4.18 mm, and the atlas pedicles of children had soft and tough sclerotin and thick periosteum, thus enabling the insertion of pedicle screw with a diameter of 3.5 mm. Group A (4–7 years old) and group C (10–12 years old) were statistically different in PW, PH, POCL, BB′ distance, and F angle and therefore were different in screw insertion mode. In group A, the atlas pedicles were too thin, so the insertion points should be 16–19 mm lateral to the midpoint of the posterior tubercle and at the midpoint of upper and lower margins of the groove for vertebral artery, and the screw should be inserted almost horizontally with a caudal angle of about 10°; the screw length was 19.0 mm according to the standard of 80% POCL full length. The parameters of children in group C (10–12 years old) were closer to adults, so the insertion point should be about 20 mm lateral

to the midpoint of the posterior tubercle and 2 mm above the lower margin of the groove for the vertebral artery, and the screw should be inserted with a cephalad angle of about 9° and caudal angle of about 12°; the screw length was 21.0 mm. Due to the significant individual variations of children atlases and the vertebral artery arrangements on them, detailed 3D observations to the atlas pedicle should be performed in operation mode selection. Assessment of the screw insertion angle before screw insertion through 3D reconstruction is very important for the insertion accuracy and safety. If necessary, 3D models should be established by rapid prototyping to guide screw insertion.

The axis is also a special cervical vertebra. Bome et al. considered that the space between the "vertebral body–fascia dentata complex" and the superior articular process was the pedicle; Yarbroush et al. believed that the connection area between superior and inferior articular processes of the axis was the pedicle, namely, the isthmus. Axis pedicle screw was inserted into the pedicle via inferior articular process and isthmus and finally fixed to the vertebral body. The axis isthmus is the necessary and narrow channel for pedicle screw fixation. This study measured the parameters of this part and found that both PW and PH of axis in children increased with age; I values in all ages were less than 1.0, namely, PW values were lower than PH values. The insertion of pedicle screw depends primarily on PW. The experiment found that the average PWs in group A (4–7 years old) and group B (7–12 years old) were for 4.23 mm and 4.62 mm, respectively, indicating the feasibility of inserting screws with minimum diameters of 3.5 mm to axial pedicle of children above 4 years old. However, the external lower part of the axial pedicle was very close to the curved vertebral blood vessels, the axial pedicle screw should be inserted upward medially and carefully, and imaging examinations should also be performed to provide sufficient evidences for screw insertion. PW and PH values in group C were statistically and significantly different from those in group A and group B. Furthermore, POCL and BB′ distance in group C was statistically and significantly different from those in group A. Therefore, different insertion modes should be adopted in various age groups. Ma Xiang-Yang et al. found in adults that the anatomic relationship between the inferior articular process of axis and axial pedicle is relatively constant; therefore, it can act as an anatomic maker for the insertion of axial pedicle screw. Observation results of the present experiments revealed that this method was also suitable for children. The axial pedicles in group A (4–7 years old) were thin, and the screw channel was almost the axis of the vertebral pedicle, so the insertion point was near the midpoint of inferior articular process and about 16 mm lateral to the central line of axis. The axial pedicles in group B (7–12 years old) were thicker; the insertion point was about 1 mm medially above the central point of inferior articular process and about 17 mm lateral to the central line of axis. The axial pedicles in group C (10–12) were close to those of adults; the cross points of the vertical line of the medial margin and the horizontal line from the point between the middle one-third and upper one-third of inferior articular process, which were about 18 mm lateral to the central line of the axis, should be used as the insertion points. POCL in various age groups showed an increasing trend and had mean values of about 26 mm. Based on the clinical standard, the inserted screw length should reach 80% of the total length of screw channel, and the screw had sufficient fixation strength, so the axial pedicle screw should had a length of about 20 mm. E and F angles also showed an increasing trend in all age groups and, however, were not statistically and significantly different between those groups. These results indicated that E and F angles of axial pedicles in children above 4 years old had small variations with individual differences.

In summary, the spines of children aged between 4 and 12 years are in development, the vertebral pedicles are thin

with different segments varying in morphology, and their arrangements are complicated with important adjacent structures. Therefore, atlantoaxial pedicle screw insertion in children at different ages should be different. The operation should be performed with high accuracy, and the application of digital technology in 3D observations to atlantoaxial pedicles of children is necessary for accurate design of pedicle screw passages.

5.2 Digitalization Research on the Pedicle Screw Internal Fixation of Lower Cervical Vertebras (C_3–C_7) in Children

Recently, the pedicle screw internal fixation technology has been widely used in treatments of spinal injuries in adults due to its advantages such as stability and fastness. Domestic and overseas scholars have attempted to apply this technology in children and archived very satisfactory results, but the operations are mainly performed in thoracic and lumbar vertebras and upper cervical spines. Basic researches on morphological characteristics of lower cervical pedicles and pedicle screw internal fixation in children at different developmental ages have been rarely performed. This study investigated the feasibility of pedicle screw internal fixation in lower cervical spines of children through morphological observations with digital technologies, thus providing basic theoretical evidences for pedicle screw internal fixation in children.

5.2.1 Materials and Methods

Imaging data of cervical vertebras of children who underwent MSCT scan were collected. After children with cervical injuries and malformations as well as obvious neurological symptoms and signs were excluded, a total of 60 patients aged 4–12 were selected and divided into three groups at an interval of 3 years of age, namely, group for 4–7 (group A), group for 7–10 (group B), and group for 10–12 (group C); 20 patients were included in each group. Parameters of both pedicles of vertebral arch of each case were measured, and 40 groups of data were obtained.

Experimental method: use GE Light QX/I 64-slice spiral CT to scan from paropia to inlet of thorax (including the scope from skull base to T_1) with the scanning line horizontal to the central axis of the body. The scanning parameters: layer thickness and interval were both 1.25 mm, reconstructed layer thickness and intervals were both 0.625 mm, Fov was 30 cm × 30 cm, and the matrix was 512 dip × 512 dpi.

1. Measured parameters:
    (a) Pedicle width (PW): the shortest distance between the exterior margins of the medial and lateral cortex of the pedicle isthmus

(b) Pedicle width (PW): the shortest distance between the exterior margins of the upper and lower cortexes of the pedicle isthmus

(c) The entire length of the pedicle osseous channel (POCL): the shortest distance from the cortex of the posterior edge of the vertebral lamina to the cortex of the anterior edge along the pedicle axis.

(d) E angle: the angle between the pedicle axis and the sagittal plane of the corresponding vertebra, namely, transverse screw angle.

(e) F angle: the angle between the pedicle axis and the horizontal plane of the corresponding vertebra at the caudal side, namely, caudal screw angle. Directing of the pedicle axis to the upper end plate and lower end plate formed positive angle and negative angle, respectively.

2. Measurement method: import original DICOM format scanning data into database by using Mimics software, select appropriate HU for 3D reconstruction, select and adjust corresponding central axis of the cervical pedicle on the reconstruction model and three axial views, and mark their cross points with the cortex of the anterior edge and the cortex of the posterior edge of the vertebral lamina (A and B, respectively). Use 3D a measurement tool of the software to measure PW, PH, and AB distances (namely, POCL) on the reconstructed 3D model. Use the cross sections and sagittal planes of vertebral pedicles to measure E angle and F angle, respectively. Alternatively, import the model into 3-Matic software and project to the cross sections and sagittal planes of vertebral pedicles to measure E and F angles by using a measurement tool (Figs. 9.38, 9.39, 9.40, 9.41, and 9.42).

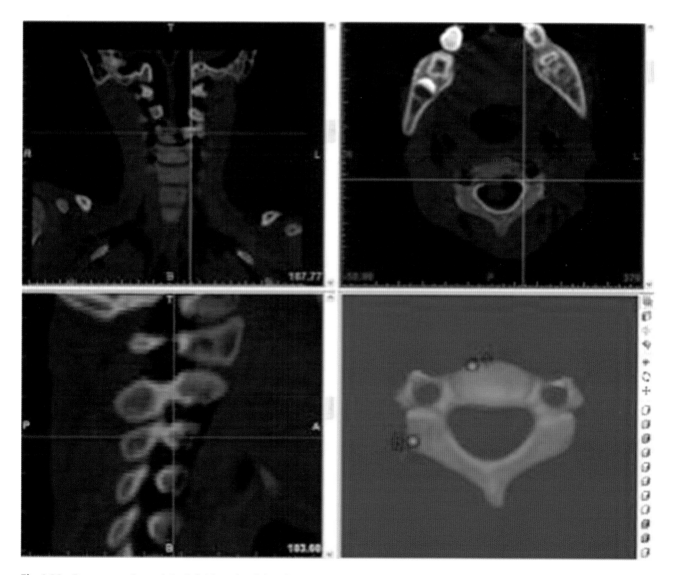

Fig. 9.38 C_3 reconstruction and the definition of pedicle axis

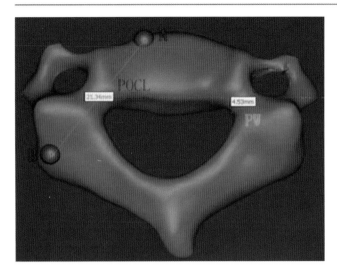

Fig. 9.39 Measurements of POCL and PW by using 3D measurement tools

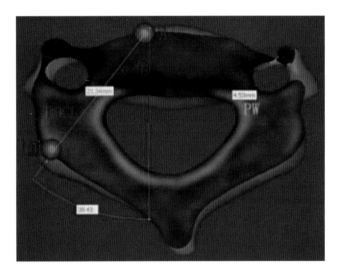

Fig. 9.40 Measurements of E angle on cross sections of vertebras

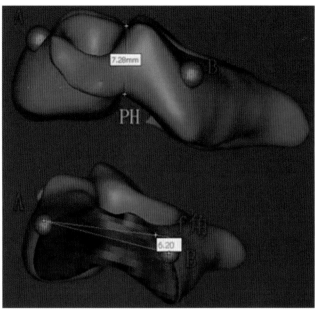

Fig. 9.41 3D measurements of PH and F angles on cross sections of pedicle axis

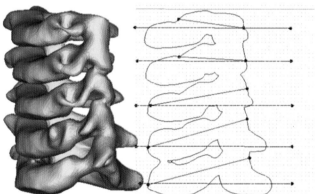

Fig. 9.42 C_3–C_7 were projected to pedicle axis pedicle planes to show the changes of F angles (C_3 and C_4 had positive angles, C_5–C_7 had negative angles)

Statistical method: the data was imported into Excel and SPSS 13.0 for summarization and statistical analysis, and the data was presented as $\bar{x} \pm s$. Changes of the same indicator in different age groups were analyzed by multiple comparisons of sample means using one-way ANOVA. Comparison between any two means was performed by using SNK method. The significant level was that $\alpha = 0.05$; $p < 0.05$ indicated a statistical and significant difference.

5.2.2 Results

Measurement Results of Pedicle Width (PW)

In general, PW showed an increasing trend with age. PW of group C was statistically different from those of group A and B ($P < 0.05$), while there was no statistical difference in group A and B ($P > 0.05$). PW in various groups increased with the vertebral sequences, and C_4 and C_7 were different in group A ($P < 0.05$); in group B, C_3 was different from C_5, C_6, and C_7, and C_4 was different from C_6 and C_7 ($P < 0.05$). C_3 and C_4 values in all groups were low (Table 9.26, Fig. 9.43).

Measurement Results of Pedicle Height (PH)

In general, PH showed an increasing trend with age. Group A and group B were statistically different in C_3, C_5, and C_6. ($P < 0.05$); all segments in group C were statistically different from those in group A and group B ($P > 0.05$). The segments within each group were not statistically different from each other (Table 9.27, Fig. 9.44).

Table 9.26 Measured values of PW in various age groups ($\bar{x} \pm s$, mm, range)

Vertebral sequences	Group A	Group B	Group C
C_3	4.06 ± 0.49 (3.24–4.65)	3.81 ± 0.51 (3.24–4.69)	4.68 ± 0.46 (4.25–5.67)$^{\#\&}$
C_4	3.75 ± 0.38 (3.01–4.35)	3.88 ± 0.44 (3.15–4.35)	4.36 ± 0.48 (3.73–5.26)$^{\#\&}$
C_5	3.92 ± 0.39 (3.21–4.34)	4.30 ± 0.47 (3.69–5.04)$^{\triangledown}$	4.89 ± 0.41 (3.96–5.40)$^{\#\&}$
C_6	4.16 ± 0.51 (3.40–5.26)	4.36 ± 0.51 (3.69–5.15)$^{\triangledown\blacktriangle}$	4.87 ± 0.46 (4.04–5.73)$^{\#\&}$
C_7	4.33 ± 0.49 (3.95–5.23)$^{\blacktriangle}$	4.37 ± 0.44 (3.59–5.12)$^{\triangledown\blacktriangle}$	5.08 ± 1.34 (4.36–6.02)$^{\blacktriangle\#\&}$

Note: $^{\triangledown}P < 0.05$ vs. C_3; $^{\blacktriangle}P < 0.05$ vs. C_4; $^{\#}P < 0.05$ vs. group A; $^{\&}P < 0.05$ vs. group B

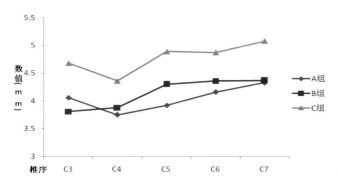

Fig. 9.43 Variation trend of average PW values in various age groups

Table 9.27 Measured values of PH in various age groups ($\bar{x} \pm s$, mm, range)

Vertebral sequences	Group A	Group B	Group C
C_3	3.53 ± 0.30 (3.12–3.96)	3.99 ± 0.26 (3.54–4.35)$^{\#}$	5.41 ± 0.50 (4.67–6.21)$^{\#\&}$
C_4	3.54 ± 0.25 (3.21–3.96)	3.73 ± 0.34 (3.27–4.32)	5.17 ± 0.53 (4.53–6.25)$^{\#\&}$
C_5	3.66 ± 0.31 (3.21–4.21)	4.02 ± 0.30 (3.56–4.57)$^{\#}$	5.41 ± 0.28 (5.06–5.80)$^{\#\&}$
C_6	3.74 ± 0.44 (3.21–4.58)	4.11 ± 0.41 (3.59–4.89)$^{\#}$	5.36 ± 0.36 (4.79–6.03)$^{\#\&}$
C_7	3.91 ± 0.44 (3.26–4.78)	4.13 ± 0.43 (3.48–4.75)	5.69 ± 0.26 (5.30–6.23)$^{\blacktriangle\#\&}$

Note: $^{\blacktriangle}P < 0.05$ vs. C_4; $^{\#}P < 0.05$ vs. Group A; $^{\&}P < 0.05$ vs. group B

Measurement Results of POCL

In general, POCL showed an increasing trend with age; various cervical vertebras had statistical and significant difference among three groups ($P > 0.05$). The segments within each group were not statistically different from each other (Table 9.28, Fig. 9.45).

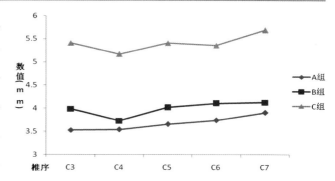

Fig. 9.44 Variation trend of average PH values in various age groups

Table 9.28 Measured values of POCL in various age groups ($\bar{x} \pm s$, mm, range)

Vertebral sequences	Group A	Group B	Group C
C_3	21.44 ± 2.78 (17.68–26.21)	25.54 ± 1.14 (23.99–27.29)$^{\#}$	27.45 ± 2.22 (24.95–31.39)$^{\#\&}$
C_4	21.89 ± 3.05 (17.43–24.56)	25.18 ± 1.23 (22.47–26.70)$^{\#}$	27.26 ± 2.45 (24.60–31.88)$^{\#\&}$
C_5	21.42 ± 1.93 (18.84–24.56)	26.46 ± 2.26 (23.64–30.26)$^{\#}$	27.76 ± 1.73 (25.46–31.05)$^{\#\&}$
C_6	22.22 ± 2.13 (19.03–24.23)	25.81 ± 1.38 (24.12–27.60)$^{\#}$	28.01 ± 2.06 (25.13–31.06)$^{\#\&}$
C_7	22.43 ± 1.87 (18.69–25.24)	25.71 ± 3.06 (22.56–31.59)$^{\#}$	28.13 ± 1.68 (26.66–31.65)$^{\#\&}$

Note: $^{\#}P < 0.05$ vs. group A; $^{\&}P < 0.05$ vs. group B

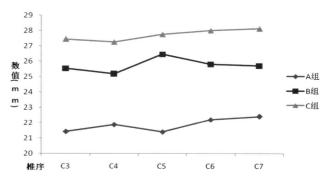

Fig. 9.45 Variation trend of average POCL values in various age groups

Measurement Results of *E* Angle

In general, *E* angle showed an increasing trend with age but had no significant difference between various age groups. C_3 and C_4 in group A were statistically different from those in group B and group C ($P < 0.05$); C_5 in group C was statistically different from those in group A and group B ($P < 0.05$). The segments within each group were not statistically different from each other (Table 9.29, Fig. 9.46).

Table 9.29 Measured values of E angle in various age groups ($\bar{x} \pm s$, mm, range)

Vertebral sequences	Group A	Group B	Group C
C_3	35.41 ± 3.25 (30.54–42.54)	40.24 ± 1.32 (37.56–42.30)$^{\#}$	41.20 ± 2.71 (36.76–44.19)$^{\#}$
C_4	35.88 ± 2.71 (33.15–41.87)	39.55 ± 3.01 (35.45–45.60)$^{\#}$	41.61 ± 2.42 (39.83–48.36)$^{\triangledown\#}$
C_5	36.77 ± 2.54 (33.77–40.35)	38.44 ± 2.33 (34.21–41.23)	41.16 ± 1.51 (39.56–44.47)$^{\#\&}$
C_6	37.92 ± 4.62 (34.26–45.51)	38.12 ± 3.34 (33.57–42.30)	39.39 ± 3.54 (32.44–44.96)
C_7	38.11 ± 4.38 (30.15–43.16)	41.17 ± 2.12 (39.47–46.20)$^{\diamond\blacklozenge}$	39.61 ± 3.37 (32.74–42.38)

Note: $^{\triangledown}P < 0.05$ vs. C_3; $^{\diamond}P < 0.05$ vs. C_5; $^{\blacklozenge}P < 0.05$ vs. C_6; $^{\#}P < 0.05$ vs. group A; $^{\&}P < 0.05$ vs. group B

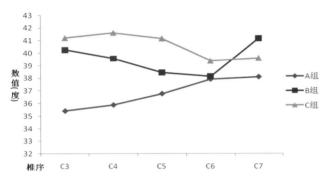

Fig. 9.46 Variation trend of E angles in various age groups

Table 9.30 Measured values of F angle in various age groups ($\bar{x} \pm s$, mm, range)

Vertebral sequences	Group A	Group B	Group C
C_3	7.28 ± 12.48 (−10.25–34.12)	4.76 ± 5.75 (−5.70–10.90)$^{\#}$	7.59 ± 3.42 (2.60–13.86)$^{\&}$
C_4	−8.93 ± 7.24 (−15.61–10.23)$^{\triangledown}$	−10.44 ± 3.63 (−15.60–3.90)$^{\triangledown}$	−9.08 ± 3.16 (−12.64–2.60)$^{\triangledown}$
C_5	−17.29 ± 3.71 (−25.12 to −10.89)$^{\triangledown\blacktriangle}$	−16.40 ± 2.63 (−19.27 to −10.60)$^{\triangledown\blacktriangle}$	−14.29 ± 3.08 (−21.34 to −10.23)$^{\triangledown\blacktriangle}$
C_6	−18.34 ± 4.61 (−25.35– 10.35)$^{\triangledown\blacktriangle}$	−18.76 ± 2.98 (−20.80 to −10.58)$^{\triangledown\blacktriangle}$	−19.39 ± 5.59 (−27.86 to −12.50)$^{\triangledown\blacktriangle}$
C_7	−20.73 ± 3.19 (−25.36 to −13.67)$^{\triangledown\blacktriangle}$	−20.79 ± 1.47 (−24.30 to −18.60)$^{\triangledown\blacktriangle}$	−22.45 ± 4.79 (−30.23 to −13.70)$^{\triangledown\blacktriangle}$

Note: $^{\triangledown}P < 0.05$ vs. C_3; $^{\blacktriangle}P < 0.05$ vs. C_4; $^{\diamond}P < 0.05$ vs. C_5; $^{\#}P < 0.05$ vs. group A; $^{\&}P < 0.05$ vs. group B

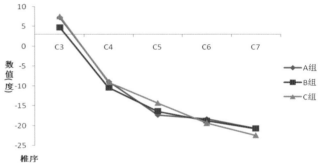

Fig. 9.47 Variation trend of F angles in various age groups

Measurement Results of F Angle

In general, F angle showed an increasing trend with age but had no significant difference between various age groups. Only C_3 in group B was statistically different from group A and group C ($P < 0.05$); C_5 in group A was statistically different from those in group C ($P < 0.05$). Various segments of cervical vertebras within each group were significantly different. F angle decreased gradually from C_3 (positive value) to C_7 (negative value), and F angle of C_7 had the most negative value (Table 9.30, Fig. 9.47).

PW/PH Ratio (I Value) of Different Age Groups

The ratio of cervical pedicle width to pedicle height is defined as I value (PW/PH). In general, I value showed an increasing trend with age. C_3 in group A was statistically different from those in group B and group C ($P < 0.05$); C_4–C_7 in group C was statistically different from those in group A and group B ($P < 0.05$); I values of C_3–C_7 in all age groups declined from the values above 1.0 to those lower than 1.0; I values of various segments within each group had no significant difference ($P < 0.05$) (Table 9.31, Figs. 9.48). In the experiments, C_3 of three children aged 4, 8, and 12 years old, respectively, were selected to observe their morphological

Table 9.31 Measured I values in various age groups ($\bar{x} \pm s$, mm, range)

Vertebral sequences	Group A	Group B	Group C
C_3	1.15 ± 0.11 (1.03–1.31)	0.95 ± 0.11 (0.81–1.14)$^{\#}$	0.87 ± 0.09 (0.68–1.14)$^{\#}$
C_4	1.09 ± 0.07 (1.01–1.22)	1.04 ± 0.12 (0.87–1.27)	0.85 ± 0.08 (0.70–0.99)$^{\#\&}$
C_5	1.13 ± 0.10 (1.01–1.30)	1.07 ± 0.65 (0.94–1.19)	0.91 ± 0.09 (0.68–0.99)$^{\#\&}$
C_6	1.12 ± 0.10 (1.03–1.28)	1.06 ± 0.07 (0.94–1.16)	0.91 ± 0.10 (0.78–1.10)$^{\#\&}$
C_7	1.11 ± 0.09 (1.01–1.30)	1.06 ± 0.04 (1.01–1.13)	0.89 ± 0.10 (0.70–1.06)

Note: $^{\#}P < 0.05$ vs. group A; $^{\&}P < 0.05$ vs. group B

characteristics through visualizing vertebral pedicle channel and projecting pedicle axis (Figs. 9.49, 9.50, and 9.51).

5.2.3 Discussions

This part will describe morphological characteristics and developmental patterns of children with lower cervical

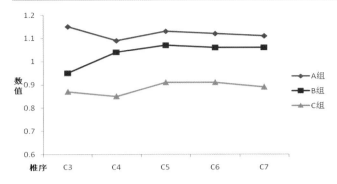

Fig. 9.48 Variation trend of average I values in various age groups

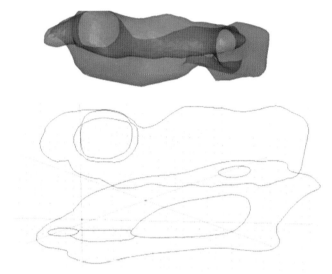

Fig. 9.49 Visualized observations of vertebral pedicles and projections of vertebral pedicle channels (transverse oval) in children aged 4

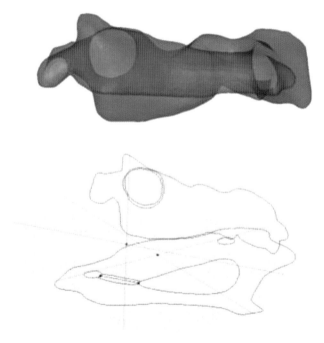

Fig. 9.50 Visualized observations of vertebral pedicles and projections of vertebral pedicle channels (suborbicular) in children aged 8

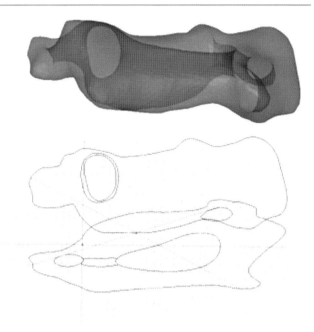

Fig. 9.51 Visualized observations of vertebral pedicles and projections of vertebral pedicle channels (longitudinal oval) in children aged 10

pedicles. In general, PW, PH, and POCL of lower cervical pedicles increase with vertebral sequence without a significant difference among different vertebral segments. They also show an increasing trend with age. PW, PH, and POCL of all vertebras in children aged 10–12 were statistically and significantly higher than those in children aged 4–7 years old and 7–10 years old, which might indicate that cervical vertebras of children aged 10–12 grew rapidly. PW and PH increased with age, but PH increased faster than PW. I value varied from the values above 1.0 to the values lower than 1.0, so PW values in children aged 4–7 were higher than PH, and their cross sections were horizontal oval or suborbicular. PW values in children aged 7–12 and aged 10–12 were lower than PH, and their cross sections were orbicular or longitudinal oval. Cross sections in elder children were closer to longitudinal oval (Figs. 9.49, 9.50, and 9.51). In general, POCL showed an increasing trend with age, and various cervical vertebras had statistical and significant difference between three groups, indicating that vertebras grew significantly with age. In general, E angle had an increasing trend with vertebral sequences without a significant difference between various vertebras. F angle varied significantly from positive angle to negative angle, and the degrees were increased, which might be related to the formation and anterior process of cervical curve in children of these ages.

This part will describe the feasibility of pedicle screw insertion in lower cervical vertebras in children. Successful pedicle screw insertion actually depends on correct determination of location, direction, and depth as well as selection of pedicle screws with appropriate diameters. The ratio of screw diameter to vertebral pedicle diameter determines their stability and safety. The holding force of pedicle screw is directly proportional to the diameter and length of inserted pedicle screw. In adults, it is generally believed that the radio between a screw diameter and pedicle diameter of 4/5 can achieve a stable internal fixation biomechanical effect. Too thick screw may break through the pedicle and injure surrounding important tissues due to increased bone fragility in adults. However, the cortical bones of children have high flexibility, so Polly et al. believed that pedicle screw diameter could be defined as 115% of transverse diameter of fixed pedicle due to its good elasticity. Rinella et al. inserted continuously various pedicle screws with gradually elevated diameters into vertebral pedicles of children aged 9, thus increasing the inner and outer transverse diameters of pedicle in children by 74% and 24%, respectively. Ideal screw diameter should be adaptable to corresponding pedicle. Furthermore, according to the characteristics of high flexibility and expansivity of pedicles of pediatric patients, slightly thicker screws should be used to maximize the resistance forces against extracting and twisting.

In group A (4–7 years old), all PW values were higher than PH values, so the pedicle screw diameters depended mainly on PH values. The average values of C_3–C_7 were 3.53–3.91 mm. Since the vertebral pedicles of children were ductile and elastic, screw insertion was feasible but had high risk and significant individual difference. Therefore, carefully and preoperatively designed insertion protocol and skilled operation technology were required. In group B (7–12 years old) and group C (10–12 years old), PW values were lower than PH values, so the diameters of inserted screws depended on the PW values with average values of 3.81–5.08 mm, wherein insertion of screws with diameters above 3.5 mm based on precise preoperative design and measurements was feasible. Fujimori et al. analyzed collected clinical data and found that pedicle screw insertion in infants and children was feasible, but the younger group (0–10 years old) had a higher incidence of complications than the older group (above 10 years old).

It is generally presumed that a pedicle screw with a length 80% of full length of pedicle channel can achieve sufficient fixation strength. C_3–C_7 POCL values of children were 25.54–28.13 mm averagely, indicating that screws with length of 20.4–22.5 mm should be used for lower cervical vertebras.

In this study, the E and F angles are measured as the intersection angles of pedicle axis with vertebral sagittal plane and horizontal plane, which do not represent the best insertion angles in clinical practices. Particularly, caudal angles of pedicle screws of the same vertebral pedicle vary significantly. Furthermore, cartilage end plates are present in upper and lower parts of cervical vertebras of children; ossification center is also present in vertebras of younger children. These important structures should be avoided in selection of insertion angle in clinical practice.

In summary, the lower cervical pedicle screw insertion in children aged between 4 and 12 years is morphologically feasible, but the spines of children are in development, the vertebral pedicles are thin and different segments vary in morphology, and their arrangements are complicated with important adjacent structures, indicating that the operation should be performed with high accuracy. Therefore, 3D observations to cervical pedicles of children are necessary for accurate design of pedicle screw channels.

5.3 A Comparative Study on the Accuracies of Freehand Cervical Pedicle Screw Insertion and the Operation Assisted by Individualized Navigation Template

Cervical vertebra injuries in children treated by conservative treatment without effects often require surgery. Recently, domestic and overseas scholars have tried to apply the pedicle screw fixation technology with good biomechanical characteristics in treating injuries of thoracic and lumbar spines in children and achieved very satisfactory effects. The cervical pedicles of vertebral arches of children are thin with large variability and complex correlation with adjacent tissues. Application of pedicle screw insertion based on adult data in children in the stage of growth and development has a high risk. Improvement of screw fixation accuracy and reduction of error rate become the key points for in-depth development of cervical pedicle internal in children. Pedicle screw internal fixation in children should lay more emphasis on individualization and digitalization and take advantage of digital orthopedics, thus improving the accuracy of screw insertion. In this study, an individualized navigation template was designed and prepared with reverse engineering software and rapid modeling technology and then applied to assist cervical pedicle screw insertion. A comparative study on the accuracies of freehand cervical pedicle screw insertion and the operation assisted by individualized navigation template was also carried out to reveal the feasibility and accuracy of cervical pedicle screw insertion assisted by individualized navigation template in children, thus providing experimental evidences for its clinical application.

5.3.1 Materials and Methods

Four child cadaver specimens (provided by the Anatomy Laboratory of Inner Mongolia Medical University) including two males and two females aged 6–9 with body length of 120.79 ± 2.70 cm were selected. All specimens were axially scanned with continuous CT (Light Speed 64, GE, USA) to exclude those specimens with cervical vertebras injuries, deformities, and tuberculosis affecting pedicle screw insertion. Four specimens were randomly and equally divided into two groups.

Experimental method:

1. Imaging data collection: MSCT scanning of those four child cadaver specimens was performed from paropia to inlet of thorax (including the scope from skull base to T_1); the scanning line was horizontal to the central axis of the body. The scanning parameters: layer thickness and interval were both 0.625 mm, reconstructed layer thickness and intervals were both 0.625 mm, Fov was 30 cm × 30 cm, and the matrix was 512 dip × 512 dpi.

2. Design and preparation of individualized navigation template of child cervical spine: MSCT image data in navigation template group were saved in DICOM format and imported into Materialise Mimics Innovation Suite 16.0 software (Materialise Company, Belgium), and then appropriate HU value was used for 3D reconstruction. The screw insertion point was defined on the 3D digital model. Atlas screw insertion point was defined according to the method by Lin et al. Axis screw insertion point was defined according to the method by Ma Xiang-Yang. Screw insertion points for C_3–C_7 cervical vertebras were marked according to the method by Wang Dong-Lai et al. Specifically, the CAD software was used to establish a cylindrical body to simulate a pedicle screw with defined diameter and length. The cylindrical body was adjusted to achieve the anastomosis of its axis to the marked points, thus looking for the best screw insertion channel for cervical pedicle screw (Fig. 9.52). Corresponding pedicle width, pedicle height, and screw channel length were measured, thus providing evidences for further selection of the diameter and length of inserted pedicle screw. The model was exported in STL format. The 3D reconstructed model was opened with 3-matic software, wherein anatomic forms of the posterior part and dorsum of spinous process base of each cervical vertebra were extracted to design a reverse template with anatomic forms which coincided

with above osseous tissues by using the software (Fig. 9.53). The optimal insertion guide posts of the screws were designed according to the axis of cylindrical bodies, and the inner diameters of the guide poles were defined according to the diameters of inserted screws. The guideposts were matched with previously designed template to form an individualized navigation template for single vertebra with guide poles of bilateral positioning. The template was fitted to the posterior part of the corresponding cervical vertebra on 3D reconstructed model of vertebra template, and then the model was turned in all directions to observe the fitting accuracy of positioning guide hole to corresponding pedicle; the real template was prepared by using stereolithography apparatus (SLA) through the SPS350B laser rapid prototyping machine (Fig. 9.54).

3. Specimen preparation and grouping: the four specimens were incised along the posterior skins of C_1–C_7 spinous processes, the posterior skins and soft tissues of cervical vertebral lamina and transverse process were cleared, and supraspinal and interspinal ligaments above the spinous process were excised to thoroughly expose the anatomic

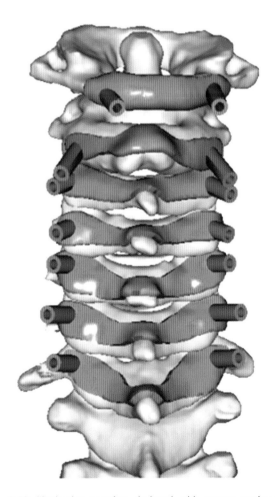

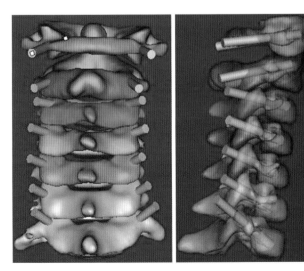

Fig. 9.52 Using CAD function of Mimics software to design an optimal screw insertion channel by simulating pedicle screw insertion

Fig. 9.53 Navigation template designed with reverse engineering software

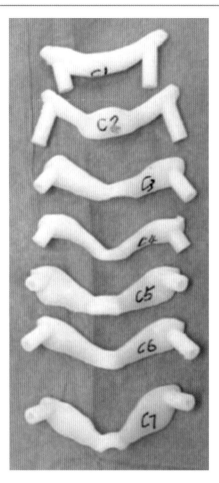

Fig. 9.54 Navigation template produced by rapid prototyping machine

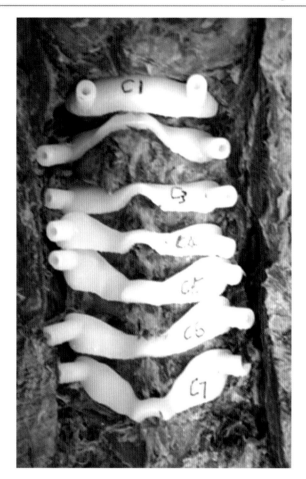

Fig. 9.55 Navigation template fitted well with cervical vertebra

structures such as the vertebral lamina, posterior part of transverse process, and dorsa of spinous process base.

4. Experimental operation methods: cervical pedicle screw insertion on the two groups of cadaver specimens was performed with navigation template method and freehand method, respectively, by the same senior experienced orthopedic chief physician. In navigation template group, the diameters and lengths of inserted screws were defined based on widths and lengths of the pedicle screw channels obtained in Materialise Mimics Innovation Suite 16.0 software. In freehand group, the diameters and lengths of inserted screws were defined, and the transverse angle (*E* angle) and caudal angle (*F* angle) were measured based on widths and lengths of the pedicle screw channels measured in preoperative CT scanning. It is generally presumed that the pedicle screw with a diameter 80% of corresponding PW and a length 80% of corresponding pedicle osseous channel length is proper. In the experiments, titanium alloy pedicle screws were used to facilitate postoperative CT evaluation; C-arm fluoroscopy and other auxiliary facilities were not used during the experiments.

5. Operation methods in navigation template group: navigation template was closely adhered to corresponding vertebral lamina of the cervical spine, posterior part of

transverse process, and spinous process (Fig. 9.55). Firstly, the fitness of navigation templates with corresponding osseous anatomic structures of the posterior part of vertebral bodies was observed, and the navigation templates were prepared from upper to lower for screw channels. The templates were held by the left hand of the operator to maintain their stabilities on the vertebral arches and spinous processes; insertion channels with lengths consistent with prepared screws were punctured along the directions defined by the guide holes at the insertion points defined on the navigation templates by the guide holes by using a drill with a bit diameter of 2.0 mm by the right hand. A spherical probe was used to ensure that the four walls were smooth and continuous sclerotins, and then screw threads were tapped by using taps with diameters 1 mm shorter than those of inserted screws. Once again, a spherical probe was used to ensure that the four walls were smooth and continuous sclerotins, and the screws with corresponding lengths and diameters were slowly screwed along the insertion channels into the vertebral pedicles (Fig. 9.56).

6. Operation methods in freehand group: screw insertion point of atlas was defined according to the methods by Lin Bin et al. Screw insertion point of the axis was defined accord-

ing to the methods by Ma Xiang-Yang et al. As for C_3–C_7 segments, the procedures were performed according to the methods by Wang Dong-Lai et al. Specifically, the surgery was started with C_1, and after the screw insertion point was defined, a rongeur was used to remove the cortical bone; the soft cancellous bone entrance of vertebral pedicle was explored based on previously measured E angle and F angle

with a cervical pedicle probe. At the beginning, the vertebral pedicle probe was inserted for a distance with the anterior curved part of facing outward, and then it was pulled out and inserted again with the anterior curved part of facing inward to a depth measured by preoperative 3D simulation measurements. After the four walls were identified as smooth and continuous sclerotins with a spherical probe, screw threads were made with a tap. Once again, the spherical probe was used to ensure that the four walls were smooth and continuous sclerotins. Any sense of penetration of indicating the penetration of cortical bone suggested reselection of screw channel. Finally, a Kirschner wire with a diameter of 2.0 mm was used to detect the screw channel depth, a screw with corresponding length, and the diameter was selected and screwed slowly into the pedicle.

7. Postoperative assessment method: postoperative MSCT scanning of the cervical segments of four child cadavers were performed (from paropia to inlet of thorax) with a thick layer of 0.625 mm, the CT image data were saved in DICOM format and then imported into Materialise Mimics Innovation Suite 16.0 software. The positions of screws within the vertebral pedicle and vertebral body from coronal view, horizontal view, and sagittal view were dynamically observed by another orthopedic chief physician. The vertebral pedicle broken by the screw should be further observed to determine whether the nerve root and spinal cord were affected.

Grading based on the extents of vertebral pedicle penetration by the screws: for the excellent screw, the screws did not penetrate the vertebral pedicle and were entirely in the vertebral pedicles; for the good screw, the screw threads slightly penetrated the cortex of the pedicle isthmus without damaging the adjacent important tissues; for the unqualified screw, the screws obviously penetrated the cortex of the pedicle isthmus and damaged adjacent tissues (Fig. 9.57). Both excellent and good screws were considered as successful insertion.

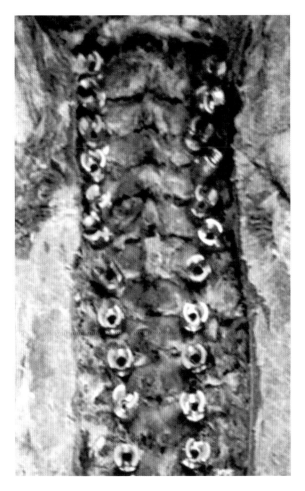

Fig. 9.56 Success screw insertion using navigation template

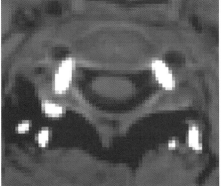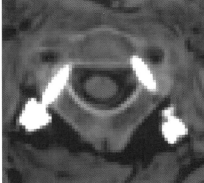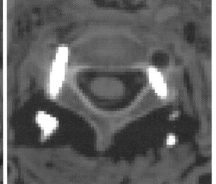

Fig. 9.57 Screws grading after operation: Grade I indicated excellent screws (both sides); grade II indicated good screw (slightly penetrating the internal wall of vertebral pedicle); grade III indicated unqualified screws (penetrating the lateral wall of vertebral pedicle)

Statistical method: the data were analyzed by using SPSS 13.0 software. Difference of screw insertion accuracies between two groups was analyzed by using chi-square test. The significant level was that $\alpha = 0.05$, $P < 0.05$ indicated a statistically significant difference.

5.3.2 Results

In group A, a total of 28 screws including 11 (39.3%) excellent, 10 (35.7%) good, and seven (25%) unqualified screws were inserted; in group B, a total of 28 screws including 19 (67.9%) excellent, six (21.4%) good, and three (10.7%) unqualified screws were inserted. Success rates of screw insertion were not significantly different between the two groups ($P > 0.05$); however, the proportion of excellent screws in group B was higher than that in group A with statistically significant difference ($P < 0.05$) (Figs. 9.57 and 9.58; Table 9.32).

5.3.3 Discussions

Pedicle screw insertion has been widely used in internal fixation of spinal disorders due to its good biomechanical properties. It is a posterior fixation method frequently used in clinical practices of cervical spine surgery, however, with a certain failure rate. With a novel digital navigation template recently proposed by Lu Sheng, Zhang Yuan-Zhi et al. have been used in internal fixation of adult spines and showed a good accuracy of screw placement, reflecting the principle of individualization in screw placement. Children are in a persistent stage of growth and development, their cervical vertebras are thinner and smaller than those of adults with complicated adjacent structures, and they have different morphological characteristics in various stages. Pedicle screw insertion in children is more complicated and dangerous than that in adults. Improvement of screw fixation accuracy and reduction of error rate become the key points for in-depth development of cervical pedicle internal in children. Therefore, adopting the concept of digital and individualized screw insertion in pedicle screw fixation in children is extremely important.

In the present experiment, 3D digital anatomic model of child cervical spine was reconstructed by using data of CT scanning. Based on this model, the optimal screw insertion channel of the vertebral pedicle was selected, and the pedicle screw insertion was simulated, thus visualizing the observations of the actual situations of the screw in the vertebral pedicle and improving the accuracy in design of screw channel. Furthermore, the reverse engineering software was used to extract the surface features of the vertebral lamina and spinous process to establish templates which is consistent with their anatomic forms, and the templates were fitted with the guide post of bilateral pedicle screw channels to establish guide templates. Finally, the templates were printed by laser rapid prototyping technology. In clinical practice, the templates should be well fitted with posterior bony structure of the cervical vertebras, and the screws should be inserted along the guide pole in the guide post, thus positioning and guiding the screw insertion for each pedicle. This approach is in compliance with the principles of individualization and accuracy for pedicle screw placement.

For 28 screws in the navigation template group, 25 screws were successfully inserted with a success rate of 89.3%, and 19 screws (67.9%) were excellent. Both success rate and excellent rate of pedicle screw placement were significantly higher than those in freehand group. Operations in both groups were carried out by the same orthopedic chief physician who operated cervical pedicle screws insertion for the first time. It was apparent that screw insertion assisted by application of navigation was less dependent on template and the surgical experience of the operators. The beginners can grasp the procedure of accurate screw insertion along the guide pole under the assistance of precisely designed navigation template. It can be seen that this method can achieve high accuracy and security in cervical pedicle screw placement in children with simpler surgical technology and shorter operative time.

Fig. 9.58 Distribution of screws of various grades in group A and group B

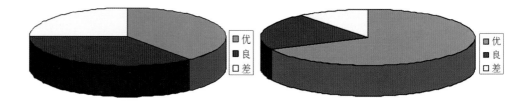

Table 9.32 A comparison of the success rates between freehand cervical pedicle screw insertion and the operation assisted by individualized navigation template, n (%)

Group	Excellent	Good	Unqualified	Total	Success rate	Excellent rate
Group A	11 (39.3)	10 (35.7)	7 (25.0)	28 (100)	21 (75.0)	11 (39.3)
Group B	19 (67.9)	6 (21.4)	3 (10.7)	28 (100)	25 (89.3)	19 (67.9)
P values					0.163	0.032

Application of individualized navigation template to assist cervical pedicle screw placement in children was a preliminary attempt. The child cervical pedicles are in the developmental stage, so they are thin and morphologically variable. Screw insertion angle has a narrow safety range, so precise design of navigation template is a key technology for successful screw insertion. Child's vertebra has a larger proportion of cartilage and relatively thicker periosteum. During the process of scanning, modeling, and template-producing, accuracy should be thoroughly promoted. An accuracy of about 1.0 mm for scanning and production should be adopted, if possible, to improve the fitness. Meanwhile, the material should be highly qualified, and soft material may lead to angle migration in drilling. In preparation of screw channel by using the navigation template, an abrasion drill or electric drill should be used, and the shaking should be minimized as far as possible to ensure that the screw is inserted exactly along the direction of guide pole as possible, thus achieving the guiding and navigating effects of designed template. When the navigation template is used during the operation, soft tissues on the posterior part of corresponding cervical vertebral lamina and spinous process base should be cleared, meanwhile avoid damaging to the bony anatomic structures of posterior part of the cervical vertebras, for fitting the template closely on the posterior part of the cervical vertebral lamina and spinous process. Base should be cleared, meanwhile damage to the bony anatomic structures of posterior part of the cervical vertebras, thus fitting the template closely on the posterior part of the cervical vertebral lamina and spinous process. Poor fitness may lead to migration of designed screw channel from actual pedicle and penetration of the screw. The operator in this experiment used this method for the first time and operation mistakes were inevitably. Surgeons with sufficient operation experience will significantly improve the success rate for insertion.

In summary, application of individualized navigation template in cervical pedicle screw placement in children is compliant with the principle of individualization screw placement. The operation is simple and easy to grasp; it can effectively reduce risk and improve the success rate.

References

1. Blondeel PN, Van Landuyt KII, Monstrcy SJ, ct al. Thc "Gcnt" consensus on perforator flap terminology: preliminary definitions[J]. Plast Reconstr Surg. 2003;112(5):1378–83. discussion 1384–1387.
2. Koshima I, Itoh S, Nanba Y, et al. Medial and lateral malleolar perforator flaps for repair of defects around the ankle[J]. Ann Plast Surg. 2003;51:579–83.
3. Masia J, Clavero JA, Larranaga JR. Multidetector-row computer tomography in the planning of abdominal perforator flap. J Plast Reconstr Aesthet Surg. 2006;59(6):594–9.
4. Phillips TJ, Stella DL, Rozen WM, et al. Abdominal wall CT angiography: a detailed account of a newly established preoperative imaging technique. Radiology. 2008;249(1):32–44.
5. Moro T, Kikuchi S, Konno S, Yaginuma H. An anatomic study of the lumbar plexus with respect to the retroperitoneal endoscopic surgery. Spine. 2003;28(5).423–8.

Finite Element Analysis in Orthopedic Biomechanics Research

10

Meichao Zhang, Zhang Hao, and Tan Tingsheng

1 Dimensional Finite Element Modeling in Orthopedics

Orthopedic dimensional finite element model is biomechanical model objects created for clinical orthopedics with finite element calculation and computer simulation technology combined, which is one of the important means of orthopedic biomechanics research. Orthopedic biomechanics is to solve problems encountered by orthopedic surgeons and use the principles and methods of mathematics, physics, and engineering in clinical orthopedics, forming a spine biomechanics, artificial joints and joint biomechanics, sports and rehabilitation medicine, and tissue engineering research.

Specimen test is a traditional orthopedic biomechanics research method, which builds different models of human bone and joint specimens for different clinical problems and simulates human activities by mechanical loading test machine or other device, and then observes and analyzes the structural stability of the model, material strength, and power conduction by means of 2D or 3D image sensors. Because of the inherent limitations and destructiveness of the experimental methods, specimen test is difficult to detect various biomechanical indicators and give multiple explanations on the multi-angle biomechanical mechanisms inside the specimen. Development of computational biomechanics timely

replenishes this deficiency, especially using finite element virtual simulation. After the establishment of effective finite element model, the biggest advantage of finite element simulation is that the model can reflect the internal stress/strain changes and analyze stress/strain conditions of structures with more complex shape, load, and mechanical properties and reflect ongoing changes in the study by repeating simulation model or changing some parameters of the mechanical conditions, which greatly reduce the cost of experiments and improve the comparability between the different parameters of the model groups. The finite element model simulation has currently been widely used in clinical applications and researched in orthopedic biomechanics, such as prosthetic implants, fracture assessment, soft tissue injury, and bone tissue reconstruction.

Orthopedic dimensional finite element model simulation cannot be done without entity model reconstruction of human bones, joints, orthopedic appliances, and artificial prosthesis. It needs to build the finite element model with structure, shape, and mechanical properties close to the actual human body and conduct for validation by reference to specimen experiments or conclusions recognized and accepted. For the researchers' point of view, establishing effective finite element model is the basis of simulation analysis and relates to the feasibility and reliability of calculation results of follow-up studies, accounting for 70–80% of the entire finite element process.

In general, finite element modeling of the basic process consists of four main steps: (1) getting the coordinates of the model structure of 2D or 3D space object, (2) 3D finite element model geometry reconstruction, (3) meshing the model and giving the material properties to determine the mechanical boundary conditions, and (4) preliminary analysis of the model and verification of its effectiveness. We make a brief introduction to the basic processes of finite element modeling in the following four aspects.

M. Zhang (✉)
Anatomy Department, School of Basic Medical Sciences, Southern Medical University, Guangzhou, China

Z. Hao
Department of Spinal Surgery, People's Hospital of LongHua District, Shenzhen City, Guangdong Province, China

T. Tingsheng
Guangdong Provincial Hospital of Integrated Traditional Chinese and Western Medicine, Foshan Shi, Guangdong Sheng, China

1.1 Obtaining the Spatial Structure Coordinates of Models

Objects of orthopedic biomechanics finite element simulation are human bones and joints, also related to the relevant prosthesis and other orthopedic devices. Establishing realistic appearance of models helps to improve the quality of finite element simulation analyses, and the main methods are as follows according to orthopedic history of finite element simulation analysis.

1.1.1 Solid Geometry Measurement

By general measure of human anatomy bone structure or orthopedic devices, we can get the approximate dimensions and geometric features of these structures. This method is easy, and finite element models are based on the method of this general measure or reference anatomical atlas in the early period, but for the objects with complex spatial structures, it can affect the fidelity of the model and the subsequent reconstruction of the mechanical reliability analysis.

1.1.2 Measurement of 3D Coordinate

Through the equipment such as 3D coordinate instruments or non-contact 3D laser scanning instruments, we can pick up the 3D coordinate information of surface position. In the method, we can do nondestructive measurement with high accuracy, but it is not suitable for the structures where contract instrument or laser cannot touch.

1.1.3 Medical Image Reconstruction

By spiral CT, magnetic resonance imaging (MRI) and other medical imaging equipment, we can scan the model object layer by layer. Or directly through cross-sectional image of the specimen, we can obtain a 2D cross-sectional image data. As long as the image-forming conditions permit, this method is not restricted to the complex structure of the model object, and the internal structure of the surface can be used with high precision. So it has become the main method of orthopedic finite element simulation modeling.

1.2 3D Reconstruction of the Finite Element Geometric Model

There are some common softwares such as AutoCAD, ProE, UG, and Solidworks for reconstruction of 3D finite element model. Such software used in engineering and industrial fields has a huge 3D modeling toolkit, and it is particularly effective for establishment of prosthetic orthopedic devices.

With the rapid development of medical imaging technology, a series of 3D medical image reconstruction software have appeared. They are compatible with medical imaging data and can quickly complete 3D model reconstruction such as 3D-Doctor, Maya, and Matlab, and later, with the promotion of the 3D reconstruction in the medical finite element simulation, the more professional software appeared such as Mimics and Simpleware software, and they directly dock with clinical CT or MRI data with merits such as convenient, small amount of data loss, and so on.

Conventional model-reconstruction is based on the basic point, lines, face, and body of geometry, and a 3D model is gradually established, which we call the forward modeling, correspondingly the inverse modeling, with which we directly access to 3D model of the structure. Reverse engineering software also plays an important role in the reconstruction of 3D finite element model.

1.3 The Finite Element Analysis Model Reconstruction

Construction of finite element analysis model consists of model meshing, giving the right material parameter, and determining the mechanical constraint and load boundary of the model for the calculation and analysis with the basis of the finite element model.

1.3.1 Finite Element Meshing

Finite element simulation modeling eventually needs to get the finite element mesh to create a numerical matrix equation. After obtaining 2D or 3D structural information of the object model, you can build finite element directly in preprocessing module of the finite element software to form the overall grid model. This method was first proposed by Kayak, although it is direct and simple and avoids the geometric modeling and the subsequent meshing process of finite element model. The information of the model coordinate has become increasingly large and complex with the development of finite element simulation technology. Instead of direct modeling method, indirect modeling method has been applied. Indirect modeling method is known as automatic mesh generation method; it needs to reestablish the 3D solid model of the object geometry and then mesh to establish finite element model, which is ideal for complex spatial structure. Finite element meshing is the key to create finite element simulation model and feasibility of appropriate quality and quantity of element related to the subsequent calculation of the simulation. Proper meshing can guarantee the convergence and stability of the model calculations, but also control the size and time of calculations. Meshing process is generally done in the finite element software. ANSYS, MSC Software, Abaqus, Adams, and other company's software products include these preprocessing functions currently. There is also specialized software, such as Hypermesh.

The feasibility meshing is directly related to the finite element model; when the narrow slit or other inappropriate geometry topology geometry appears, it will produce poor quality element or cannot mesh at all, and the poor elements will pose a threat to the convergence of calculation and analysis. Therefore, in the finite element modeling process, it needs to modify the mode due to difficulty in meshing, especially in the situation of completely adaptive meshing. In addition to providing a reasonable geometric model, the accuracy of grid is also guaranteed to the convergence of calculation. However, this approach would be a way to increase the number of finite elements and nodes, thereby increasing the time of the subsequent analysis calculated. Therefore, under the premise of convergence, we also need to pay attention to the number of elements and nodes to save computing time and computer resources.

In orthopedic finite element model, many body structures, such as ligaments, cartilage, and other end-plate structure are established based on the bone structure completed. For example, ligament structure is simulated by adding link unit or cable unit; articular cartilage or cortical bone is generated by adding shell element on the surface of bone structure; cortical bone or end plate is established by changing the material properties of elements and in joint model; and the nonlinear contact of different articular cartilage surface is achieved by defining reasonable contact elements.

1.3.2 Material Properties Assignment

Biomechanics materials of human tissue show the diversity. Cortical bone, cancellous bone, cartilage end plate, intervertebral disk fibers, nucleus, various ligaments, and other mechanical parameters of the material are very different. Even bone mineral densities in different parts of the same piece of bone are significantly different, this suggests that their mechanical properties are different and the results of mechanical testing in biological materials also prove this point. Osteoporosis is a typical example.

Besides, compared with conventional construction materials, the material properties of human tissue have the nonlinear characteristics, and the material of tissue tested in the human motor system expresses the nonlinear properties of plastic, viscoelastic, and super elasticity, in addition to the classic elastic properties.

Therefore, not only is the selection of appropriate materials important in establishing the finite element model, but it also ensures the authenticity and reliability of analytical results in finite element model.

1.3.3 Constraints and Load Boundary Conditions

Proper boundary conditions and loading constraints are also the elements which guarantee finite element analysis. Bones, joint bearing, and muscle movement are inseparable from the surrounding tissue and other related support and cooperation, and we cannot establish a complete finite element structural model because of the complexity of modeling. Orthopedic finite element model established is often the skeleton joint model of the partial human body. In this case, the mechanical effect of defects in the structure of the model needs to be loaded by mechanical constraints and boundary conditions to truly reflect the role of bones and muscles in the finite element analysis model. Simulating the strength of changes in muscle

and body mass is the key of the success of the finite element analysis, especially in the dynamic analysis.

1.3.4 Preliminary Analysis of the Model and Validation

As for a final step necessary for finite element modeling, validity of the model is to summarize and validate the previous three steps which can reflect the degree of the simulation model. Only by establishing an effective finite element model can the results of computer simulation experiment in the follow-up study have the reliability and credibility.

Under normal circumstances, the result of specimen test is the gold standard in orthopedic biomechanics experimental studies. The effectiveness of the finite element model is to verify by comparing the experimental results of specimen test such as the classic results of biomechanics experiments. Specimen test is fit for obtaining macroscopic mechanical indicators of models; therefore, the common mechanical indicators include the results of 3D activity, structural rigidity, mechanical strength, and three- or four-point bending test model. Of course, comparison with simulation data of finite element model reported in the literature is also one of the important means of validation, which has gradually been adopted with the increase in the development of finite element techniques and related literature.

By comparison with the experimental specimens in the macrobiomechanical experiment indicators, the apparent validity of the finite element model has been verified, and the subsequent microscopic biomechanical findings of model are authentic in the absence of continued contrast. Therefore, finite element simulation experiment is a good supplement and sublimation of conventional experimental method and can observe and measure indicators which cannot be obtained by traditional biomechanical test. The wider range and angle of contrast, the more apparent the validation is and the more reliable the conclusion of simulation research is.

In recent years, with the rise and growth of digital medicine, digital orthopedic technologies are evolving; 3D finite element model is also increasingly becoming an important research tool in digital orthopedic and finite element modeling, and simulation in orthopedic will develop with the clinical research and software development.

2 Finite Element Modeling and Examples (1–22)

2.1 Example 1: Influence from Different Assigned Gradients of Material Attributes on Mechanical Properties of the Vertebral Finite Element Model

2.1.1 Purpose

It is to study the effects of gray scale in different material properties on the mechanical properties of vertebral finite element model.

2.1.2   Methods

Establishment of Finite Element Model

We collected the CT data of a normal male volunteer (T12–L5), which was scanned by a computerized tomography scanner with 0.5 mm intervals, and the image data were stored in DICOM format.

The CT data were imported into the Mimics 10.0, and 3D outline of images was extracted by regional growth and cavity filling, and the characteristics of the vertebrae were simulated and saved in stl. format.

The files were imported into the reverse engineering software Geomagic Studio11 where better 3D model was generated by relaxing and smoothing the grids, and then it was imported into Mimics in stl. format where better surface mesh model was produced by using remesh tool (Fig. 10.1a). Then it was imported into finite element analysis software ANSYS in lis. format to generate body meshing by FVMESH method (Fig. 10.1b). The images of prep7 nodes and elements were stored for backup.

The files were imported into Mimics, and the material properties were assigned by CT gray value. The models were separated into 2, 4, 8, 10, 50, 100, 200, and 400 gradients to assign the material attribute, and the assignment formula was from the empirical formula provided by Mimics:

$$Density = 47 + 1.122 \times Gray\ value$$

$$E - Modulus = -172 + 1.92 \times Density$$

$$Poisson's\ ratio = 0.3$$

Finally, the finite element model of the vertebrae after assignment was imported into ANSYS for analysis in lis., node, and element format.

Finite Element Analysis

Each vertebrae of different segments was loaded, respectively, and the specific loading conditions were as follows: (1) 600N compression load was applied on the surface of each vertebral body in the vertical downward direction and (2) each vertebral surface was fixed with degree of freedom zero. The main outcome measures were as follows: we select four paths in each section of the vertebral—Path 1 was the line with the midpoint of up/down vertebrae; Path 2 was along the central horizontal peripheral vertebral; Path 3 was the line with the midpoint of anteroposterior vertebrae; and

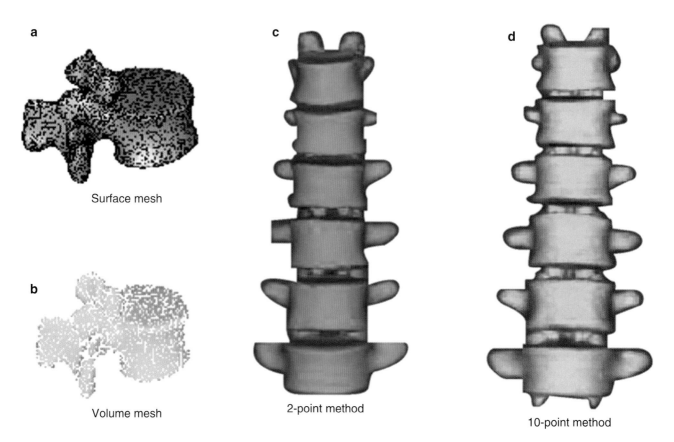

a

Surface mesh

b

Volume mesh

c

2-point method

d

10-point method

Fig. 10.1 FE Model

Path 4 was the left and right sides of the vertebral central surface. Finally, we solved and compared the stress conditions under the 2, 4, 8, 10, 50, 100, 200, and 400 kinds of material properties on the four paths.

2.1.3 Results

Corresponding von Mises stress with four paths of six vertebral was analyzed in the distribution of different material properties. Stress conditions of eight kinds of material properties were compared under the same path (Fig. 10.11). Von Mises stress values were measured by analysis of variance using SPSS software. It was shown that the von Mises stress from 2 copies, 4 copies, and 400 copies was significantly different from the datasets of other number of copies, while 8, 10, 50, 100, and 200 copies had little deviation.

2.1.4 Conclusion

Finite element model of the material properties should not be too much or too little. Gradient of about ten parts can not only guarantee the accuracy of the calculation but increase the speed relatively which is especially suitable for clinical personalized finite element modeling.

2.2 Example 2: Establishment of the 3D Finite Element Model of the Human Thorax

2.2.1 Purpose

It is to provide the biomechanical simulation foundation of clinical effect and mechanism of human chest compressions by establishing 3D finite element model of the human thorax.

2.2.2 Methods

Test Object

One healthy volunteer (male) was scanned by a computerized tomography scanner ranging from T1 to T12 segment.

Reconstruction

CT images were stored in DICOM format and imported into Mimics 10.1, where 3D models of bony thorax that contained the spine, sternum, and ribs were established. Then the surface-meshed model was produced in finite element analysis software. By corresponding interface, the volume-meshed model was performed and imported into the Mimics 10.1 where 3D thoracic models were assigned material properties for each unit. A variety of materials and organizations of the model was considered as isotropic linear elastic material in this study. The thorax was divided into six kinds of

Table 10.1 Material parameters and FE mesh of thorax

Material property	Modulus of elasticity (Pa)	Poisson's ratio	Number of element (pcs)	Number of nodes (pcs)
Cortical bone 1	1.0×10^{10}	0.30	500	2595
Cortical bone 2	8.0×10^{9}	0.30	10,687	39,804
Cancellous bone 1	1.0×10^{9}	0.25	61,174	177,333
Cancellous bone 2	2.0×10^{8}	0.25	130,687	305,253
Cartilago costalis 1	5.0×10^{7}	0.30	63,193	161,288
Cartilago costalis 2 (including nucleus pulposus)	2.5×10^{7}	0.30	3474	12,222

material properties according to the CT from the bone cortex to the nucleus (Table 10.1). Then a complete finite element mesh model of the human thorax was established.

2.2.3 Results

We obtained a precise human thorax spiral CT tomography and image data and reconstructed 3D model of the human thorax by using Mimics 10.1 software. 3D finite element model of the human thorax contained 1,158,085 nodes and 736,022 elements, which were intuitive and impressive including clavicle, ribs, spine, and other structures (Fig. 10.12).

2.2.4 Conclusion

3D finite element model of the human thorax has high authenticity and accuracy built by high authenticity and accuracy, which can meet the needs of biomechanical analysis of the human thorax and provide the basis for further analysis of finite element model of the human thorax.

2.3 Example 3: The Impact of Different Length Distal Locking Screw on the Unstable Distal Radial Fracture Fixation Systems

2.3.1 Purpose

It is to compare the postoperative stability of unstable distal radius fractures fixed by distal locking screws with different length, analyze the stress distribution of internal fixation systems and callus at different healing periods, and investigate the effect of distal locking screws with different length on stability of the whole internal fixation systems and fracture healing after operation.

2.3.2   Methods

Acquisition of Original CT Data
The forearm of a 25-year-old healthy male volunteer was scanned by a computerized tomography scanner with 0.5 mm intervals, and the CT data was stored in DICOM format.

Reconstruction of Unstable Distal Radius Fracture Model
Reconstruction of 3D geometric model of ulna and radius was as follows: The CT data (DICOM format) was imported into Mimics 14.11 software. First, we set the proper gray threshold, and then graphics division, regional growth, and cavity filling were performed to build a 3D model of the radial ulnar bone, and they were stored in stl. format, and the saved file was imported into reverse engineering software

Geomagic Studio 2012 to denoise and smooth, cut triangular facets, graphic scaling processing, and fit the NURBS surface to establish 3D geometric models of radius and ulna which contain cortical and cancellous bone (Fig. 10.2b).

Reconstruction of 3D geometric model of distal radius fracture was as follows: (1) We established oblique T-shaped plates and screws with different lengths by plane sketching, drawing, and rotation characteristics in 3D drawing software ProE5.0 (Fig. 10.3), and they were stored as iges format files. (2) The 3D model of the radius and ulna containing cortical and cancellous bone and volar locking fixation system was imported into ANSYS workbench14.0 where a 3D model that contains cortical and cancellous bone and fracture section was established in DM module (DesignModeler) by face fusion and Boolean operation (Fig. 10.4). (3) We simulated the membrane and distal radioulnar ligament in DS module (Design Simulation) with link10 element. (4) We made the following assumptions without affecting the final conclusions: Cortical bone, cancellous bone screws, and plates

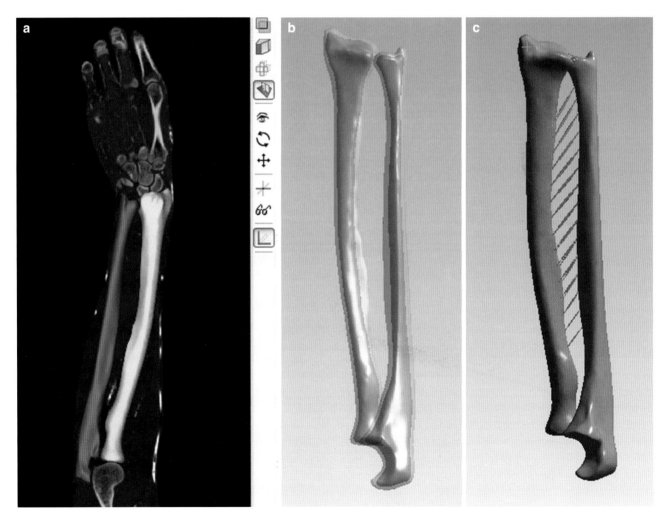

Fig. 10.2 3D geometric models of radius and ulna: (**a**) initial model established in Mimics; (**b**) model with cortical and cancellous bones; (**c**) model with the interosseous membrane and distal radioulnar ligament

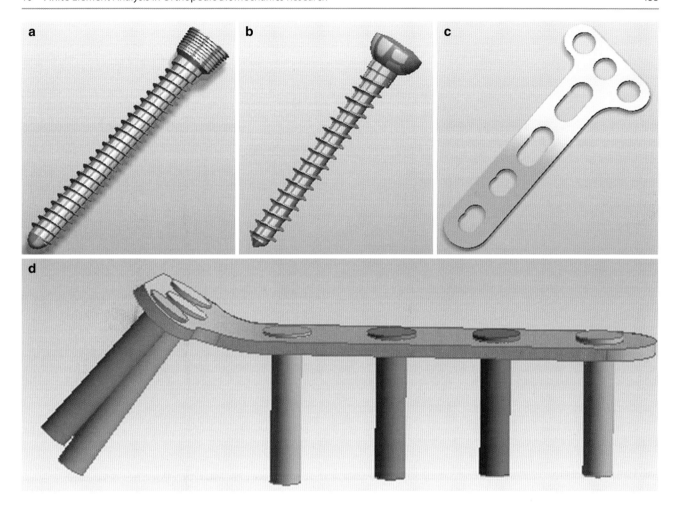

Fig. 10.3 The geometric model of internal fixator: (**a**–**c**) screws and T-shaped plate established in ProE; (**d**) internal fixation system simplified

were assumed to be homogeneous, isotropic linear elastic materials. Material properties of titanium plate and screw were from the library in ANSYS workbench, and bones and callus from different healing period were from literatures (Table 10.2). The tetrahedron method (Patching Conforming) was used to mesh for cortical bone, cancellous bone screws, and plates, which retained intermediate nodes and adjusted the parameters of overall grids.

Establishment of the Boundary Loading Conditions

The proximal radial head and olecranon were fully constrained, while the distal radius were applied 50–250N axial compression load with 1NM torque, and the distal radius volar or dorsal pressure exerted 0–50N vertical loads.

Finite Element Analysis

The maximum displacement of the fracture cross section, clinical failure load to 2 mm displacement of fracture section and stress distributions of callus from different healing periods were analyzed under physiological load conditions using ANSYS 14.0 general finite element software, and the aver-age stiffness values under different fixation of the fracture were calculated according to load displacement curve. Statistical analyses were performed in professional software SPSS20.0.

2.3.3   Results

Stress concentration appeared on the plating fixation system, and the stress value near the distal radius fracture line was also higher. With the screw length increasing, the maximum stress of callus was decreased gradually during the period of early healing, while the maximum stress of distal screws was increasing gradually with the increase of screw length at middle and last period of fracture healing, and the stress of distal bicortical screw was the largest. As with axial compression stiffness, there was no statistically significant difference between 75% length unicortical and bicortical fixation group ($p > 0.05$), while the stiffness of 50% length unicortical fixation decreased significantly and differences were statistically significant with 75% length unicortical and bicortical fixation group ($p < 0.01$). As for volar, dorsal, and torsional rigidity, differences between

Fig. 10.4 The fixation of unstable distal radius fracture: (**a**, **b**) unstable fracture model with fracture section and callus; (**c**) meshing of the whole internal fixation system

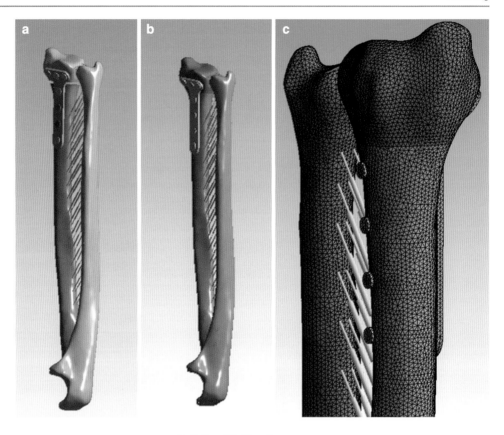

Table 10.2 Material properties of 3D models

Types of material	Modulus of elasticity/Mpa	Poisson's ratio
Cortical bone	13,800	0.3
Cancellous bone	690	0.3
Early callus	0.2	0.167
Later callus	1000	0.3
Plate and screw	96,000	0.36
Membrane	135.29	0.3

three kinds of fixation group were no statistical significance ($p > 0.05$).

2.3.4 Conclusion

The internal fixation system plays an important role in shelter effect, and the unicortical distal locking screws with at least 75% length can not only sustain the stability of the whole fixation system to avoid extensor tendon injuries due to dorsal screw prominence but also make for early postoperative fracture healing.

2.4 Example 4: Finite Element Analysis of Anterior Cervical Butterfly Plate

2.4.1 Purpose

It is to analyze the stress and strain distributions of anterior cervical plate and predict the breakable parts after fatigue test.

2.4.2 Methods

Finite Element Model of Anterior Cervical Plate
The actual geometry of the anterior plate can be seen in Fig. 10.5. We used the powerful preprocessor of the finite element software ANSYS 5.3 to create a finite element model which can be seen in Fig. 10.6.

We added four bases near the nail holes in order to perform the loading condition, and the base was hexahedral which was suitable for adding different load or torque in different directions, and the plate modified was shown in Fig. 10.6 (Table 10.3).

Meshing of Finite Element Model
We used automatic meshing capabilities with solid 92, and the material properties were assigned as follows: modulus of elasticity $E = 1.13e10$ N/m^2; Poisson's ratio = 0.15, and this model was divided into a total of 16,026 units (Fig. 10.7).

Constraints, Loading, and Solving
After meshing, we simulated the loading conditions of fatigue test (Fig. 10.8). In ANSYS solver, we performed constraints, loading, and solving to analyze stress and strain variations under the loading conditions.

Postprocessor of the Solving Results
In Fig. 10.9, the different colors represent different values of stress and strain. Right in the figure shows a scaling

Fig. 10.5 The actual geometric dimension of anterior cervical plate

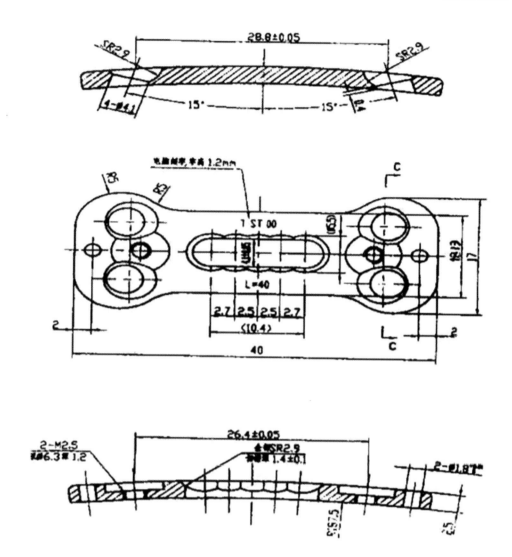

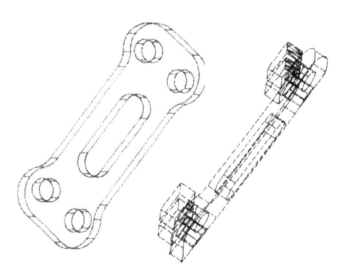

Fig. 10.6 Finite element solid model

value, and with this value, we can probably understand the value of the size. The stress and strain values at the center of the plate edges and four corners of the plate were larger than the surrounding areas from the two figures. These were the places where strain and stress concentration appeared (Fig. 10.10).

Fatigue Testing of Plate

Fatigue testing of MAPI was performed in materials testing machine named MTS-858 (MTS Systems Corporation, Minneapolis, MN). The plate is fixed to the upper and lower ends in polymethyl methacrylate block, making up a model similar to the removal of vertebral. This model was upright on MTS-858 material testing machine and the loading conditions were compression load of 100N and frequency of 1 Hz, the times of fatigue test was 1,000,000 with load ratio of 10. We recorded the parameters once every 2000 cycles including the changes of amplitude and load. The test is stopped

Table 10.3 Validation of the finite element model of the upper cervical spine

	Panjabi et al. [32]		Normal model		Unstable model	
	C_0–C_1	C_1–C_2	C_0–C_1	C_1–C_2	C_0–C_1	C_1–C_2
Moment (Nm)	1.5		1.5		1.5	
Flexion	3.5 ± 0.6	11.5 ± 2.0	3.1	11.7	6.7	14.2
Extension	21.9 ± 1.9	10.9 ± 1.1	20.5	9.5	21.2	12.7
Later bending	5.6 ± 0.7	4.0 ± 0.8	5.1	4.1	6.1	6.2
Axial rotation	7.9 ± 0.6	38.3 ± 1.7	7.6	38.7	9.5	45.1

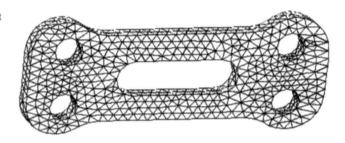

Fig. 10.7 Meshing of finite element meshing solid model

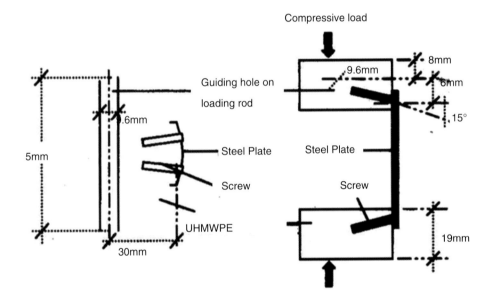

Fig. 10.8 Schematic diagram of fatigue test

when plate or a screw breaks and record the times of loading and place of breakage. If there is no break after the completion of the fatigue test, loose of plates and screws will be observed (Fig. 10.13).

2.4.3 Results

Two cracks appeared in the outer steel plates near the three nail holes after fatigue test, and the fracture plane was in nail holes. Junction with plate and screws was loosening, and there was no fracture and crack on screws. The results of finite element analysis: stress distribution area was larger around the nail holes which were through the outer diameter of the plate. This result was consistent with the fatigue test, which means that the construction of finite element model is reliable; meanwhile, greater stress distribution can be seen at both ends of the nails. In addition, stress and strain concentration can be firstly seen at outer edge of the plate through a phased simulation of the loading process, and then this area gradually extended to the nail holes' edge with the load increasing. Stress and strain concentration can always be seen at outer edge of the plate in the whole process.

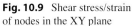 **Fig. 10.9** Shear stress/strain of nodes in the XY plane

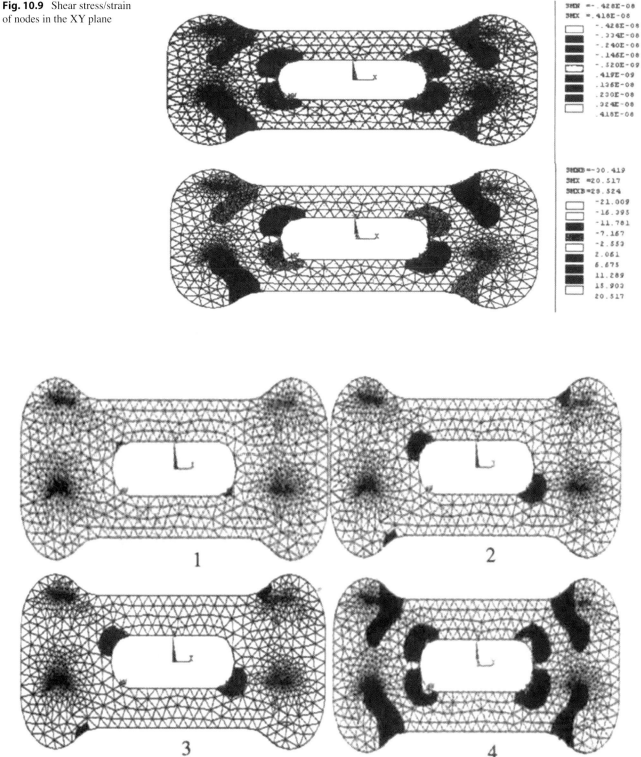

Fig. 10.10 Stress and strain nephogram in the direction of shear stages

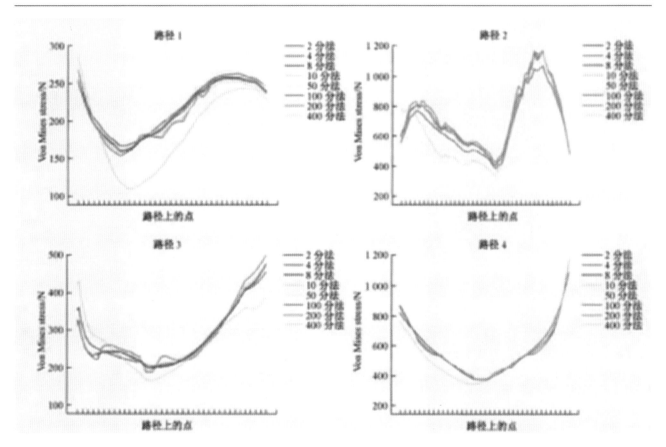

Fig. 10.11 Comparison of von Mises stress with different material properties division method on the four paths of same vertebral. 路径1 Path 1, 路径2 Path 2, 路径3 Path 3, 路径4 Path 4, 路径上的点 Points on path,

2分法 2-point method, 4分法 4-point method, 8分法 8-point method, 10分法 10-point method, 50分法 50-point method, 100分法 100-point method, 200分法 200-point method, 400分法 400-point method

Fig. 10.12 Finite element meshing model of human thorax

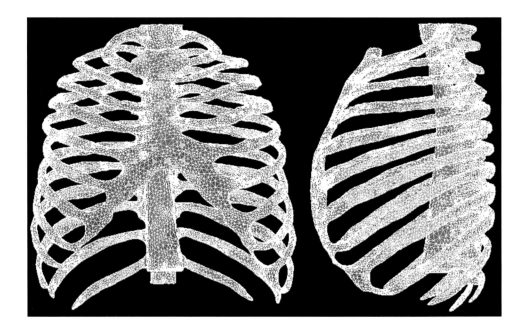

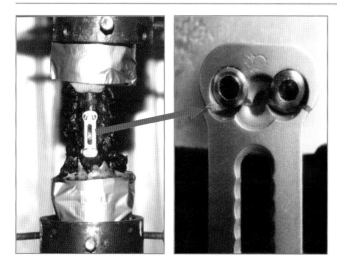

Fig. 10.13 The peak displacement of two implants

2.4.4   Conclusion

The results of fatigue test and finite element analysis are consistent, and the stress concentration appears near the nail holes of the plate where it is the weakest place of plates and prone to breakage.

2.5   Example 5: 3D Finite Element Analysis of Anterior Atlantoaxial Transarticular Locking Plate System

2.5.1   Purpose

It is to analyze the mechanical stability of a new anterior atlantoaxial locking plate system, so as to provide theoretical basis of biomechanics for the internal fixation of the cervical spine in clinic.

2.5.2   Methods

Design of Anterior Atlantoaxial Transarticular Locking Plate System

The anterior atlantoaxial transarticular locking plate system includes a titanium plate, several screws, an atlantoaxial reduction device, and other supporting surgical instruments. The plate is 2 mm in thickness and composed of medical titanium alloy. There are two oval-shaped locking screw fixation holes in the upper part of the plate used for inserting screws through the atlantoaxial joint. In addition, there are two round locking screw fixation holes in the lower part of the plate used for inserting screws into the axis body. A round hole is located at the center of the plate for reduction.

Finite Element Model of the Upper Cervical Spine

A 21-year-old healthy male volunteer, 171 cm tall and weighing 61 kg, was selected as our cervical spine model

after open mouth and lateral cervical spine X-rays excluded any congenital cervical spinal malformation or lesions. Spiral CT scanning was performed from the base of the occipital bone to C3 vertebrae using 1 mm thick slices, and the scanning data were collected and stored in DICOM format for the reconstruction of 3D bone structure using Mimics 13.0 software (Materialise, Leuven, Belgium). The geometric model was imported into Freeform Plus software (Geomagic Sensable group, Wilmington, MA, USA) for sanding, filling, and denoising to form a geometric solid model which approximated a normal human cervical spine.

The geometric solid model was imported into ANSYS 10.0 software (ANSYS, Inc. Canonsburg, PA, USA) for meshing and ligament loading according to start and end points of ligaments and cross-sectional area. This model consisted of 55,371 elements and 86,050 nodes. The model data are summarized in Table 10.4. Bone structures (including facet) and transverse ligaments were simulated using the eight-node tetrahedral elements. Other ligamentous structures were simulated using a two-node cable element. At the articular surface of the lateral atlantoaxial joint, the generated thickness of the dens and transverse ligament both consisted of 0.5 mm articular cartilage. They possessed an elastic modulus of 10.4, Poisson's ratio of 0.4, and an articular surface coefficient of friction of 0.1. The definition of screw–bone interface in our model was close contact that ignored the micromotion between the screw and bone.

The range of motion at the base of the C2 vertebra was defined in all directions as 0. Forty Newton (N) of vertical downward pressure were imposed on the surface of the occipital condyle to simulate the weight of the head due to gravity. Approximately 1.5 Nm torque was imposed on the model from various directions to produce flexion, extension, lateral bending, and axial rotation. The range of motion at the atlantoaxial joint was calculated and compared with the results in vitro tests performed by Panjabi et al. [32] The results from this comparison are shown in Table 10.3.

Finite Element Model with Two Different Anterior Implants

All units representing the transverse ligament were removed from the cervical spine model to establish a finite element model of atlantoaxial instability. This established a finite element model to treat atlantoaxial instability with atlantoaxial transarticular locking plate. The elastic modulus of the medical titanium was 110,000 MPa and Poisson's ratio was 0.30. All units of the titanium plate were then removed to establish a finite element model for the treatment of atlantoaxial instability using simple anterior transarticular screw fixation system.

Table 10.4 Material properties used for various components of the model

Material	Young's modulus (Mpa)	Poisson's ratio
Bone[a]		
Cortical bone	12,000	0.29
Cancellous bone	450	0.29
End plates	500	0.4
Posterior element	3500	0.29
Annulus	3.4	0.4
Nucleus	1	0.49
Ligaments[a]		
ALL	30	0.3
PLL	20	0.3
ISL, LF	10	0.3
CL (C_0–C_1)	1	0.3
CL (C_1–C_2)	1.0	0.3
AIL	5	0.3
TL	20	0.3
ApL	20	0.3
NL	20	0.3

ALL anterior longitudinal ligament, *PLL* posterior longitudinal ligament, *ISL* interspinous ligament, *LF* ligamentum flavum, *CL* capsular ligament, *AIL* alar ligament, *TL* transverse ligament, *ApL* apical ligament, *NL* nuchal ligament

[a]Values were taken from Table 1 in Zhang et al. [30], which were derived from the literature Ng and Teo [29]

Boundary and Loading Conditions

Displacements of all the nodal points in the inferior margin of the axis on the X, Y, and Z axes were constrained to 0. Forty Newton of vertical downward pressure were imposed on the surface of the occipital condyle to simulate the weight of the head. Approximately 1.5 Nm torque was imposed on the model from various directions to produce flexion, extension, lateral bending.

Finite Element Analysis

Stress diagrams and displacement diagrams were analyzed and compared. The quantitative method calculated the maximum displacement of the anterior transarticular screw, maximum paradigm of stress, and maximum paradigm stress of the screw–bone interface. Our model used a cylinder to represent the screw. The interface between screws and surrounding bone was defined as "close contact without movement" in our finite element analysis, and their micromovements were ignored.

2.5.3 Results

The maximum displacement of the anterior transarticular screw is shown as it appeared during extension in both internal fixation devices. Maximum values of screw displacement were located at the screw tail. The anterior atlantoaxial transarticular locking plate system produced less displacement compared to the simple anterior atlantoaxial transarticular screw fixation; the anterior atlantoaxial transarticular lock-

ing plate system produced less stress on the screw compared to the simple anterior atlantoaxial transarticular screw fixation. The two axial vertebral screws bore relatively less stress at the junction of the screw and plate and the screw body. There was no significant stress concentration. The maximum von Mises stresses at the screw–bone interface of the transarticular screw were less than those measured at the simple screw fixation group.

2.5.4 Conclusion

The anterior atlantoaxial transarticular locking plate system not only provided stronger fixation but also decreased screw-bearing stress and screw–bone interface stress compared with simple anterior atlantoaxial transarticular screw fixation.

2.6 Biomechanical Effects of Vertebroplasty on the Adjacent Intervertebral Levels Using a 3D Finite Element Analysis

Abstract

Vertebroplasty is therefore gaining popularity for the treatment of patients with osteoporotic vertebral fractures (Heini et al., Eur Spine J 9:445–450, 2000; Hodler et al., Radiology 227:662–668, 2003). But Recently, vertebroplasty has been suggested to be the cause for a higher incidence of adjacent vertebral fractures observed clinically (Lindsay et al., JAMA 285:320-323, 2001; Uppin et al., Radiology 226:119–124, 2003). Many studies have been undertaken to examine the effects of augmentation procedures (Belkoff et al., Spine 26:1537–1541, 2001), but the results were controversial. To investigate effects caused by cement volume, distribution and leakage of bone cement in vertebroplasty on the adjacent intervertebral bodies by 3D osteoporosis finite element model of lumbar. L4–L5 motion segment data is from an old man cadaver. 3D model of L4–L5 was established with Mimics software, and finite element model of L4–L5 functional spinal unit (FSU) was established by ANSYS 7.0 software. The effect of different loading conditions and distribution of bone cement after vertebroplasty on the adjacent vertebral body was investigated.

This study presents a validated functional spinal unit (FSU) L4–L5 finite element model with a simulated vertebroplasty augmentation to predict stresses and strains of adjacent non-treated vertebral bodies. The findings from this FSU study suggest that the end plate and disk stress of the adjacent vertebral body were not influenced by bone cement filling volume but unipedicle injection and leakage to the disk of bone cement improving the stress of adjacent end plate. Asymmetric distributions and leakage of cement into intervertebral disk can improve the stress of end plate in adjacent vertebral body.

These results suggest that biomechanical optimal configuration should have symmetric placement and avoid leakage of cement in operation.

Osteoporotic vertebral compression fractures have traditionally been treated conservatively, but these fractures are sometimes responsible for persistent pain with impaired quality of life. Vertebroplasty with polymethyl methacrylate (PMMA) has been accepted as a viable treatment option for osteoporotic vertebral compression fractures. Early clinical results were very encouraging since relief from pain was immediate and reliable, and the complication rate was low. Vertebroplasty is therefore gaining popularity for the treatment of patients with osteoporotic vertebral fractures [23, 24]. But recently, vertebroplasty has been suggested to be the cause for a higher incidence of adjacent vertebral fractures observed clinically [25, 26]. Many studies have been undertaken to examine the effects of augmentation procedures [27], but the results were controversial. It remains unclear whether adjacent vertebral body fractures are related to the natural progression of osteoporosis or if adjacent fractures are a consequence of augmentation with bone cement. This study presents a validated functional spinal unit (FSU) L4–L5 finite element model with a simulated vertebroplasty augmentation in L4 to investigate the biomechanical effects of volume and distribution of bone cement on the adjacent vertebra.

2.6.1   Establishment of the L4 L5 3D Finite Element Models

L4–L5 motion segment data were obtained from computed tomography (CT) scans of the lumbar spine from an old man cadaver who had no abnormal findings on roentgenograms, taken at 1 mm intervals. The slices were preserved in computer, and 3D model of L4–L5 bone structure was established with Mimics software. Depending on the L4–L5 bone structure, the others such as end plate, annulus, nucleus, anterior longitudinal ligament, and posterior longitudinal ligament were established; different ligaments were orientated along the respective ligament directions obtained from anatomic textbooks. A solid model of the two vertebral bodies and the posterior elements was built. The finite element mesh model of L4–L5 was established by ANSYS 7.0 software. At last, FE model of the functional spinal unit consisted of 31,714 elements (Fig. 10.14a). The ratio between the surface areas of the nucleus pulposus and the annulus ground-substance was defined such that the area of the nucleus occupied on average 43% of the total disk area. The thickness of end plate and cortical bone is 0.35 mm. The assigned material properties were adapted from previous finite element studies and were assumed to be linear and isotropic. Model of osteoporosis FSU reduced 30% of Young's modulus compared with the normal structure. Their values and the chosen element-specific actions are presented in Table 10.5.

2.6.2   Vertebroplasty Simulation

Establishing 3D finite element models of FSU with vertebroplasty was generated. One FSU of each pair was augmented with PMMA bone cement in the unipedicle and unilateral distribution in vertebra (Fig. 10.14b, c), while the other in the bipedicle served as a control (Fig. 10.14d). The percent of volume age of bone is about 40% in unipedicle injection and 80% in bipedicle injection. We also simulated the leak cement in which the bone cement occupied the 20% disk (Fig. 10.14e). Axial compressive load of 260 N represented the weight of upper body, and 7.5 N in the other direction included flexion, extension, and bending which simulated various posture of the body under physiological loads. Von Mises stress distribution on the end plate in different condition had been analyzed.

According to the von Mises stress results of FE analysis, different filling volume of cement affecting the stress and strains in the adjacent vertebra is minimal at flexion and bending. But bending to the lateral side of augmented in unipedicle injection, the stress of inferior end plate increases. So the filling volume has minimal influence on the adjacent level, and asymmetric distribution of the cement has a little effect on the levels above and below an augmented vertebra at bend. Leak of cement into intervertebral disk improves the stress and strains on adjacent levels at every direction (Fig. 10.15).

2.6.3   Effects of Bone Cement Volume on Adjacent Vertebrae After Vertebroplasty

In the previously biomechanical study on the vertebroplasty, most aim is to investigate the effects of volume and distribution of bone cement on stiffness recovery of the vertebral body. But the adjacent vertebra fracture after vertebroplasty has been emphasized, because osteoporosis is a systemic disease; if augmented vertebra leads to the adjacent vertebra fracture, the vertebroplasty will be considered as benefit less than the harm. So the effect of the bone cement augmenting the osteoporosis vertebra on the adjacent vertebrae must be studied. Berlemann et al. [7] found that there was a trend toward lower failure loads with increased filling with cement by FE model study. The current practice of maximum filling with cement to restore the stiffness and strength of a vertebral body may provoke fractures in adjacent, non-augmented vertebrae. Further investigation is required to determine an optimal protocol for augmentation. Baroud et al. [8] found that vertebroplasty may induce subsequent fractures in the vertebrae adjacent to the ones augmented and hypothesized that adjacent fractures may result from a shift in stiffness and load following rigid augmentation. A finite element (FE) model of a lumbar motion segment (L4–L5) was used to quantify and compare the pre- and post-augmentation stiffness and loading of the intervertebral disk adjacent to the augmented vertebra in response to quasi-static compression. The results showed that the rigid cement augmentation underneath the end plates acted as an upright pillar that

Fig. 10.14 (**a**) 3D finite element model; (**b**) distribution of cement in vertebral; (**c**) distribution of cement unipedicular injection (40% cement filling volume) volume model; (**d**) distribution of cement bipedicular injection (80% cement filling volume); (**e**) leakage of cement into intervertebral disk.

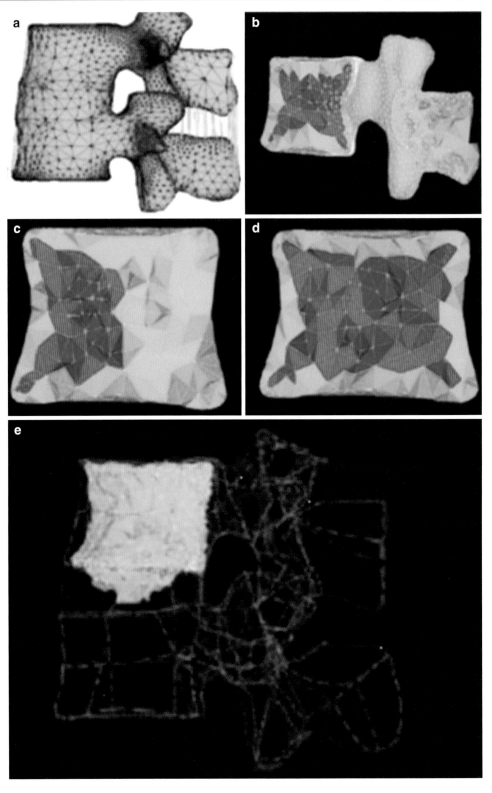

severely reduced the inward bulge of the end plates of the augmented vertebra. The inward bulge of the end plate adjacent to the one augmented (L4 inferior) increased considerably, by approximately 17%. This increase up to 17% in the inward bulge of the end plate adjacent to the one augmented may be the cause of the adjacent fractures.

The influence of augmentation level as well as uni- and bipedicular filling with PMMA has been investigated. Augmentation increased the pressure in the nucleus pulposus and the deflection of the adjacent end plate. The stresses and strains in the vertebrae next to an augmentation were increased, and their distribution was changed. Larger areas were subjected to higher stresses and strains. This supports the hypothesis that rigid cement augmentation may facilitate the subsequent collapse of adjacent vertebrae. Further study is required to determine the optimal reinforcement material and filling volume to minimize this effect [28]. But Villarraga et al. [10] found that changes in stresses and strains in levels adjacent to a kyphoplasty-treated level are minimal. Furthermore, the stress and strain levels found in the treated levels are less than injury tolerance limits of cancellous and cortical bone. Therefore, subsequent adjacent level fractures may be related to the underlying etiology (weakening of the bone) rather than the surgical intervention. Our experimental result found that the bone cement volume has little influence on the adjacent vertebrae, so we concluded that the bone cement volume had no obvious biomechanical effect on the adjacent vertebrae.

2.6.4   Effects of Bone Cement Distribution on Vertebral Stiffness

Though the effect of bone cement volume is little on the adjacent vertebra, we found that the unipedicle injection bended to the same lateral as the augment, and the stress of adjacent vertebra increased more than bipedicle injection. We think it is because the asymmetric distribution of bone cement leads to the stress improvement on the adjacent vertebra, which is same as the result of Liebschner et al. [11]. They found that the unipedicular distributions exhibited a comparative stiffness to the bipedicular or posterolateral cases, and it showed a medial-lateral bending motion ("toggle") toward the untreated side when a uniform compressive pressure load was applied. Asymmetric distributions with

large fills can promote single-sided load transfer and thus toggle. The most biomechanically optimal configuration and an improvement might be achieved by use of lower cement volume with symmetric placement. Our results suggest if the goal is to avoid adjacent vertebra fracture, the cement may be best injected via bipedicular approach because they should have symmetric placement of the cement. Additional fractures and partly patient may also be provoked by an adjacent rigid asymmetric cement distribution. We think the different conclusion from different author may be related to the different model of FE, so it is very important that there is an accurate model of FE as clinical practice.

The bone cement can leak into the disk in the vertebroplasty; we found the stress of end plate of adjacent vertebrae increased in the leakage FE model of cement, so maybe the leakage of cement is the major reason of adjacent vertebra fracture. Lin et al. [33] found patients successfully treated with vertebroplasty often returns with new pain caused by a new vertebral body fracture. The new fractures are often adjacent to the vertebral bodies that were initially treated. This study was based on 38 patients with painful compression fractures treated with vertebroplasty. Patients who returned with new pain after initial successful vertebroplasty were evaluated by repeat MR imaging. Fourteen patients developed new fractures during the follow-up period. In ten patients, the new fractures were associated with cement leakage into the disk, whereas four patients had new fractures that were not associated with cement leakage into the disk. This difference was statistically significant. A detailed analysis showed that 58% of vertebral bodies adjacent to a disk with cement leakage fractured during the follow-up period compared with 12% of vertebral bodies adjacent to a disk without cement leakage. So the author concludes that Leakage of cement into the disk during vertebroplasty increases the risk of a new fracture of adjacent vertebral bodies. Our result is same as the clinical observation.

The model of FE is not very accurate with the practical vertebroplasty, so our FE experiment was not able to accurately predict the numerical value of the biomechanics with

Table 10.5 Material properties of different components

Components	Young's modulus (MPa)	Poisson's ratio
Cortex	8040	0.3
Trabeculae	34	0.2
End plate	670	0.4
Bone cement composite	2160	0.2

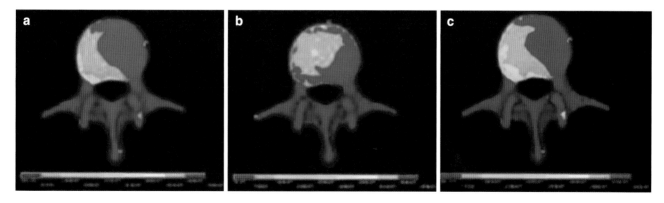

Fig. 10.15 Von Mises stress distribution in different condition. (**a**) Bipedicular injection; (**b**) unipedicular injection; (**c**) leakage of cement

respect to loading. But it can predict the obvious current. Though plenty of biomaterials have been used in the vertebroplasty, presently the PMMA cement is best in the biomaterials, so it is important to study the methods of injection of bone cement, reduce the syndrome, and improve the clinical result. According to the result of biomechanics, we emphasize that the bone cement volume could have little impact on adjacent vertebra, but the bone cement distribution might be on the adjacent vertebrae and effect especially leakage of bone cement into disk. Thus, we suggest that biomechanically optimal configuration should have symmetric placement in operation and avoid leakage of cement.

References

1. Shizhen Z. New progresses in fundamental research of traumatic orthopedics. Chin J Orthop Trauma. 2002;4:81–3.
2. Ruokun H, Ming X, Wusheng K, et al. Research progress in digital orthopedics. Orthop J China. 2010;18:1003–5.
3. Hodler J, Peck D, Gilula LA. Midterm outcome after vertebroplasty: predictive value of technical and patient-related factors. Radiology. 2003;227:662–8.
4. Lindsay R, Silverman S, Cooper C, et al. Risk of new vertebral fracture in the year following a fracture. JAMA. 2001;285:320–3.
5. Uppin AA, Hirsch JA, Centenera LV, et al. Occurrence of new vertebral body fracture after percutaneous vertebroplasty in patients with osteoporosis. Radiology. 2003;226:119–24.
6. Belkoff SM, Mathis JM, Jasper LE, et al. The biomechanics of vertebroplasty. The effect of cement volume on mechanical behavior. Spine. 2001;26:1537–41.
7. Berlemann U, Ferguson SJ, Nolte LP, et al. Adjacent vertebral failure after vertebroplasty. A biomechanical investigation. J Bone Joint Surg (Br). 2002;84:748–52.
8. Baroud G, Nemes J, Heini P, et al. Load shift of the intervertebral disc after a vertebroplasty: a finite-element study. Eur Spine J. 2003;1:421–6.
9. Polikeit A, Nolte LP, Ferguson SJ. The effect of cement augmentation on the load transfer in an osteoporotic functional spinal unit: finite-element analysis. Spine. 2003;28:991–6.
10. Villarraga ML, Bellezza AJ, Harrigan TP, et al. The biomechanical effects of kyphoplasty on treated and adjacent nontreated vertebral bodies. J Spinal Disord Tech. 2005;18:84–91.
11. Liebschner MA, Rosenberg WS, Keaveny TM. Effects of bone cement volume and distribution on vertebral stiffness after vertebroplasty. Spine. 2001;26:1547–54.
12. Keyak JH, Meagher JM, Skinner HB, et al. Automated three-dimensional finite element modeling of bone: a new method. J Biomed Eng. 1990;12:389–97.
13. Panjabi MM, Crisco JJ, Vasavada A, et al. Mechanical properties of the human cervical spine as shown by three-dimensional load-displacement curves. Spine. 2001;26:2692–700.
14. Nolte LP, Panjabi MM, Oxland TR. Biomechanical properties of lumbar spinal ligaments. In: Heimke G, Soltesz U, AJC L, editors. Clinical implant materials, advances in biomaterials, vol. 9. Heidelberg: Elsevier; 1990. p. 663–8.
15. Shizhen Z. Digitization of medical biomechanical parameters and digital medicine. J Med Biomech. 2006;21(3):169–71.
16. Meichao Z, Hong X, Jihong F. Reconstruction of the human skeleton finite element model. Chin J Clin Anat. 2003;21(5):531–2.
17. Lengsfeld M, Schmitt J, Alter P, et al. Comparison of geometry-based and CT voxel-based finite element modeling and experimental validation. Med Eng Phys. 1998;20(7):515–22.
18. Hazinski MF, Nadkarni VM, Hickey RW, et al. Major changes in the 2005 AHA Guidelines for CPR and ECC: reaching the tipping point for change. Circulation. 2005;112(24 suppl):IV206.
19. He Z, Guo X, Dong C, et al. Oxygen metabolism during CPR in critically ill patients. Chin J Emerg Med. 2001;10(6):376.
20. Cai XH, Liu ZC, Yu Y, et al. Evaluation of biomechanical properties of anterior atlantoaxial transarticular locking plate system using three-dimensional finite element analysis[J]. Eur Spine J. 2013;22(12):2686–94.
21. Kim YH, Khuyagbaatar B, Kim K. Biomechanical effects of spinal cord compression due to ossification of posterior longitudinal ligament and ligamentum flavum: a finite element analysis [J]. Med Eng Phys. 2013;35(9):1266–71.
22. Rohlmann A, Burra NK, Zander T, Bergmann G. Comparison of the effects of bilateral posterior dynamic and rigid fixation devices on the loads in the lumbar spine: a finite element analysis. Eur Spine J. 2007;16:1223–31.
23. Heini PF, Walchli B, Berlemann U. Percutaneous transpedicular vertebroplasty with PMMA: operative technique and early results. A prospective study for the treatment of osteoporotic compression fractures. Eur Spine J. 2000;9:445–50.
24. Wei Q, Wei L, Yabo Y. Three dimensional finite element analysis of stress distribution on continuously varying of length of pedicle screw [J]. J Med Biomech. 2010;25(3):206–11.
25. Qin L. Mechanical stimulation enhances osteogenesis and bone generation [J]. J Med Biomech. 2012;02:129–32.
26. Jin D, Chen J, Jiang J, et al. The application of Orion lock anterior cervical plate system in cervical surgery [J]. Chin J Orthop Trauma. 1999;19(6):328–31.
27. Tian W, Liu B, Hu L, et al. Cervical disease treatment by titanium plate with coral artificial or autogenous bone anterior fixation [J]. Traumatol Orthop Q. 1997;26(4):201–4.
28. Yuan W, Jia L, Dai L, et al. AO titanium locking plate in anterior cervical fixation: a preliminary report [J]. Chin J Spine Spinal Cord. 1996;6(4):161–3.
29. Ng HW, Teo EC. Nonlinear finite-element analysis of the lower cervical spine (C4–C6) under axial loading. J Spinal Disord. 2001;14:201–10.
30. Zhang QH, Teo EC, Ng HW, Lee VS. Finite element analysis of moment-rotation relationships for human cervical spine. J Biomech. 2006;39:189–93.
31. Panjabi MM. Cervical spine models for biomechanical research. Spine. 1998;23:2684–700.
32. Panjabi M, Dvorak J, Duranceau J, et al. Three-dimensional movements of the upper cervical spine. Spine. 1988;13:726–30.
33. Lin EP, Ekholm S, Hiwatashi A, et al. Vertebroplasty: cement leakage into the disc increases the risk of new fracture of adjacent vertebral body. Am J Neuroradiol. 2004;25:175–80.

Digital Fracture Classification

11

Dan Wang and Guoxian Pei

1 Significance of Digital Fracture Classification

Bone and joint trauma occur frequently. Accurate, timely, and comprehensive diagnosis and treatment of these injuries are critical for a favorable prognosis. The purpose of imaging is to elucidate the fracture location, understand the fracture anatomy, distinguish between fractures and dislocations, determine whether the fracture involves the joint surface or epiphyseal plate cartilage, and visualize the adjacent viscera for the presence of lesions. Most fractures can be definitively diagnosed by plain radiographs; however, it can be difficult to visualize some minor fractures, obscured parts of the fracture, or complex anatomical sites on x-ray film. For high-resolution images of soft tissue, magnetic resonance imaging (MRI) may be used in the diagnosis of joint trauma; however, the imaging time is lengthy and the bone cortex is poorly visualized, so MRI is not routinely used for bone trauma. Conventional computed tomography (CT) axial scanning is also problematic because it is a two-dimensional image that lacks realism.

With the development of imaging and computer technology, CT scanning and three-dimensional reconstruction have been increasing in popularity, allowing for stereoscopic observation of fractures and improving the accuracy of diagnosis. Multislice spiral CT (MSCT) has played an important role in the diagnosis of bone and joint trauma. Four-layer spiral CT was launched in 1998, after which the software and hardware for MSCT rapidly improved. At present, 320-layer spiral CT can be used in the clinic. A remarkable feature of MSCT is the ability to scan thin layers, which improves the z-axis resolution. Using FireVoxel imaging software, every element in the

coronal, sagittal, and transverse positions in three directions are equal, which ensures an accurate reconstruction of the spatial resolution image on any level; this is truly high-resolution isotropic imaging. Isotropic voxel data processing can provide coronal, sagittal, slope, and surface resolution at or near the original cross-sectional images. This can overcome the usual problems with volume CT imaging, including the perception of a ladder on the axis and numerous shortcomings when viewing subtle structures. With MSCT, a wide range of the volume scan can be completed within seconds, with high longitudinal resolution and powerful post-processing functions. Commonly used post-processing techniques for fractures include multiplanar reconstruction (MPR), surface shaded display (SSD), and volume rendering (VR).

MSCT and its post-processing techniques have the following benefits for the diagnosis of bone and joint trauma:

1. *Suspected fractures*: MSCT scanning and three-dimensional reconstruction (using coronal, sagittal, and oblique MPR reconstruction combined with VR or SSD technology) can visualize areas with hidden or tiny fractures.
2. *Complex anatomical sites*: When complex anatomical structures overlap bone or severe trauma has occurred (e.g., shoulder, spine, pelvis, maxillofacial bones), MSCT post-processing technology can accurately show fracture lines, the direction of the fracture, its length and width, the configuration of the broken bone, its size and spatial location, and other details.
3. *Adjacent soft tissues and organs*: The biggest advantage of MSCT is that a scan not only shows fractures clearly, but also adjacent anatomical structures (whether or not the patient has a compound injury). For example, in spinal fractures, cross-sectional MPR images can show whether the broken bone extends into the vertebral canal and at what depth, as well as whether there is spinal cord or nerve compression. In pelvic fractures, MSCT can also show any compound injury of the pelvic cavity viscera.
4. *Treatment planning*: VR and SSD technology allow for arbitrary axial and angle rotation, adjustments to the

D. Wang (✉)
The First Affiliated Hospital of Zhengzhou University, Zhengzhou, China

G. Pei
The Fourth Military Medical University, Xi'an, China

fracture orientation, and elucidation of the spatial relationship. MPR can also show fractures from the coronal, sagittal, or any other angle in layers to visualize every detail, showing surgical indications such as fracture instability and involvement of broken bones or joints. The use of VR or SSD combined with MPR can fully display fracture details and spatial relationships. Physicians can view any area for observation when making a treatment plan and choosing a surgical approach, simulate the reset procedure, determine the fixation, determined where the nail plate should be placed parts, and position screws, which will shorten the operation time, improve the success rate of surgery, and reduce complications.

5. *Postsurgical evaluation*: MSCT reconstruction after surgery can help to determine fracture reduction, articular face leveling, the position of the steel plate, the direction of the screw, and whether it extends into the joint cavity. It can also determine bone and metal structure variations and threshold values for internal fixation through the observation of complex fractures.

A good fracture classification system accurately describes fracture characteristics, provides robust fracture data, and serves as a methodical and systematic guide for the selection of treatment interventions, and helps to predict therapeutic effects. An important reference tool for the classification of fractures is a fracture map. At present, fracture maps are still a two-dimensional expression of a three-dimensional fracture. When two-dimensional graphics are used to render a three-dimensional structure, errors can sometimes occur, especially for physicians who lack clinical experience. Therefore, we established a fracture classification using a three-dimensional fracture "map" to help solve this problem, with an aim to deepen a physician's understanding of all types of fracture classifications.

In the development of our fracture classification system, we used a leading expert and robust data of normal adult bones from 64-row CT scans according to other common international fracture classification methods. Three-dimensional reconstruction was performed using Mimics, UG, and other modeling software. To simulate some clinically challenging fractures, we used the Neer classification for proximal humeral fractures, the Tile classification for pelvic fractures, the Schatzker classification for tibial plateau fractures, and the Lange-Hansen classification for ankle fractures. Fracture classification using digital images and animations allows for 360°, multiangle, dynamic views of the fracture, which is conducive to a quick and accurate assessment of a fracture.

Compared with a traditional fracture map, a three-dimensional map has many advantages:

1. *From two-dimensional to three-dimensional, from plane to solid*: Fracture characteristics can be more accurately described, allowing for more effective treatment of patients, increased reliability, and improved decision-making.
2. *From static to dynamic*: Each type of fracture can be rotated 360° in a dynamic, three-dimensional view that can be played again and again.
3. *From simulation to reality*: A traditional fracture map is a hand-painted simulation diagram. Three-dimensional mapping is derived from real bone reconstruction, thus improving the authenticity of the fracture simulation.
4. *From paper to electronic*: The old hard-copy method has improved to more portable and sharable electronic data, thus meeting the demands of modern work.

The three-dimensional digital model of fracture classification also has some disadvantages:

1. Due to technical problems in the reconstruction, it is not possible to distinguish between cancellous bone and cortical bone.
2. A three-dimensional map has obvious advantages for viewing the surface of the bone. However, visualization of the interior of some bones is inferior to a CT scan, such as with compression fractures. A CT scan and MPR reconstruction show this condition more clearly.
3. Certain soft tissues cannot be viewed well, such as for reconstruction of ligaments.

The three-dimensional map is not a panacea—you may sometimes need to combine the two-dimensional map and the three-dimensional map to more accurately visualize certain fractures. However, with the continued development of computer hardware and software technology, the three-dimensional digital fracture classification model will keep improving until it can stand alone.

Compared with conventional methods (e.g., radiographs, CT, MRI), digital fracture classification can greatly help the physician in teaching, diagnosis, surgical planning, and treatment by providing a clear, dynamic, three-dimensional, multiangle image of bone and joint structures and fracture types. In the next section, we illustrate some of the typical fracture classifications using the digital method.

2 Shoulder and Upper Limb Digital Fracture Classification

2.1 Scapula Fractures: AO Classification

For scapula fractures, the AO classification can be divided into scapula extra-articular fractures and scapula intra-articular fractures [2, 3].

Type A: Scapula extra-articular fracture
   A1: Acromion fracture
      A1.1 Acromion, non-comminuted
      A1.2 Acromion, comminuted
      A1.3 Coracoid fracture
   A2: Coracoid
      A2.1 Coracoid, non-comminuted
      A2.2 Coracoid, comminuted
      A2.3 Scapular neck fracture
   A3: Complex fractures
      A3.1 Scapular neck + Body fractures
      A3.2 Scapular neck + Simple clavicle fracture
      A3.3 Scapular neck + Comminuted clavicle fracture
Type B: Scapula intra-articular fractures
   B1: Glenoid cavity intra-articular embedded fracture
      B1.1 Anterior rim
      B1.2 Posterior rim
      B1.3 Lower edge
   B2: Glenoid cavity intra-articular non-embedded fracture
      B2.1 Anterior rim, free

B2.2 Posterior rim, free
B2.3 Anterior/posterior rim fracture with scapular neck fractures
B3: Complex fractures
   B3.1 Intra-articular comminuted fracture
   B3.2 Comminuted fracture of the scapular neck and (or) body
   B3.3 Comminuted clavicle fracture

2.1.1 Three-Dimensional Simulation Fracture Images

Figures 11.1, 11.2, 11.3, 11.4, 11.5, 11.6, 11.7, 11.8, 11.9, 11.10, 11.11, 11.12, 11.13, 11.14, 11.15, 11.16, 11.17, and 11.18.

2.2 Clavicle Fractures: Craig Classification

In 1990, the Craig Classification was proposed using the comprehensive Allman classification and Neer classification, which contained many rare types of clavicle fractures [2–4].

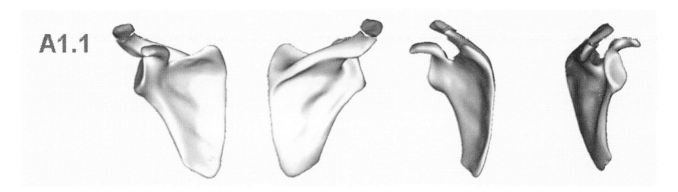

Fig. 11.1 A1.1

Fig. 11.2 A1.2

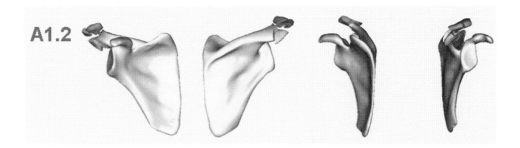

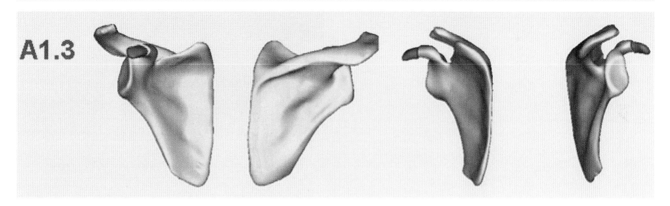

Fig. 11.3 A1.3

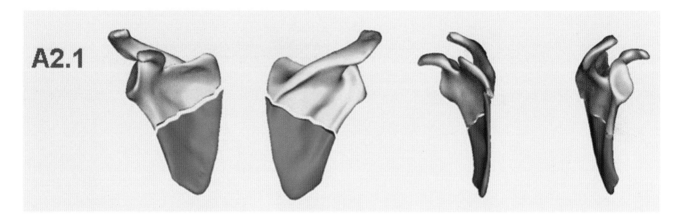

Fig. 11.4 A2.1

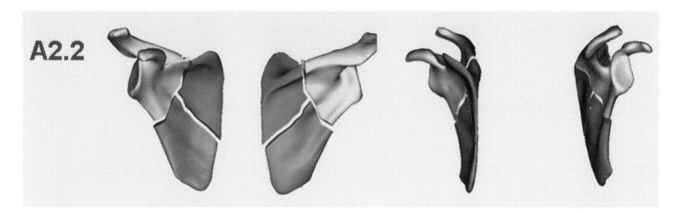

Fig. 11.5 A2.2

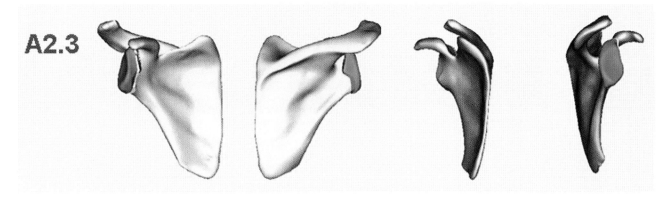

Fig. 11.6 A2.3

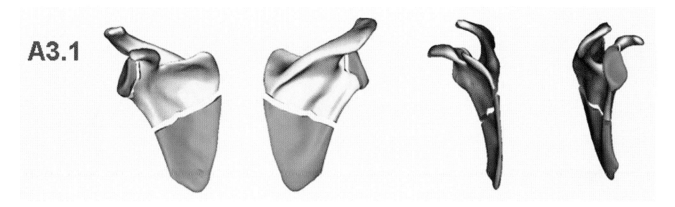

Fig. 11.7 A3.1

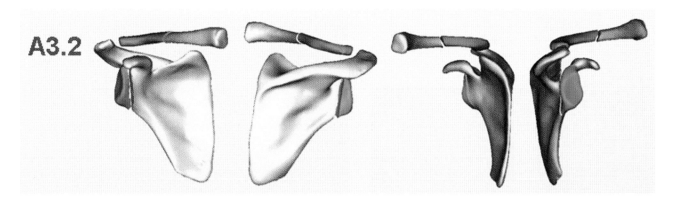

Fig. 11.8 A3.2

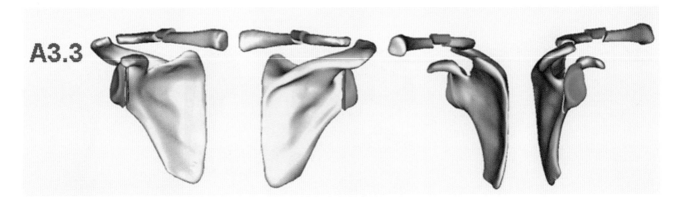

Fig. 11.9 A3.3

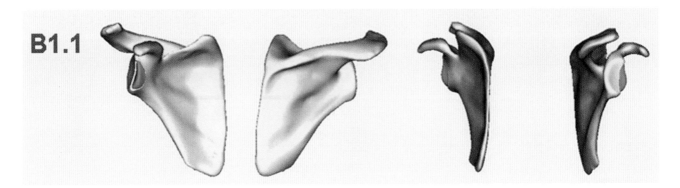

Fig. 11.10 B1.1

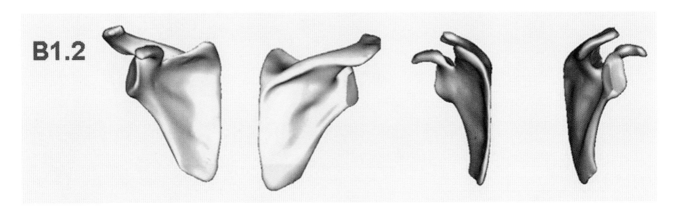

Fig. 11.11 B1.2

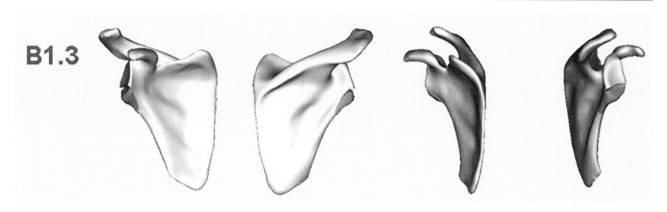

Fig. 11.12   B1.3

Fig. 11.13   B2.1

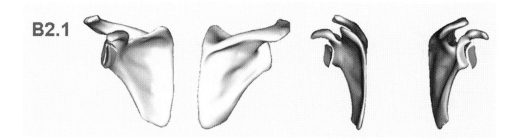

Fig. 11.14   B2.2

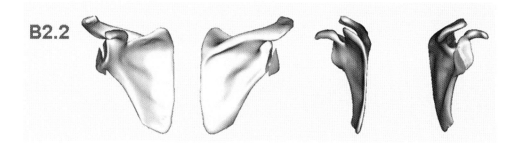

Fig. 11.15   B2.3

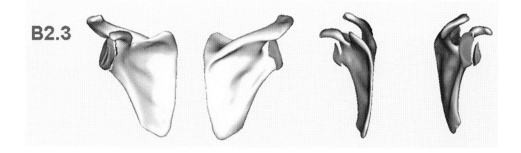

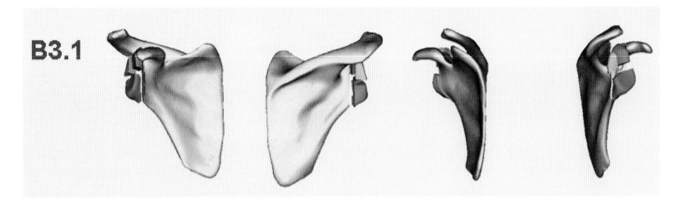

Fig. 11.16 B3.1

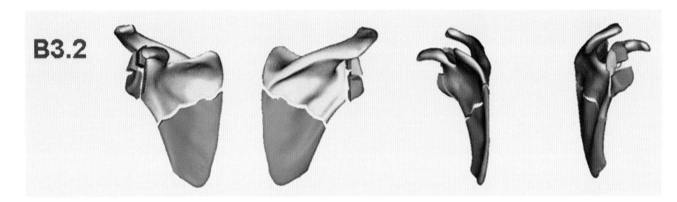

Fig. 11.17 B3.2

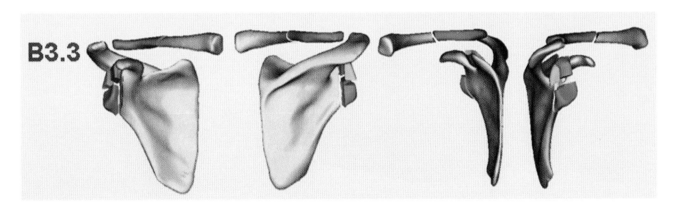

Fig. 11.18 B3.3

Group I: Fracture of the middle third.

Group II: Fracture of the distal third. Subclassified according to the location of coracoclavicular ligaments relative to the fracture as follows:

    Type I: Minimal displacement: interligamentous fracture between conoid and trapezoid or between the coracoclavicular and acromioclavicular ligaments;

    Type II: Displaced secondary to a fracture medial to the coracoclavicular ligaments (higher incidence of non-union);

        IIA: Conoid and trapezoid attached to the distal segment;

        IIB: Conoid torn, trapezoid attached to the distal segment;

    Type III: Fracture of the articular surface of the acromioclavicular joint with no ligamentous injury (may be confused with first-degree acromioclavicular joint separation).

    Type IV: Periosteal sleeve fracture (children);

    Type V: Comminuted fracture, coracoclavicular ligament and fracture block below are linked together, but the inside and outside of the main fractures are not connected.

Group III: Fracture of the proximal third

    Type I: Minimal displacement;

    Type II: Significant displaced (ligamentous rupture);

    Type III: Intraarticular;

    Type IV: Epiphyseal separation (children and adolescents);

    Type V: Comminuted.

2.2.1 Three-Dimensional Simulation Fracture Images

Figures 11.19, 11.20, 11.21, 11.22, 11.23, 11.24, 11.25, 11.26, 11.27, 11.28, 11.29, and 11.30.

2.3 Acromioclavicular Dislocations: Rockwood Classification

In 1984, acromioclavicular joint dislocations were divided into three types by the Rockwood fracture treatment team, increasing to six types in 1996 [3, 4]. The classification is widely used in the clinic.

Type I

    Sprain of the acromioclavicular (AC) ligament. AC joint tenderness, minimal pain with arm motion, and no pain in coracoclavicular interspaces. No abnormality on radiographs.

Type II

    AC ligament tears with joint disruption and sprained coracoclavicular ligaments. Distal clavicle is slightly

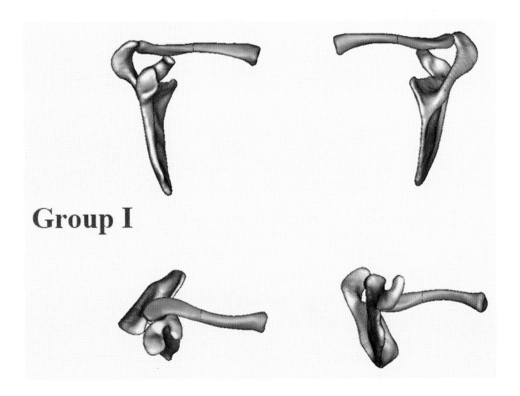

Fig. 11.19 Group I

Fig. 11.20 Group II Type I

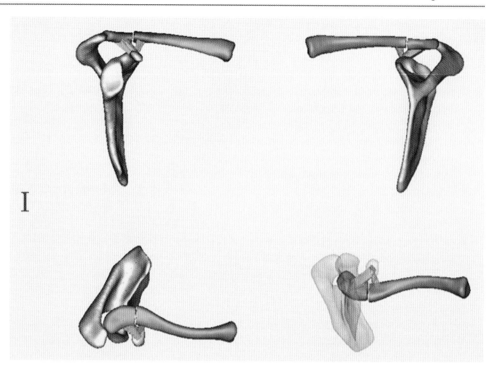

Fig. 11.21 Group II Type IIA

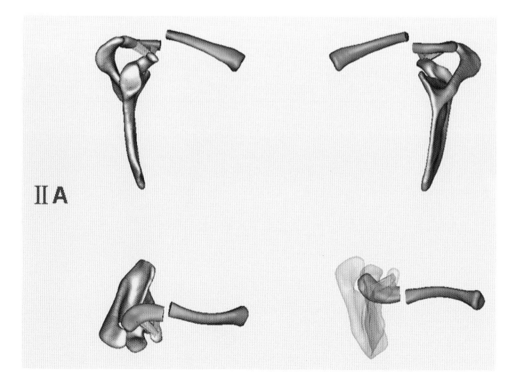

Fig. 11.22 Group II Type
IIB

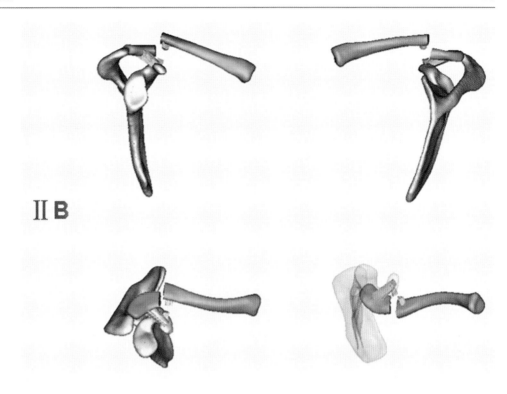

Fig. 11.23 Group II Type III

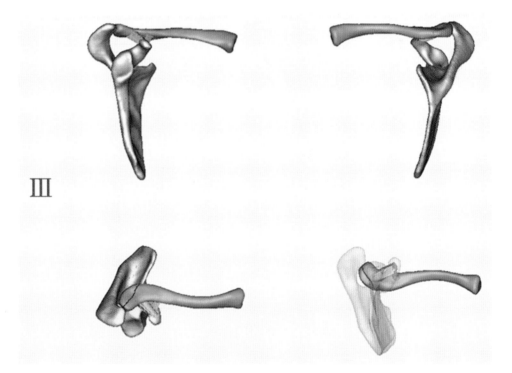

Fig. 11.24 Group II Type IV

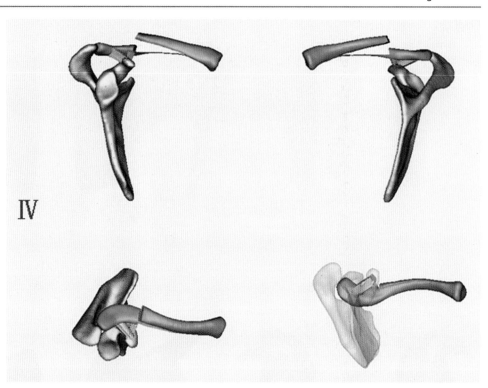

Fig. 11.25 Group II Type V

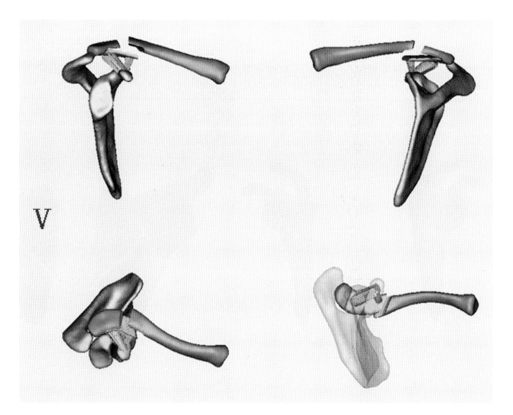

Fig. 11.26 Group III Type I

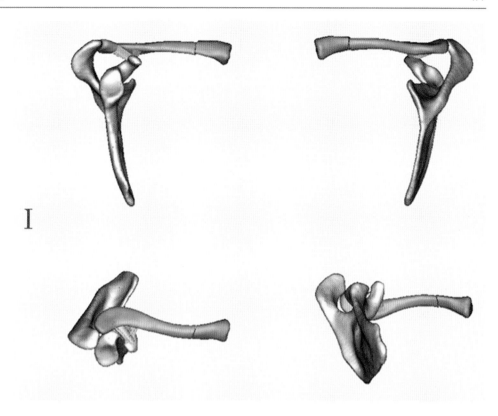

Fig. 11.27 Group III Type II

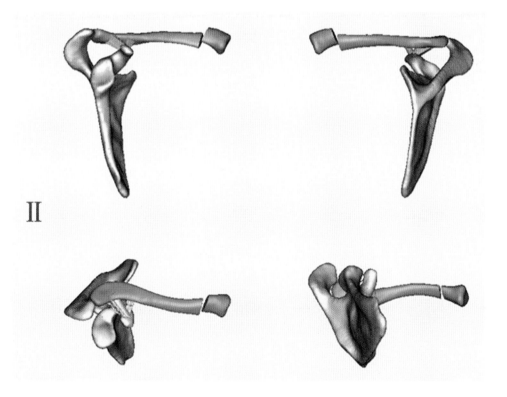

Fig. 11.28 Group III Type
III

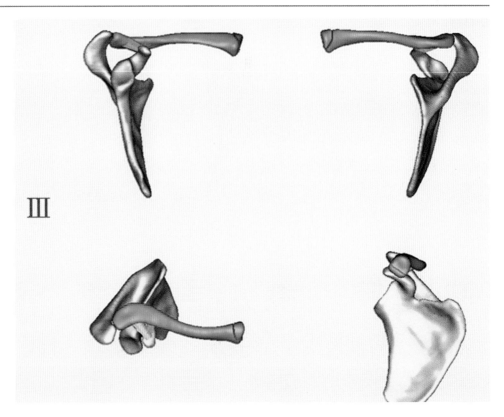

Fig. 11.29 Group III Type
IV

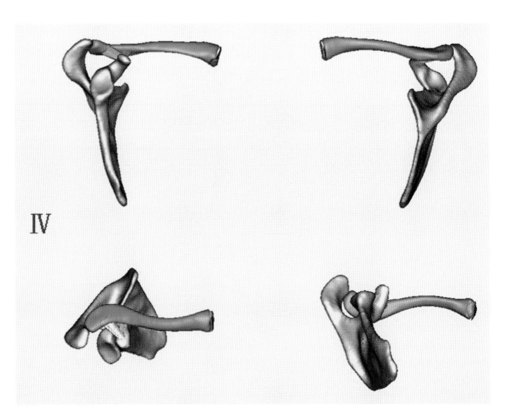

Fig. 11.30 Group III Type V

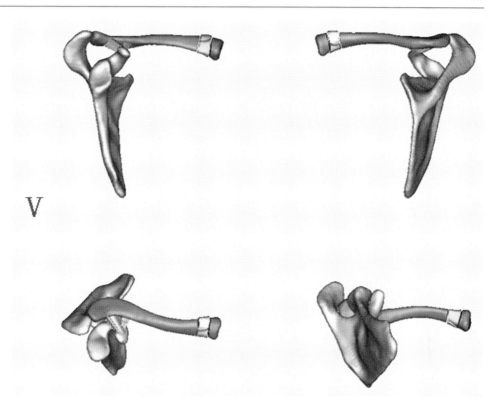

superior to acromion and mobile to palpation; tenderness is found in the coracoclavicular space. Radiographs demonstrate slight elevation of the distal end of the clavicle and AC joint widening. Stress films show the coracoclavicular ligaments are sprained but the integrity is maintained.

Type III

AC and coracoclavicular ligaments torn with AC joint dislocation; deltoid and trapezius muscles usually detached from the distal clavicle. The upper extremity and distal fragment are depressed, and the distal end of the proximal fragment may tent the skin. The AC joint is tender, and coracoclavicular widening is evident. Radiographs demonstrate the distal clavicle superior to the medial border of the acromion; stress views reveal a widened coracoclavicular interspace 25–100% greater than the normal side.

Type IV

Type III with the distal clavicle is displaced posteriorly into or through the trapezius. Clinically, more pain exists than in type III; the distal clavicle is displaced posteriorly away from the clavicle. Axillary radiograph or computed tomography demonstrates posterior displacement of the distal clavicle.

Type V

Type III with the distal clavicle is grossly and severely displaced superiorly. This type is typically associated with tenting of the skin. Radiographs demonstrate the coracoclavicular interspace to be 100–300% greater than the normal side.

Type VI

AC dislocated, with the clavicle displaced is inferior to the acromion or the coracoid; the coracoclavicular interspace is decreased compared with normal. The deltoid and trapezius muscles are detached from the distal clavicle. The mechanism of injury is usually a severe direct force onto the superior surface of the distal clavicle, with abduction of the arm and scapula retraction. Clinically, the shoulder has a flat appearance with a prominent acromion; associated clavicle and upper rib fractures and brachial plexus injuries are due to high energy trauma. Radiographs demonstrate one of two types of inferior dislocation: subacromial or subcoracoid.

2.3.1   Three-Dimensional Simulation Fracture Images

Figures 11.31, 11.32, 11.33, 11.34, and 11.35.

Fig. 11.31 Type II

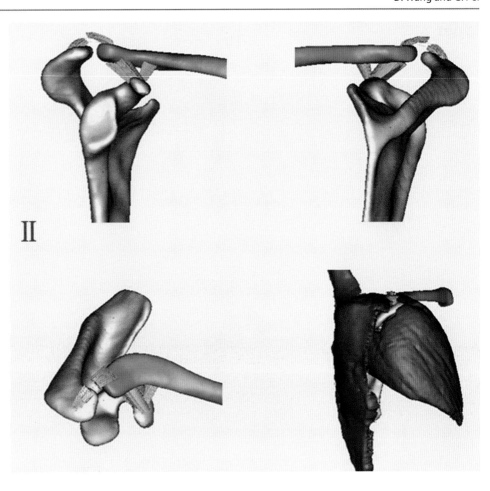

Fig. 11.32 Type III

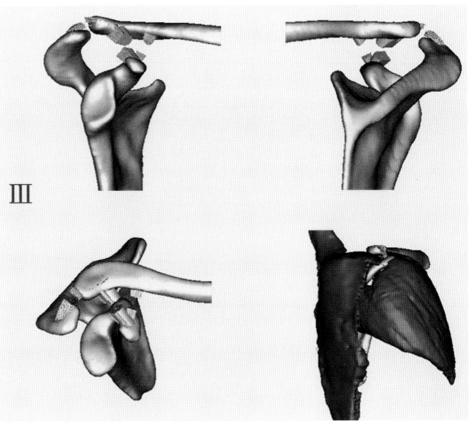

Fig. 11.33 Type IV

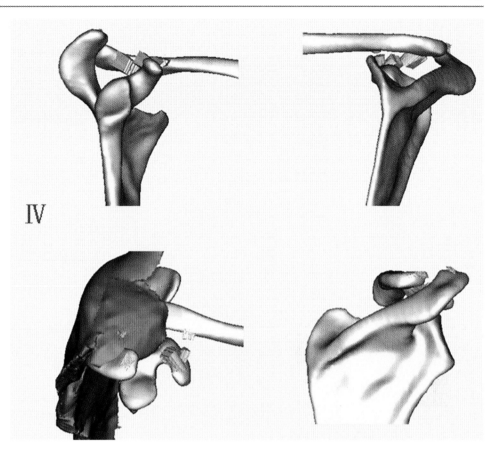

Fig. 11.34 Type V

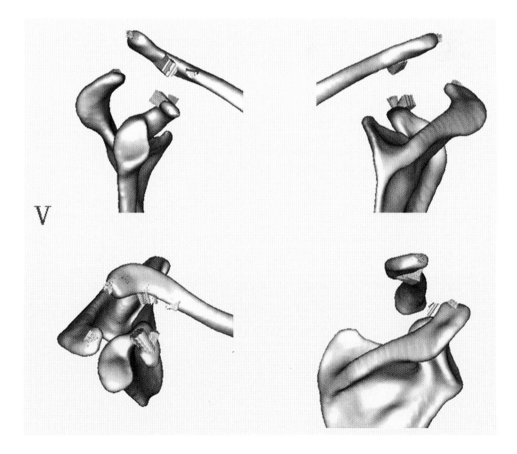

Fig. 11.35 Type VI

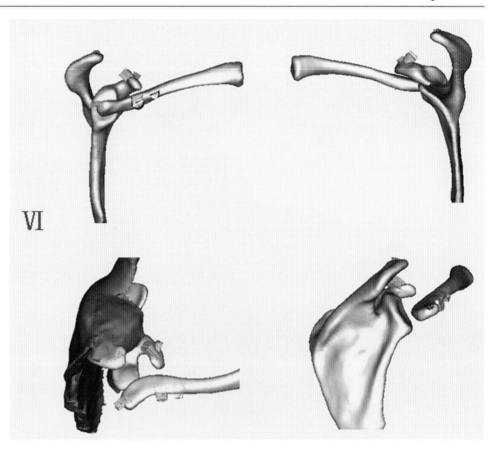

2.4 Shoulder Joint Dislocations: Anatomical Classification

Shoulder joint dislocations can be divided into anterior dislocations and posterior dislocations, according to the anatomical classification [3–5].

An anterior dislocation can be divided into four types:

Type I: Subcoracoid dislocation, dislocation of the humeral head to below the coracoid;
Type II: Infraglenoid dislocation; the humeral head under forward dislocation in the lower edge of glenoid;
Type III: Dislocation of clavicle, after the humerus head dislocation to the inside of the shift, to the inside of the rostrum, down to the bottom of the clavicle;
Type IV: Intrathoracic dislocation; humerus head dislocation through the ribs into the chest. This type is rarer with lungs and blood vessel involvement, nerve damage.

Posterior dislocations can be divided into three types:

Type I: Under the acromion dislocation, accounting for 98% of the dislocation, joints, oriented nodules occupied shoulder socket with humerus head in front of the fracture;
Type II: Glenohumeral subluxation;

Type III: Under the shoulder blade, dislocation, head of the humerus in the acromion medial, shoulder is below.

2.4.1 Three-Dimensional Simulation Fracture Images

Figures 11.36, 11.37, 11.38, 11.39, 11.40, 11.41, and 11.42.

2.5 Humerus Fractures: Neer Classification

Codman was the first to observe that there were four major fracture fragments when a proximal humerus fracture occurred. Neer modified and improved on Codman's classification by emphasizing the patterns and degrees of displacement rather than the location of fracture lines. He believed this gave important insight into humeral articular segment viability by providing evidence of the likelihood of soft-tissue disruption and vascular integrity to the head. Neer's classification scheme is the system most widely used by orthopedic surgeons today [2–5]. It groups fractures based on the number of parts and their displacement from each other. In this system, the criteria for displacement are 45° of angulation or more than 1 cm of displacement between fracture parts. If displacement is less than this, then the fracture is considered to be minimally displaced regardless of the number of fracture lines (Table 11.1).

Fig. 11.36 Anterior dislocation Type I

Fig. 11.37 Anterior dislocation Type II

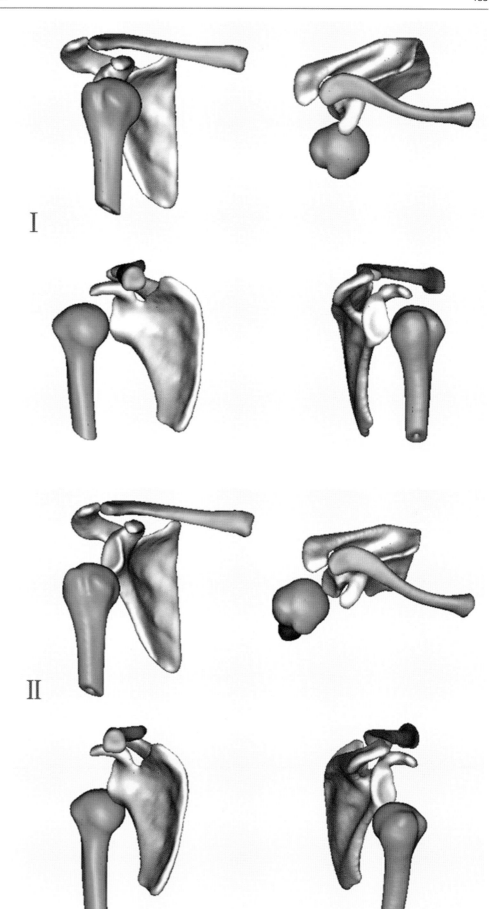

Fig. 11.38 Anterior
dislocation Type III

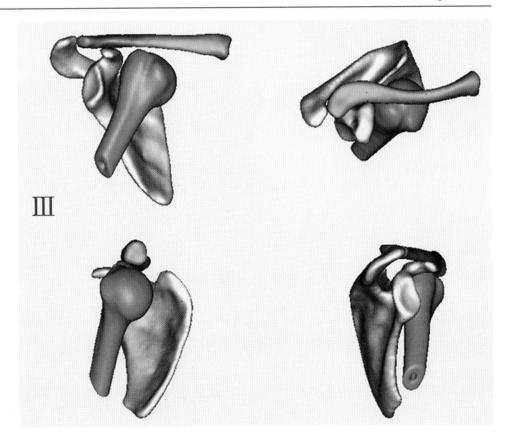

Fig. 11.39 Anterior
dislocation Type IV

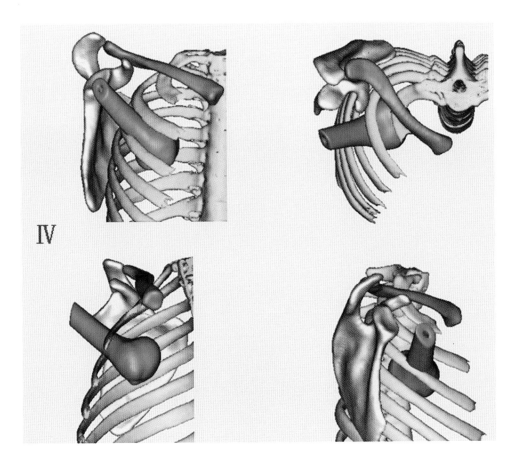

Fig. 11.40 Posterior
dislocation Type I

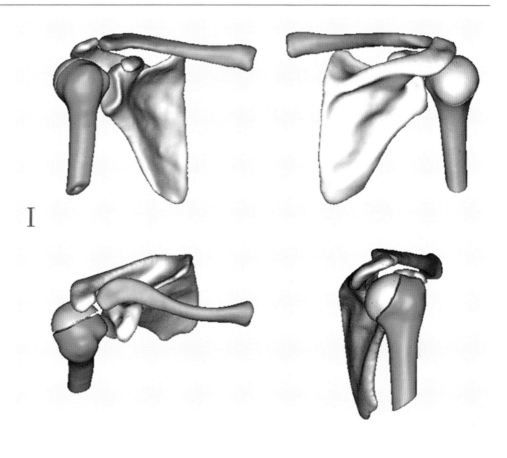

Fig. 11.41 Posterior
dislocation Type II

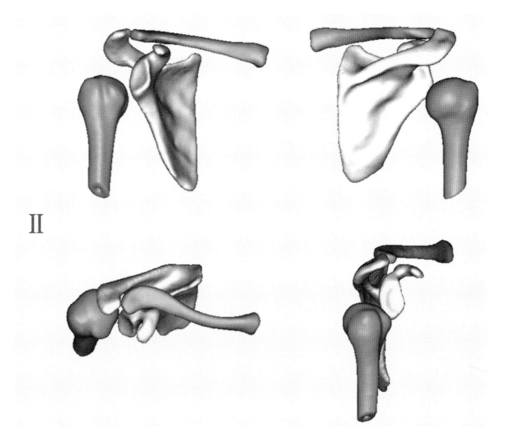

Fig. 11.42 Posterior
dislocation Type III

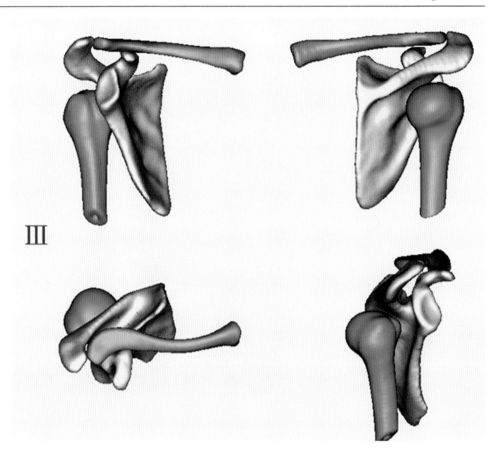

Table 11.1 Neer classification of proximal humeral fractures

One-part fracture (no or slight displacement)	1. Single line: anatomic neck fractures, surgical neck fractures, fracture of the greater tuberosity, small nodule fractures
	2. Two fracture lines: greater tuberosity and surgical neck fracture, small nodule and surgical neck fractures
	3. Several fracture lines: anatomic neck fracture, greater tuberosity fractures, small nodule fractures, surgical neck fracture
Two-part fracture	1. Anatomic neck fracture
	2. Surgical neck fracture: Angulation, displacement, comminuted fracture
	3. Greater tuberosity fracture
	4. Small nodules fracture
Three-part fracture	1, Surgical neck + greater tuberosity (small nodules and the humeral head together)
	2. Surgical neck + small nodules (greater tuberosity and the humeral head together)
Four-part fracture	Anatomic neck + greater tuberosity + small nodules + Humeral shaft
Humeral head articular surface fracture	1. Collapse
	2. Splitting
Dislocation of shoulder joint	1. Anterior dislocation (often associated with greater tuberosity)
	2. Posterior dislocation (often associated with small nodules)

2.5.1   Three-Dimensional Simulation Fracture Images

Figures 11.43, 11.44, 11.45, 11.46, 11.47, 11.48, 11.49, 11.50, 11.51, 11.52, 11.53, 11.54, and 11.55.

2.6   Elbow Dislocations: AO Classification

In the AO classification, elbow dislocations are coded as 20-D [2, 3]. The specific classifications are as follows:

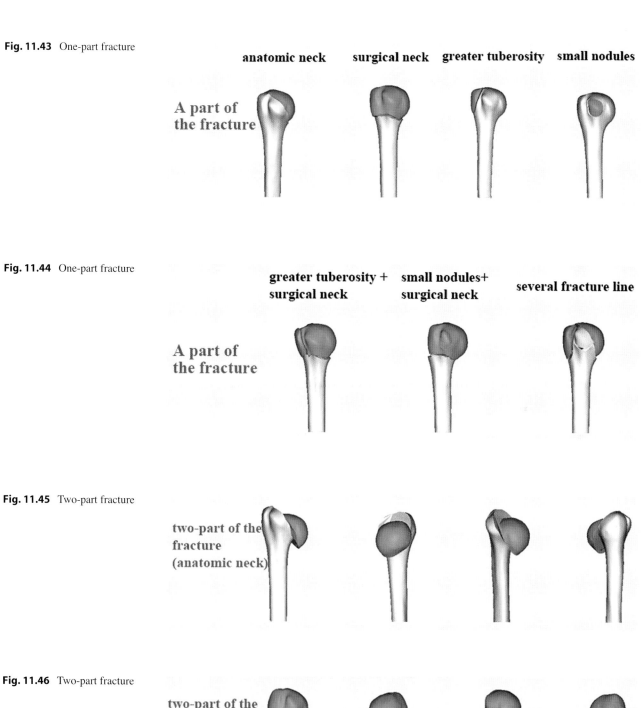

Fig. 11.43 One-part fracture

Fig. 11.44 One-part fracture

Fig. 11.45 Two-part fracture

Fig. 11.46 Two-part fracture

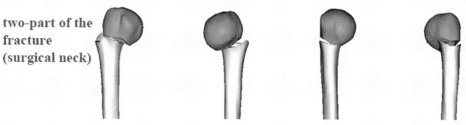

Fig. 11.47 Two-part fracture

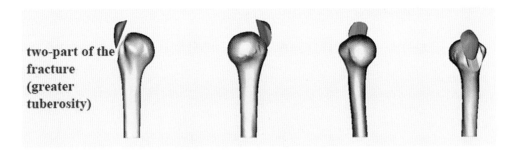

two-part of the fracture (greater tuberosity)

Fig. 11.48 Two-part fracture

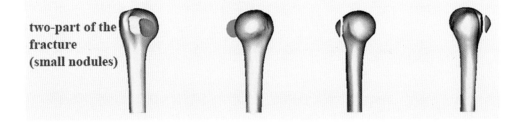

two-part of the fracture (small nodules)

Fig. 11.49 Three-part fracture

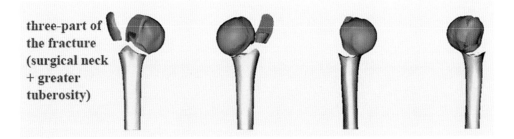

three-part of the fracture (surgical neck + greater tuberosity)

Fig. 11.50 Three-part fracture

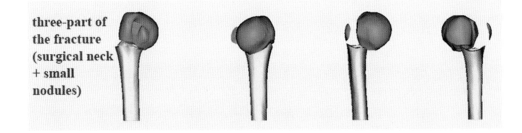

three-part of the fracture (surgical neck + small nodules)

Fig. 11.51 Four-part fracture

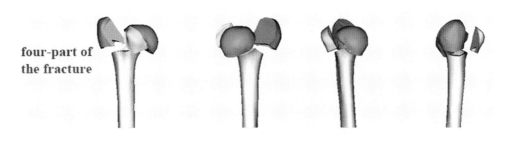

four-part of the fracture

Fig. 11.52 Humeral head articular surface fracture

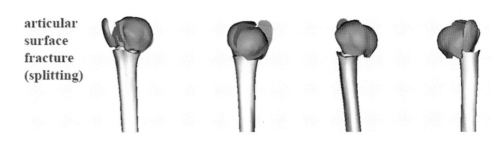

articular surface fracture (splitting)

Fig. 11.53 Humeral head articular surface fracture

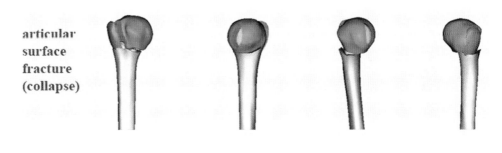

articular surface fracture (collapse)

Fig. 11.54 Dislocation of the shoulder joint

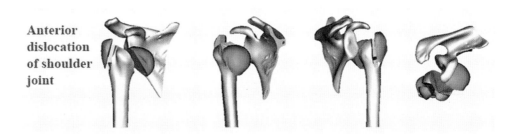

Anterior dislocation of shoulder joint

Fig. 11.55 Dislocation of
the shoulder joint

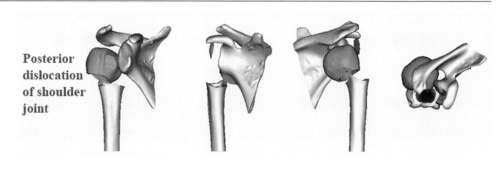

Fig. 11.56 20-D10

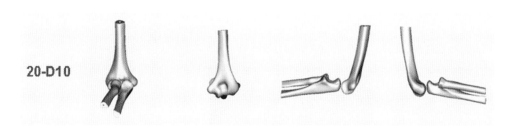

Fig. 11.57 20-D11

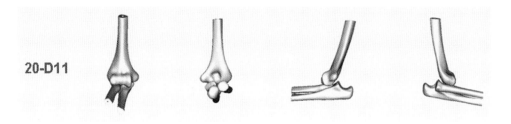

Fig. 11.58 20-D12

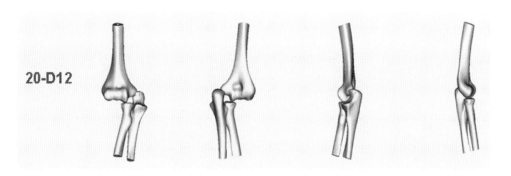

20-D10: Anterior dislocation;
20-D11: Posterior dislocation;
20-D12: Inside dislocation;
20-D13: Lateral dislocation;
20-D16: Posterior internal dislocation;
20-D17: Posterolateral dislocation;
20-D18: Separation dislocation.

2.6.1 Three-Dimensional Simulation Fracture Images

Figures 11.56, 11.57, 11.58, 11.59, 11.60, 11.61, and 11.62.

Fig. 11.59 20-D13

Fig. 11.60 20-D16

Fig. 11.61 20-D17

Fig. 11.62 20-D18

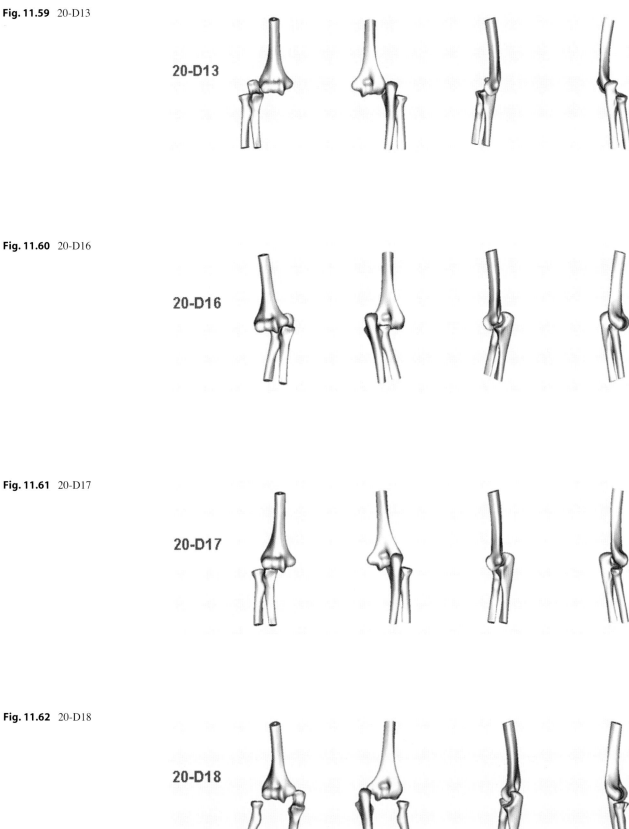

2.7 Ulnar and Radial Fractures: AO Classification

In the AO classification, ulnar and radial proximal fractures are coded as 21. They are divided into ulnar and radial proximal, extra-articular fractures (21-A); ulnar and radial proximal, articular surface, one bone (21-B); and ulnar and radial proximal, articular, both bones (21-C) [2–5].

Type A: ulnar and radial proximal, extra-articular fracture
    Type A1 is pure ulnar fracture, radial integrity.
        A1.1 Avulsion of triceps insertion from olecranon
        A1.2 Metaphyseal, simple
        A1.3 Metaphyseal, multi-fragmentary
    Type A2 is pure radial fracture, ulnar integrity.
        A2.1 Avulsion of bicipital tuberosity of radius (21-A2.1)
        A2.2 Neck, simple (21-A2.2)
        A2.3 Neck, multi-fragmentary (21-A2.3)
    Type A3 is ulnar and radial fracture.
        A3.1 Simple fracture of both bones
        A3.2 Multi-fragmentary fracture of one bone and simple fracture of other bone
          1. Multi-fragmentary, ulna
          2. Multi-fragmentary, radius
        A3.3 Multi-fragmentary, both bones
Type B: Ulnar and radial proximal, articular surface one bone
    Type B1 is pure ulnar fracture, radial integrity.
        B1.1 Single fracture
        B1.2 Simple double fracture
        B1.3 Crushing double fracture

Type B2 is pure radial fracture, ulnar integrity.
    B2.1 Simple fracture
    B2.2 Multi-fragmentary without depression
    B2.3 Multi-fragmentary with depression
Type B3 is articular fracture of one bone, extra-articular fracture of other bone.
    B3.1 Ulna, articular simple fracture
    B3.2 Radius, articular simple fracture
    B3.3 Articular multi-fragmentary fracture
Type C: Ulnar and radial proximal, articular both bones
    Type C1 is articular both simple fracture.
        C1.1 Ulnar olecranon and radial head simple fracture
        C1.2 Ulnar coronoid process and radial head simple fracture
    Type C2 is one articular simple fracture, the other articular multi-fragmentary fracture.
        C2.1 Ulnar olecranon multi-fragmentary fracture, radial head simple fracture
        C2.2 Ulnar olecranon simple fracture, radial head multi-fragmentary fracture
        C2.3 Ulnar coronoid process simple fracture, radial head multi-fragmentary fracture
Type C3 is articular multi-fragmentary fracture of both bones.
    C3.1 Three fragments, both bones
    C3.2 Ulna, more than three fragments
    C3.3 Radius, more than three fragments

2.7.1 Three-Dimensional Simulation Fracture Images

Figures 11.63, 11.64, 11.65, 11.66, 11.67, 11.68, 11.69, 11.70, 11.71, 11.72, 11.73, 11.74, 11.75, and 11.76.

Fig. 11.63 Type A1

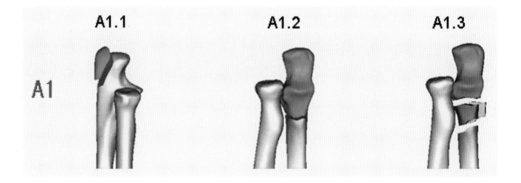

Fig. 11.64 Type A2

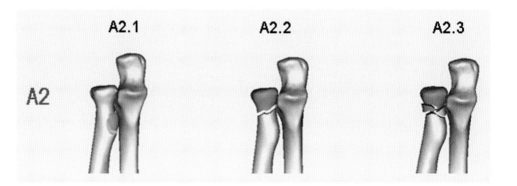

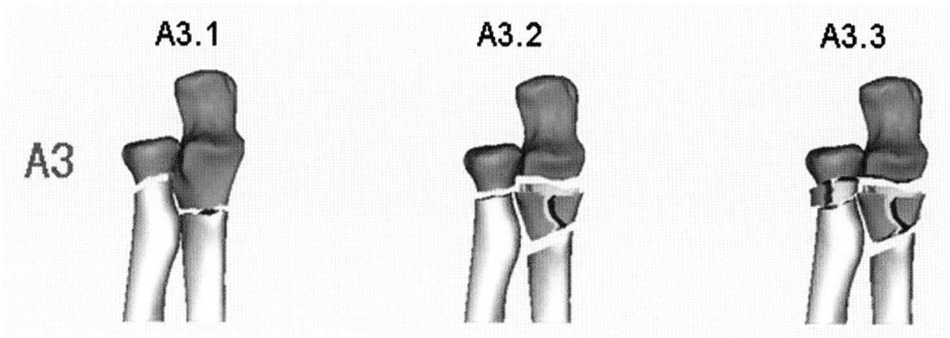

Fig. 11.65   Type A3

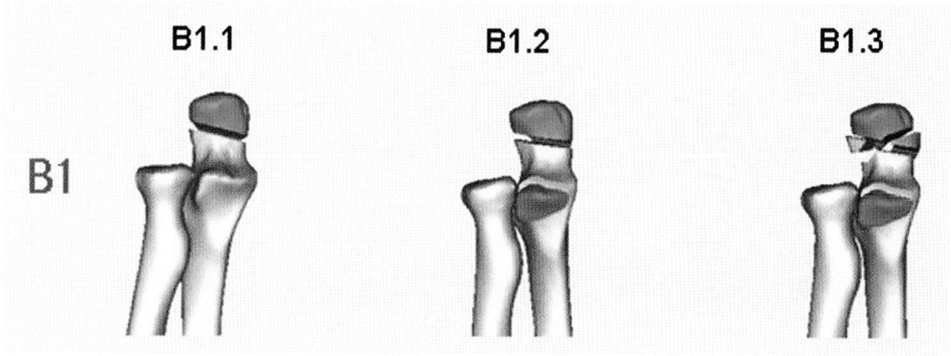

Fig. 11.66   Type B1

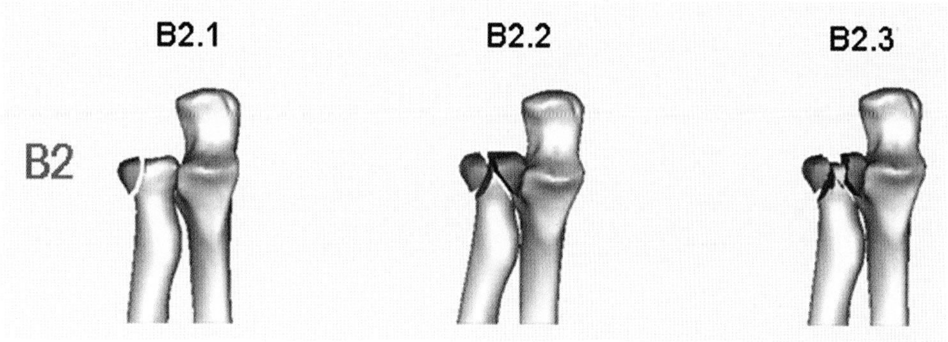

Fig. 11.67   Type B2

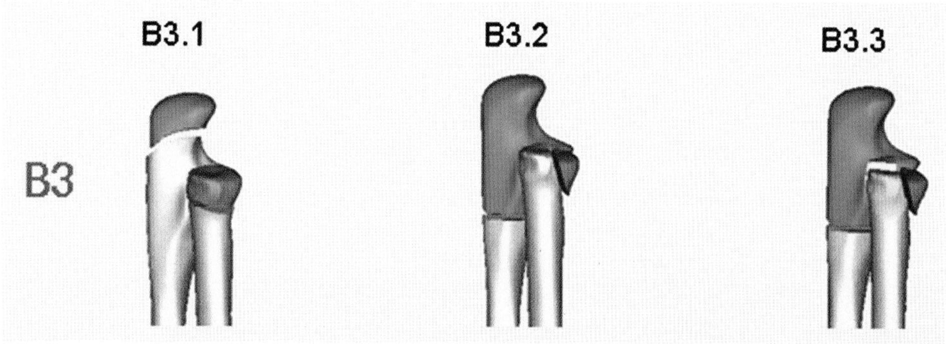

Fig. 11.68   Type B3

Fig. 11.69   Type C1.1

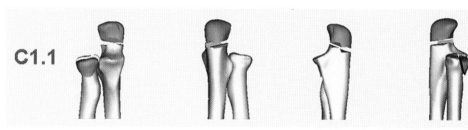

Fig. 11.70 Type C1.2

Fig. 11.71 Type C2.1

Fig. 11.72 Type C2.2

Fig. 11.73 Type C2.3

Fig. 11.74 Type C3.1

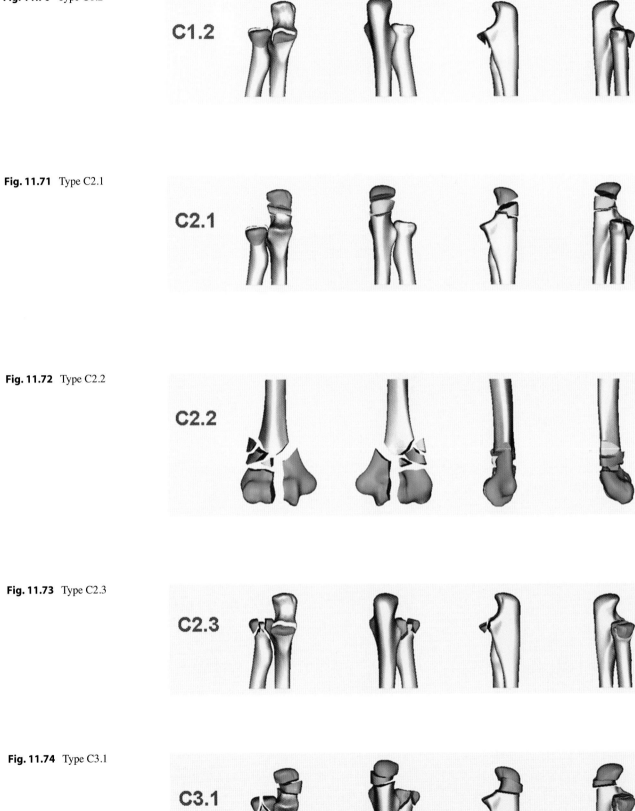

Fig. 11.75 Type C3.2

Fig. 11.76 Type C3.3

Fig. 11.77 Type I

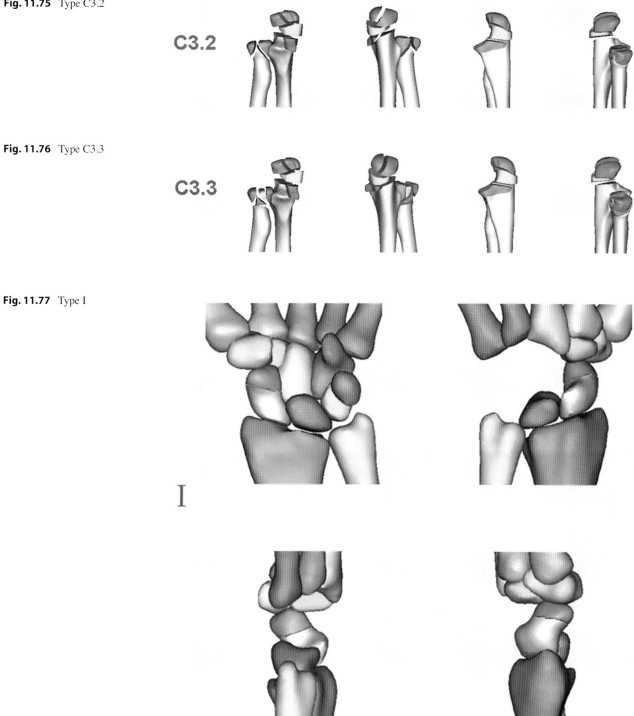

2.8   Wrist and Hand Fractures

2.8.1   Scaphoid Fractures: Russe Classification

In 1960, wrist scaphoid fractures were divided into three types by Russe, according to the fracture line relationship with the long axis of the wrist scaphoid [4, 5].

Type I: Horizontal oblique fracture line
Type II: Transverse fracture line
Type III: Vertical oblique fracture line

Three-Dimensional Simulation Fracture Images
Figures 11.77, 11.78, and 11.79.

Fig. 11.78 Type II

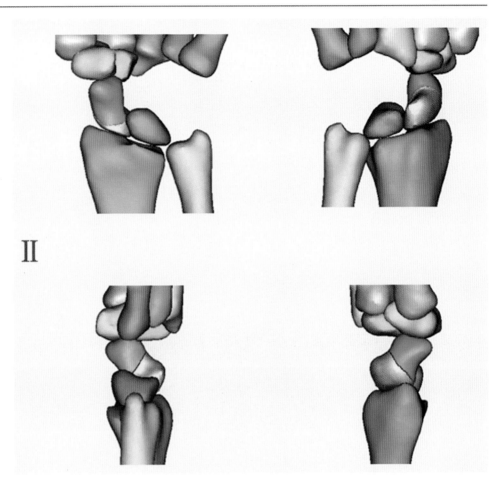

Fig. 11.79 Type III

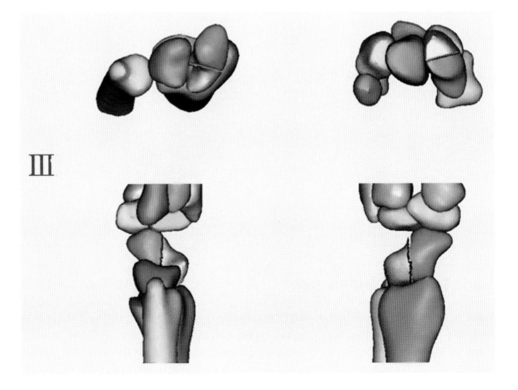

2.8.2   First Metacarpal Fractures: Green Classification

In 1972, first metacarpal base fractures were divided into four types by Green [4–6].

Type I: Bennett fracture—fracture line separates the major part of the metacarpal from volar lip fragment, producing a disruption of the first carpometacarpal joint; first metacarpal is pulled proximally by the abductor pollicis longus.

Type II: Rolando fracture—requires greater force than a Bennett fracture; presently used to describe a commi-nuted Bennett fracture, a "Y" or "T" fracture, or a fracture with dorsal and palmar fragments.

Type III: Extraarticular fractures
 Type IIIA: Transverse fracture
 Type IIIB: Oblique fracture

Type IV: Epiphyseal injuries seen in children

Three-Dimensional Simulation Fracture Images

Figures 11.80, 11.81, 11.82, 11.83, and 11.84.

Fig. 11.80   Type I

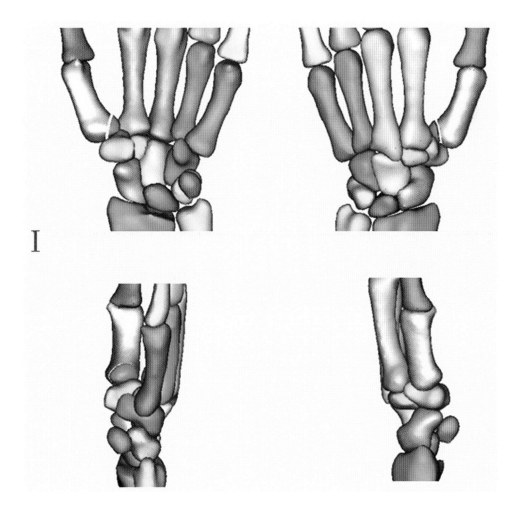

Fig. 11.81 Type II

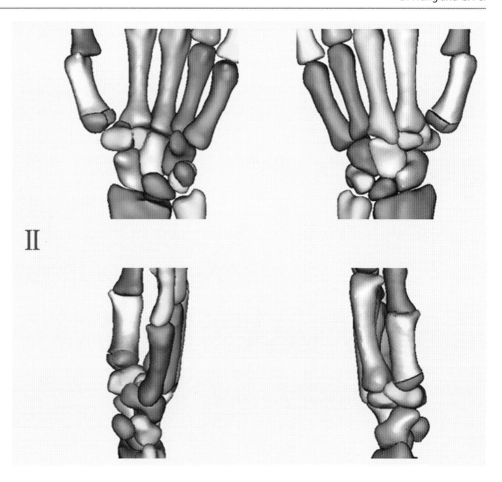

Fig. 11.82 Type IIIA

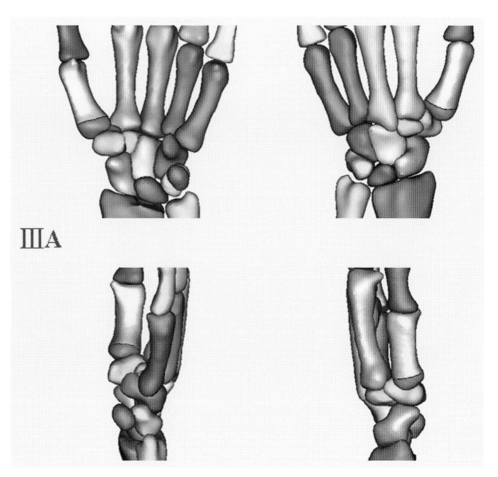

Fig. 11.83 Type IIIB

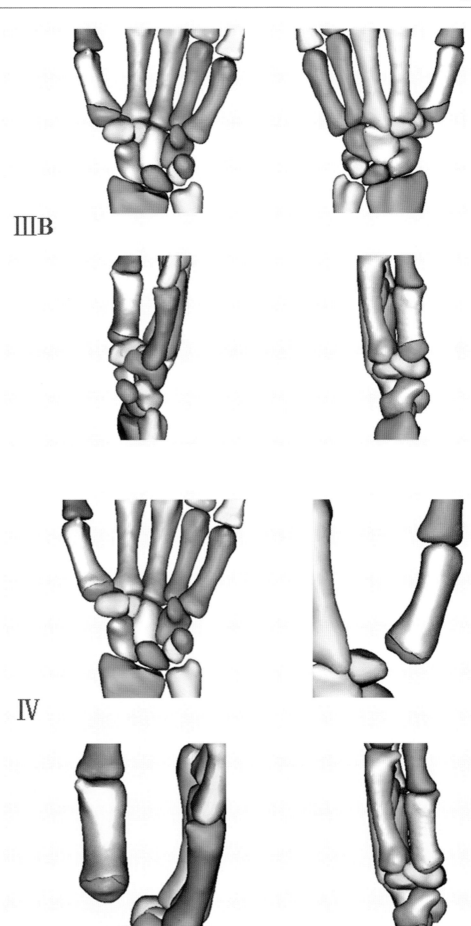

Fig. 11.84 Type IV

3 Spine Digital Fracture Classification

3.1 Cervical Spine Fractures

3.1.1 Atlantoaxial Injuries: AO Classification

The spine is coded as 5, atlantoaxial as 50, atlas fractures as (50-A), axis fractures as (50-B), and atlantoaxial associated injury as (50-C) [4–6].

Type A: Atlas fracture
  A1: Single arch of atlas fracture
    A1.1: Posterior arch fracture
    A1.2: Anterior arch fracture
  A2: Atlas anterior arch and posterior arch fracture
  A3: The lateral mass of atlas fracture
    A3.1: One side of lateral mass crushing
    A3.2: Bilateral lateral mass crushing
Type B: Axis fracture
  B1: Axis isthmus fracture
    B1.1: Minimal shift
    B1.2: Obvious shift
    B1.3: A large shift in flexion
  B2: Axis odontoid fracture
    B2.1: Odontoid process dentate fracture
    B2.2: Base of odontoid process or axis fracture
    B2.3: Odontoid process neck fracture
  B3: Axis complex fractures
    B3.1: Axis isthmus, the base of odontoid process and axis body fracture
    B3.2: Axis isthmus and odontoid process neck fracture
    B3.3: Odontoid process fracture with the axis rotation and crushing
Type C: Atlantoaxial injury
  C1: Fracture
    C1.1: Atlas posterior arch and axis isthmus fractures
    C1.2: Atlas posterior arch, axis isthmus, the base of odontoid process and axis fracture
    C1.3: Atlas posterior arch and odontoid process neck fracture
  C2: Bone and ligament injury
    C2.1: Base of odontoid process fracture and atlanto-axial dislocation (Dislocation gap less than the width of the odontoid (11 mm))
    C2.2: Base of odontoid process fracture and atlanto-axial dislocation (Dislocation gap greater than the width of the odontoid (11 mm))
    C2.3: Atlas fracture combined with lateral mass shift outward >7 mm
  C3: Ligament injury
    C3.1: Severe sprain, atlantoaxial anterior dislocation
    C3.2: Rotary subluxation
    C3.3: Atlantoaxial posterior dislocation

Three-Dimensional Simulation Fracture Images
Figures 11.85, 11.86, 11.87, 11.88, 11.89, 11.90, and 11.91.

3.1.2 Lower Cervical Spine Injuries: AO Classification

For lower cervical spine injury, the AO classification is divided into anterior injuries of the cervical spine (51-A), posterior injuries of the cervical spine (51-B), and compound injuries of the anterior and posterior cervical spine (51-C) [4–6].

Type A: Anterior injuries of the cervical spine
  A1: Fracture
    A1.1: Vertebral body uniform collapse fractures
    A1.2: Vertebral edge fractures with no obvious ligament injury
    A1.3: Wedge fracture with no obvious ligament injury
  A2: Bone and ligament injury
    A2.1: Vertebral comminuted fracture, involving one disc
    A2.2: Vertebral comminuted fracture, involving two discs
    A2.3: Vertebral comminuted fracture, the posterior wall is displaced by <3 mm or the posterior is not obviously damaged
  A3: Ligament injury
    A3.1: The anterior longitudinal ligament and intervertebral disc to tear off
    A3.2: Disc herniation
Type B: Posterior injuries of the cervical spine
  B1: Fracture
    B1.1: Posterior simple fracture
    B1.2: Non-displaced intervertebral joints fractures
    B1.3: Intervertebral joints fractures and posterior non-displaced fracture
  B2: Bone and ligament injury
    B2.1: Posterior fracture complicated with subluxation
    B2.2: Articular surface fracture
    B2.3: Broken of articular process
  B3: Ligament injury
    B3.1: Posterior ligament complex rupture with intervertebral joint subluxation (bilateral)
    B3.2: Posterior ligament complex rupture with intervertebral joint asymmetric subluxation (unilateral)
Type C: Compound injury of the anterior and posterior cervical spine
  C1: Fracture
    C1.1: Comminuted fracture of vertebral body with posterior fracture
    C1.2: Horizontal fractures of vertebral body with posterior fracture
  C2: Bone and ligament injury
    C2.1: Complete fracture dislocation with posterior fracture

Fig. 11.85 Type A

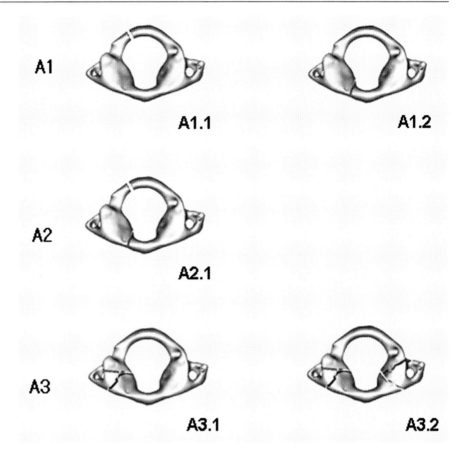

Fig. 11.86 Type B1

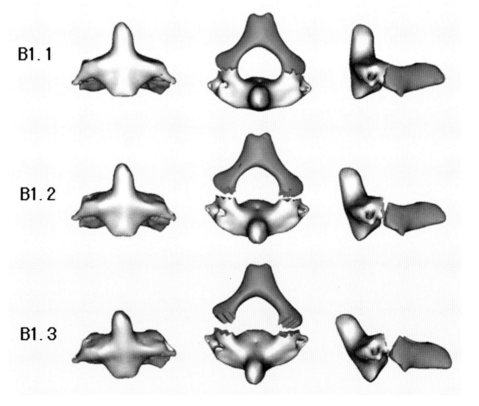

Fig. 11.87 Type B2

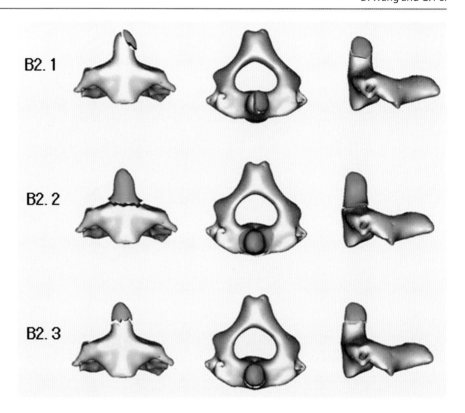

B2. 1

B2. 2

B2. 3

Fig. 11.88 Type B3

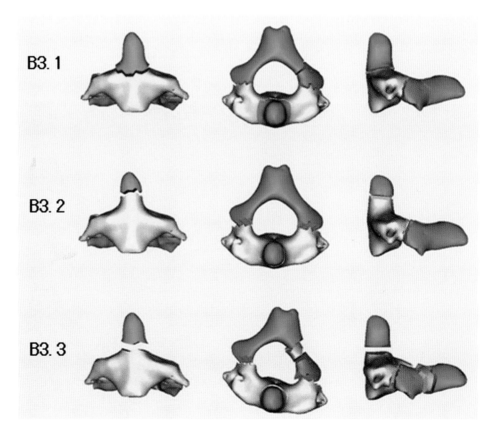

B3. 1

B3. 2

B3. 3

Fig. 11.89 Type C1

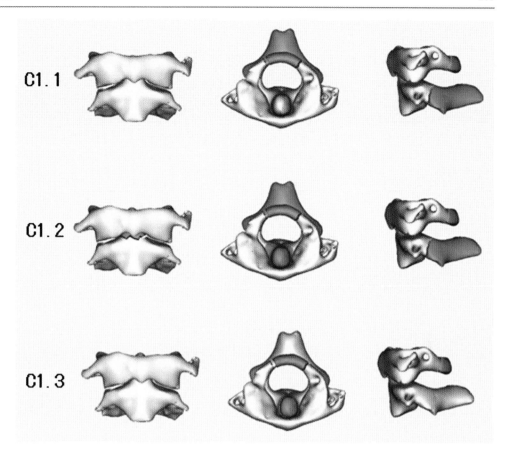

Fig. 11.90 Type C2

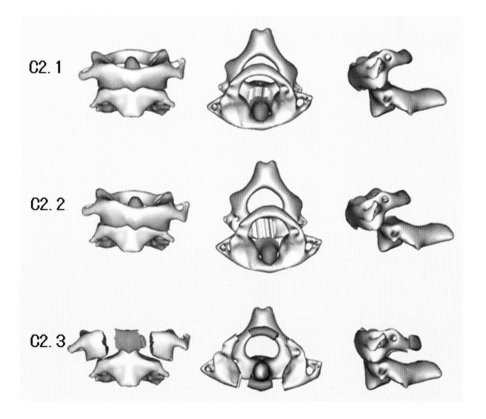

Fig. 11.91 Type C3

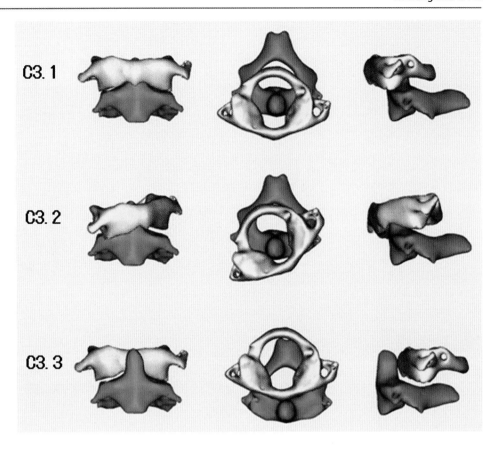

C2.2: Wedge fracture (>11°) and posterior ligament complex avulsion

C2.3: Spinal fracture (splitting up and posterior bone to the spinal canal >3 mm)

C3: Ligament injury

  C3.1: Simple dislocation, side locking (disc and posterior ligament complex avulsion)

  C3.2: Simple dislocation, double locking (disc and posterior ligament complex avulsion)

  C3.3: Posterior dislocation with disc and posterior ligament complex avulsion

Three-Dimensional Simulation Fracture Images

Figures 11.92, 11.93, and 11.94.

3.2 Thoracolumbar Vertebral Fractures: AO Classification

For thoracolumbar vertebral fractures, the AO classification can be divided into compression injuries of the body, distraction injuries of the anterior and posterior elements, and multidirectional injuries with translation affecting the anterior and posterior elements [2–4].

Type A: Compression injuries of the body

  A1: Impaction fractures

    A1.1 End plate impaction

    A1.2 Wedge impaction

    A1.3 Vertebral body collapse

Fig. 11.92   Type A

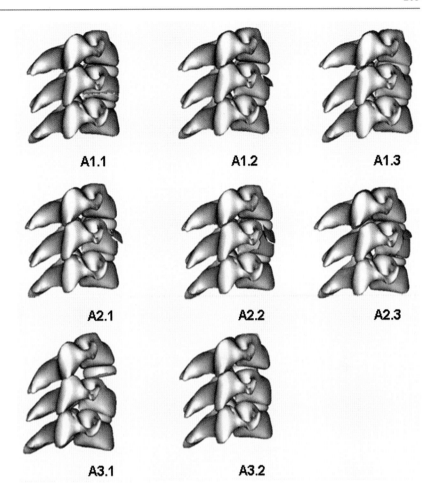

A1.1   A1.2   A1.3

A2.1   A2.2   A2.3

A3.1   A3.2

A2: Split fractures
    A2.1 Sagittal
    A2.2 Coronal
    A2.3 Pincer
A3: Burst fractures
    A3.1 Incomplete burst
    A3.2 Burst-split
    A3.3 Complete burst
Type B: Distraction injuries of the anterior and posterior elements (tensile forces)
    B1: Posterior disruption predominantly ligamentous (flexion-distraction injury)
        B1.1 With transverse disruption of the disc
        B1.2 Vertebral body compression fracture
    B2: Posterior disruption predominantly osseous (flexion-distraction injury)

B2.1 Transverse bicolumn fracture
B2.2 With transverse disruption of the disc
B2.3 With vertebral body compression
B3: Anterior disruption through the disc (hyperextension-shear injury)
    B3.1 Hyperextension-subluxation
    B3.2 Hyperextension-spondylolysis
    B3.3 Posterior dislocation
Type C: Multidirectional injuries with translation affecting the anterior and posterior elements (axial torque causing rotation injuries)
    C1: Rotational wedge, split, and burst fractures
        C1.1 Rotational wedge fractures
        C1.2 Rotational split fractures
        C1.3 Rotational burst fractures

Fig. 11.93 Type B

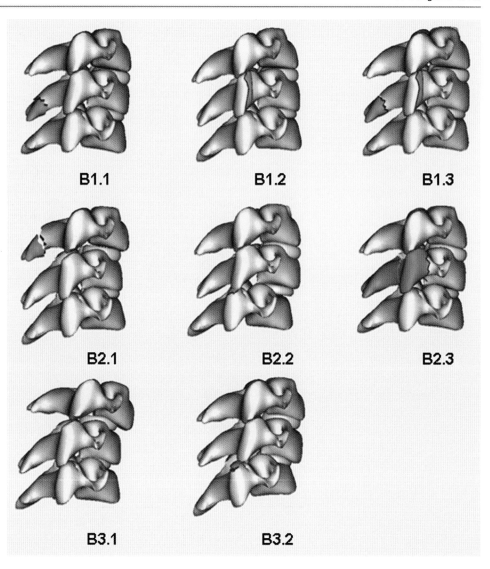

B1.1 B1.2 B1.3

B2.1 B2.2 B2.3

B3.1 B3.2

C2: Flexion subluxation with rotation
   C2.1 Flexion-distraction injuries with rotation
   C2.2 B2 with rotation
   C2.3 Hyperextension-shear-rotation of spine
C3: Rotational shear injuries (Holdsworth slice rotation fracture)
   C3.1 Slice
   C3.2 Oblique

3.2.1 Three-Dimensional Simulation Fracture Images

Figures 11.95, 11.96, 11.97, 11.98, 11.99, 11.100, 11.101, 11.102, 11.103, 11.104, 11.105, 11.106, 11.107, and 11.108.

Fig. 11.94 Type C

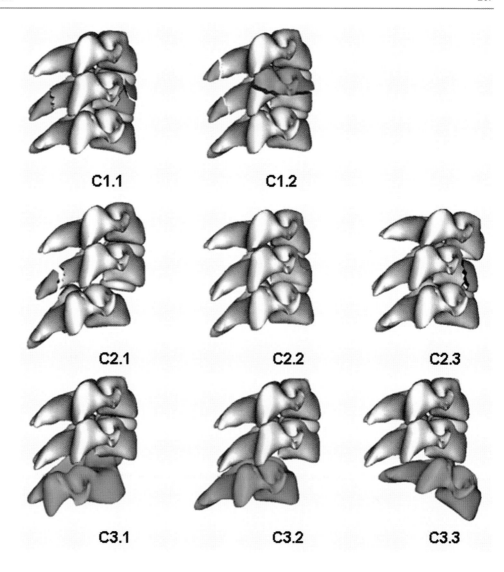

C1.1 C1.2

C2.1 C2.2 C2.3

C3.1 C3.2 C3.3

Fig. 11.95 A1

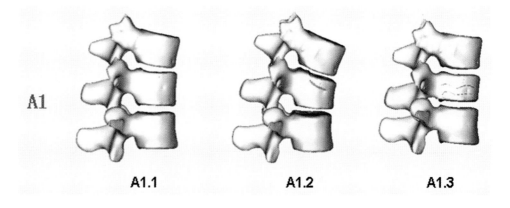

A1

A1.1 A1.2 A1.3

Fig. 11.96 A2

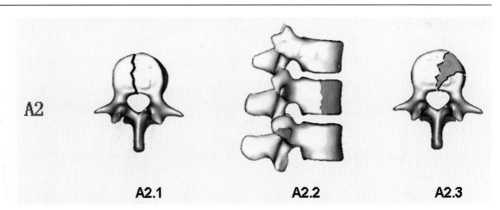

Fig. 11.97 A3

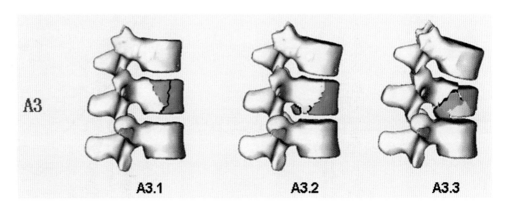

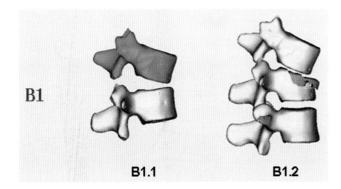

Fig. 11.98 B1

Fig. 11.99 B2

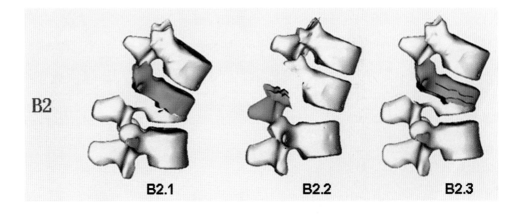

Fig. 11.100 B3

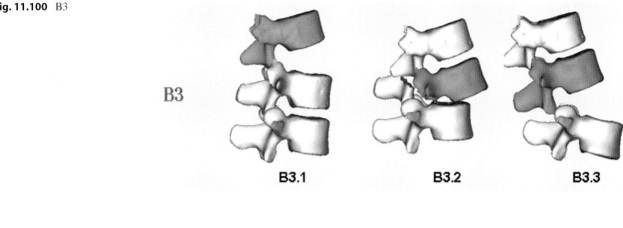

Fig. 11.101 C1.1

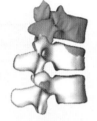

Fig. 11.102 C1.2

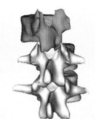
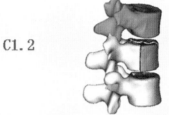
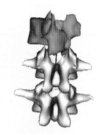
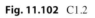

Fig. 11.103 C1.3

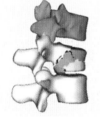
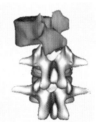

Fig. 11.104 C2.1

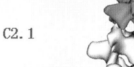
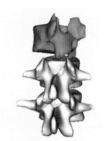

Fig. 11.105 C2.2

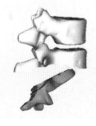
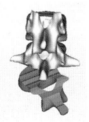

Fig. 11.106 C2.3

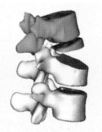
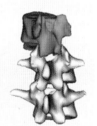

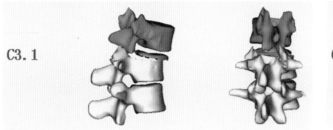

Fig. 11.107 C3.1

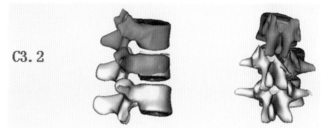

Fig. 11.108 C3.2

---

4 Pelvis and Acetabulum Digital Fracture Classification

4.1 Pelvic Fractures: Tile Classification

The pelvis is a ring structure, with three pieces of bone (two pieces of hip and one piece of sacrum) and three joints (on both sides of sacroiliac joint and pubic symphysis). The pelvic ring relies on ligaments for internal stability; the rear of sacroiliac ligament is the most important, being responsible for load-bearing functions. Pelvic stability refers to resisting deformation from normal physiological stress without exception, including vertical stability and rotational stability. Perpendicular to the direction of the ligaments against vertical shear force, the lateral lines of ligaments are against rotation. In 1988, the Tile classification was proposed based on the injury mechanism and pelvic stability from radiology to determine prognosis and treatment options [2–5].

Type A: Stable
  Type A1: Fractures of the pelvis not involving the ring; avulsion injuries
  Type A2: Stable, minimally displaced fractures of the ring
Type B: Rotationally unstable, vertically stable
  Type B1: Open-book
  Type B2: Lateral compression; ipsilateral
  Type B3: Lateral compression; contralateral (bucket handle)
Type C: Rotationally and vertically unstable
  Type C1: Unilateral
  Type C2: Bilateral; one side rotationally unstable, with contralateral side vertically unstable
  Type C3: Associated acetabular fracture

4.1.1 Three-Dimensional Simulation Fracture Images

Figures 11.109, 11.110, 11.111, 11.112, 11.113, 11.114, 11.115, 11.116, and 11.117.

4.2 Acetabulum Fractures: Letournel–Judet Classification

For acetabulum fractures, the Letournel–Judet classification is widely applied in the clinic. Judet put forward the concept of the two-column acetabulum fracture and its classification in 1964. Letournel made further improvements in 1980, then created the current classification system. The classification of acetabulum fractures can be divided into five simple types and complex types (joint). The simple types include posterior wall fractures, posterior column fractures, anterior wall fractures, anterior column fractures, and transverse fractures. The complex types include posterior column and posterior wall fractures, transverse and posterior wall fractures, T-shaped fractures, anterior column fractures, posterior hemitransverse fractures, and two-column fractures [2–4].

Elementary patterns
  1. Posterior wall
  2. Posterior column
  3. Anterior wall
  4. Anterior column
  5. Transverse
Associated patterns
  1. Posterior column and posterior wall
  2. Transverse and posterior wall
  3. T-shaped
  4. Anterior column: Posterior hemitransverse
  5. Both columns

Fig. 11.109   Type A1

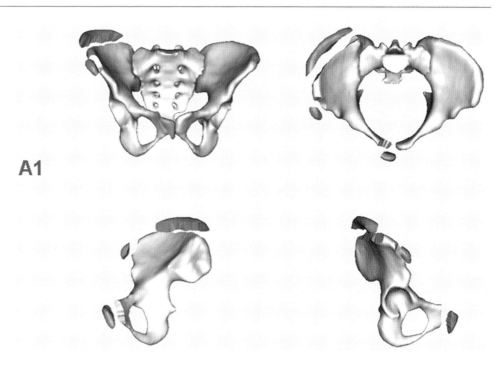

A1

Fig. 11.110   Type A2

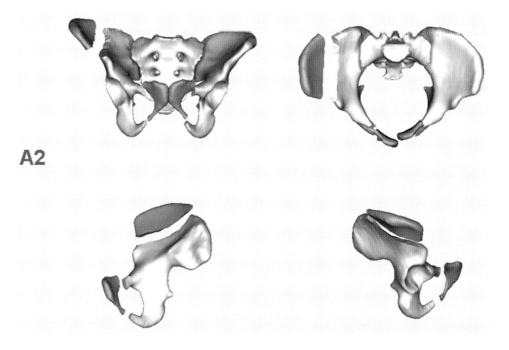

A2

Fig. 11.111 Type A3

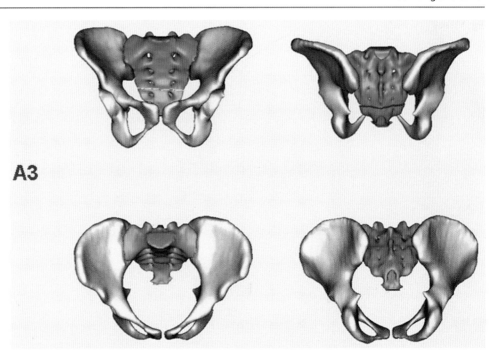

Fig. 11.112 Type B1

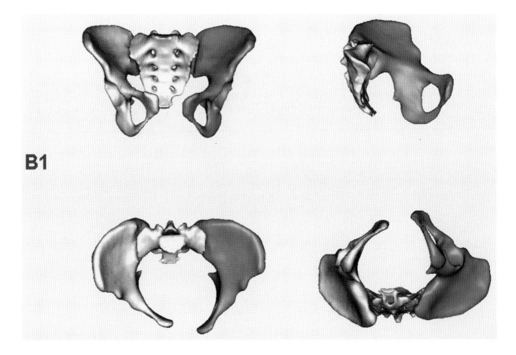

Fig. 11.113 Type B2

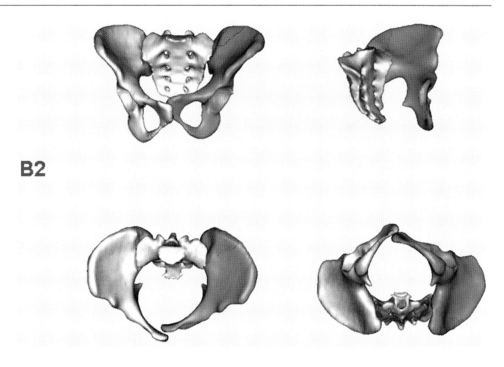

B2

Fig. 11.114 Type B3

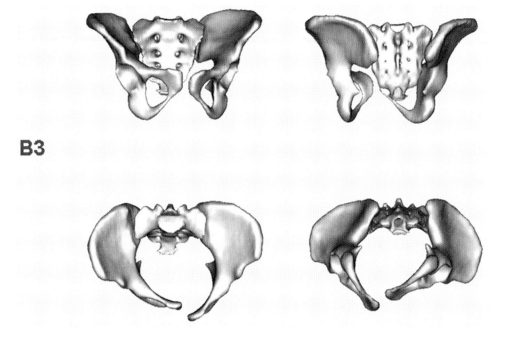

B3

Fig. 11.115 Type C1

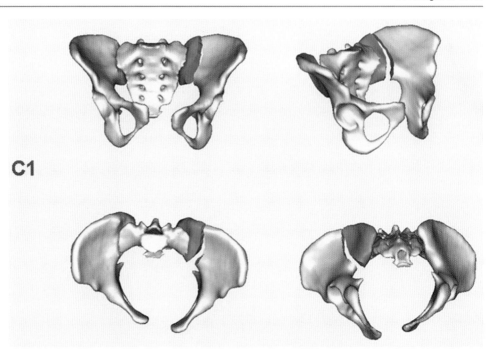

Fig. 11.116 Type C2

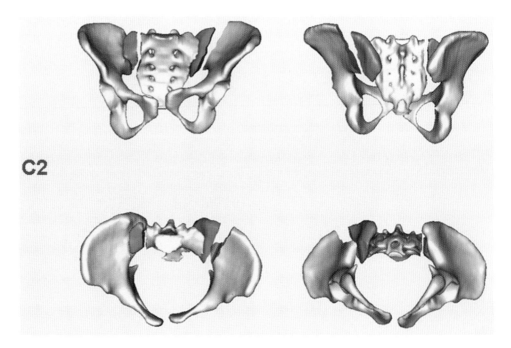

Fig. 11.117 Type C3

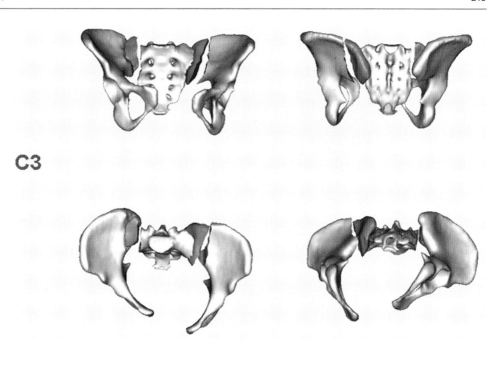

Fig. 11.118 Posterior wall
fracture

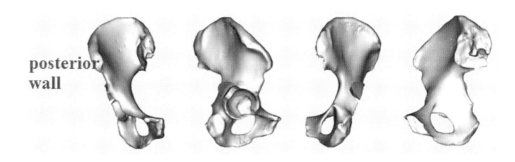

4.2.1   Three-Dimensional Simulation Fracture Images
Figures 11.118, 11.119, 11.120, 11.121, 11.122, 11.123, 11.124, 11.125, 11.126, and 11.127.

4.3   Sacral Fractures: Denis Classification

In 1988, sacrum fractures were divided into three types according to their different anatomical locations by Denis. The system is relatively simple, practical, and very helpful to determine whether sacral nerve injury has occurred. It has been recognized as a typing method [4–6].

Type I: Fracture of sacrum wing area. Fracture through the sacral wing, no sacral foramen and sacral canal injury

Type II: Fracture of sacral foramen. Fracture through one or a plurality of sacral foramina, involving the sacral wing, but not involving the sacral canal

Type III: Sacral canal fractures, fracture through the sacral canal, involving the sacrum wing and sacral foramen, transverse sacral fractures also belong to the type, fracture line through the three districts

4.3.1   Three-Dimensional Simulation Fracture Images
Figures 11.128, 11.129, and 11.130.

Fig. 11.119 Posterior column fracture

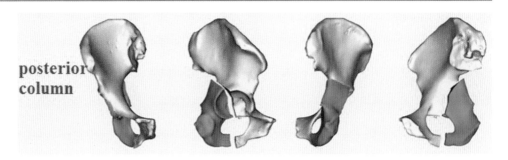

Fig. 11.120 Anterior wall fracture

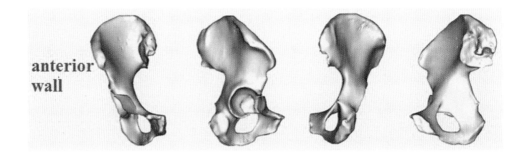

Fig. 11.121 Anterior column fractures

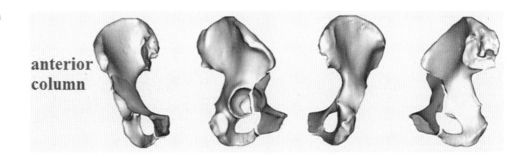

Fig. 11.122 Transverse fracture

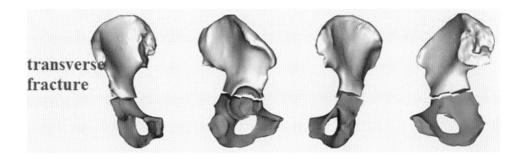

Fig. 11.123 Posterior column and posterior wall fracture

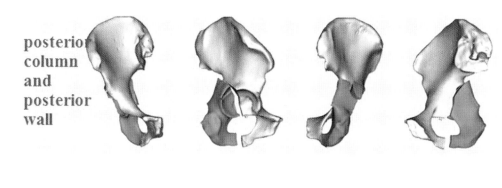

Fig. 11.124 Transverse and posterior wall fracture

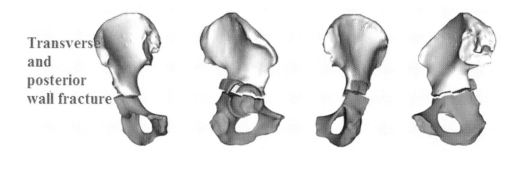

Fig. 11.125 T-shaped fracture

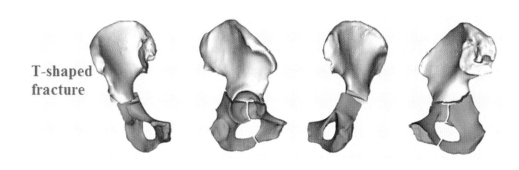

Fig. 11.126 Anterior column and posterior hemitransverse fracture

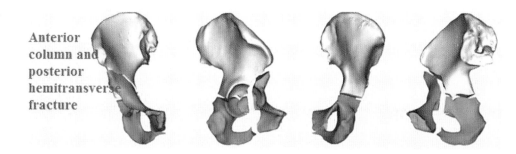

Fig. 11.127 Two-column fracture

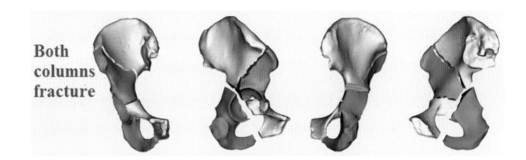

Fig. 11.128 Type I

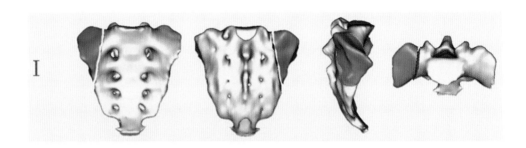

Fig. 11.129 Type II

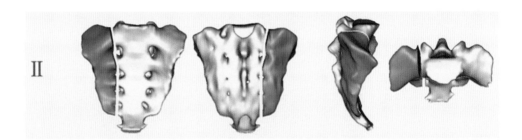

Fig. 11.130 Type III

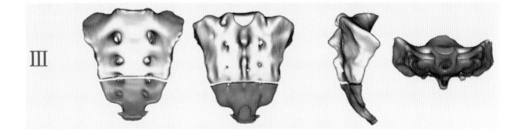

5   Lower Limb Digital Fracture Classification

5.1   Femoral Fractures: AO Classification

Femoral neck fractures were classified into slightly displaced subcapital femoral neck fractures (31-B1), transcervical fractures (31-B2), and significantly displaced subcapital femoral neck fractures (31-B3) [2, 4, 5].

Type B1: Slightly displaced subcapital femoral neck fractures
B1.1: Impacted in valgus ≥15°, (1) posterior tilt <15°, (2) posterior tilt >15°

B1.2: Impacted in valgus <15°, (1) posterior tilt <15°, (2) posterior tilt >15°

B1.3: Nonimpacted

Type B2: Transcervical fracture

    B2.1: Basicervical

    B2.2: Midcervical adduction

    B2.3: Midcervical shear

Type B3: Significantly displaced subcapital femoral neck fractures

    B3.1: Moderate displacement in varus and external rotation

B3.2: Moderate displacement with vertical translation and external rotation

B3.3: Marked displacement: (1) in varus; (2) with translation

5.1.1   Three-Dimensional Simulation Fracture Images

Figures 11.131, 11.132, 11.133, 11.134, 11.135, 11.136, 11.137, 11.138, and 11.139.

Fig. 11.131 Type B1.1

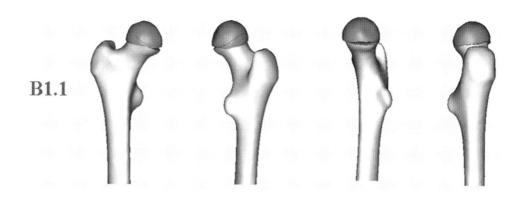

Fig. 11.132 Type B1.2

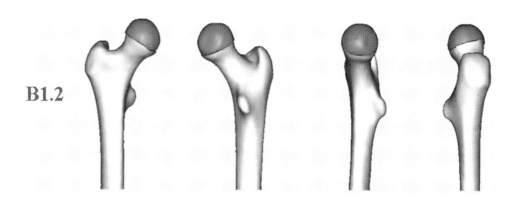

Fig. 11.133 Type B1.3

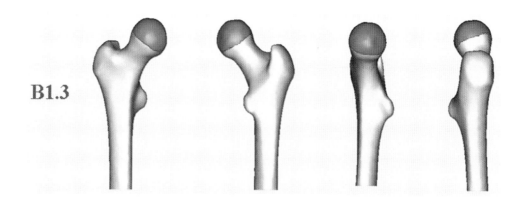

Fig. 11.134 Type B2.1

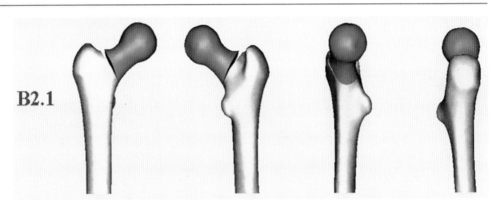

Fig. 11.135 Type B2.2

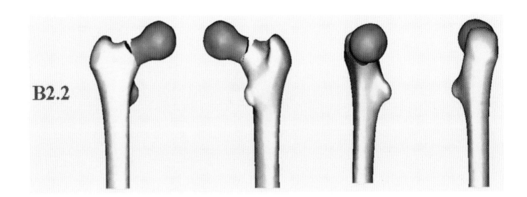

Fig. 11.136 Type B2.3

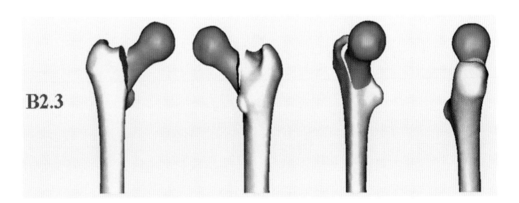

Fig. 11.137 Type B3.1

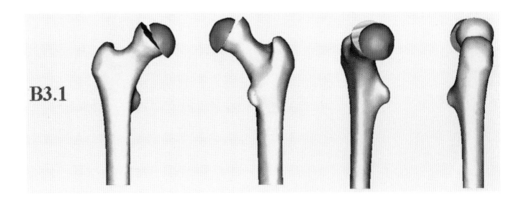

Fig. 11.138 Type B3.2

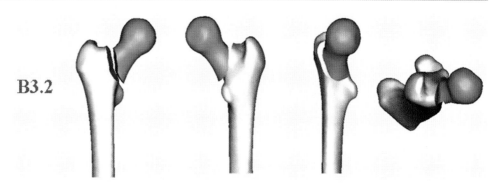

Fig. 11.139 Type B3.3

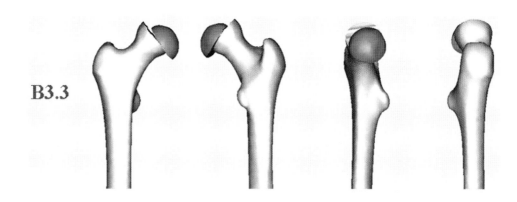

5.2 Tibia and Fibula Fractures: Schatzker Classification

For tibial plateau fractures, the Schatzker classification was proposed by Schatzker and other scholars in 1979. It is simple and practical, emphasizing the accuracy of local feature changes in tibial plateau fractures. Each type corresponds to a clear surgical option and clinical practicality is very strong. According to the type of fracture, physicians can determine a surgical approach, reduction method, and internal fixation. The Schatzker fracture classification of tibial plateau fractures is divided into six types based on the degree of injury, which increases from type I to type VI [1, 3, 5].

Type I: Lateral plateau, split fracture
Type II: Lateral plateau, split depression fracture
Type III: Lateral plateau, depression fracture
Type IV: Medial plateau fracture
Type V: Bicondylar plateau fracture
Type VI: Plateau fracture with metaphyseal-diaphyseal dissociation

5.2.1 Three-Dimensional Simulation Fracture Images

Figures 11.140, 11.141, 11.142, 11.143, 11.144, and 11.145.

5.3 Ankle Fractures: Lauge-Hansen Classification

Ankle fractures can be divided into according to their anatomical classification: medial malleolus fractures, lateral malleolus fractures, and posterior malleolus fracture. In addition, according to the severity of the fracture, they can be divided into single ankle fractures, double ankle fractures, and triple ankle fractures. In 1950, Lauge-Hansen classified ankle fractures based on cadaver studies, combined with clinical and X-ray observations. According to the position of the injured foot and direction of the talus in the ankle by external force, ankle joint fractures can be divided as follows: supination-external rotation (SER), pronation-external rotation (PER), supination-adduction (SA), and pronation-abduction (PA). The Lauge-Hansen classification method

Fig. 11.140 Type I

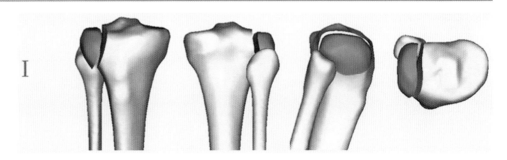

Fig. 11.141 Type II

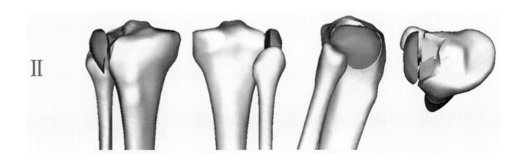

Fig. 11.142 Type III

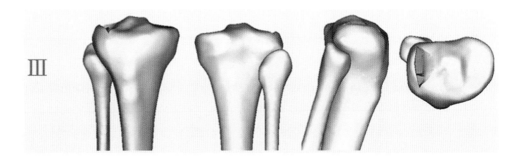

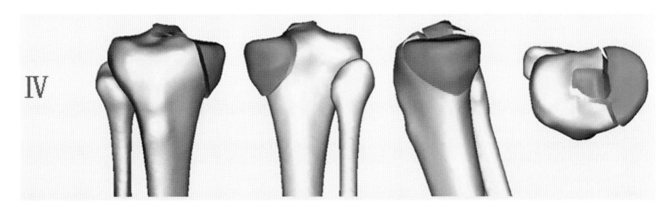

Fig. 11.143 Type IV

Fig. 11.144 Type V

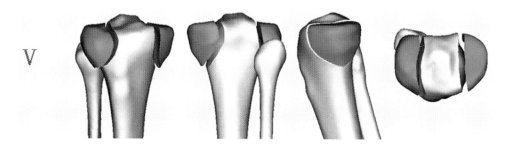

Fig. 11.145 Type VI

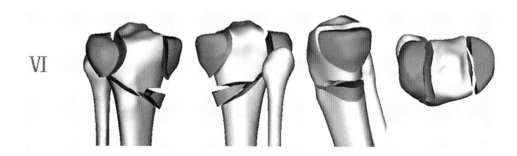

can be used in the treatment of the fracture. Because it emphasizes ligament damage and correctly estimates the severity of the injury, it is conducive to choosing a clinical treatment. Approximately 95% of clinical ankle fractures can be classified using this system [2–5].

Type I: Supination-external rotation (SER)
  Stage I: Disruption of the anterior tibiofibular ligament with or without an associated avulsion fracture at its tibial or fibular attachment
  Stage II: Spiral fracture of the distal fibula, which runs anteroinferiorly to posterosuperiorly
  Stage III: Disruption of the posterior tibiofibular ligament or a fracture of the posterior malleolus
  Stage IV: Transverse avulsion-type fracture of the medial malleolus or a rupture of the deltoid ligament
Type II: Pronation-external rotation (PER)
  Stage I: Transverse fracture of the medial malleolus or a rupture of the deltoid ligament
  Stage II: Disruption of the anterior tibiofibular ligament with or without an avulsion fracture at its insertion sites
  Stage III: Short oblique fracture of the distal fibula at or above the level of the syndesmosis
  Stage IV: Rupture of the posterior tibiofibular ligament or an avulsion fracture of the posterolateral tibia
Type III: Supination-adduction (SA)
  Stage I: Transverse avulsion-type fracture of the fibula distal to the level of the joint or a rupture of the lateral collateral ligaments

Stage II: Vertical fracture of medial malleolus
Type IV: Pronation-abduction (PA)
  Stage I: Transverse fracture of the medial malleolus or a rupture of the deltoid ligament
  Stage II: Rupture of the syndesmotic ligaments or an avulsion fracture at their insertions
  Stage III: Transverse or short oblique fracture of the distal fibula at or above the level of the syndesmosis

5.3.1   Three-Dimensional Simulation Fracture Images
Figures 11.146, 11.147, 11.148, and 11.149.

5.4   Foot Fractures

Talus fractures can be divided into central compartment fractures (head, neck, and body) and peripheral fractures. The blood supply of a central compartment fracture of the talus is larger if accompanied by dislocation; it almost always has ischemic necrosis of the bone.

5.4.1   Talar Neck Fractures: Hawkins Classification
In 1970, Hawkins proposed a classification system according to the location of the talus fracture, displacement of the ankle, and subtalar joint degree to determine the level of fracture of the talus neck (using three levels). In 1978, Canale and Kelly added a fourth type [2, 5, 6].

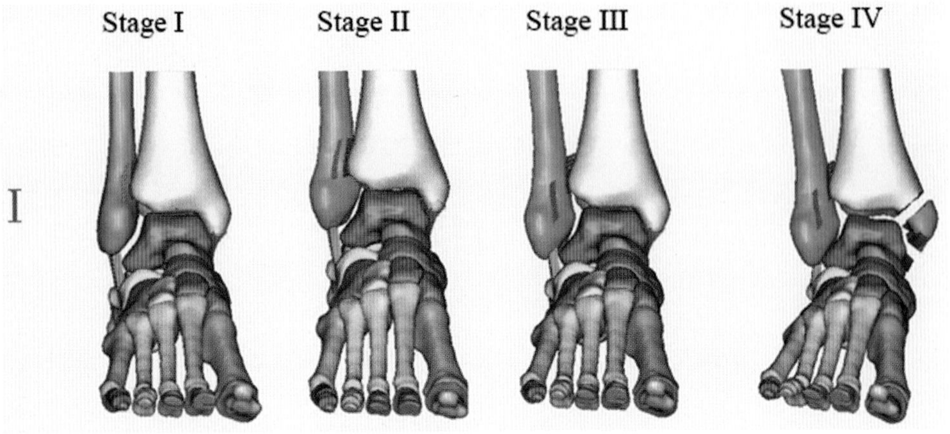

Fig. 11.146 Type I

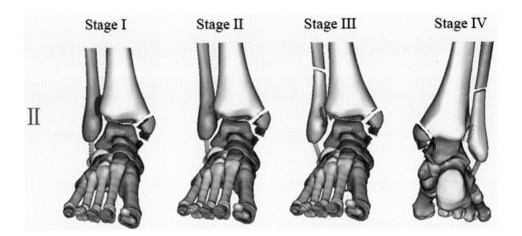

Fig. 11.147 Type II

Fig. 11.148 Type III

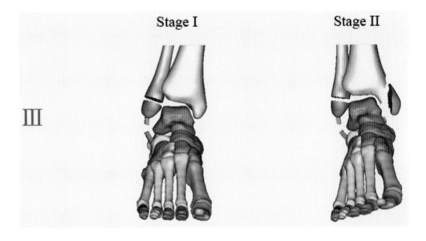

Fig. 11.149   Type IV

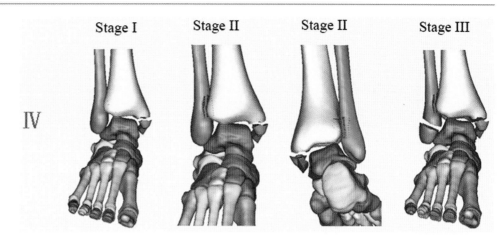

Fig. 11.150   Type I

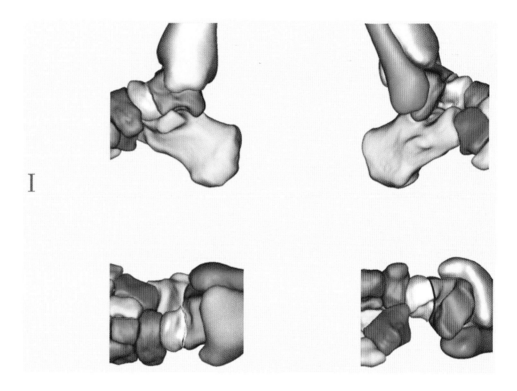

Type I: Vertical talus neck fracture, no displacement, mild blood circulation disorders, ischemia necrosis rate is less than 10%.

Type II: Vertical talus neck fracture, talus from subtalar joint subluxation or dislocation, ischemia necrosis rate is less than 40%.

Type III: Vertical talus neck fracture, the talus body dislocation from the ankle and subtalar joint, open injury, ischemic necrosis occurred rate is more than 90%.

Type IV (Canale and Kelley): Type III with associated talonavicular subluxation or dislocation, open injury; ischemic necrosis occurs in 100%.

Three-Dimensional Simulation Fracture Images

Figures 11.150, 11.151, 11.152, and 11.153.

Fig. 11.151 Type II

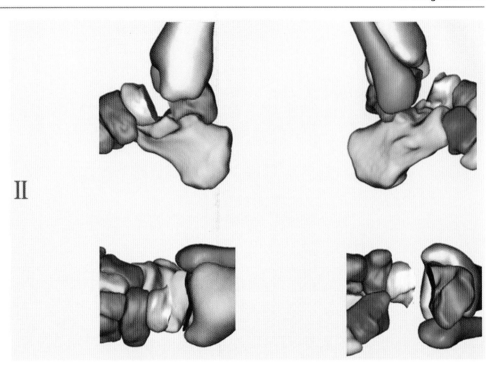

Fig. 11.152 Type III

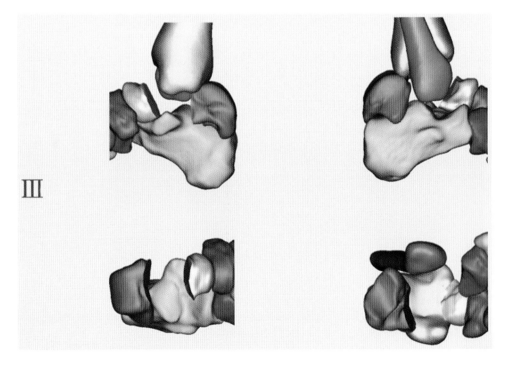

Fig. 11.153 Type IV

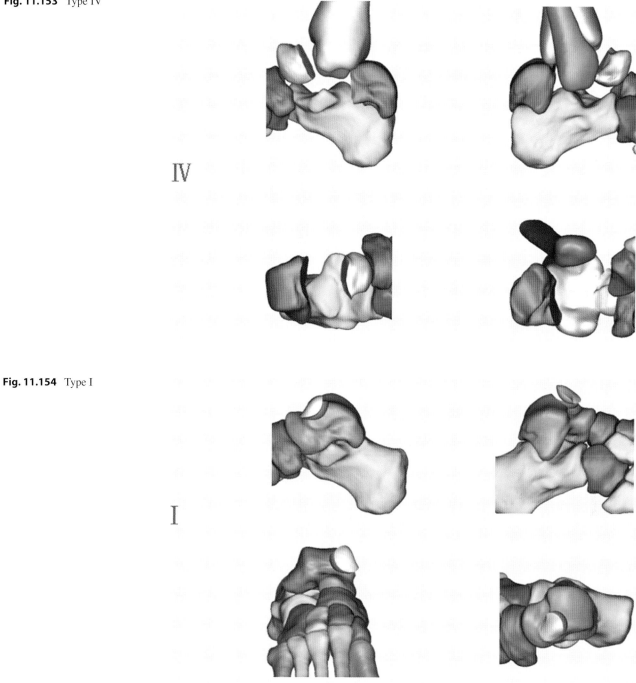

Fig. 11.154 Type I

5.4.2   Talar Body Fractures: Sneppen Classification

In 1977, Sneppen divided talus body fractures into six types according to location and fracture line direction. Talus body fractures are intra-articular fractures involving the tibiotalar joint and talocalcaneal joint [4–6].

Type I: Superior articular surface of talus body compression fractures

Type II: The talus body coronal shear fractures
Type III: The talus body sagittal shear fractures
Type IV: Posterior tubercle of talus fracture
Type V: Processus lateralis of talus fracture
Type VI: Compression comminuted fracture of talus body

Three-Dimensional Simulation Fracture Images
Figures 11.154, 11.155, 11.156, 11.157, 11.158, and 11.159.

Fig. 11.155 Type II

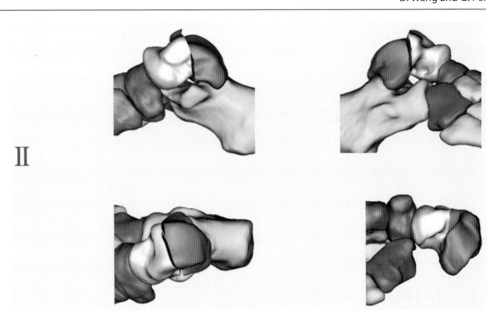

Fig. 11.156 Type III

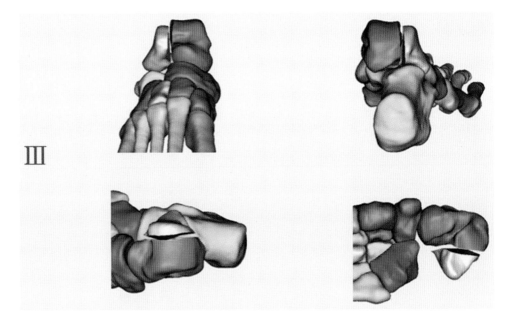

Fig. 11.157 Type IV

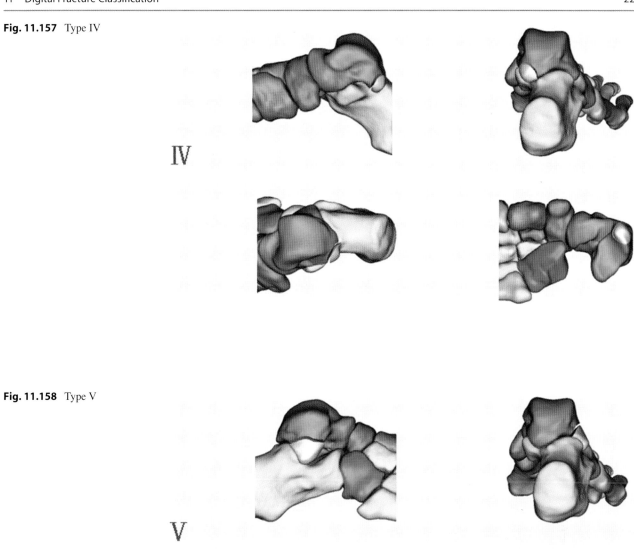

IV

Fig. 11.158 Type V

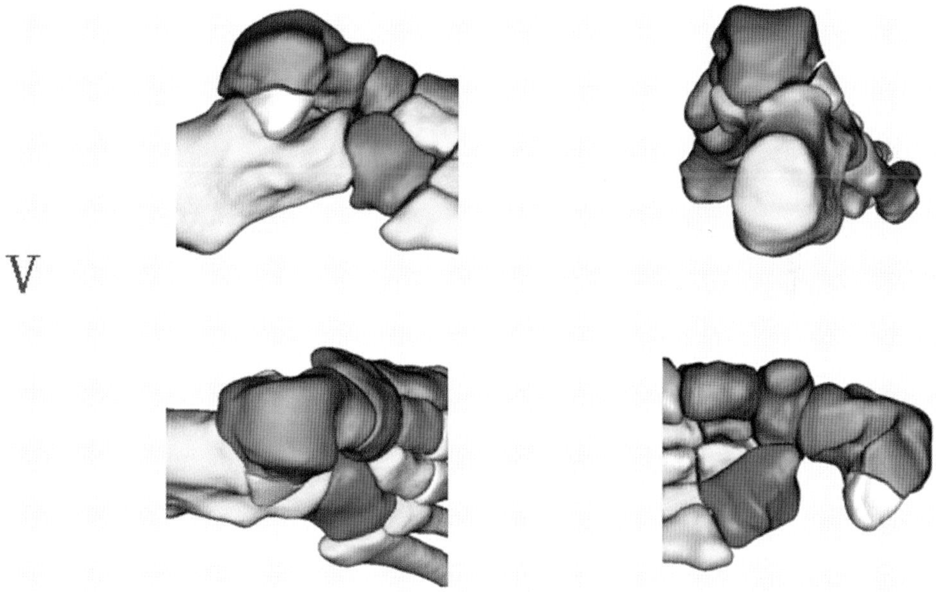

V

Fig. 11.159 Type VI

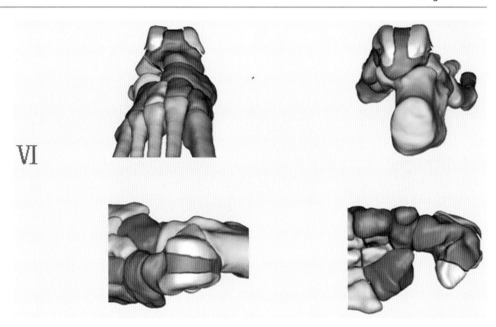

References

1. Schatzker J, McBroom R, Bruce D. The tibial plateau fracture: the Toronto experience. Clin Orthop Relat Res. 1999;138:94–104.
2. Pei G. Digital fracture classification. 1st ed. Beijing: People's Medical Publishing House; 2010. p. 1–2.
3. Seyed BM. Fracture classifications in clinical practice. 6th ed. London: Springer; 2005. p. 10–13, 19, 35, 38, 58, 62, 67
4. Zhang S, Li H, Huang Y. Fracture classification and functional evaluation. 1st ed. Beijing: People's Military Medical Press; 2008. p. 41–98, 143, 205
5. Zhang C, Shi H. Fracture classification manual. 1st ed. Beijing: People's Medical Publishing House; 2008. p. 28–30, 130–132
6. Zhixiong L. Common diagnostic classification methods and functional evaluation criteria in orthopedics. 1st ed. Beijing: Beijing Science and Technology Press; 2005. p. 53–7, 139–41

Xie Le, Guolin Meng, Long Bi, Jian Liu, Yuanzhi Zhang,
Sheng Lu, Yongqing Xu, Zhigang Wu, Jun Fu, and Zhi Yuan

1 Concept of Rapid Prototyping

Guolin Meng

The traditional manufacturing model concerns a single species in large quantities with long production cycles. With the progress of modern scientific technology, manufacturing model transfer to more species in small quantities with short production cycles becomes possible. How to satisfy the demands of the market quickly has become one of the important directions of modern manufacturing. With the development of computer, microelectronics, informatization, automation, new materials, and modern enterprise management technology, many new manufacturing techniques and models have been produced. Rapid prototyping (RP) technology, which was born in the 1960s, has made its progress under such kind of background.

1.1 The Development of RP Technology

Rapid prototyping technology is one kind of manufacturing methods of accumulating the materials layer by layer or point by point. The early thoughts of layered manufacturing first appeared in the nineteenth century, at which time the manufacturing technology was much underdeveloped. Blanther suggested that 3D map models could be produced layer by layer in 1892. 1n 1979, Nakagawa of Tokyo University produced metal blanking mold, model dies, and injection mold using layered techniques. The development of lithography technology has the catalytic effect on the appearance of modern rapid prototyping. From the end of 1970s to early 1980s, Alan J. Hebert of 3M company of the USA in 1978, Kodama of Japan in 1980, Charles W. Hull of UVP company of the USA in 1982, and Maruya of Japan in 1983 put forward the concept of rapid prototyping independently, i.e., the idea of using selection of continuous layers to produce three-dimensional entities. Charles W. Hull successfully developed one complete system, stereolithography apparatus (SLA-1), which could construct parts automatically. This was one milestone in the development of RP technology. Charles W. Hull together with shareholders of UVP established 3D system company in the same year. Many new concepts and technologies associated with RP were developed gradually, and many other kinds of prototyping principles and machines also developed at the same period. In 1984, Michael Feygin put forward the method of laminated object manufacturing (LOM). He then established Helisys Company in 1985 and developed the first business model LOW-1015 in 1990. Since the first SLA prototyping model developed in the 1980s to now, many RP technologies have been enabled, but SLA, LOM, selective laser sintering (SLS), and fused deposition modeling (FDM) are still the mainstream of RP technology.

1.2 Basic Prototyping Principles of RP Technology

RP technology is the integration of computer-aided design (CAD) and related manufacturing technology, reverse engineering technology, solid freeform fabrication (SFF), and

X. Le (✉)
The National Center of Digitizational Manufacture Technique, Shanghai Jiaotong University, Shanghai, China

G. Meng · L. Bi · J. Liu · Z. Wu · J. Fu · Z. Yuan
Department of Orthopedics, The First Affiliated Hospital of Air Force Military Medical University, Shaanxi, China
e-mail: menggl@fmmu.edu.cn; bilong@fmmu.edu.cn

Y. Zhang
Department of Orthopedics, Affiliated Hospital of Inner Mongolia Medical University, Hohhot, China

S. Lu · Y. Xu
Department of Orthopedics, Kunming General Hospital of Chengdu Military Area Command, Kunming, China

material removal process (MRP) or material augmentation process (MAP). Simply, RP technology is the kind of technology of producing entity prototype by accumulating the materials layer by layer using 3D CAD data.

There are many kinds of prototyping techniques in RP technology. SLA, SLS, LOM, FDM, and 3D printing (3DP) are the many kinds of methods much more used. These techniques are based on material accumulation prototyping principles, connected with the physiochemical characteristics of the material and advanced technology methods. The development of these techniques is also closely related with other subjects.

1.2.1 Stereolithography Apparatus (SLA)

Stereolithography apparatus (SLA) is one kind of RP technique that is most widely used at the moment, with most mature technology and most thorough research. Photosensitive resin is always used as the material in SLA. The computer-controlled ultraviolet laser scans alone the orbit of the contour of each cross section of the predetermined parts point by point. Light polymerization occurs at the thin layer resin at the scanned area, and the thin layer cross section of the parts is formed. When one layer cross section is solidified, the workbench is moved so that a new layer of liquid resin could be attached to it, waiting for the next scan and solidification. The new solidified layer is tightly adhered to the front layer. The process is repeated until the production of the prototype parts is finished.

1.2.2 Laminated Object Manufacturing (LOM)

In the technique of LOM, papers coated with hot glue were adhered tightly using heat rolls. The laser beam irradiated from the laser generator cut the paper into the contour of the determined parts according to the cross-sectional model's CAD data. Another layer of paper was then added and tightly adhered to it using a hot-press device. The laser beam cut the paper and then adhered again. The process is repeated until the production of the total parts model is finished.

1.2.3 Selective Laser Sintering (SLS)

CO_2 laser is always used as the energy in the technique of SLS. A thin layer of powder could be spread evenly over the working bench. Laser beam sinters the powder according to the section contour of each layer of the parts controlled by the computer. One layer sintered after the other. When the total sintering is finished, the redundant powder could be cleaned; after polishing and drying, part models could be acquired. The materials used in mature technology are always wax powder and molding powder at the moment.

1.2.4 Fused Deposition Modeling (FDM)

In the technique of FDM, filamentous materials could be placed in the spray through feeding devices and then heated to melting state. The melting filamentous materials could be sprayed on the workbench according to the contour of the

cross sections of the parts that were predetermined and then be cooled and solidified rapidly. The spray increased one layer's height after one time spraying to the next spraying until the total parts prototype is finished.

1.2.5 Three-Dimensional Printing (3DP)

The operational principle of 3DP is just like ink jet printing. Liquid agglomerant could be sprayed on special area prespread with powder according to cross-sectional data of the parts predetermined. The workbench then decreased a height, and the powder is spread again, and agglomerant is sprayed according to the cross-sectional data. The process is repeated until the needed 3D geometry is acquired. The acquired 3D geometry then could be solidified using high-sintering methods and the needed parts could be achieved.

1.3 Characteristics of RP Technology

1.3.1 Rapidity

RP technology has overcome many shortcomings of traditional manufacturing, such as too many intermediate links, too long period, and high cost. The manufacturing period could save 70% compared with that of traditional techniques. It is especially true when manufacturing complex parts, which is incomparable.

1.3.2 Lower Cost

The cost of the RP product has nothing to do with the complexity. The manufacturing cost could be decreased about 50%. It is especially suitable to the development of new products and the production of small batch parts.

1.3.3 Wide Selection of Materials

Material selection is not limited in RP technology. Not only metallic materials but also lots of nonmetallic materials could be selected accordingly. Prototypes made of resins, plastics, papers, paraffin wax, compounded materials, metals, and ceramics all could be acquired.

1.3.4 High Adaptability

Parts with different figures could be produced using RP technology. The manufacturing technique has nothing to do with the complexity of the parts and is not limited by the facilities. The prototype has high interconvertibility and could be copied.

1.3.5 High Modifiability

In RP technology, the producing method of noncontact processing is selected without any kinds of tool clips. Parts and prototypes with much precision and strength, which could be satisfied with certain function, could be prototyped rapidly. If the parts waiting to be produced need to be repaired, the CAD data needs to be fixed. This is especially suitable to the production of small batch parts.

1.3.6   Highly Integrated

RP technology is one kind of integrated developed manufacturing technology including computer, digital control, laser, material, and mechanics. The total manufacturing processing has realized automation and digitization. What you see is what you get. Parts could be repaired or produced at all times. The design and manufacturing integration has been realized under RP technology.

2   Applications of Rapid Prototyping Technology

Long Bi

2.1   Applications of Rapid Prototyping Technology in Manufacturing Individualized Graft Materials

Rapid prototyping technology (RP technology) was applied in computer-assisted manufacturing engineering of solid models. After it was otherwise applied in biomedicine, the three carriages—modern computer-assisted design (CAD), computer-assisted manufacturing (CAM) and rapid prototyping-based solid model (RPSM)—are going hand in hand, playing an important role in complicated fracture diagnosis, surgical-aided design and manufacturing of materials for prosthesis implantation, and other aspects. In recent years, along with the constant updating and improvement of hardware and software systems, the superiority of RP technology in individualized graft manufacturing has been increasingly apparent.

In the fields of orthopedic surgery as well as oral and maxillofacial surgery and neurosurgery, individualized grafts mainly refer to those prosthetic grafts used to replace the structure of damaged or diseased tissues and organs to restore the appearance or function. Compared with the current conventional methods to manufacture prosthetic grafts, RP technology may formulate the appearance and structure features of the tissues and organs to be replaced more accurately, and the RP-constructed prostheses and local structures may fit more in the anatomic aspects. Meanwhile, since the structure fits more, it may simplify the processing to local structures and reduce operation time and operational injuries to normal tissues. Concerning orthopedic and cosmetic operations, it is easier to control sizes of RP-based prostheses to improve postoperative aesthetics and reduce postoperative complications.

On the other hand, since most damaged or diseased tissues and organs requiring prostheses have lost their original anatomic structures or deformed or worn, it is impossible to obtain the raw data and information for PR-based prostheses. To this end, we usually adopt digital modeling and other methods with the mirroring-transferred data of the unaffected side and local structure of the affected side to repair the data of damaged or worn structures of the affected side for previously normal local anatomic structure of the affected side. To achieve the above goal, we need to complete an individualized reverse engineering (RE) design for prosthetic grafts based on morphological data obtained to provide the data for the subsequence process of RP-based prosthesis manufacturing. Therefore, to an extent, the process of individualized RP-based graft manufacturing is actually a combination of RE technology and RP technology.

For now, individualized RP-based grafts are mainly manufactured in the following three ways: individualized RP-based grafts by solid modeling of bones, individualized RP model-based grafts, and direct individualized RP-based grafts. The three ways are supplement and complement each other, which have provided important technical support for the design, construction, and clinical transformation of individualized grafts. Here are introductions to these ways.

2.1.1   Individualized RP-Based Grafts by Solid Modeling of Bones

The so-called individualized RP-based grafts by solid modeling of bones is, firstly, to produce the solid models for the bones and surrounding tissues of the site to be grafted with a RP-based molding machine; secondly, to define the anatomic structure features of the solid part based on the measurements of the solid model; thirdly, to construct the prototype of the grafts in line with the anatomic features of the solid part of the site to be grafted by way of perfusion, sintering, forging, grinding, and other conventional methods; and, finally, to observe how well the prototype fits the solid model and make final adjustments to the graft so as to obtain individualized grafts satisfying the treatment of different clinical patients. Antony et al. have constructed prosthesis models for hip joints in the way of individualized RP-based grafts by solid modeling of bones. It is proved by experiments that the model may well adapt anatomical features of the graft site. Meanwhile, due to the presence of the solid model which allows simulation of the operative procedure, it also improves the accuracy of operation and reduces the rate of accidental injuries to nonsurgical sites. Studies show the superiority of this way lies in the simulation of solid-based model of the site to be grafted, and the structure features of grafts produced this way may better meet the requirements of individualized treatment. Owing to the presence of the solid model, we can adjust and experience the product, predict the clinical effects, and avoid postoperative risks by continuous implantation experiments. Meanwhile, owing to the conventional methods used in the manufacturing process, the product strength this is stronger than direct PR technology-manufactured products—prostheses that are more applicable to weight-bearing parts. Without doubt, the way is limited to the assistance of conventional construction methods. Therefore, it also presents the same drawbacks as conventional construction methods—longtime, large demand for raw materials—and repeats attempts to achieve individualized features.

2.1.2 RP Model-Based Grafts

The so-called RP model-based grafts is actually a way of indirect molding method, that is, firstly, to conduct a contralateral imaging scan to the site to be grafted and obtain the bone structure of the affected site by software; secondly, to make the prototype with manufacturing-friendly materials by using RP technology; thirdly, to construct the model required by metal grafts using the prototype as the master pattern or mold core by conventional molding technologies; and, finally, to construct the individualized grafts in line with site features of patients by pouring metal raw materials in the grinding tools. Teng Yong et al. have designed artificial articular surface based on data obtained by spiral CT scan of external surface of femoral condylar of patients with bone tumor and hemi-articular surface of other people. They made the resin model by RP technology first, then built the master mode, and finally molded the prosthesis based on the master mode with titanium alloy and applied the bulk recombination of the allogeneic bone graft to distal femur for limb reconstruction after excision of tumor. The results showed that individualized artificial femoral condyle prosthesis fitted allograft bone and contralateral joint well and significantly improved the keen joint functions of patients with semi-allogeneic transplant; and the wearing of the contralateral unaffected joint caused by lateral replacement and the tendency to osteoarthritis due to allogeneic replacement of joints were also significantly solved. This way is actually a RE technology, that is, to interpret and draw the design elements such as processing procedure, tissue structure, function features, and technical specifications by reverse analysis and study of a target product to make a product of similar but not exactly the same functions. RE technology roots from hardware analysis in the commercial and military fields. The main purpose is to analyze based on the finished product directly and obtain its design principles when it is not easy to obtain the necessary production information. See Chaps. 7 and 8 of this book for more descriptions and practical applications of the RE. The superiority of this way rests on the higher molding accuracy compared with the first way provided by the standard mold manufactured by RP equipment and molding based on the said mold; controllable production strength may be applied to the construction of grafts with lower elasticity modulus, such as titanium alloy and cobalt-nickel alloy. It remains limited to the use of conventional construction methods and high accuracy requirements; since the grafts' surface are to be grinded and polished in later phase, it is bound to impose impacts on the shape and structure.

2.1.3 Direct Individualized RP-Based Grafts

The so-called direct individualized RP-based grafts, as the name implies, is to establish the structure data of the affected side by RE technology based on imaging data of the unaffected side and finally construct the grafts in line with clinical applications by RP equipment. With respect to the first two indirect construction methods, the third way is more direct;

therefore, it is also known as the three-dimensional printing (3DP) individualized graft. This way is mainly to scan the conventional graft and establish critical technical parameters based on RE and then print in specific machine. Commonly used methods include selective laser sintering (SLS), selective laser melting (SLM), stereolithography appearance (SLA), laminated object manufacturing (LOM), laser cladding forming (LCF), and laser engineering net shaping (LENS). The superiority of the above methods is that it can print directly the required graft products, which are molded with one take, consume short preparation time, and have high degree of simulation. There are also shortcomings in the following aspects:

Firstly, extremely demanding on the material properties in line with RP preparation in particle size, molding technology, and other aspects—they are often at the expense of the mechanical strength of the alternative raw materials. Therefore, the processed products are far inferior to conventional products in terms of strength, stiffness, etc.

Secondly, it is the accuracy problem, because layered manufacturing exists in all constructing methods, and there is a step effect in layered manufacturing—each layer is thin, but "steps" with a certain thickness remain formed at a certain microscopic scale. In case of a circular arc-shaped product surface, deviation in accuracy will be caused.

Thirdly, extremely demanding on materials. Currently, limited metallic materials can be applicable in 3DP, mostly are rare metals and nonferrous metals because the finished products of 3DP are quite "fragile," and some are even broken by a pinch and unable to resist any large move. Therefore, many products require repeated print, greatly increasing the production costs. Because of the shortcomings, there is no clinical application of 3DP individualized grafts for structure reconstruction of weight-bearing parts in non-tumor patients reported.

In summary, because of the respective superiorities and limitations of these three ways, for example, an individualized graft product with the first and second is finally produced by conventional processing ways involving complicated preparation processes, and the structural simulation of the final product is limited; however, the two ways retain the strength advantages of the conventional method, so that the graft may better adapt to clinical needs of high-strength fixation. The third way is constructed by simple steps and controls the product shape precisely, but it is applied to sites with low demand of strength only due to poor mechanical strength. None of the three ways is an alternative way for the other two. They complement each other and enrich the means used for individualized RP-based orthopedic grafts.

Due to the poor mechanical strength, current individualized RP-based prostheses remain in the phase of manufacturing solid models for mode and making final grafts with conventional methods. When designing individualized prostheses made of titanium and other materials, the finished product may have the identical external contour and local anatomic structures, but there are certain internal differences due to the limitations of conventional processes. These methods also reduce the convenience to produce individualized RP-based prosthetic grafts. Therefore, it is necessary to conduct further studies to improve the mechanical strength of RP-based prosthesis so that PR technology may be used to produce individualized prostheses directly, to enhance the convenience and individualized prostheses better fit the external contour and internal structures of patients' local anatomic structures.

2.2 RP Technology in Applications of Scaffold Manufacturing of Tissue-Engineered Bone

Different with individualized metal grafts, RP technology may construct biodegradable and eventually absolvable grafts by means of (bone) tissue engineering technologies, which are highly praised. Tissue-engineered bone technology uses seed cells of porous scaffolds for tissue engineering and growth factors to constitute bone substitutes and bone graft for absences so as to restore, maintain, and improve tissue functions. The porous scaffolds for tissue engineering are the environment for seed cells to infiltrate, nutrients to penetrate, and tissues' ingrowth; the porous structures shall be similar to the site to be grafted for the ingrowth of vessels and satisfy the demands of internal nutrient supply and exchange. There are many ways for conventional tissue-engineered bone scaffolds, such as bonding by fibrous bone bonding, emulsion freeze-drying, solution casting, leaching, gas foaming, thermally induced phase separation, and electrostatic spinning. However, regardless of the method used, no internal or external structure of the scaffold may perfectly match the anatomic structure of the patients' bone defect, which causes the manufacturing and production of individualized scaffolds unavailable.

The RP technology based on CT or MRI data may be available to design and produce scaffolds for tissue-engineered bone that matches the external contour of patients' bone defects, in which seed cells may survive, tissue may penetrate, and blood vessels may grow into the internal porous, internal structure, and internal channels. Artificial bones manufactured with RP technology are prominently featured by controllable porous numbers, sizes, distributions, and shapes. Such artificial bone is a scaffold with the shape of the bone to be replaced, it also has excellent biocompatibility and biodegradability; thus the bone defects may gradually be replaced by the regenerated bone tissues. Owing to its internal microporous structure, tissue fluid, and ingrowth tendency, cells, the carrier framework, may create a microenvironment that is conducive to cell adhesion, pro-

liferation, and functioning, in order to achieve a parallel growth of tissue-engineered bone, accelerate degradation of materials and osteogenesis, and promote the repair of bone tissues. Some scholars have designed and made evenly distributed and interconnected scaffolds for tissue engineering, respectively, with polycaprolactone and polycaprolactone/hydroxyapatite, with porosity rate of 60–70%; hydroxyapatite effectively improved the anti-compression performance. Co-cultured with fetal bovine osteoblasts for 11d showed cell adhesion and proliferation on the surface and superficial canaliculus of the scaffold. Hollander et al. made titanium (Ti-6Al-4 V) porous scaffolds for tissue-engineered bone by means of RP technology. It showed better biomechanical properties; Young's modulus reached (118.000 ± 2.300) MPa; co-cultured with human osteoblasts for 14d, adhesion and proliferation of a large number of good-morphological cells were observed on the surface and in the micropores.

Currently, there are three commonly used study methods for CAD-guided bone scaffold molding, which are medical computer-assisted design (MedCAD), stereolithography (STL), and reverse engineering (RE).

MedCAD is to establish a direct interface through the medical image database within Mimics, which is each and fast; however, not all bone imaging information can be input in the CAD system, and the only way is to embody the basic characteristics of the bone with a cylindrical, spherical, and other geometries performance. Precise and complex modeling of bone scaffolds is not available. STL is to influence the STL triangle-format documents between Mimics and Geomagics or Magics. For example, process local spiral CT/MRI scans (DICOM) by Mimics for 3D reconstruction of the geometric model of bone defects and converts the reconstruction date into RP-recognizable STL format to construct the bone defect substitute in RP machine. With this method, it is quite fast to build bone scaffold models; however, such models can be used for surface reconstruction only. It is not applicable to the reconstruction of complex structures and the scaffold model is not editable. RE modeling method is by far the best method. Firstly, it builds the 3D reconstruction based on image data of patients, extracts necessary data for the bone scaffold, and establishes the anatomic model; then it designs internal porous model with CAD software, orderly arranges these micropores' units to form microporous space, and determines the microporous structure with required rate of porosity, inter-pore communication, and mechanical performances; finally, it applies Boolean operations to form a biomimetic scaffold with both internal porous structure and external contour.

After a successful modeling of bone scaffold, the data may be input into RP equipment for any solid processing and manufacturing of the bone scaffold. Currently, commonly used methods for porous scaffolds for tissue-engineered bone include gas foaming, molten casting/particle suction and filtration, lyophilized emulsion/phase separation, sintering, hydrothermal hot pressing, fiber bonding, 3DP, organic filling degradation, etc. The following describes the progress and several most commonly used processes and related applications.

2.2.1 Fused Deposition Modeling (FDM)

The technology makes scaffolds with heating nozzles. Scaffold materials are in liquid form when heated in the nozzle to slightly above the melting state. FDM nozzle is controlled by the stratified data of bone scaffold to perform X-Y 2D motions, so that the semimobile scaffold materials may be squeezed out from the nozzle and rapidly cooled and solidified to form a thin layer as the contour and shape of the target scaffold; then the nozzle raises up. The entire bone scaffold is formed by overlaying. FDM was developed by the American scholar Scoa Crump in 1988, and the commercialized machine was launched by Stratasys. Rohner et al. made polycaprolactone (PCL) bone scaffold using FDM and the scaffold and marrow-coated scaffold to repair pig skull defect. They found the molded scaffold matched the bone defect accurately; and compared with the control group, significantly improved performances in bone repair were obtained in the scaffold and marrow-coated scaffold groups. Sawyer et al. used FDM-molded PCL-tricalcium phosphate (TCP)/collagen scaffold loaded with rhBMP-2 to repair skull defects in rats. The results suggested that the bone healing rate was significantly higher than the control group; and for the expressions of osteogenic protein, collagen I and osteocalcin were all up-regulated. However, there are also some problems in FDM-based scaffolds: (1) Because of the metaling of PCL and other materials in the manufacturing process, the choice of biological materials are greatly limited; (2) FDM-based manufacturing defects include extremely small processing space, such as the nozzle design, which is a serious problem for material processing and techniques. In addition, there is water in various tissues of the body; hydrophilic property is also a requirement for materials that cannot be ignored. Therefore, the use of hydrogels, etc. is also quite important. Apparently, this is not available in FDM.

2.2.2 Three-Dimensional Printing (3DP)

The 3DP nozzle "prints" powers and binders for bone scaffolds under the instructions of computer, and the powders and binders bond to each other to form a layer and print layer by layer according to the molding data of the computer and finally form a 3D bone scaffold. This scaffold forming method is similar to the principle of printers, so it is vividly described as the "printing" technology. The 3DP was first reported by Emanual Sachs et al., Massachusetts Institute of Technology, in 1989, and it was soon used to make scaffolds for tissue-engineered bone. The 3DP is applicable to a variety of powder materials forming bone scaffolds, including polymers, such as polycaprolactone/polyethylene oxide (PCL/PE),

poly-L-lactic acid (PLLA), and ultrahigh molecular polyethylene/maltodextrin; various ceramics, such as ß-TCP, TCP/tetracalcium phosphate, and CPC; and various complex compounds, such as ß-TCP/bio-glass, hydroxyapatite (HA)/starch, and HA/maltodextrin. Fierz et al. made three kinds of cylindrical hollow bone scaffolds using HA and the water-soluble binders by 3DP technology, scaffold diameter of 3.9–4.2 mm, the center tube diameter of 0.70–0.87 mm, and microporous contents in all scaffolds of 70%; and histological analysis showed that stimulation of osteoblast progenitor cells could be well attached to the scaffold.

2.2.3 Selective Laser Sintering (SLS)

The steps of SLS are as follows: A thin layer of scaffold powders is evenly spread on the table, then the powers will be selectively sintered by infrared laser under the control of a computer according to the hierarchical outline data layer by layer until the bone scaffold is established based on the data of the computer. The high temperature generated during SLS-based molding limits its applications in preparation of biologically active bone scaffolds. Zhou et al. dissolved carbonated hydroxyapatite (CHAp) nanoparticles in PLLA to produce nan-microspheres and made porous bone scaffolds by SLS technology in SLS machine. The scan showed that CHAp was widely distributed on the porous surfaces.

2.2.4 Three-Dimensional Bioplotting (3DBP)

The 3DBP was firstly reported by Landers in 2000 in the way of extruding bone scaffold materials in a solution containing crosslinking agents to form bone scaffold layer by layer under the control of computer; due to the compensation of liquid buoyancy, no temporary support was required in the molding process. Studies on 3DBP-based and 3DP-based molding polyurethane bone scaffolds show both technologies may be used for molding of polyurethane bone scaffolds; however, 3DBP is superior to 3DP mainly manifested in better mechanical properties, saving molding materials, sharing molding time, smoothing surface of the scaffold, conducive to cell adhesion, and other aspects.

2.2.5 Low-Temperature Deposition Manufacturing (LDM)

Low-temperature deposition manufacturing (LDM), also known as low-temperature rapid prototyping (LRP), was a novel RP technology firstly proposed by Laser RP Research Center, Tsinghua University. It has developed rapidly since the early 2000s. Owing to the simple operation, high controllability of parameters, maintainable biological activities of materials, and other superiorities, it is quickly applied to scaffold molding for tissue-engineered bone. LDM is placing liquid materials for bone scaffolds into a storage tank, extruding the liquid materials from the nozzle at the bottom under the control of computer according to the predesigned bone scaffold model in the way of X-Y 2D scanning; after accumulation of a layer, the workbench drops the height of a layer; the 2D layers shall form the bone scaffold finally by accumulating layer by layer. The technology is low-temperature extrusion of liquids and room temperature molding to make treatment of the materials effective to obtain a frozen bone scaffold; and finally the scaffold shall be used after it has been freeze-dried and lyophilization solvent has been removed. LDM extrudes polymer/injects polymer solutions into a low temperature (below 0 °C) for molding, which requires not much for materials, is easy to form graded porous structures, and may maintain the biological properties of materials. LDM-based molding equipment may deposit and manufacture bone scaffolds for tissue-engineered bone with a single nozzle, two nozzles, three nozzles, and four nozzles as different processes may require.

In conclusion, in the bone tissue engineering, RP-based production of bio-bone scaffolds, bio-bones with growth factors, target cell technologies, etc. are widely referred to in many literatures; from the current situation, people focus on 3D, FDM, and LDM methods. Taking into account the principle of SLS technology, we may find it difficult to select biological materials due to the use of laser. Moreover, local overheating processing is likely to cause modification of materials and other toxicological reactions.

2.3 Applications of RP Technology in Orthopedic Trauma

Long Bi and Jian Liu

RP technology is an emerging engineering and manufacturing technology, which may manufacture models for human tissues and organs after obtaining the data of tissues and organs by medical imaging technologies, with 3D reconstruction, and based on progresses in computer-aided design (CAD), computer-aided manufacturing (CAM), and other applications. The models may be applicable to clinical diagnosis, determination of complex surgical plans, creation of individualized prostheses, and medical teaching. The organization where the author worked since 2003 applied RP technology in clinical orthopedic trauma in an earlier phase; the author has experienced a lot in this regard from over a decade's practice.

2.3.1 Applications of RP Technology in Teaching of Orthopedic Trauma

The use of RP-based 3D models in clinical teaching may help students (young doctors) grasp the anatomical characteristics of bones, gradually develop a 3D imagination, and deepen their understanding of the characteristics of different fractures, so as to enhance interests in learning and improve learning efficiency.

Take pelvis with complex anatomic structures as an example; it is connected by joints and ligaments to sacrococcyx; there are three bones (two hips and one sacrococcyx), five joints (two sacroiliac joints, two acetabula, and one pubic symphysis), and eight ligaments (two anterior and posterior sacroiliac ligaments, two sacrospinous ligaments, and two tuberososacral ligaments). The main blood vessels include iliac vein, external iliac artery and vein, and internal iliac artery and vein; and the main nerves include bone nerves (lumbar plexus) and the sciatic nerves (sacral plexus). These complex anatomical structures may make beginners deter. RP is featured by 3D and dynamic factors which may provide tremendous help for beginners, be easy for them to understand, and deepen their memories. For example, when learning acetabular fractures (Fig. 12.1) with conventional X-rays, it is required to analyze and identify complex structures such as posterior lip line, anterior lip line, acetabular roof line, iliopubic line, ilioischial line, and tear line on X-rays. These are extremely important for the diagnosis of pelvic fractures; however, the knowledge is too difficult for medical students to learn and understand. The learning curve is quite long. However, the actual RP-based model for teaching may easily visualize complex structures of the acetabulum to the students, so that they may grasp the characteristics and difficulties of acetabular fractures more effectively. In short, the application of RP technology can make clinical teaching of orthopedic trauma more intuitive and efficient.

2.3.2 Applications of RP Technology in Preoperative Preparation of Orthopedic Trauma Surgeries

Injury judgment is especially important for trauma orthopedists. But sometimes it is difficult to judge patients' injuries, especially patients in emergency treatment of trauma. For example, tension pneumothorax due to blunt chest trauma, pancreas fracture due to blunt abdominal trauma, and complex bone fractures of limbs are the tests for physicians. Due to overlap of bones and poor imaging position of patients, sometimes conventional X-ray examination may be insufficient to help us make accurate judgments on the actual injuries. Pelvic acetabular fractures, for example, due to the interference of organs, intestinal gases, and overlapping bones, are difficult for physicians to judge their neighboring relationships and pitting fractures; moreover, pelvic ring fracture is easily missed. In this case, underestimation that may cause serious consequences may occur. CT, for the overlapping of the fracture line, non-displaced fracture line, occult fracture, compression depressed fractures, and intra-articular fracture tablets, has better recognition rate, thus reducing the rate of misdiagnosis. However, it is 2D image after all and there is no 3D sense; the overall understanding of fractures and fracture lines is always not displayed in parallel to the fault plane. Sometimes the radiologist also

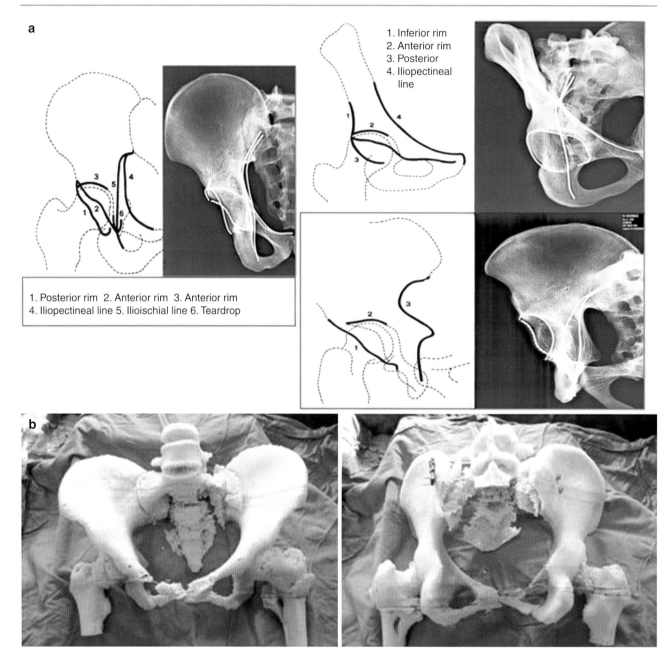

Fig. 12.1 RP-based acetabular fracture modeling used for teaching. (**a**) The traditional use of X-rays in the teaching of acetabular fractures, which is obscure and hard to understand. (**b**) Using RP technology to create a solid model can make teaching more intuitive and easy to understand

displays 3D reconstruction data to us, but this reconstructed image is often not the biggest help for diagnosis. Based on the author's more than 10 years of clinical experience, computer-aided integration of CT data for a reconstructed 3D image is required for the comprehensive assessment of acetabular fractures, and in such a 3D image, five locations are extremely important. (see Fig. 12.2)

For particularly complex fractures, we can create solid model of the fractures with RP technology and clearly evaluate each fracture line and understand the size, displacement, and relations to neighboring structures of each fracture flat,

especially articular surfaces or load-bearing parts (acetabulum top) involved, through observations of the models (Fig. 12.3). Access to the information is extremely important for the accurate development and treatment protocols of the injuries!

In acetabular surgeries, the surgical field is deep, operational difficulties, irregular shapes, and complex injuries leading to difficulties in restoration and fixation; hence, acetabular fractures are praised by "expert-level operation" in orthopedic trauma. Preoperative use of 3D image reconstruction on a computer for operation protocol design may provide

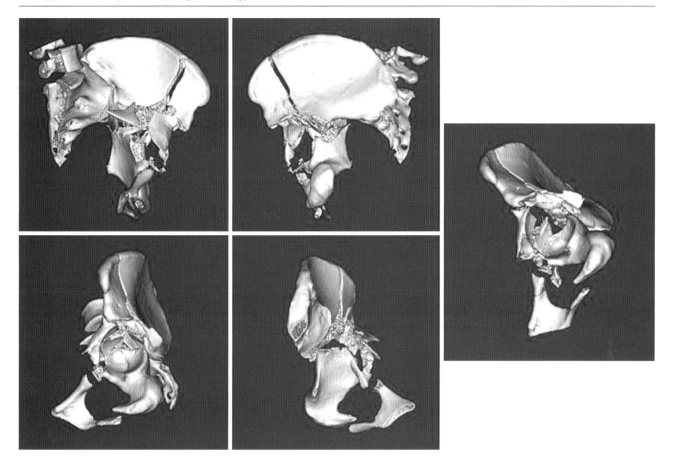

Fig. 12.2 Five critical 3D reconstruction images in the assessment of acetabular fracture. (**a**) Similar to the iliac oblique position in X-ray projection (*anterior view*). (**b**) Similar to the iliac oblique position (*dorsal view*) in X-ray projection (*posterior view*). (**c**) Similar to obturator oblique position in X-ray projection (anterior view). (**d**) Similar to obturator oblique position in X-ray projection (posterior view). (**e**) Anterior view of overall acetabular bone (including acetabular *bottom*)

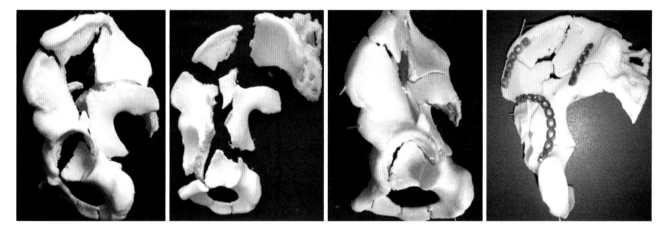

Fig. 12.3 Use RP technology to make complex model of acetabular fractures, conduct operation design, preoperation on the model, and prebending of steel plate

a great help to orthopedic surgeons; the method is also applied to a considerable amount of cases in the author's working organization. However, the computer-aided image is different with the actual situation after all, and it makes it difficult for complex acetabular fractures—a slight sense of being "engaged in idle theorizing." At this time, RP technology may show its unique advantages. It may create the 1:1 real models with RP technology of fractures; and preoperative restoration and fixation to fractures may provide actual experiences for surgeons, or surgeons even provide prebent steel plates according to models and use such steel plates in operation directly. This greatly improves the efficiency, shortens operation time, and reduces the injury possibility and bleeding tendency in operations (Fig. 12.3).

Typical Case 1

The patient, Ms. Cheng, female, has multiple injuries caused by car accident: pelvic fractures (61-c2.2), fracture of femoral neck, fracture of left femoral trochanter, urethral rupture, and vaginal laceration. To obtain a more complex model of the patient's pelvis through RP technology (Fig. 12.4), in the intuitive guidance of the model, the physician shall fully display the wealth of knowledge and experience and conduct an internal and open fixation within the restoration of pubis, percutaneous fixation and close restoration of the right sacroiliac joint, internal fixation and close restoration of the left sacroiliac joint, and open internal fixation and restoration of proximal femur. Detailed preoperative planning significantly shortened the operation time and significantly reduced blood loss, improved the success rate of

operation, reduced the risk of operation, and achieved good therapeutic effects (Fig. 12.4).

In short, RP technology has become the diamond in the hands of surgeons and makes them may easily grasp complex injuries and enter the advanced preoperative drill. Full preoperative preparation may simplify complex procedures, shorten operation time, reduce operative injuries, and lower patients' bleeding to obtain a satisfactory outcome.

2.3.3   Surgical Templates

Design and Application of Surgical Navigation for Sacral Fractures

Establishing pelvis stability is largely dependent on the stability with the posterior pelvic ring. Owing to the unstable posterior pelvic ring caused by sacral fractures, the treatment of sacral fractures seems particularly important in the treatment of pelvic fractures. With the development of transport and construction, patients with pelvic fractures are increasing in the clinic. For unstable sacral fractures, most scholars

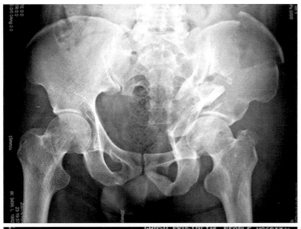

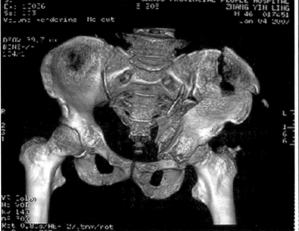

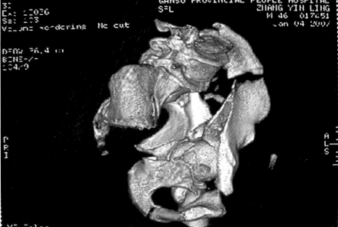

Fig. 12.4 Typical case I. (**a**) Basic conditions and X-rays of patient. (**b**) 3D CT reconstruction image of the patient. (**c**) Use RP technology to make physical model of fractures, conduct operation design, preop-

eration on the model, and prebending of steel plate required for use. (**d**) The prebent steel plate is used directly in the operation and the effect is good

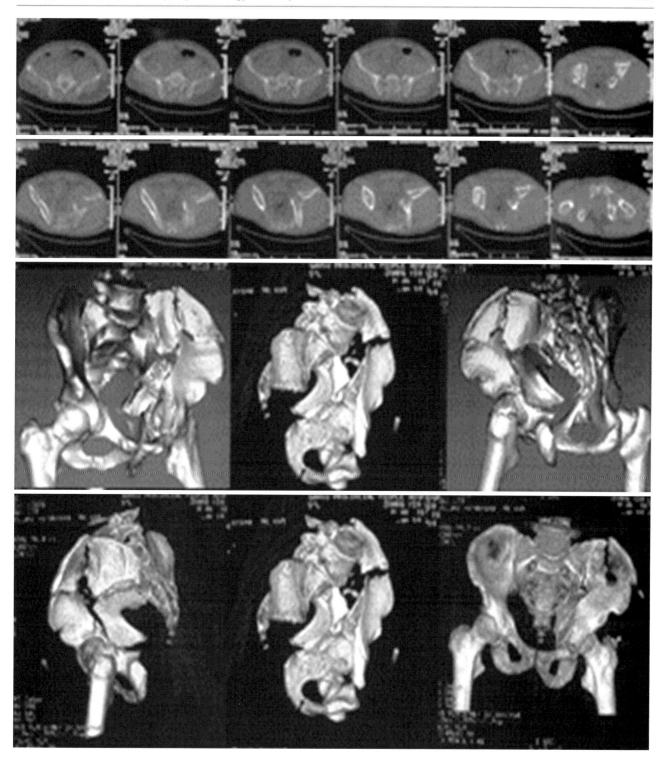

Fig. 12.4 (continued)

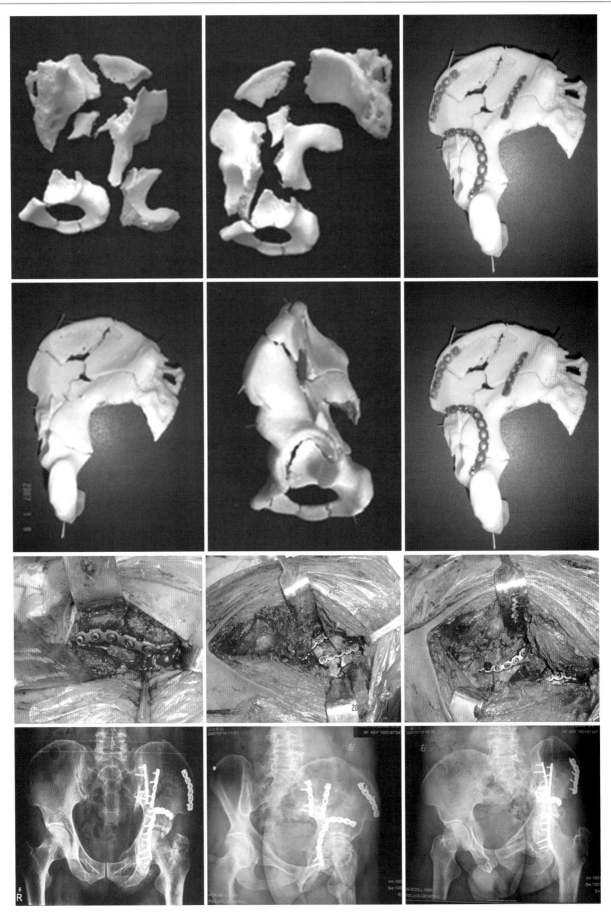

Fig. 12.4 (continued)

advocate operative treatment. Common operative procedures for sacral fractures may include sacrum rod, pelvis anterior plate, sacroiliac lag screws, etc. Biomechanical studies show that sacroiliac lag screws maximally stabilize the pelvis and thus become the preferred option of operation. However, owing to the risk of accidental injury to sacral nerve and cauda equina, a 3D navigation template reconstructed by RE may provide a simple, accurate, and minimally invasive approach for fixation of sacrum lag screws:

1. Method of continuous spiral CT tomography of pelvis, import DICOM-format images scanned into Amira software for 3D surface reconstruction with SSD, and then save the reconstructed pelvic model in stl. Format and import it in Imageware surfacer 10.0, simulate the restoration on the pelvis model and design tracks for lag screws, extract iliac rear surface morphology and anatomy and model of screw tracks, and import them in RapidForm software to establish a navigation template consistent with the iliac rear anatomic morphology, and generate the template by RP technology.
2. In clinical application, fit the template and the rear ilium according to the predesigned method, drive two Kirschner needles into the navigation tracks, insert lag screws after inspection that the positions are satisfactory, and conduct X-ray and CT examinations to assess the positions of screws.

Sacral fracture has a low incidence rate but tends to be missed in clinical diagnosis and treatment. The bone ligament structure posterior to the pelvic ring serves as the hub for load transfer between the body and lower extremities, and its functions account for 60% of the entire pelvis. As an important component of the pelvic ring, sacral fractures may produce damages to the stability of the pelvis, its therapeutic effect plays an importation role in recovery of pelvic functions, and its treatment includes restoration of pelvic stability and relief and avoidance of nerve compression, fixed appropriately according to the type of fractures.

Kraemer et al. conducted studies on the biomechanical strength of pelvis specimens in fresh-frozen corpses, and their findings show that long-threaded screws shall be used in sacroiliac screw fixation provided that the safety is ensured; at the same time, biomechanical tests confirm no difference in effects between two screws with one fixed at S1 and the other at S2; however, fixation with two screws provides better stabilization effects compared with fixation with one screw. Clinical and biomechanical studies have shown that lag screw inserted from the facies lateralis of iliac wing through the sacroiliac joint into S1 is a better way of fixation. Sacroiliac lag screws provide good fixation strength and stability. Studies have confirmed that the fixation strength of sacroiliac lag screw is greater than front-approach steel plate

fixation, and percutaneous fixation is feasible and applicable to most patients—small incision, less blood loss, mild trauma, and extremely beneficial to postoperative recovery of patients. Garcia et al. concluded by 3D finite element simulation of pelvic fractures that only internal fixation of pubic symphysis and two-screw sacroiliac fixation may achieve adequate stable fixation. Therefore, for patients with fractures of the anterior ring, they may be fixed with support lag screws through a small incision at the pubis accompanied by fixation in anterior and posterior rings. Sacral lag screw technology also has drawbacks, mainly including complex local anatomic structure, important adjacent structures, surgical risks, and injuries to sacral nerve, cauda equina, and pelvic large vessels or organs that may be caused by inaccurate screw directions, etc.

The advent and unceasing development of digital 3D reconstruction technology and RE software has provided many novel means for modern orthopedic operations, such as intuitive insight of features of surgical sites based on CT data-based 3D models and digital analysis of structures of surgical sites; in this way, both the accuracy of internal fixation and operative safety may be further enhanced. Therefore, with the purposes of the positioning of the sacroiliac lag screw tracks, we have designed and simulated fixation tracks as per surgical requirements and designed the navigation template accordingly. The template is individually designed and greatly matched to ensure an exact match between lag screws and the posterior ilium, providing accurately determined positions and directions, which may not only avoid accidental injuries but also make the operative procedures quicker and easier.

Syndesmotic Separate Navigation Template

1. Method continuous spiral CT tomography of ankle joint, import DICOM-format images scanned into Amira software for 3D surface reconstruction with SSD, and then save the reconstructed pelvic model in stl. Format and import it in Imageware sufacer10.0 to determine the direction and angle of screw, extract ankle rear surface morphology and anatomy and model of screw tracks and import them in RapidForm software to establish a navigation template, and generate the template by RP technology.
2. In clinical application, fit the navigation template and the lateral ankle according to the predesigned method, drive one Kirschner needle into the navigation tracks, insert lag screws after inspection that the positions are satisfactory, and conduct X-ray examination to assess the positions of screw. The syndesmosis is closely constituted by inferior tibiofibular ligament, posterior ligament, lower transverse ligament, and inter-bone ligaments. The separation of syndesmosis is always caused by strong violence to ankle joint, such as external ectropion and external rotation. It may occur in isolation, but mostly it is accompanied by

other ankle ligament inquiries or fracture and dislocation. If not treated promptly or properly, it often leaves chronic pain, joint instability, and traumatic arthritis, seriously affecting the ankle functions. There are many fixation methods for syndesmosis separation, such as screw, bio-absorbable grafts, fibula hook, and line-buckle fixation. In China, screws, inferior tibiofibular hook plate, and absorbable screws are commonly used. In an operation, after confirmation and restoration under by C-arm fluoroscopy, one cortical bone screw (diameter of 3.5 mm) forward forming a 30° angle with the horizontal plane, parallel to the tibial articular surface shall be inserted into three layers of cortex at about 2–3 cm from the proximal tibial articular surface and the screw top shall reach the medullary cavity of tibia to adapt to the micro-movement of syndesmosis when ankle moves. The navigation template fully reflects this requirement. It is also minimally invasive.

2.3.4 Production of Prostheses

Using the RP technology, we produce equal proportional, personalized, precise, and strong biological fusion prosthesis, and for precise correction of deformity of joint, personalized design and production of total knee, total hip and half pelvic, complex fractures and intra-articular fracture anatomical reduction (especially for difficult, complex and special cases), we can try, the technology improves the operation efficiency, and ensure the safety of operation.

There are different types in case of radial head fracture:

Type I: Fracture without displacement.

Type II: Fracture with separation and displacement. The fracture block is in different size; sometimes small fracture fragments are embedded in the joint space or separated from the outer edge of the humeroradial joint.

Type III: The radial head comminuted fracture. Radial head was in comminution, displacement, or without displacement.

Type IV: Capitulum radii fracture and dislocation of the elbow. Improper treatment of Mason III type and Type IV capitulum radii fracture can lead to elbow pain, elbow instability, and rotation dysfunction. The surgical incision in traditional radial head replacement therapy, due to the large metal prostheses, may be longer, leading to the occurrence of elbow subluxation and femoral head wearing. Moreover, since the traditional metal prosthesis is not proper, only a few radial head can get anatomical reduction.

Use RP technology and 3D CT scanning to output joint anatomical model in STL format and to produce the bone joint prototype. Through the physical observation of bone joint prototype and comparing with the mirror image of contralateral joints and accurate analysis of joint damage, we can create a truly suitable prosthetic model. In addition,

the end of slot type, ladder, and other various shapes can be made according to the surgical needs.

2.3.5 RP Technology in the Diagnosis and Treatment of Other Complex Fractures

Andreas Schweizer et al. conducted outside-in correction osteotomy in six patients with intra-articular fractures of distal radius and malunion longer than 2 mm, using 3D technology for guidance and precise incision. Postoperative X-ray plain film showed no collapse of articular surface and degenerative changes; all the patients' wrist activity and grip strength were improved. And they believed that this technology can help physicians to handle complex articular osteotomy safely, reducing such remedial program as part/full wrist arthrodesis as much as possible.

Tricot M et al. performed a CT scanning in three patients with distal humerus deformity (two of elbow valgus, one of cubitus varus), using RP technology to produce a 3D model to guide operation, eventually receiving satisfactory correction results, and all the activities of the elbow were restored. In view of the author, the RP technology has several advantages: It reduces the time of operation and shortens the incision. Its disadvantages include increased time of planning, modulation guidance, need for a CT scanning, and cost.

Hsieh MK et al. performed osteotomy reduction in 12 patients with intra-articular fractures of distal radius (accompanying radiocarpal joint and proximal radioulnar joint subluxation) and follow-up evaluation (the average time is of 3.6 months). Preoperative RP model is regarded as part of the preoperative plan. Finally, the entire bone cutting site healed, and all radiocarpal joint and proximal radioulnar joint subluxation have been corrected. And they all believe that the RP technology is a very useful tool, which can be used as physical model for osteotomy and joint replacement simulation actually before the operation.

2.4 Rapid Prototyping Technology in Hip Resurfacing Arthroplasty

Yuanzhi Zhang

2.4.1 Introduction

Total hip resurfacing arthroplasty, viewed by many as representing an evolution from the mold arthroplasty procedure of Smith-Petersen, has been considered as an alternative to total hip replacement for adult patients diagnosed with osteoarthritis of the hip or congenital hip dysplasia. It has been performed with a variety of materials, designs, operative approaches, techniques, and fixation methods. Many advantages of hip resurfacing arthroplasty have been suggested, including bone conservation, improved function as a consequence of retention of the femoral head and neck and more

Guolin, Meng, Long Bi, Jian Liu, Yuanzhi Zhang, Sheng Lu, Yongqing Xu, Zhigang Wu, Jun Fu, Zhi Yuanl, precise biomechanical restoration, decreased morbidity at the time of revision arthroplasty, reduced dislocation rates, normal femoral loading, and reduced stress shielding. In hip resurfacing arthroplasty, the prosthetic location is a key to postoperative joint stability. In conventional hip arthroplasty, the neck-shaft angle is determined by the design of the prosthesis itself, whereas in hip resurfacing it is determined by valgus or varus placement of femoral prosthesis arthroplasty. When the prosthesis is inserted by conventional positioning, some positioning devices are needed; however, accuracy cannot always be achieved with the devices currently in use. Successful positioning thus depends largely on the surgeon's experience. With the development of computer-aided design (CAD) and computer-aided engineering (CAE), the trends in medical technology have been toward individualization, fidelity, and mini-invasion with the results of safe, enhanced surgical procedures and more easy dealing with complicated surgery by clinical doctors. In this study, novel locating navigation templates were both introduced and validated in clinical settings. Design of the templates is based on the reverse engineering (RE) principle. With the patient-specific design of the template, close contact with acetabular and femoral features is established, hopefully providing the best possible stability in hip resurfacing arthroplasty.

2.4.2   Design of the Navigation Template

The 3D CT scan pelvis image data was obtained from ten healthy volunteers through a spiral 3D CT scan (Light Speed VCT, GE, USA) with 0.625 mm slice thickness and 0.35 mm in-plane resolution. The data was transferred via a DICOM network into a computer workstation. The 3D models of the hips were reconstructed using Amira 3.1 (TGS) software and saved in STL format. The 3D models were then imported into Imageware 12.0 (EDS, USA) software. The center of rotation being measured is that of the hip and femoral head being determined, and the extract location of the best channel of the cup and stem of femoral component were defined using reverse engineering. First, data of the transaction planes (1.0 mm thickness) of the acetabular and femoral head surfaces were extracted, and the correctly fitting globe was produced, respectively. The global center could be considered as the rotation center of both acetabulum and femoral head. Second, the presumed ideal acetabular location should be about 45° of abduction and 18° of anteversion, and the best location of the femoral head implant has 140° of abduction along with the axis of the formal neck. Finally, the specific navigation templates were designed according to the anatomical features of the acetabular contour and the femoral head (Figs. 12.5 and 12.6).

2.4.3   Clinical Application

Twenty patients with pathological changes in one hip, aged from 24 to 37 years, 11 males and 9 females, were scheduled for total hip resurfacing arthroplasty. The twenty patients

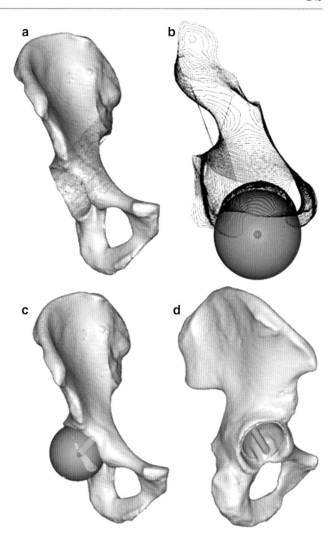

Fig. 12.5 Determine the center of rotation and the navigation template design of acetabulum: (**a**) 3D reconstruction of hip and dissection of acetabulum, (**b**) construction of the center of rotation of acetabulum (*small ball*), (**c**) the channel of navigation, (**d**) navigation template

were randomly assigned to undergo either conventional implantation of resurfacing prosthesis (control group) or navigation template implantation (NT group). The navigation templates were made by the abovementioned method. Navigation template models were exported in STL format and produced by acrylate resin (Somos 14,120, DSM Desotech Inc., USA) using the stereolithography rapid prototyping (RP) technique (Fig. 12.7). Operative time and operative blood loss in the navigation template group and the control group were compared. The deviation between the ideal abduction angles and the actual angles of the implanted acetabular cup was calculated, as well as the deviation of the cup anteversion angles. The deviation between the neck-shaft angle (NSA) and the actual implanted short stem-shaft angle (SSA) and that between the anteversion angle of femoral neck and the anteversion angle of the actual implanted short stem were measured. Angle deviations in the navigation template group were compared with those in the control group. All surgeries were performed by the senior author through a posterior approach, as in the usual procedure. In the NT group, after dislocation of the hip and insertion of the template into the acetabulum, a 3.2 mm diameter guide pin

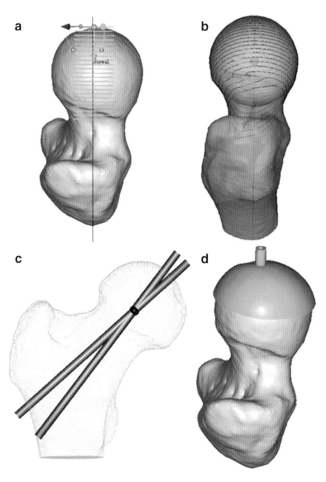

Fig. 12.6 Design of femoral head navigation template: (**a**) determine the axial ray neck of femur and dissection of femoral head, (**b**) construct the center of femoral head (*small ball*), (**c**) the channel of navigation, (**d**) navigation template

was placed in the template hole. The acetabular reamer followed the guide pin to drill and shape the prosthetic socket which should be about 45° of abduction and 18° of anteversion. When the femoral head was dislocated and correctly exposed, we matched the locating template to the surface of femoral head as well as possible. A Kirschner wire was inserted into the femoral neck according to the template. We evaluated the axial location of the femoral component (shown by the K wire) with anteroposterior (A-P) and lateral position photographs in operation by C-arm machine (Fig. 12.8). All patients have received an X-ray during the 7–10-day postoperative period. The radiographic analysis included an anteroposterior view of the pelvis, anteroposterior, and lateral views of the hip. In A-P radiographs, the stem-shaft angle was measured between the axial line of femur and the extension line of the component stem with a measuring tool from software Adobe Photoshop.

2.4.4 Statistical Analysis

Analysis was performed by SPSS 10.0. Data were all displayed in normal distribution. The level of significance was defined as P values <0.05 with 95% confidence intervals. Every group data was compared with setting certified value by single sample T-test. There was no difference in each group with regard to abduction angle and anteversion angle of acetabular and femoral component stem-shaft angles.

2.4.5 Results

The navigation templates were found to be highly accurate (Fig. 12.9). The average operative time of the NT group procedures was 118.6 min, shorter than those with conventional procedures 140.2 min ($P < 0.05$). The average operative blood loss in NT group was 410.9 ml, less than the 480.6 ml with the conventional procedures ($P < 0.05$). The deviation of the cup abduction angle ($1.2° \pm 0.9°$) was significantly lesser in NT group than those in the control group ($5.4° \pm 3.2°$) ($P < 0.05$). The deviation of the cup anteversion angle was ($2.1° \pm 1.2°$) significantly lesser in NT group than those in

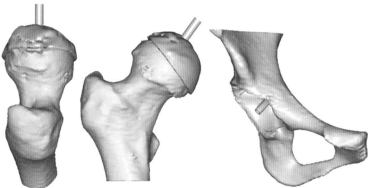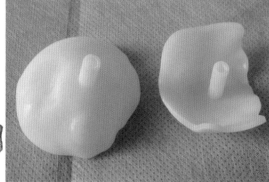

Fig. 12.7 Template models of acetabular and femoral head

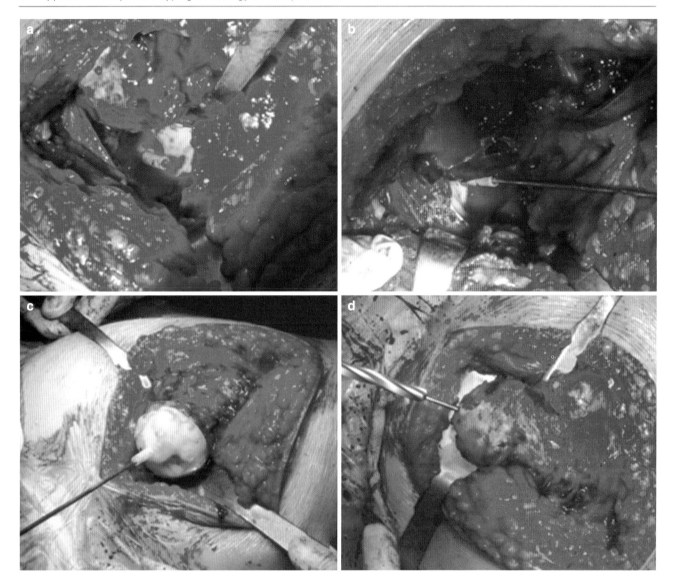

Fig. 12.8 Procedure of operation in NT group: (**a**) locating of acetabular, (**b**) inserting guide pin, (**c**) matching navigation template and inserting Kirschner wire, (**d**) enlargement of canals

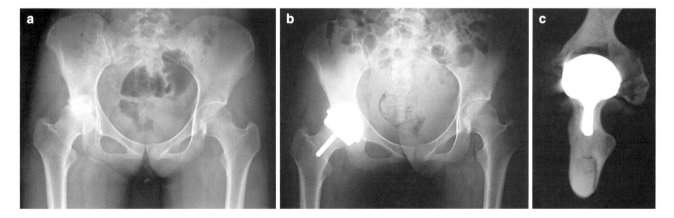

Fig. 12.9 X-ray and CT show the position of the prosthesis in NT group. (**a**) A-P radiograph shows the pathological hip before operation, (**b**, **c**) A-P radiograph and CT image show the position of the prosthesis postoperation

Table 12.1 Evaluation between two groups

Group	Operative time	Operative blood loss	Deviation of cup angle Abduction (°) anteversion (°)	Deviation of FSS angle (°)
NT	116.8 ± 25.1	410.9 ± 130.7	1.2 ± 0.9	2.1 ± 0.9
Control	130.5 ± 30.1	480.6 ± 135.9	5.4 ± 3.2	4.1 ± 2.8
P value	<0.05	<0.05	<0.05	<0.05

control group (4.1° ± 2.8°) ($P < 0.05$). The deviation of the femoral stem-shaft angle was (1.3° ± 1.0°) significantly lesser in NT group than in control group (10.2° ± 1.5°) ($P < 0.05$) (Table 12.1).

2.4.6 Discussion

Metal-on-metal hip resurfacing arthroplasties represent an alternative to total hip arthroplasties for young and active patients, enabling the preservation of the intact femoral bone and therefore improving the prognosis for future hip joint replacements. One goal of hip resurfacing arthroplasty is to closely mimic the normal anatomy of the proximal part of the femur and the hip joint, and it has been suggested that implant positioning may have a greater impact on implant survival and patient function than it does in a conventional hip replacement. "Normality" applies to the position of the center of rotation of the hip, anteversion (femoral and acetabular components), overall offset, and leg length. Careful preoperative planning, templating, and choice of implant should ensure that after total hip replacement the center of rotation is restored to its pre-disease position. Lewinnek suggests that the position of the acetabular cup relative to the body's axis is important. The "safe" range of the cup orientation was anteversion of 15 ± 10 and lateral opening of 40 ± 10 . Some authors think the main reason for instability of the hip postoperation is the poor accuracy of cup positioning during operation. Several studies now show that cup inclination should be 45° or less because inclination greater than that is directly related to accelerated wear. The goal of cup implantation is to achieve stable fixation of the cup in a position that provides hip stability by avoidance of impingement, provides correct combined anteversion, and is favorable for wear. Restoration of the center of rotation (COR) of the hip with the COR of the cup has been an important goal of the cemented cup technique because of reports of the relationship of this to wear. Finite element studies promoted this solution by showing that inclination of 45–55° was best to avoid impingement. Freeman and other authors emphasize the importance of a valgus orientation of the femoral component relative to the native femoral neck. A valgus angle of approximately 140°, anatomically anteverted could minimize lateral neck and head interfacial stress.

The modern concepts of computer-assisted orthopedic surgery (CAOS) create intraoperative problems with additional technical system components that are necessary for the intraoperative registration of bone structures and the spatial arrangement of displays, sensors, and robot systems. Only a few hospitals can bear the costs of the sensor or robot-based systems. Individual templates eliminate the need for complex equipment and time-consuming procedures in the operating room. A preoperative CT scan is mandatory to generate the individual templates and for a precise spatial correspondence between the individual bones structure in situ and the intended position of the tool guide. According to these theories, we designed the patient-specific templates of the hip resurfacing arthroplasty. Our study was to evaluate practicability and accuracy of the image-based patient-specific templates. These templates are a simple and low-cost solution that provides exact, safe, and fast implementation of elective surgery on bone structures. This technique also has potential sources of error. Since 3D model of hip is constructed by manual or automatic segmentation, there is potential error on the procedure. Furthermore, the RP model can deviate from the computer 3D model, but present RP technology can control the preciseness within 0.1 mm. Finally, however, geometric accuracy alone does not insure the accurate prosthesis placement. During operation, the template should be able to be used as in situ drill guide, and any movement between the bones will affect the accuracy.

A novel navigational template designed for the use in the hip resurfacing arthroplasty was introduced in this study, and the clinical application suggested its good applicability and high accuracy. The procedure of generating a medical model can be broken down into the following three major steps: the CT scan for data acquisition, the image segmentation combined with data processing, and the building of the model itself. The availability of high-resolution CT scanner and advanced technologies used in the present study provides the possibility for high geometric accuracy of the drill template. The software which is used to segment the CT scan images and perform data processing can provide fast, easy, and powerful 3D image processing and editing. The advantage of the individual template is as follows: First, the surgeon can choose the placement and the size of cup based on the unique morphology of the acetabular component before surgery. Second, the advantage of the individual template is its uncomplicated applicability and requires no surgeon-derived registration step. The preoperatively prepared drill template is used intraoperatively to assist with surgical navigation and the placement of instrumentation. Third, in contrast to the image-guided technique, individual template technique eliminates the need for complex equipment and time-consuming procedures in the operating room, and the techniques reduce the time of surgical procedures. Finally, individual template technique eliminates the need for fluoroscopy, and significantly reduces radiation exposure to the members of the surgical team as a result.

However, some aspects are insufficient in our study, such as the premise that all acetabular and femoral component positions with resurfacing arthroplasty should be the same may be not suitable for all patients. We think the ideal acetabular and femoral component position could be determined by the patient's healthy hip using a mirror image, when there is a single pathological hip. It would have been preferred to accurately compare the postoperative component abduction and anteversion and femoral component abduction to the desired angles by use of postoperative CT scans for both the control and navigated groups to confirm the reliability. However, this would add the patient costs. We will attempt to use this method in our future research, if possible.

2.5 Application of a Novel Patient-Specific Rapid Prototyping Template in Spinal Surgery

Sheng Lu, Yongqing Xu, and Yuanzhi Zhang

Abstract Spinal pedicle screw fixation systems provide three-dimensional (3D) fixation in the spine. Compared with conventional hook instrumentation, the clinical advantages of such systems include enhanced correction and stabilization of various deformities, shorter fusion length, more solid and reliable fixation, and no encroachment into the spinal canal. Therefore, pedicle screw fixation systems have gained popularity for internal fixation of fractures, tumors, and deformities of the spine. Manual placement has a high associated rate of unplanned perforation, which is the major specific complication of pedicle screw placement and causes a high risk of bone weakening or lesions of the spinal cord, nerve roots, or blood vessels. Successful placement of pedicle screws in the spine requires a thorough 3D understanding of the pedicle morphology in order to accurately identify the ideal screw axis. The authors have developed a novel patient-specific navigational template for pedicle screw placement with good applicability and high accuracy. The potential use of navigational templates to place pedicle screws is promising. The methodology appears to provide an accurate technique and trajectory for pedicle screw placement in the spine.

2.5.1 Introduction

Conventional surgical handwork requires competences such as dexterity or fine motor skills, which are complemented by visual and tactile feedback. Computer-assisted orthopedic surgery aims at improving the perception that a surgeon has of the surgical field and the operative manipulation. Bony manipulation such as drilling, chiseling, or sawing can be performed more accurately and implants can be placed more exactly. This reduces the risk of harming the patient intraoperatively by damaging sensitive structures.

CT scans are very suitable for surgical navigation, especially in orthopedics. The bones can be easily distinguished from any other tissue and can be easily segmented out. The bones are also the least deformable parts of the body, and therefore the most stable references for navigation, making it possible for different phases of surgical planning and execution to be performed well after the patient imaging. Preoperative planning is typically done in three orthogonal cross-sectional views made through the CT scan volume.

A Novel Computer-Assisted Rapid Prototyping Drill Guide Template for Spinal Pedicle Screw Placement

Spinal pedicle screw fixation systems provide 3D fixation in the spine. Compared with conventional hook instrumentation, the clinical advantages of such systems include enhanced correction and stabilization of various deformities, shorter fusion length, more solid and reliable fixation, and no encroachment into the spinal canal. Therefore, pedicle screw fixation systems have gained popularity for internal fixation of fractures, tumors, and deformities of the spine. In spinal pedicle screw insertion, it is important both to select the correct size of screw and to place it properly within the pedicle to ensure good anchoring. Manual placement has a high associated rate of unplanned perforation, which is the major specific complication of pedicle screw placement and causes a high risk of bone weakening or lesions of the spinal cord, nerve roots, or blood vessels.

Successful placement of pedicle screws in the cervical spine requires a thorough 3D understanding of the pedicle morphology in order to accurately identify the ideal screw axis. Several methods have been explored for precise cervical pedicle screw placement including anatomic studies, image-guided techniques, computer-assisted surgery system, and drill templates. These techniques can be broadly classified into five types: (1) techniques relying on anatomical landmarks and averaged angular dimensions; (2) techniques with direct exposure of the pedicle, e.g., by laminaminotomy; (3) CT-based computer-assisted surgery (CAS); (4) fluoroscopy-based CAS techniques; and (5) drill template techniques.

The principle of image guidance is to register the patient's preoperative computed tomography (CT) scans, thus permitting the surgeon to navigate simultaneously within the patient and the CT scan volume. Such navigation systems have shown good clinical results. There are, however, several disadvantages associated with navigation systems. In cases where screws are to be placed in more than one vertebra, it is necessary to perform a separate registration step for each vertebra. Intraoperative registration of bone structures takes up to several minutes, and thus the time taken for the overall procedure is increased compared with a conventional approach. The navigation equipment often requires additional personnel to be presented during surgery, and this, together with the increased operating time, leads to a higher risk of intraoperative infection. The navigation equipment is cumbersome and occupies a lot of space in the operating room. Finally, only a few hospitals can bear the costs of sensor or robot-based systems. One way to overcome these drawbacks is the production of personalized templates. These are designed using preoperative CT to fit in a unique position on the individual's bone, and they have carefully designed holes to guide the drill through a preplanned trajectory.

A Novel Patient-Specific Navigational Template for Cervical Screw Placement

Successful placement of pedicle screws in the cervical spine requires a thorough 3D understanding of the pedicle morphology in order to accurately identify the ideal screw axis. The accuracy of computer-assisted screw insertion has been demonstrated recently. The rate of pedicle perforations was 8.6% in the conventional group and 3.0% in the computer-assisted surgery group in 52 consecutive patients who received posterior cervical or cervicothoracic instrumentations using pedicle screws. Another group has also reported similar results, in which the rate of pedicle wall perforation was found to be significantly lower in the computer-assisted group (1.2%) than in the conventional group (6.7%). However, despite advances in instrumentation techniques and intraoperative imaging, successful implementation of posterior cervical instrumentation still remains a challenge.

Considered these difficulties, this study introduces an ingenious, custom-fit navigational template for the placement of pedicle screws in the cervical spine and further validates it in the clinical settings. Based on this technique, the trajectory of the cervical pedicle screws was first identified based on the preoperative CT scan model. The drill template was then patient specifically designed so that it can keep in close contact with the postural surface of the cervical vertebra in order to provide the best stability for drilling.

Twenty-five patients (14 males, 11 females, age of 17–53 years) with cervical spinal pathology including 10 patients with destabilizing cervical spine injuries, 4 patients with cervical spondylitic myelopathy, and 11 patients with basilar invagination requiring instrumentation underwent cervical pedicle screw placement using a novel, patient-specific navigational template technique. According to this technique, a spiral 3D CT scan (LightSpeed VCT, GE, USA) was performed preoperatively on the cervical spine of each patient with a 0.625 mm slice thickness and 0.35 mm in-plane resolution. The images were stored in DICOM format

and transferred to a workstation running MIMICS 10.01 software (Materialise, Belgium) to generate a 3D reconstruction model of the desired cervical vertebra.

The 3D cervical vertebral model was then exported in STL format to a workstation running reverse engineer software UG imageware12.0 (EDS, USA) for determining the optimal screw size and orientation. Using the UG Imageware software, the pedicles (left and right pedicle) were projected toward the vertebra and lamina. As the thickness and cross section of the pedicle vary along its length, the smaller diameter of the elliptical inner boundary of the pedicle's projection was used in determining the maximum allowable dimension for screw diameter. This diameter was further used to draw a circle and projected between the vertebra and the lamina to obtain the optimal pedicle screw trajectory. A 3D vertebral model was reconstructed with a virtual screw placed on both sides.

Following the determination of the optimal pedicle screw trajectory, a navigational template was constructed with a drill guide on either side. The template surface was created as the inverse of the vertebral posterior surface, thus potentially enabling a near-perfect fit. It was also made sure that there was no overlapping of the template onto adjacent segments.

The bio-model of the desired vertebra as well as its corresponding navigational template were produced in acrylate resin (Somos 14,120, DSM Desotech Inc., USA) using stereolithography—a rapid prototyping (RP) technique (Hen Tong Company, China). The accuracy of the navigational template was examined by visual inspection before surgery. The bio-model of the vertebra and its corresponding template were placed together, and a standard electric power drill was used to drill the screw trajectory into the bio-model of the vertebra through the template navigation holes. Visual inspection was performed for identifying any violation.

The template was sterilized and used intraoperatively for navigation and for confirming anatomic relationships. For safety reasons, fluoroscopy was performed intraoperatively during drilling and insertion of the pedicle screw on the first three patients. For the remaining cases, fluoroscopy was performed only after the insertion of all the pedicle screws, thus considerably reducing the exposure time to radiation. After surgery, the positions of the pedicle screws were evaluated using X-ray and CT scan. An axial image, including the whole length of each screw was obtained, and the medial and lateral deviation of the screw was classified into four grades 6:

Grade 0, no deviation: the screw was contained in the pedicle.
Grade 1: the deviation is less than 2 mm or less than half of the screw diameter.
Grade 2: the deviation is more than 2 mm and less than 4 mm or half to one screw diameter.
Grade 3: the deviation is more than 4 mm or complete deviation.

The accuracy of the navigational template was examined before operation by drilling the screw trajectories into the vertebral bio-models. Each navigational template was found to be fitting to its corresponding vertebral bio-model appropriately without any free movement, and the K wires were found to be inserted through the drill hole and the pedicle and into the desired vertebra without any violation as found by visual inspection.

During the operation, it was easy to find the best fit for positioning the template manually, as there was no significant free motion of the template when it was placed in position and pressed slightly against the vertebral body. As such, the navigational template fulfilled its purpose for use as in situ drill guide.

A total of 88 screws were inserted into levels C2–C7 with 2–6 screws on each patient. Of these pedicle screws, 71 were in Grade 0, 14 in Grade 1, 3 in Grade 2, and no screw in Grade 3. None of the cases had complications caused by pedicle perforation, and especially there were no injury to the vertebral artery or to the spinal cord, nor was there a need for revision of pedicle perforation in any of the cases.

In this study, cervical pedicle abnormality existed in five patients. The pedicles (four C2 and one C7) of these patients were very narrow with a minimum diameter of 3.5 mm. Screws of relatively smaller diameter (3 mm) were chosen for these patients accordingly and were placed inside pedicles accurately using navigational templates.

In another case, the pedicle was extremely narrow in level C2 with a minimum diameter of only 1.5 mm, and therefore the C2 cervical fixation was not performed. The CT data showed congenital fusion between C2 and C3, and therefore pedicle screw fixation was successfully performed on level C3 using the drill template.

By using this novel, custom-fit navigational template, the operation time had been considerably reduced. On an average, each vertebral pedicle screw insertion took about 80 s. Fluoroscopy was required only once after the insertion of the entire pedicle screws, which has considerably reduced the duration of radiation exposure to the members of the surgical team. Currently the production time for RP model is about 2 days and the cost is about $50 per vertebral level. The production time can be brought down to 1 day, and the cost can be reduced to $20 if the RP model of the vertebra is not needed.

A Novel Patient-Specific Navigational Template
for Thoracic Pedicle Placement

Most studies have shown that the rates of misplacement for the free-hand technique are usually between 28% and 43%, while only a few studies have shown rates of less than 5%. Hence, the screw breach rate may be dangerously high when the anatomy is altered as in scoliosis. Lonner et al. [1] suggested that there should be a considerable learning curve for

using the pedicle screws in scoliosis surgery to avoid complications. The need for improved accuracy and consistency in the placement of thoracic pedicle screws has led to investigations on the application of computer-navigated spine surgery. Computer-assisted pedicle screw installation allows an increased accuracy in using screws, thus decreasing the incidence of misplaced screws. Considering these difficulties, surgeons must use whatever techniques they find helpful to create a safe environment when placing thoracic pedicle screws into the deformed pediatric spine.

Sixteen patients (12 females, 4 males, age of 5–18 years) with scoliosis (14 of adolescent idiopathic scoliosis, 2 two of congenital scoliosis) undergoing spinal deformity correction surgeries using posterior pedicle screw instrumentation of the thoracic spine formed the study group. Before the operation, a spiral 3D CT scan (LightSpeed VCT, GE, USA) was performed on the thoracic spine of each patient with 0.625 mm slice thickness and 0.35 mm in-plane resolution. The images were stored in DICOM format and transferred to a workstation running MIMICS 10.01 software (Materialise Company, Belgium) to generate a 3D reconstruction model for the desired thoracic vertebra. The 3D vertebral model was then exported in STL format and opened in a workstation running reverse engineering (RE) software UG imageware12.0 (EDS, USA) to determine the optimal screw size and orientation. A screw with a diameter of 5 mm was placed virtually into the 3D spinal model on both sides. The virtual screw's entry point and the trajectory were placed at the center of the pedicle without violating the cortex.

2.5.2 Preoperative Planning

According to the type of scoliosis, the fusion level is determined, and the instrumentational vertebra is chosen. The design and development of the drill template for each vertebra are also made according to the instrumentational vertebra. The vertebral rotation, axes, length, and diameter of the pedicle were measured from the preoperative CT scan. Thus, the length and diameter of every pedicle screw were decided upon before operation. The concave periapical (T5–8) pedicles are often deformed and are considered to be the most difficult area to work on during pedicle screw placement [2–5]. If the pedicle is very narrow, an in-out-in technique can be chosen.

2.5.3 Operation Procedure

The spine was exposed subperiosteally on both sides, up to the tips of the transverse processes. For the thoracic spine, the soft tissues on the facet joints were thoroughly cleaned off to ensure better visualization of the bony landmarks. The drill template was then placed on the spinous, lamina, and transverse processes. The drill template and the corresponding spinous process were fitted well. A high-speed drill was used along the navigational channel to drill the trajectory of each pedicle screw. Using a hand drill, the trajectory of the pedicle screw was carefully drilled to a depth in accordance with the preoperation plan. The pedicle screw, the diameter and length of which had been chosen preoperatively, was carefully inserted along the same trajectory. After screw placement and correction of deformity, all exposed laminar surfaces were decorticated, and the autologous iliac crest bone was grafted.

A total of 168 screws were placed from T2–T12 in the 16 cases, and postoperative CT scans were obtained in all 16 patients. About 157 screws were considered intrapedicular, while 11 screws were considered to have a 0–2 mm breach (one medial, ten lateral in which eight belonged to the planned in-out-in screws). No pedicle screw breached was more than 2 mm, and the overall screw accuracy (<2 mm breach is safe) was 100%. No screw penetrated the inferior or superior cortex in the sagittal plane.

A Novel Patient-Specific Navigational Template for Laminar Screw Placement

Instability of the occipitocervical junction requiring surgical stabilization may be treated with a variety of techniques. The objective is to obtain solid fusion of the involved segments, which is best achieved by minimizing motion between them. Older methods such as the Brooks-Jenkins or modified Gallie wiring techniques are simpler procedures, have been known for a long time, and are associated with failure rates of fusion up to 25%, primarily in cases with rotational instability. Newer techniques have been described that effectively limit motion along all axes. The addition of transarticular screw fixation, according to Magerl and Seemann, offers a better biomechanical stability. But, Magerl screw fixation must be very precise point of placement to make screw fixation in the lateral mass of atlas, which can result in a significant risk to the vertebral artery. The size of the C2 pedicle can limit the ability to safely place these screws, particularly taking into account the anomalous position of the vertebral artery in relation to the isthmus of C2 in up to 20% of the population. Leonard and Wright [6] described a new technique of C2 laminar screw for rigid screw fixation of the axis and incorporation into atlantoaxial fixation or subaxial cervical constructs, and subsequent cases have shown good clinical results with this technique. C2 laminar screws are appealing due to the reduced risk of injury to the vertebral artery and biomechanical stability. The present method of C2 laminar screw placement relies on anatomical landmarks for screw placement. Placement of C2 laminar screws using drill template has not been described in the literature. A novel computer-assisted drill guide template for placement of C2 laminar screws is designed to simplify and shorten the surgical act and at the same time further enhance the accuracy of screw positions in the C2 laminar.

Before the operation, a spiral 3D CT scan (LightSpeed VCT, GE, USA) was performed on cervical spine of each patient with 0.625 mm slice thickness and 0.35 mm in-plane resolution. The images were stored in DICOM format and transferred to a workstation running MIMICS 10.01 software (Materialise Company, Belgium) to generate a 3D reconstruction model for the desired C2 vertebrae. The 3D vertebral model was then exported in STL format and opened in a workstation running reverse engineering (RE) software UG imageware12.0 (EDS, USA) for determining the optimal screw size and orientation. A screw with a diameter of 4 mm was placed virtually into the 3D spinal model on both sides. The virtual screw's entry point and the trajectory were placed centered on the lamina without violating the cortex, and two screws would not interfere with each other.

The optimal screw size was determined according to the size of laminea as well. Afterward, a navigational template was constructed with one drill guide on either side. The template surface was created to be the inverse of C2 spinous process and laminar, thus potentially enabling a fit in a lock-and-key fashion similar to a physical casting of the vertebral surface, and specifically avoided overlap onto adjacent segments. The inner diameter of the hollow cylinder was created to accommodate the preplanned trajectory for drilling. Once these had been done, a drill template was constructed with a surface designed to be the inverse of the vertebral surface.

The computer model was then exported in STL format. The bio-model of the C2 vertebra as well as its corresponding navigational template were both produced by acrylate resin (Somos 14,120, DSM Desotech Inc., USA) using stereolithography rapid prototyping (RP) technique. The accuracy of the navigational template was examined by visual inspection before surgery. The bio-model and its corresponding template were placed together, and a standard electric power drill was used to drill screw trajectory into the bio-model at the predefined placement, and visual inspection was taken for any violation of C2 laminar.

From June 2006 to September 2008, nine patients (four males, five females, age of 17–53 years) with basilar invagination requiring the posterior instrumentation were performed occipitocervical fusion surgery by C2 laminar screw fixation. There are eight cases with occipitalization of the atlas, and six cases accompanied by C2–C3 vertebral fusion. In three patients a transoral surgery was performed firstly, followed by posterior surgery. The anatomy of C2 pedicle was observed by preoperative X-ray and CT scan; if the pedicle is very narrow, thin, or vertebral artery high riding, it would be inappropriate placement of pedicle screw, and the lamina screw fixation can be chosen.

Using tracheal intubation general anesthesia, patients are placed in the prone position with the head and cervical spine maintained in the neutral position using the Mayfield head holder. The spinous process, laminae, and lateral masses of C2 are then exposed as needed. Then the drill template was placed on the spinous process and laminae of C2. Template and the corresponding spinous process were fitted well. The high-speed drill is used along the navigational channel to drill the trajectory of laminar screw. Using a hand drill, the trajectory of laminar screw is carefully drilled to a depth of preoperative plan. A 4.0 mm screw is carefully inserted along the same trajectory. Using the same technique as above, a 4.0 mm screw is placed into the other lamina. After screw placement, all exposed laminar surfaces are decorticated with the high-speed drill. Autologous iliac crest bone grafts are wedged under the rods between the occipital bone and the spinous process and lamina of C2.

Using the virtual 3D model, the optimal entry point for the bore can be chosen, thus determining the entry point and direction for the C2 laminar screw. The drill template was created to fit the postural surface of C2 spinous process very well. The accuracy of the drill template was examined before operation by drilling K wire trajectory into the vertebra bio-model. Each navigational template fits its corresponding vertebral bio-model perfectly, and K wire was found to be inserted through the drill hole into the C2 lamina, and no violation was found by visual inspection.

Nine patients with basilar invagination were performed occipitocervical fusion surgery, the bilateral cross laminar screw fixation was performed in eight patients, and unilateral laminar screw fixation and the other side of pedicle screw fixation was performed in a patient. Average follow-up was 9 months (range 4–13 months). Preoperative and postoperative functional comparisons were made using the ASIA grading scale for all cases. Seven of the patients (77.8%) improved at least one ASIA grade. Two patients have not improved. No patient suffered from neurological deterioration as a result of the procedure.

Seventeen C2 laminar screws were inserted using drill template. No screw inserted with complications, such as spinal cord, nerve, and vertebral artery injury, appeared in this group. The mean operative time between fixation of the template to the lamina and placement of the screw was 1–2 min. Operative time was reduced through the use of the navigational template. No additional computer assistance was needed during surgery, and fluoroscopy was used only once after all the C2 laminar screws had been inserted. The method thus significantly reduced radiation exposure for the members of the surgical team.

It takes about 16 h to manufacture the RP model, and the price of each RP model of the vertebra and navigational template is about $20. Postoperative CT scans showed that the individual template had a higher precision. No laminar screw misplacement occurred using the individual template.

A Novel Patient-Specific Navigational Template for Hangman Fracture

In 1965, after noting a similarity between certain C2 fractures and injuries sustained in judicial hanging, Schneider et al. adopted the phrase "hangman fracture," which is also called atlantoaxial traumatic spondylolisthesis. The occipital base bends the posterior structures of the axis, which results in a bipedicular fracture. Although nonoperative management is the primary management paradigm, internal fixation should be considered in several situations. An in-depth understanding of hangman fracture led to the improvement of surgical techniques, the development of internal fixation devices, and an increase in the number of accepted spine surgeons for early surgical fixation. The posterior C2 pedicle single- or double-paragraph segment fixation is the treatment for hangman fracture. Despite the effectivity of the pars screw for the treatment of hangman's fracture, the risk injuring the vertebral artery and spinal cord remains a potential risk for this procedure. The size of the C2 pedicle can limit the ability to place safely these screws, particularly taking into account the anomalous position of the vertebral artery in relation to the isthmus of C2 in up to 20% of the population. Computed tomography (CT)-based navigation in the presence of unstable fracture is not ideal because the intervertebral anatomy alters between the supine position in which the CT scan is performed and the prone position in which the surgery is performed. Minor inaccuracies in this region may also be unacceptable, and the chance of injury to vital structures is higher. Intraoperative Iso-C3D navigation acquires fluoroscopic images after patient positioning and completion of surgical exposure, thereby avoiding registration-related errors. Real time navigation with Iso-C3D also helps in the accurate and safe placement of cervical pedicle screws. In this paper, we report the successful performance of pedicle screw fixation of C2 vertebra in hangman fracture using a computer-assisted drill guide template.

Before the operation, a spiral 3D CT scan (LightSpeed VCT, GE, USA) was performed on the cervical spine of each patient with 0.625 mm slice thickness. The images were stored in DICOM format and then transferred into a workstation running MIMICS 10.01 software (Materialise Company, Belgium) to generate a 3D reconstruction model for the desired hangman fracture vertebrae. A screw with a diameter of 4 mm was placed virtually into the 3D spinal model on both sides. The entry point and the trajectory of the virtual screws were centered on the pedicle without violating the cortex. Afterward, a navigational template was constructed with one drill guide on either side. The template surface was created to be the inverse of the C2 spinous process and lamina, thereby potentially enabling a fit in a lock-and-key fashion similar to a physical casting of the vertebral surface. The inner diameter of the hollow cylinder was created to accommodate the preplanned trajectory for drilling. Once these steps were done, a drill template was constructed with a surface designed to be the inverse of the vertebral surface. We also observed the reduction of fracture along the pedicle screw during the simulation of fracture reduction.

The computer model was exported in STL format. The bio-model of the hangman fracture vertebra and its corresponding navigational template were both produced by acrylate resin (Somos 14,120, DSM Desotech, Inc., USA) using stereolithography rapid prototyping (RP) technique. Before surgery, the accuracy of the drill template was examined by visual inspection. The bio-model and its corresponding template were put together, and then a standard electric power drill was used to drill the screw trajectory into the bio-model at the predefined placement. Visual inspection was taken for any violation of C2 pedicle screws.

Skull traction with extension was used in all patients after admission to reduce the fracture. This partial reduction was confirmed fluoroscopically. Under tracheal intubation and general anesthesia, patients were placed in prone position, with the head and cervical spine maintained in the neutral position by using skull traction. The spinous process, lamina, and lateral masses of C2 were exposed as needed. This partial reduction was confirmed fluoroscopically as well. Then, the drill template was placed on the spinous process and lamina of C2. The template and the corresponding spinous process fitted well. The high-speed drill was used along the navigational channel to drill the trajectory of the pedicle screw. The trajectory of the pedicle screw was carefully drilled to a depth of the preoperation plan. Cannulated, self-drilling, self-tapping, and end-threaded lag screws were inserted over the Kirschner wires to reduce the fracture completely. A 4.0 mm screw was carefully inserted along the same trajectory. With the same technique, a 4.0 mm screw was placed into the other pedicle.

With the virtual 3D model, the optimal entry point for the drill can be chosen, which determines the entry point and direction for the C2 pedicle screw. The drill template was created to fit the postural surface of the C2 spinous process quite well. Each navigational template fitted its corresponding vertebral bio-model perfectly, and K wire was inserted through the drill hole into the C2 pedicle. No violation was found by visual inspection.

During the operation, the best fit for positioning the template can easily be found manually because no significantly free motion of the template occurred when pressed slightly against the C2 spinous process and lamina. The individual navigational template technique has the ability to customize the placement and size of each screw based on the unique morphology of the C2 pedicle of each patient, which can be used to prepare preoperatively the surgical plan. To achieve this step, exact preparation of the bone surface is essential, which includes the thorough removal of the attached muscle and fat tissue without damaging the bony surface. No pedicle screw misplacement occurred using the individual template. The mean operative time between the fixation of the template to the lamina and placement of the screw was 1–2 mins. No additional computer assistance was needed during surgery, and fluoroscopy was used only two times: before the operation to ascertain the reduction of fracture and after all the C2 pedicle screws were inserted. The method reduced radiation exposure for the members of the surgical team.

2.5.4 Conclusion

The authors have developed a novel patient-specific navigational template for spinal pedicle screw placement with good applicability and high accuracy. The potential use of navigational templates in spinal surgery is promising. Our methodology appears to provide an accurate technique and trajectory for spinal surgery.

2.6 Osteoarticular Allograft Reconstruction After Bone Tumor Resection with the Assist of Preoperative 3D Planning and Surgical Navigation

Zhigang Wu and Jun Fu

Abstract Objective: This study aims to describe the preoperative planning of tumor resection and allograft reconstruction based on 3D models that include the selection of the allograft from a digital bone bank and the subsequent intraoperative application of this procedure assisted by navigation. Methods: From November 2011 to June 2013, operative treatments based on 3D preoperative planning and intraoperative assistance of computer navigation technology were performed in 14 patients with malignant tumors. The average age of 14 patients was (21.8 ± 5.9) years. The malignant tumor types included osteosarcoma (8), Ewing sarcoma (3), Giant cell tumor of bone (GCT) (2), and chondrosarcoma (1). The tumor locations included distal femur (2), proximal tibia (6), distal tibia (2), pelvic (2), distal radius (1), and scapula (1). The local recurrence of tumor and functional results were postoperatively followed up. Results: Establishment of the digital bone bank shortened the selection time of allograft osteoarticular materials before surgery and improved the selection accuracy compared with routine preparations of osteoarticular allograft. Tumor resection and allograft osteoarticular reconstruction were performed assisted by computer navigation. The dissection register spot during surgery matched with the 3D CT images before surgery well. Postoperative images showed that the tumor resection territory and allograft osteoarticular cutting region were in complete agreement with the preoperative design. Joint reconstruction was stable, limb isometry was achieved, and joint malformation was absent. The average follow-up was (16.1 ± 8.2) months. Local recurrence or remote metastasis was not reported except one pulmonary metastasis. No screw loosening, breakage, or joint collapse occurred in any of the patients at last follow-up. The average MSTS93 functional score was 25.7 ± 1.1. Conclusion: Establishment of a digital bone bank provides accurate information for allograft bone material selection before surgery. The individual design of bone resection and reconstruction may be achieved with computer navigation, thereby improving the safety and effectiveness of salvage limb operation.

Keywords Digital bone bank; Bone tumor; Allograft bone; Preoperative planning; Computer-assisted navigation

Osteoarticular allograft transplantation is a useful method used to reconstruct joint defects after bone tumor resection in limb salvage treatment of bone tumors. With the establishment of bone banks and development of allograft bone processing technology, the risks of immunity rejection and disease transmission have been significantly reduced. However, the selection of allograft bone materials, especially amorphous joint ends, remains a problem among clinicians. Unsatisfactory matching between allograft bone and host bone negatively affects the results of reconstruction [7]. Application of digital technology in the orthopedics field allows the quick acquisition of accurate information of banked bone [8]. Using digital technology, we established a digital system for the management and analysis of allografts. This system is called the digital bone bank. The accurate matching function of the digital bone bank allows the selection of proper allografts and preoperative designs of individual allograft osteoarticular cutting and trimming. During surgery based on the preoperative design, precise en bloc resection and individual allograft bone reconstruction can be achieved with the aid of a navigation guide. This study aims to describe the preoperative planning of tumor resection and allograft reconstruction based in 3D models that include the selection of the allograft from a digital bone bank, and the subsequent intraoperative application of this procedure assisted by navigation.

2.6.1 Materials and Methods

General Information
Massive bone allografts in the *FMMU*-Xijing Hospital bone bank were classified by anatomical site, including scapula, clavicle, proximal humerus, distal humerus, ulna, radius, pelvis, proximal femur, distal femur, proximal tibia, distal tibia, fibula, and calcaneus. Allografts were then scanned by 64-row computer tomography (CT) and analyzed. The three-dimensional (3D) information of each allograft, including length, width, and height, was saved in digital imaging and communications in medicine (DICOM) file format. Important data, such as articular surface and osseous mark, were also noted. All of the information related to the massive bone allografts were coded and saved

to establish a digital system for the management and analysis of allografts; this system was called the digital bone bank. In choosing, firstly bone allografts were selected by the size of bone and distance of osseous mark, and then, the definite curve was matched.

From November 2011 to June 2013, operative treatments assisted by the digital bone bank and tumor resection reconstructions with computer navigation technology were performed in 14 patients with malignant tumors. The average age of 14 patients was (21.8 ± 5.9) years. The malignant tumor types included osteosarcoma (8), Ewing sarcoma (3), GCT (2), and chondrosarcoma (1). The tumor locations included distal femur (2), proximal tibia (6), distal tibia (2), pelvic (2), distal radius (1), and scapula (1). (Table 12.2) All of the patients underwent needle biopsy before surgery and obtained clear pathological diagnoses. Adjuvant chemotherapy was performed on all cases except GCT and chondrosarcoma.

Prior to surgery, X-ray, CT, magnetic resonance imaging (MRI), and single-photon emission computed tomography/CT (SPECT/CT) scan were performed on all patients to determine the tumor boundary, tumor stage, and resection territory. We simulated joint defection after tumor resection on a computer and selected the optimum matching bone remodeling segments from the digital bone bank. The allograft bone segments were trimmed according to 3D information of the defection, and the position and direction of internal fixation were decided. Local recurrence and metastasis of the tumor, functional results, and complications were followed up postoperatively.

2.6.2 Surgical Navigation
The CT and MRI scanning data of tumor part and the CT scanning data of the selected allograft bone were imported into the navigation system (Cart II navigation system, Stryker, USA). For a better show of tumor border, the MRI images were infused into CT images in the software with a navigation system.

The preoperatively designed cutting plane and fixation implant position were marked on the 3D model. Then the register spots (3–5 points) were marked on the 3D model according to the surgical approach and exposure range.

The tracker was installed by surgery and the register spot was exposed. Patients' anatomy marks and 3D models were registered and then surface correction was performed. After registration, the tumor was resected and the allograft bone was cut to repair the defect using the navigation guide based on the preoperative design. The internal fixation implant position was determined according to the navigation guide. Proper alignment and joint angles were also examined by the navigation system. Finally, the effect of operation was evaluated by the postoperative photograph and MSTS93 [9] functional score.

Table 12.2 Details of 14 cases with tumor operative treatments based in 3D preoperative planning and intraoperative navigation

Case	Gender	Age(yrs)	Location	Diagnosis	Operation time (mins)	Amount of bleeding (ml)	Follow-up (myhs)	Function (MSTS score)	Local recurrence and distant metastasis
1	F	20	Right proximal tibia	Osteosarcoma	280	300	23	26	DFS
2	F	27	Left distal radius	GCT	85	150	27	25	DFS
3	F	22	Left proximal tibia	Osteosarcoma	135	300	23	26	DFS
4	M	15	Right proximal tibia	Osteosarcoma	220	700	10	25	Living with pulmonary metastasis at 5th month postoperatively
5	M	22	Right distal tibia	Osteosarcoma	330	600	6	27	DFS
6	M	11	Right ilium and peri-acetabulum	Ewing's sarcoma	215	2100	5	24	DFS
7	M	18	Left distal femur	Ewing's sarcoma	235	500	31	27	DFS
8	M	11	Right proximal tibia	Osteosarcoma	170	150	14	26	DFS
9	F	31	Left distal femur	Osteosarcoma	160	300	23	27	DFS
10	M	13	Right peri-acetabulum	Ewing's sarcoma	310	3000	11	25	DFS
11	M	16	Left distal tibia	Osteosarcoma	180	300	17	27	DFS
12	M	19	Right proximal tibia	Osteosarcoma	300	300	10	26	DFS
13	F	20	Right proximal tibia	GCT	250	300	19	24	DFS
14	M	60	Right scapula	Chondrosarcoma	160	500	7	25	DFS

2.6.3　Case 1

A 19-year-old male patient was diagnosed with osteosarcoma at the right upper tibia. He developed right knee pain for 5 months. Radiological investigations of right knee showed an osteoblastic destruction (Fig. 12.10a). The biopsy revealed an osteosarcoma. Preoperatively a computer design was performed and the border of tumor and the plane of osteotomy were described. A compatible allograft was found from digital bone bank by shape matching (Fig. 12.10b), and the osteotomy for this allograft was described (Fig. 12.10c). All design data were inputted into the navigation system. After preoperative chemotherapy and routine preparation, we ensured tumor resection plane by navigation which was designed preoperatively. (Fig. 12.10d, e) After osteotomy, the allograft was trimmed by navigation guidance. Then a plate was used to fix the allograft to the rest of tibia (Fig. 12.10f). Postoperative and 6-month follow-up radiograph was given and good resection and reconstruction were seen (Fig. 12.10g).

2.6.4　Case 2

An 11-year-old male patient was diagnosed with Ewing's sarcoma at the right acetabular. He developed right hip pain for 9 months. Radiological investigations of pelvic showed an osteolytic destruction at ilium and acetabular (Fig. 12.11a). The biopsy revealed an Ewing's sarcoma. Preoperatively a computer design was performed and the border of tumor and the plane of osteotomy were described. There was no suitable allograft for child. An adult allograft pelvic was found and the osteotomy for this allograft was designed (Fig. 12.11b). All design data were inputted into Navigation system. With these data, a guide plate was designed and made by rapid prototyping technology (Fig. 12.11c). After routine preparation, we ensured tumor resection plane by navigation which was designed preoperatively (Fig. 12.11g). After osteotomy, the allograft was trimmed by the guidance of guide plate and computer navigation. Then a plate and screws were used to fix the allograft to the rest of pelvic (Fig. 12.11e). Postoperative radiograph and 3 month follow-up CT were given and good resection and reconstruction were seen (Fig. 12.11f).

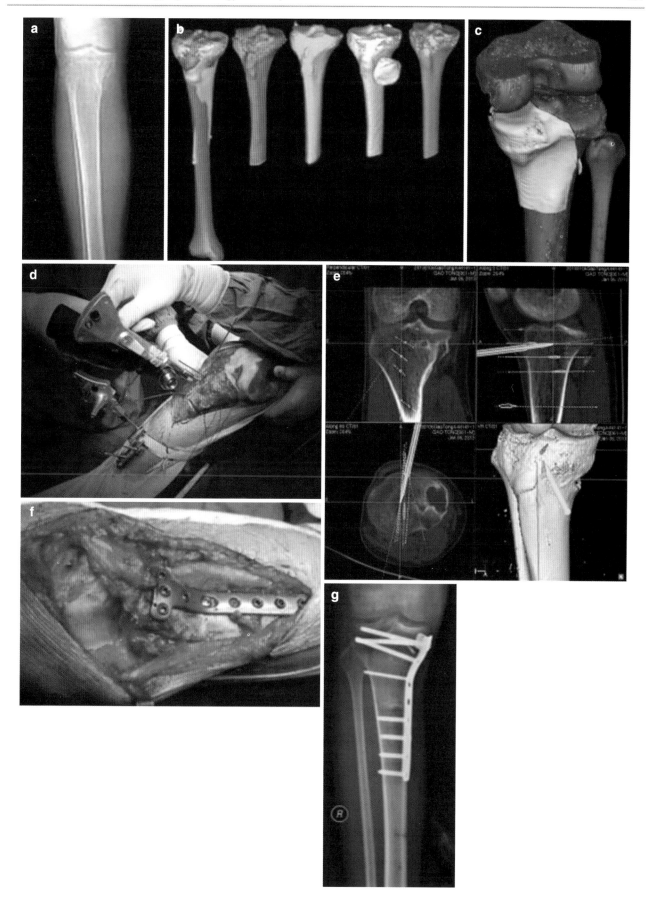

Fig. 12.10 (a) Radiological investigations of right knee showed an osteoblastic destruction. (b) A compatible allograft was found from the digital bone bank by shape matching. (c) The osteotomy for this allograft was described. (d) Operation with navigation guidance. (e) Navigation operation system. (f) A plate was used to fix the allograft to the rest of tibia. (g) 6-month follow-up radiograph

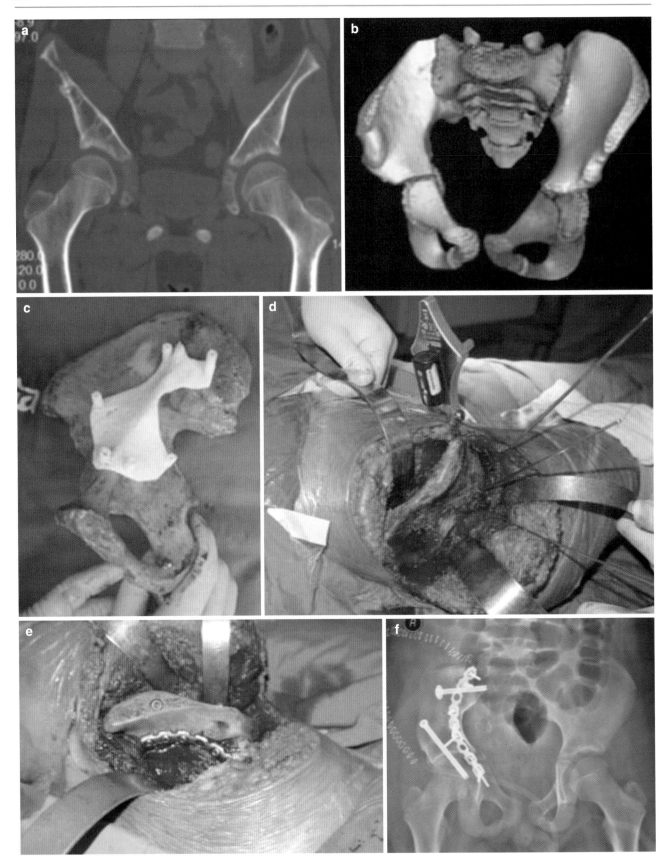

Fig. 12.11 (**a**) Radiological investigations of pelvic showed an osteo-lytic destruction at ilium and acetabular. (**b**) An adult allograft pelvic was found, and the osteotomy for this allograft was designed. (**c**) A guide plate was designed and made by rapid prototyping technology. (**d**) Operation with navigation guidance. (**e**) A plate and screws were used to fix the allograft to the rest of pelvic. (**f**) Postoperative radiograph

2.6.5 Results

Establishment of the digital bone bank could shorten the selection time of the allograft osteoarticular material before surgery and improve selection accuracy compared with the routine preparation of allograft. Tumor resection and allograft osteoarticular cuts were performed with the aid of computer navigation. The dissection register spot during surgery matched the 3D CT images before surgery well. Postoperative images (X-ray and CT) showed that the tumor resection territory and allograft osteoarticular cutting region were in agreement with the preoperative design. Joint reconstruction was stable, limb isometry was achieved, and no joint malformation was observed. No important nerve or vascular damage occurred during surgery. The operation time ranged from 85 min to 300 min, averaging about 216 min. The bleeding volume ranged from 150 ml to 3000 ml, averaging about 678 ml.

The average follow-up was 16.1 ± 8.2 months. Local recurrence or remote metastasis did not occur except pulmonary metastasis in one case at 5 months after operation. No screw loosening, breakage, or joint collapse occurred in any of the patients. The average MSTS93 functional score was 25.7 ± 1.1 at a recent follow-up.

2.6.6 Discussion

Limb salvage has become the most common option of bone tumor surgery. Massive allograft osteoarticular and artificial joints are usually necessary for bone reconstruction after en bloc tumor resection. The major complications after limb salvage operations, aside from local recurrence and remote metastasis, include screw loosening, hydrops, dislocation, nonunion, immunity rejection, internal fixation fatigue, fracture, and infection [10, 11]. For allograft bone transplantation, the most significant concern is providing not only a holder with suitable strength, shape, and size but also a good articular surface and attachment point of muscle, ligament, and joint capsule [7]. The bone end can achieve satisfactory biological healing and induce important soft tissues to easily meet biomechanical demands. The long-term function is better compared with artificial prosthesis [12]. The emergence of normalized bone banks ensures stationary sources and scientific preparation methods for allograft bone [13]. However, accuracy of allograft bone transplantation, especially partial osteoarticular transplantation, and the methods of selecting banked bones are still inadequate. The core problem lies in the quick selection of optimum matching bone remodeling segments.

With the application of digital technology in the medical field, establishment of an accurate and efficient selecting system can help improve the clinical results of allograft osteoarticular transplantation.

Through the establishment of a digital bone bank, accurate information for selecting allograft osteoarticular materials can be achieved prior to surgery. With computer navigation, the individual design of resection and reconstruction can be achieved during surgery. The safety and effectiveness of the bone bank were evaluated through practical application. As the earliest transplant material, the clinical results of allograft osteoarticular materials have been validated, but much room for further development remains [14, 15]. At present, many regions in China have established normalized bone banks, so stable sources and scientific storage methods are ensured. The bone bank in FMMU-Xijing hospital is the earliest to be established at 2010 in China.

The resources for this study were acquired from the bone bank in FMMU-Xijing Hospital. Massive bone allografts near the joint were classified by anatomical site, including scapula, clavicle, proximal humerus, distal humerus, ulna, radius, pelvis, proximal femur, distal femur, proximal tibia, distal tibia, fibula, and calcaneus. After distinguishing by side, allografts with similar classes were scanned by 64-row CT and analyzed. The 3D information of each allograft, including length, width, and height, was saved in DICOM file format. Important data, such as articular surface and osseous mark, were also marked. All of the information of the massive bone allografts was coded and saved to establish a digital system for the management and analysis of allografts. This system was called the digital bone bank. Information from patients and the bone bank can be accurately and efficiently matched according to clinical requirements to obtain individual allograft osteoarticular materials. Our digital bone bank has been practically proven to possess the following features: (1) convenient management of the bone bank and determination of necessary bone materials, (2) accurate matching of osteoarticular defection, (3) shortened preoperative preparation times, (4) promotion of the development of computer navigation-assisted surgery, and (5) bone allograft salvage.

Digital anatomy is enhanced by ever-changing computer technologies, and digitization of the surgical field has seen major growth. Modern surgery has entered a new era that features a digital, individual, microscopic, accurate, and artificially intellectual development trend. For instance, the application of computer navigation has extended from the neurosurgical field to other areas, such as joint prosthesis selection, prosthesis implantation, and oral and maxillofacial deformity correction [16]. Some application studies have shown that computer navigation systems or imaging navigation can provide real-time information of anatomy sites, implants, and relative instruments for surgeons [17–19]. Thus, the accuracy of implants and intraoperative feedback are improved and the exposure time to radiation is shortened.

Computer-aided 3D reconstruction technique can help build anatomical models of osteoarticular materials. The models are imported into computer-aided design (CAD) software to obtain accurate analysis. Information of matching allografts is then extracted from the bone bank and imported into the computer. The design and simulation of surgery, selection of internal fixation materials, development of a surgery-assisted template based on CAD rapid prototyping technology, and production of individual implants are conducted in the computer. Surgery based on the preoperative design is finally performed precisely. Limb salvage assisted by computer navigation technology can overcome the shortcomings of previous conventional surgeries and result in more accurate preoperative design, surgery simulation, accurate allograft bone cutting, and precise implantation of internal fixation during surgery [20].

In this clinical study, 3D reconstructed CT image data of the bone tumor before surgery were compared with allograft osteoarticular data in the digital bone bank to select optimum matching bone remodeling segments. Information from DICOM data were imported into the navigational system to accurately scale the territory of tumor resection and allograft osteoarticular cutting. During surgery based on the preoperative design, the tumor was resected, and the allograft bone was cut with the aid of the navigation guide to achieve allograft bone structural reconstruction. Accurate reconstruction was further validated by the navigational system. Establishment of the digital bone bank significantly shortened the selection time of allograft osteoarticular materials before surgery and improved the selection accuracy compared with routine preparation of allograft osteoarticulation. Tumor resection and allograft osteoarticular incision were performed with the aid of computer navigation. The dissection register spot during surgery matched the 3D CT images before surgery well. Compared with operations based on surgeon experience, the technique presented in this study showed less injuries, higher accuracy, more reasonable matching, and shorter operation time. Follow-up showed that the bones healed and functioned well. Only one patient was found a pulmonary metastasis at 5th month postoperatively then a second-line chemotherapy was given. Except this case, local recurrence or remote metastasis did not occur.

In conclusion, establishment of the digital bone bank provided accurate information for selecting allograft bone materials before surgery. The individual design of resection and reconstruction was achieved with the aid of computer navigation, thereby improving the safety and effectiveness of the salvage limb operation. Although this single-center study was small in scale and the follow-up time was short, the results clearly demonstrate the advantages of this technology.

Acknowledgments We acknowledge the great assistance of Prof. Luis Aponte Tinao (Ortopedia Oncologica, Hospital Italiano de Buenos Aires, Argentina) in the digital bone bank setup and paper modification.

2.7 Application of RP to Sport Injury Surgery

Zhi Yuanl

(Whether the title can be changed into: Exploration of RP for Articular Cartilage Injury Repair?)

Articular cartilage injury is very common in sport injury surgery. However, there is no feasible method to repair articular cartilage injury at present; thus it remains a great clinical problem, and the development of tissue engineering technology brings a new thought to deal with it.

2.7.1 Prepare Tissue Engineering Cartilage Bracket with PR

Bracket material plays a critical role in tissue engineering: (1) It is the carrier to which the cells and growth factors adhere; (2) It can provide temporary support in the process of tissue repair, guide the regenerated tissue to grow into the designated form and form the shape of targeted tissue. The following criteria shall be contained in ideal bracket materials for repairing cartilage defect: (1) excellent biocompatibility; (2) vivo degradability matched with regenerated tissues; (3) favorable plasticity and mechanical strength; (4) appropriate 3D pore structures; (5) favorable hydrophilicity; and (6) favorable performance of compound growth factors.

In the past, people mainly focused on the use of tissue engineering cartilage. Some scholars prepared tissue engineering cartilage with RP, and research reports had been published regarding preparing tissue engineering cartilage bracket with RP for cartilage injury repair abroad. However, at the time the tissue engineering cartilage is implanted into in vivo defect area, the integrated interface formed is cartilage-bone and cartilage-cartilage. In case of cartilage defect, retrogression including sclerosis etc. will frequently occur on subchondral bone, and it is hard to integrate the interface of cartilage-bone, while the process of integration between transplant and recipient site will be accelerated if the integrated interface of cartilage-bone is transformed to bone-bone. Based on this principle, more importance has been attached to osteochondral tissue engineering, and osteochondral compound is designed and prepared to repair osteochondral lesion. When implanted into recipient site, it can not only help to accelerate the process of its integration with recipient site, but also bring convenience to fix the bracket on recipient site, which contributes to reduce the whole transplant's potential to shed due to the stress of articulation, thus the success rate is improved.

2.7.2   Prepare Osteochondral Tissue Engineering Material Containing Calcified Layer with RP

So far, however, the research of osteochondral tissue engineering is still on its initial stage. Existing osteochondral composite bracket has poor biomechanical property. When implanted into the body, it cannot fully bear the shear force created by the articulation movement particularly, thus breakage tends to appear between the cartilage bracket and bone bracket of osteochondral composite bracket. In addition, the seed cells' capacity of proliferation and differentiation is insufficient to meet clinical demands. We hold that it is partly resulted from that most scholars have limited understanding toward the organization structure of articular cartilage, the living environment of cells, the integration function of calcified layer between the cartilage and the subchondral bone, and the isolation function of calcified layer to chondrocytes and osteoblasts in order to provide an independent and distinct living environment for both of them. Ideal osteochondral tissue engineering bracket shall simulate the osteochondral structure of normal articulation and prepare a structure equivalent to calcified layer in osteochondral composite bracket to improve the biomechanical property of osteochondral composite bracket and accelerate the repair of articular cartilage in a better way.

The Department of Orthopaedics of Xijing Hospital creates compact layer made from PLGA/β-TCP with RP, through which the cartilage bracket and the bone bracket can be integrated to form a new type of osteochondral composite bracket (Fig. 12.12). The integration and isolation function of compact layer is equivalent to calcified layer, which equips this new osteochondral composite bracket with better

biomechanical characteristics. When implanted into the body, it can isolate chondrocytes and osteoblasts into different living environments, thus the seed cells can proliferate and differentiate better to achieve the functions above. The design of compact layer shall (1) contain pores as small as possible and appropriate thickness, (2) contain appropriate degradation velocity to match the velocity of tissue regeneration and compact layer degradation, and (3) contain sufficient mechanical property to allow the cartilage bracket and bone bracket to be integrated, so that they cannot be mutilated easily after being implanted.

The reason why the author selected PLGA/TCP as the material of compact layer is that by the mixed use of PLGA and TCP, the material can be equipped with favorable formability, and its degradation velocity as well as mechanical property is adjustable. Moreover, TCP can meet the calcified layer's demands for calcium and phosphorus, and Ca ions contained in the degradation products of TCP may neutralize acidic products resulted from PLGA degradation. Liu Li et al. from Tsinghua University observe that their optimal proportion is 7:3. In this proportion, the best formability, degradation velocity, and mechanical property can be achieved.

For the preparation of compact layer, manufacturing process of low-temperature deposition is adopted, through which the materials do not need heating and melting, while intrinsic physicochemical and biological properties remain with micropores on the surface, and any complicated shapes can be formed. Dissolve PLGA/TCP in 1,4-dioxane, the organic solvent, with the proportion of 7:3 in normal temperature. Prepare them into 25% homogeneous solution for standby application after intensive dissolving. Inject the pre-prepared material organic solution into the container above sprayer. Translate the layered tablet files in the computer into corresponding NC code in order to control the horizontal scanning motion and spraying velocity of each sprayer and the descending motion of workbench. Temperature in the plastic room is −40 °C. The material organic solution will solidify into solid state immediately after being sprayed from the sprayer to the workbench. When a row of solution is formed, the sprayer will translate for a certain distance directed by the computer and begin to spray on the next row. The translation distance of the sprayer minus the width of one row of solid material is the preset distance between two adjacent rows, i.e., the diameter of the macropore's aperture of compact layer is 0 in this subject. When the accumulation of one layer is completed, the workbench will descend to form the next layer and spray with a sprayer rotating 90° directed by the computer. The material organic solution sprayed out by the sprayer uses the waste heat to melt the little parts of bracket which it contacted in the former layer and has formed in solid state. The contact surface will be adhered,

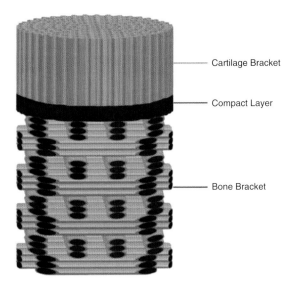

Fig. 12.12 Schematic diagram of new osteochondral composite bracket containing compact layer. Top, cartilage bracket material; middle, compact layer; bottom, bone bracket material

mixed together, and back to normal. Conduct the process above repeatedly, and finally the frozen bracket with the same form as the target will be accumulated. Place the formed frozen bracket in the freezer dryer for 12 h to allow sublimation to occur on the organic solvent 1,4-dioxane and get the tissue engineering bracket with micropores on material surface. When manufacturing the compact layer, PLGA/TCP organic solution is sprayed onto the surface of tissue engineering bone bracket with a 3D core-spun structure, and the thickness is controlled to be 0.5 mm. This will help to conduct the manufacturing process of low-temperature deposition and the one-batch forming of

the bone bracket. Then prepare the osteochondral composite bracket using pre-prepared cartilage bracket and compact layer-bone bracket with the fabrication processing of "melting adherent" (Fig. 12.13).

Vivo experiments on animals show that due to the compact layer, mechanical property of osteochondral composite bracket has been improved significantly. The bracket is able to adapt to complicated mechanical environments in particular and guarantee the repair of osteochondral tissue to be conducted smoothly (Figs. 12.14 and 12.15).

In general, osteochondral composite bracket with compact layer has favorable biomechanical property. When implanted into the body, it will help chondrocytes and osteoblasts to further differentiate and proliferate and accelerate the repair of full thickness defect of articular cartilage, thus has an important prospect in clinical practical application. However, the application of this technology is only limited to animal experiments rather than clinical stage, thus its actual effect is to be verified over time.

2.7.3 Application of Bioprinting Technology to Cartilage Repair

Bioprinting is one of the most attractive technologies in tissue engineering and regenerative medicine areas in recent years, through which cells, cell factors, etc. can be arranged in a predesigned 3D space structure in proportion accurately. Therefore, creating real living tissues can be achieved theoretically. However, this technology is still in its initial stage. The prototype of the first 3D bioprinter has been manufactured in the end of 2009 for testing. Researches concerning artificial livers, kidneys, vessels and skins have been

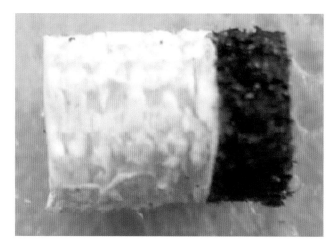

Fig. 12.13 Osteochondral composite bracket with compact layer prepared by RP. Black, cartilage bracket material; white, bone bracket material, though it is not easily perceived because of thin compact layer

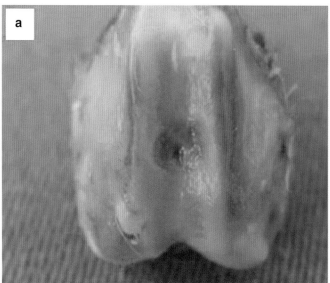

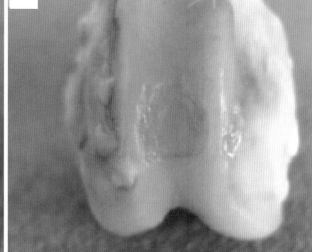

Fig. 12.14 Micro-CT observation on the effect of osteochondral composite bracket material with compact layer in repairing cartilage defect. (**a**) Control group after 3 months of operation (where the osteochondral bracket material has no compact layer); (**b**) control group after 6 months of operation (where the osteochondral bracket material has no compact layer); (**c**) experimental group after 3 months of operation (where the osteochondral bracket material has compact layer); (**d**) experimental group after 6 months of operation (where the osteochondral bracket material has compact layer)

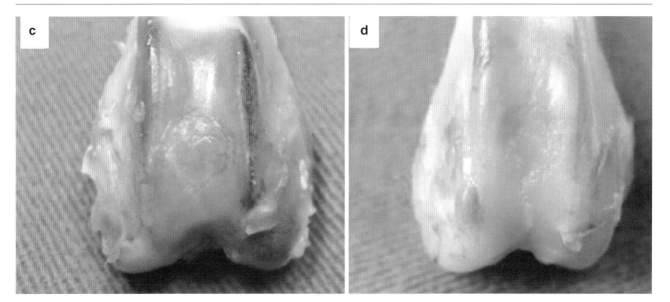

Fig. 12.14   (continued)

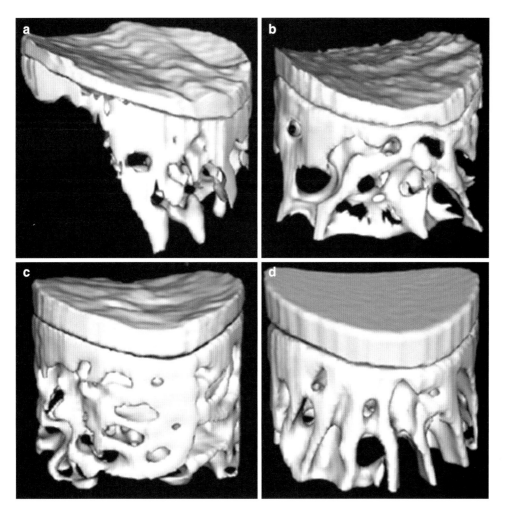

Fig. 12.15   Micro-CT observation on the effect of osteochondral composite bracket material with compact layer in repairing cartilage defect. (**a**) Control group after 3 months of operation (where the osteochondral bracket material has no compact layer); (**b**) control group after 6 months of operation (where the osteochondral bracket material has no compact layer); (**c**) experimental group after 3 months of operation (where the osteochondral bracket material has compact layer); (**d**) experimental group after 6 months of operation (where the osteochondral bracket material has compact layer)

conducted widely home and abroad. For example, American scientists have successfully printed out the "micro liver" layer by layer in lab through bioprinter.

Recently, some scientists are endeavoring to repair cartilage defects with bioprinting technology. Cui X et al. manufactured artificial biomimetic with chondrocytes and bracket material polyethylene glycol 200 diacrylate through bioprinter, and the result indicated that the artificial cartilage made showed favorable biological activity and had a prosperous prospect. This technology, however, is still in its laboratory stage and far from clinical application.

In summary, repairing cartilage defects through RP has an attractive prospect, yet all researches are limited to laboratory stage at present and far from clinical application.

References

1. Lonner BS, Auerbach JD, Estreicher MB, et al. Thoracic pedicle screw instrumentation: the learning curve and evolution in technique in the treatment of adolescent idiopathic scoliosis. Spine. 2009;34:2158–64.
2. Amstutz HC, Beaulé PE, Dorey FJ, et al. Hybrid metal-on-metal surface rthroplasty of the hip. Oper Tech Orthop. 2001;11(41):253–62.
3. Birnbaum K, Schkommodau E, Decker N, et al. Computer-assisted orthopedic surgery with individual templates and comparison to conventional operation method. Spine. 2001;26:365–70.
4. Radermacher K, Portheine F, Anton M, et al. Computer-assisted orthopedic surgery with image based individual templates. Clin Orthop. 1998;354:28–38.
5. Lu S, Xu YQ, Zhang YZ, Xie L, Guo H, Dong PL. A novel computer-assisted drill guide template for placement of C2 laminar screws. Eur Spine J. 2009;18(9):1379–85.
6. Leonard JR, Wright NM. Pediatric atlantoaxial fixation with bilateral, crossing C-2 translaminar screws. Technical note. J Neurosurg. 2006;104:59–63.
7. Enneking WF, Campanacci DA. Retrieved human allografts. A clinicopathological study. J Bone Joint Surg Am. 2001;83-A:971–86.
8. Ritacco LE, Seiler C, Farfalli GL, et al. Validity of an automatic measure protocol in distal femur for allograft selection from a three-dimensional virtual bone bank system. Cell Tissue Bank. 2013;14(2):213–20.
9. Enneking WF, Dunhmn W, Gebhardt MC, et al. A system for the functional evaluation of reconstructive procedures after surgical treatment of tumors of the musculoskeletal system. Clin Orthop Relat Res. 1993;286:241–6.
10. Ozger H, Bulbul M, Eralp L. Complications of limb salvage surgery in childhood tumors and recommended solutions. Strategies Trauma Limb Reconstr. 2010;5(1):11–5.
11. Blacksin MF, Benevenia J, Patterson FR. Complications after limb salvage surgery. Curr Probl Diagn Radiol. 2004;33(1):1–15.
12. Farfalli GL, Aponte-Tinao LA, Ayerza MA, Muscolo DL, Boland PJ, Morris CD, Athanasian EA, Healey JH. Comparison between constrained and semiconstrained knee allograft-prosthesis composite reconstructions. Sarcoma. 2013;2013:489652.
13. AATB. American association of tissue banks-standards for tissue banking. Viginia: AATB McLean; 2001.
14. Gebert C, Wessling M, Hoffmann C, et al. Hip transposition as a limb salvage procedure following the resection of periacetabular tumors. J Surg Oncol. 2011;103(3):269–75.
15. Biau D, Faure F, Katsahian S, Jeanrot C, Tomeno B, Anract P. Survival of total knee replacement with a megaprosthesis after bone tumor resection. J Bone Joint Surg Am. 2006;88(6):1285–93.
16. Wong KC, Kumta SM, Chiu KH, et al. Precision tumour resection and reconstruction using image-guided computer navigation. J Bone Joint Surg (Br). 2007;89(7):943–7.
17. Grunert P, Darabi K, Espinosa J, Filippi R. Computer-aided navigation in neurosurgery. Neurosurg Rev. 2003 May;26(2):73–9.
18. Viceconti M, Lattanzi R, Antonietti B, Paderni S, Olmi R, Sudanese A, Toni A. CT-based surgical planning software improves the accuracy of total hip replacement preoperative planning. Med Eng Phys. 2003;25(5):371–7.
19. Meyer U, Wiesmann HP, Runte C, Fillies T, Meier N, Lueth T, Joos U. Evaluation of accuracy of insertion of dental implants and prosthetic treatment by computer-aided navigation in minipigs. Br J Oral Maxillofac Surg. 2003;41(2):102–8.
20. Konyves A, Willis-Owen CA, Spriggins AJ. The long-term benefit of computer-assisted surgical navigation in unicompartmental knee arthroplasty. J Orthop Surg Res. 2010;5:94–6.

The Application of Reverse Engineering Technology in Orthopaedics

13

Qin Lian and Yaxiong Liu

1 Reverse Engineering in the Design of Customized Prosthesis

For patients with bone defects, the traditional repair methods are bone graft and implant general prosthesis. Nevertheless, the bone graft is poorly moulded, cannot correct the deformity and is prone to complications. Without bone shape, general prosthesis needs processing adjustment according to the demands of the patient during the operation, which is dependent on the surgeon's experience, and the adjustment mostly doesn't match with the autologous bone of the patient, which not only affects the appearance but also causes the decreases of bearing capacity, inaccurate positioning and unstable connection. All these problems easily cause the failure of the bone defect repairing and serious impact on physical and psychological rehabilitation of patients after operation. A fundamental way to solve the problem is to design a tailored customized prosthesis for patient. With the development of medical image processing technology, it has become an important prosthesis reconstruction method to design customized prosthesis by reverse engineering, through which patients with bone defects will get customized repair. In this way, the prosthesis can match the original bone of patients with bone defects very well, and it can well restore the bone morphological function, mechanical function and physiological function.

1.1 The Customized Prosthesis Design Process Based on Reverse Engineering

Here, we take the mandibular reconstruction a typical case as an example to introduce the design method of customized prosthesis that is designed for the patient to externally match its

Q. Lian (✉) • Y. Liu
State Key Laboratory for Manufacturing System Engineering,
School of Mechanical Engineering, Xi'an Jiaotong University,
Xi'an, 710054, Shaanxi, China

physical characteristic and physiological feature. In the reverse engineering, CT, Mimics and Geomagic Studio are powerful tools. Here are the advantages. Firstly, the design uses the original data from start to end, and so the prosthesis designed has the property of original data and can match the original bone. The STL file format during the entire design progress effectively avoids the tolerance caused by format conversion. The visual interface helps designers to operate easily in the design progress. Figure 13.1 shows the modelling flow.

1.1.1 Date Acquisition of the Bone

Customized prosthesis is supposed to match the skeletal shape of the patient, and so we use the method of reverse engineering in which we get the bone data with the help of medical spiral CT. Since the CT acquisition is planar picture, which not only contains the skeletal data but also an image data of other organizations, we must adopt a reasonable image processing method to separate the skeletal data from the other data. Mimics developed by a Belgian company named Materialise can deal with various CT images. By setting different thresholds, we can extract skeletal data shown in Fig. 13.2. Then, we can separate the mandible data from other skeletal data and convert each layer of bone data into 3D data in STL format, as a reference for the doctor to determine the position of osteotomy in surgical project.

1.1.2 Mirror Repairing

By the medical CT scan, we can only get the incomplete mandible data, and so it's necessary to obtain the missing data in a certain way. We can reconstruct the defect and get the missing data by mirror method based on the nature that a human skeleton is basically symmetrical from left to right. That is to say, we can obtain the missing data by mirror method based on STL files. For image processing using Geomagic Studio software, we can use three-point method and select the intermediate points of left first and right first teeth and mental spine vertices as points of reference to establish the mirror plane. For the defect cases nearby the mandibular midline, select the point nearby the skull midline

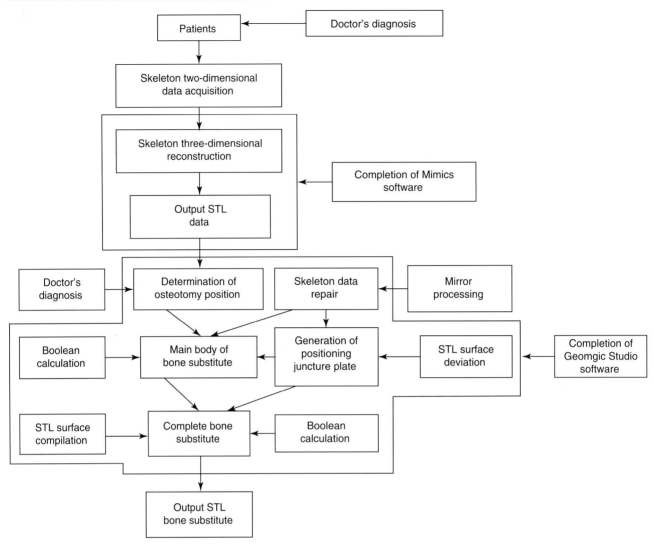

Fig. 13.1 Modelling process of customized prosthesis

point as a point of reference for image processing. The skeleton of human is substantially symmetrical from left to right, but not completely symmetrical, which is especially common for those who have incomplete or deformed craniofacial skeleton. Considering the fact above-mentioned, it cannot perfectly make the mirror data match up with the losing part by using midline to create the mirror image. In this paper, we use the registration function in Geomagic Studio to solve the problem. In the registration function, we fix the original craniofacial skeleton data on the three-dimensional system of coordinate and keep the mirror data movable in the three-dimensional system of coordinate. By matching some key points on the two data model, we can adjust the relative position between the original data and the mirror data to make them coincide. After that, we use Boolean operation between models which include basic set operations, namely, union, intersection and complement, instead of constructing the surface directly to get the prosthesis model. Using subtraction Boolean operation, we can subtract the original craniofacial

data from the mirror data to obtain the prosthesis model that is perfectly fit with the original craniofacial section. Figure 13.4 show the model without repairing and the model repaired. The model repaired is generally symmetrical from left to right.

1.1.3 Location and Connection

To achieve the contact, joint and fixation between the prosthesis and the mandible fracture, doctors usually locate the prosthesis by fitting extending plate to outside surface of the mandible and fix it stably with the screws. The mandible surface is a free one, so the concavo-convex features on the surface can be used to locate the prosthesis, and the key to locate is to fit the extending plate on the outside surface of the mandible perfectly somehow. By using the special function in Geomagic Studio, we can create the junction plate with the mandible playing a role as matrix and its surface as interarea. If the internal surface of the junction plate coincides with the outside surface of the matrix, we can

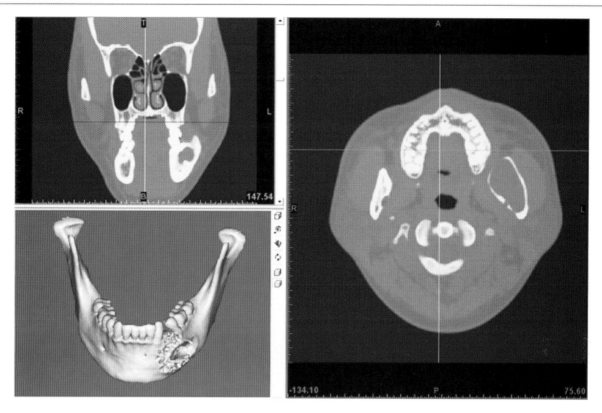

Fig. 13.2 Extraction of mandible data from the patient

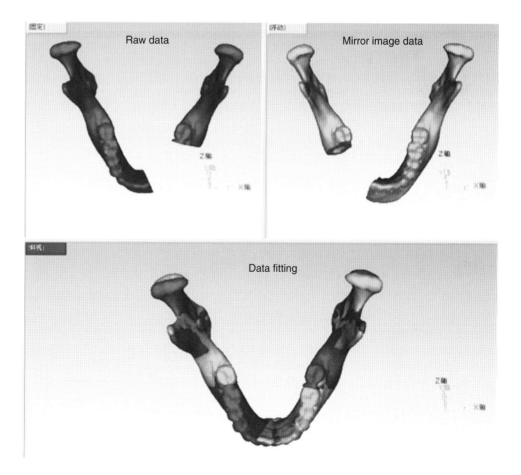

Fig. 13.3 Mirror data and data fitting

Fig. 13.4 Comparison between repaired and unrepaired

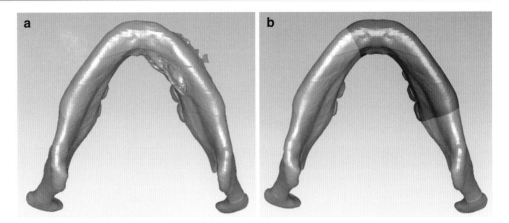

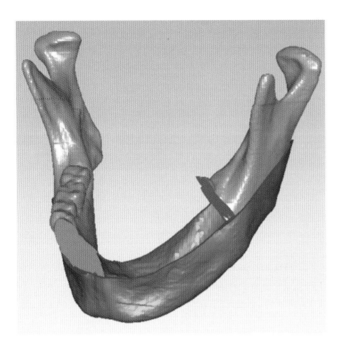

Fig. 13.5

guarantee that the junction plate for customized prosthesis will be attached to the mandible very well. Then we can combine the junction with the data reconstructed by Boolean operation. The method above-mentioned can not only guarantee the effectiveness of the connection but also has little influence on the patient's facial appearance (Fig. 13.5).

The Application of Reverse Engineering in Customized Prosthesis

The customized prosthesis model designed through reverse engineering must be machined before applied in clinic. The main method of manufacturing customized prosthesis is quick casting. We make the prototype of customized prosthesis by rapid prototyping based on the CAD data and models designed through reverse engineering and then manufacture the cast based on the prototype and obtain the titanium alloy prosthesis by investment casting. After some post-processing, we will get the prosthesis that can be used in clinic.

The Application of Reverse Engineering in Customized Cranio-Maxillofacial Prosthesis

Here are some successful examples produced by the Institute of Advanced Manufacturing Technology, Xi'an Jiaotong University.

The world's first customized titanium alloy prosthesis designed through reverse engineering and manufactured by rapid prototyping that is used to repair the mandible defect after tumour operation was applied in clinic on October 18, 2001 at Stomatological Hospital, Xi'an Jiaotong University (Fig. 13.6). The world's first customized upper jaw prosthesis designed through reverse engineering and manufactured by rapid prototyping that is used to repair the upper jaw bone defect after tumour operation was applied in clinic successfully on July 13, 2005 at Stomatological Hospital, Xi'an Jiaotong University (Fig. 13.7). China's first customized skull prosthesis designed through reverse engineering and manufactured by rapid prototyping was applied in clinic successfully in June 2007 at the Fourth Military Medical University (Fig. 13.8).

The Application of Reverse Engineering in Other Customized Implants

At present, reverse engineering has also been widely used for other customized medical service, such as composite customized hemi-knee joint, customized sternum correction, jaw correction, malformation correction, false teeth, artificial limbs and ocular prosthesis. Combining reverse engineering with rapid prototyping, the Institute of Advanced Manufacturing Technology, Xi'an Jiaotong University, designed and manufactured the composite customized hemi-knee joint, which was applied in clinic to treat the osteosarcoma on the upper part of left tibia on August 27, 2004, at the Department of Orthopaedic Surgery, Xijing Hospital of Fourth Military Medical University. Four weeks after the surgery, the patient could walk slowly and 5 months later recovered well. The joint prosthesis has not only customized titanium alloy articular surface but also biodegradable ceramics which constructs microchannel to help degrade and promote bone formation. In that way, the problem that

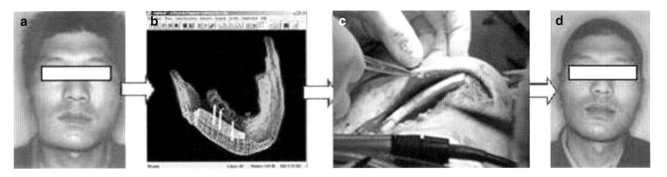

Fig. 13.6 Effect of customized mandible prosthesis. (**a**) Patient condition. (**b**) Design of customized implant. (**c**) Operation process. (**d**) Recovery

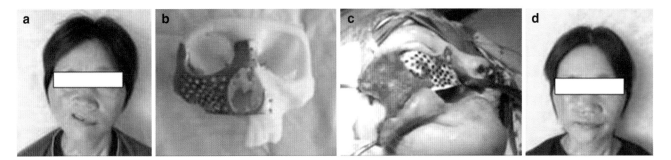

Fig. 13.7 Effect of customized upper jaw prosthesis. (**a**) Patient condition. (**b**) Design of customized implant. (**c**) Operation process. (**d**) Recovery

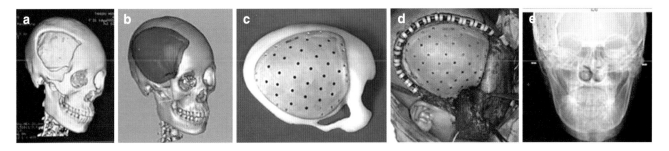

Fig. 13.8 Manufacturing and application of customized skull prosthesis. (**a**) CT three-dimensional reconstruction. (**b**) Model of skull prosthesis. (**c**) Implant product. (**d**) Operation process. (**e**) Observation after 6 months

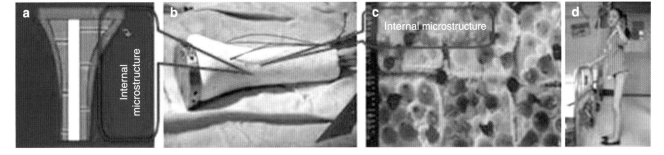

Fig. 13.9 The application of composite hemi-knee joint. (**a**) Internal microstructure design of the joint. (**b**) Composite implant. (**c**) The main microchannel and natural holes. (**d**) Recovery

traditional total knee arthroplasty will impede the development of teenagers' leg was solved well. On the other hand, Xi'an Jiaotong University completes China's first customized titanium alloy hemi-knee joint repairing using reverse engineering to design and rapid prototype to manufacture (Fig. 13.10). This customized hemi-knee joint can not only closely contact with allograft bone transplantation but also match the surface of the lateral tibial cartilage.

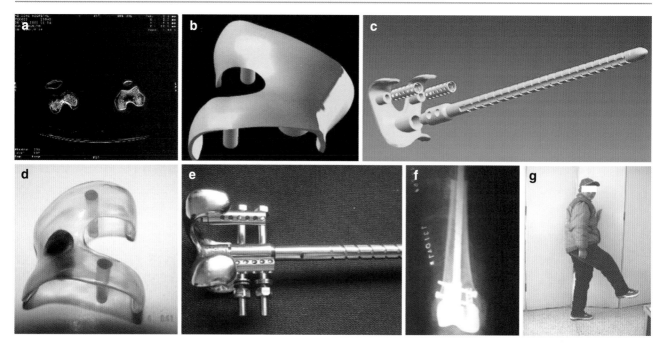

Fig. 13.10 Digitized design, manufacturing and effect of customized hemi-knee joint. (**a**) CT image. (**b**) Joint design. (**c**) Assembly of customized hemi-knee joint. (**d**) Prototype of joint. (**e**) Components of tita-nium alloy hemi-knee joint. (**f**) X-ray after 1 week. (**g**) Good recovery after 12 months

Fig. 13.11 Customized three-dimensional curve distraction osteogenesis artefact and animal experiment

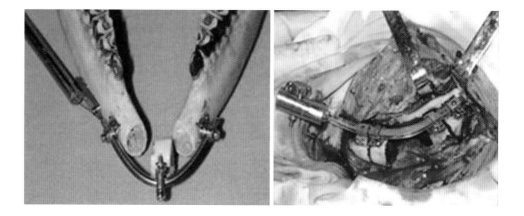

Combining with reverse engineering used in prosthesis design, we can design and manufacture the customized distraction osteogenesis artefact according to the principle of distraction osteogenesis, which will facilitate bone growth, and the shape function is highly adopting. In this way, we can avoid to pick up bone from other part of the patient which effectively reduces the damage to the patient. The Institute of Advanced Manufacturing Technology, Xi'an Jiaotong University, and School of Stomatology, the Fourth Military Medical University, cooperated in the goat animal experiment whose result proved that the distraction osteogenesis artefact works well (Fig. 13.11).

2 Bone Repair Based on Reverse Engineering Techniques

2.1 Introduction

The bone is a complex, living, constantly changing tissue [1]; bone lesions and injuries can seriously affect the quality of patient's life; large bone defect caused by bone tumour and tuberculosis cannot repair itself [1], so clinical treatment of bone defects is mainly focused on reconstruction of large-size bone defect. Current treatment methods including autologous or allograft bone with bone growth factors have been used for bone regeneration and defect healing. Autologous bone graft is still the preferred fracture therapy [1], but there are limitations of rare source, while there is allergenic bone graft rejection and mortal problems [2]. Therefore, the development and application of artificial bone to repair large bone defects have become a new direction of biomedical engineering research.

Anatomically, natural joint bone and cartilage tissues have the complex physical structure; in their interior, there are complex and interconnected microtubule structures to ensure the blood circulation and nutrient transplantation within, maintaining the metabolism organization and exchanging cell activity for new tissue regeneration. So the porous structure of artificial scaffolds is important in bone regeneration in case of large bone and cartilage defect repairing. Reasonable three-dimensional microstructures are premise for manufacturing tissue engineering scaffolds with the shape of the replaced bone and cartilage.

In this section, the anatomical structures of the joints, bone, cartilage and bone-cartilage interface were in-depth evaluated using clinical image data, and reverse engineering techniques, microstructural parameters of bone tissue (such as microtubules of direction, angle, size, proportion) and bone-cartilage interfacial integration means were explored for designing and fabrication of biomimetic bone, and osteochondral composites of in vitro and in vivo experiments were carried out for reverse engineering-based repairing.

2.2 RE for Bone and Joint Structure Characterization

Fabrication methods of bone and joint tissue engineering scaffolds are based on combination of clinical and practical methods; computer-aided tissue engineering is used to get the actual size and structure of bones and joints, which is essential for designing and manufacturing biomimetic scaffold with integrative internal microstructure and matched external contour.

2.2.1 Skeletal Contour Reconstructions

Existing bone reconstructions are mostly concentrated in the inside microstructure of the bone; simple geometric structures like cylindrical one are the most acceptable. However, most of the bone defects in clinical practice are found with complex curved structure. Based on biomaterial clinical application, many researches are not only limited to small pieces, simple cylindrical or square structure, they also focus on large-size bone or osteochondral defects with complex contour structure. Therefore, customized scaffolds with matched external design consistent with the defect area are really important. Reverse engineering can meet the needed customized design in following human distal femur cases.

To obtain complex contour of bone defect, CT data (shown in Fig. 13.12a–c) were obtained by computed tomog-raphy (computerized tomography, CT) scanning of the bone defect area and then imported into the reverse engineering software such as Mimics software; the contour of the distal femur point cloud data (Fig. 13.12d) was stored in IGES format and inputted into Geomagic software for three-dimensional surface reconstruction. Due to the complex contour of the distal femoral articular surface and curvature change, traditional 3D reconstruction methods, such as Loft, Sweep, Through Curve and Through Curve Mesh, etc., are not able to obtain effectively the high-quality joint surfaces. Therefore, two kinds of three-dimensional reconstruction methods of free-form surfaces (fit free form) and boundary curves (fit free form with cloud and boundary curve) were combined to complete the whole joint surface reconstruction and stored in IGES format. The data was further processed in the CAD software to make the solid models (Fig. 13.12e) with 2 mm of shell thickness (Fig. 13.12f), which were finally shelled to build the distal femur contour models.

2.2.2 Bone Microarchitecture Reconstruction

As the activities of the body to maintain the basic functional requirements, the ability of bones to load and disperse stress not only depends on the joint-specific physiological external contour but also on the multilayer structure of articular cartilage, cortical bone and cancellous bone. Based on cancellous bone porosity or average porosity parameters, most scaffolds contain porous structure because it is necessary for bone repair, but the high strength cortical bone microstructure was ignored. In this section, the cortical bone samples from human, dogs, rabbits and tigers were analysed, and reverse engineering techniques were applied as shown in Fig. 13.13a. The long bone cortical bone 2D and 3D microstructure model and characteristics were analysed, and the impact of microstructural parameters on tissue regeneration was studied, and bone scaffold based on cortical bone microstructure [4–6] was established with biomimetic porous structure.

Specific methods were processed as follows: sampling, fixation, histological degreasing treatment and then cutting the distal femur into continuous sections with 30 μm of thickness using hard tissue microtome (LEICA SP1600); after staining, the hard tissue slices were optically observed to obtain the two-dimensional cortical bone microstructure image (Fig. 13.13b) under the microscope (KEYENCE VH-Z450), and then the two-dimensional size of Haversian canal and Volkmann canal was measured and statistically analysed to obtain the basic law of bone canals; MATLAB (MathWorks, USA) graphics software was used for image registration by build-in processing toolbox; the registered images were input into the Mimics software sequentially for three-dimensional microstructure reconstruction (Fig. 13.13c), and the obtained three-dimensional microstructure point cloud data were stored in Initial Graphics Exchange Specification (IGES) storage format; the cloud point data were imported into CAD software to acquire three-dimensional solid model of bone microtubules, and the topological

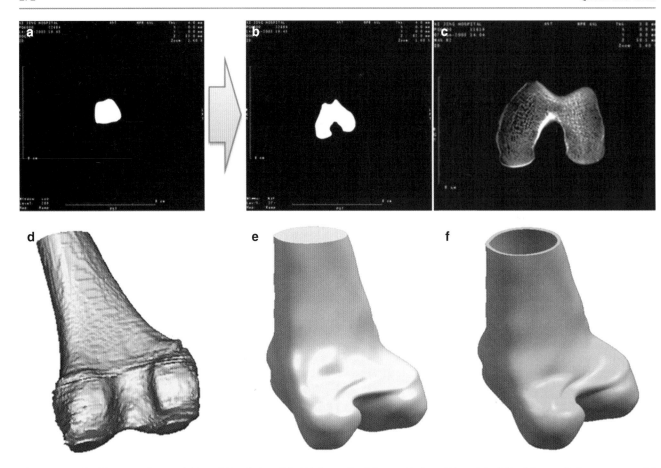

Fig. 13.12 Distal femur surface model from RE technique [3]. (a) The initial distal femur CT image, (b) the middle of distal femur CT image, (c) the enlargement of distal femur CT image, (d) point cloud model of distal femur, (e) the solid model of distal femur, (f) the contour model of distal femur

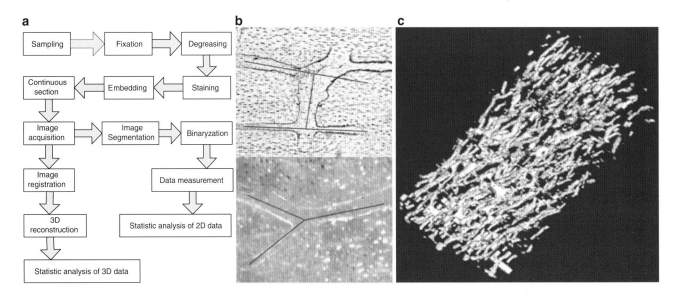

Fig. 13.13 Microstructure of the natural bone [4–6]. (a) Technical route, (b) stained image of internal bone micro-canal, (c) three-dimensional solid model of micro-canal structure

structure was obtained and analysed statistically for the representative extracted features, such as the distribution of microtubules, angle, direction, etc., which was a guideline for the design of internal microstructure based on biomimetic bone scaffolds. Meanwhile, regular structures were useful for cell attachment, and neo-bone ingrowth was also involved in the internal structure design, including the size of the internal micro-canal, shape, direction, branch connectivity, etc.

Two kinds of microtubule connectivity structures were found in the 20-year-old and 60-year-old human distal femur samples (Fig. 13.13b): (a) H-type connectivity structure (two Haversian canals connected by one Volkmann canal) and (b) Y-type connectivity structure (one Haversian canal with two branches) [4]. Connectivity structures of rabbit femur and tiger tibia bones were in line with the classical theory of microtubules, mainly orthogonal connectivity structure.

The angle between the Haversian canal and Volkmann canal in H-type structure is about 70–80°, with a mean angle of 75°, which is in line with the result of microfluidics simulation model: maximum liquid flow rate at the branching canal structure [5] and Y-type connectivity structure. The angle of Haversian canal and the two branched canals are basically the same: between 45 and 55° [4]. The numbers ratio of H- and Y-type connectivity structure is 3: 2 [4].

2.2.3   Bone-Cartilage Interface Microstructure Reconstruction

Traditional treatments such as cartilage debridement and microfracture are difficult to repair large-size cartilage defect [7–11]. Osteochondral tissue engineering is expected to restore large-size defects in situ regeneration by combining different materials for cartilage and bone scaffolds.

Current problems for osteochondral tissue-engineered cartilage are delamination, poorly controlled blood flow at osteochondral interface, limited function of repaired cartilage, etc., and these problems might be related to the limited understanding of natural osteochondral interface microstructure in the osteochondral scaffold design and poor material selection [11–13]. Full understanding of the microscopic structure of osteochondral interface is indeed important for osteochondral tissue engineering [13]. Microstructural studies of osteochondral interface are analysed intensively using scanning electron microscopy (SEM) and histological continuous section methods in human knee osteochondral composite, to provide support for biomimetic gradient osteochondral scaffolds [12–16].

Quantitative Study of Structural Characteristics

SEM

After oxidation and ultrasonic vibration treatment, cartilage layer was peeled off over the surface of subchondral bone. Then subchondral bone samples underwent drying and sprayed gold processing and were processed for scanning electron microscopy observation.

A number of holes and hollow structures were found on the subchondral bone surface, with no uniform size (Fig. 13.14a), and the hole structures were regular with nearly circular hole wall, and granular-like structures were found on the surface of hole wall and subchondral

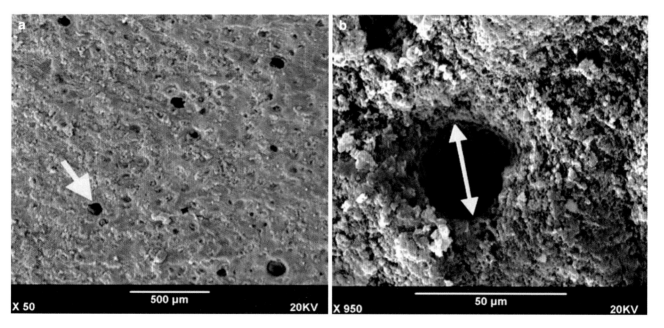

Fig. 13.14 SEM image subchondral bone surface [14, 15], (**a**) the hole-like structure distribution on subchondral bone surface, (**b**) enlargement of hole-like structure on subchondral bone

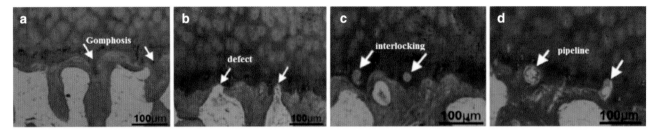

Fig. 13.15 Osteochondral interface structures [15]. (**a**) Gomphosis, (**b**) defect, (**c**) interlocking, (**d**) pipeline (100×)

Fig. 13.16 Continuous
section process [15]. (**a**)
Paraffin-embedded tissue, (**b**)
a series of continuous sections

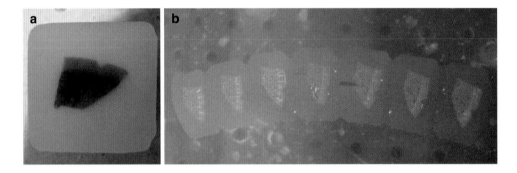

bone (Fig. 13.14b); these structures might increase the contact area between the cartilage and the subchondral bone surface.

The long diameter of each hole was seen as the approximate diameter of the hole. The hole diameter on the upper surface of subchondral bone plate distributed in 10–50 µm interval and 20–40 µm accounted for 61.96% of the total number of holes, with the average pore diameter of 34.08 µm, and the proportion of the total area of hole structure on the subchondral bone surface is 7%.

Histological Experiment

As observed on the Safranin O/Fast green-stained sections, there is a clear interface between subchondral bone and calcified cartilage, and the subchondral bone plate surface is uneven. There is a lot of hollow structures on the subchondral bone, and the subchondral bone integrates intensively with cartilage tissue through outstretched protuberance structures (Fig. 13.15a), named as "gomphosis". Part of calcified cartilage tissue communicates directly with the marrow cavity via some kind of defects (Fig. 13.15b), named as "defect". Some bone tissue is surrounded by cartilage from both sides and connected at bottom part (Fig. 13.15c) as "interlocking". As cartilage tissue was generally considered like avascular tissue, our study found that some vascular tissue containing blood contents extends from the subchondral bone to the calcified cartilage part and ends in calcified cartilage (Fig. 13.15d), named as "pipeline".

Cartilage Histological Structure Reconstruction

Preparation of Continuous Sections

The osteochondral tissue blocks were processed for continuous sections (Fig. 13.16), stained with Safranin O/Fast green, observed with a digital microscope (LEICA DMLA, Germany) at a magnification of 40 times, and a series of continuous sections on the target area were obtained with a resolution of 1600 × 1200.

Semiautomated Image Registration

One hundred continuous sections were obtained for each tissue block and then input into MATLAB software for image registration. A semiautomated registration method was explored with combination of manual operation and computer-aided registration. The adjacent two images were marked with three points (not on a straight line) separately (Fig. 13.17a) and then registered by the registration procedure (Fig. 13.17b).

Automatic Segmentation of Continuous Images

After image registration, all the corrected images yield some displacement or rotation of different extents, and relatively stable morphological structures were manually determined as the target area, and any broken/twisted/folded sections were discarded. The process was completed using MATLAB software, and then continuous sections were obtained with consistent size and pixel numbers (Fig. 13.18).

Fig. 13.17 Schematic of paired semiautomated image registration [15]. (**a**) Manual selection of the anatomical points, (**b**) automated registration

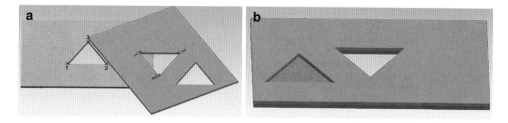

Fig. 13.18 Continuous section automatic segmentation [15]. (**a**) The manual selection of targeted area, (**b**) automated segmented image (×40)

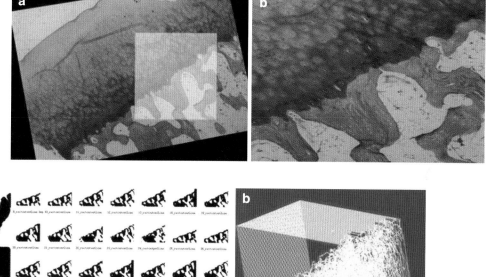

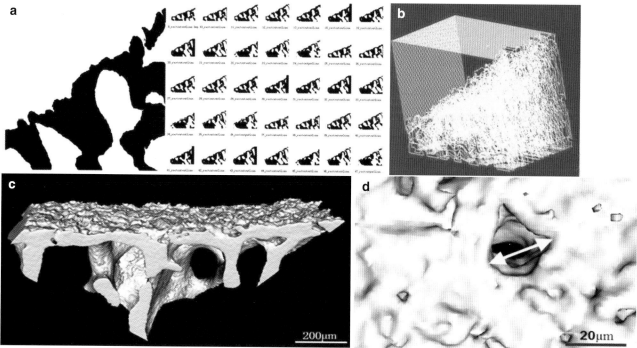

Fig. 13.19 Binarization histological sections and three-dimensional structural reconstruction [15]. (**a**) The binarization process, (**b**) alignment of binarized sections, (**c**) reconstructed three-dimensional solid model of subchondral bone, (**d**) defect structure on the surface of subchondral bone plate

3D Bone Microstructure Reconstruction

All images were processed for binarization, the structure of the bone was set to "1", the other structure was set to "0" and the "0" area was removed with only bone structure left (Fig. 13.19a). All images were input into the Mimics software (Materialise, Belgium) for bone structure contour reconstruction, with layer spacing of 5 μm. Then the subchondral bone plate was three-dimensional reconstructed (Fig. 13.19b).

The reconstructed subchondral bone plate (Fig. 13.19c) was a whole structure supported by columnar-like sponge trabecular structure. The surface of the subchondral bone was filled with uneven and hollow structures, and a lot of protuberance and hollow structures could be found on the cross section; some defect or pipeline structures also exist on some part of the bone plate structure (Fig. 13.19d).

3 Design and Application of Bone and Osteochondral Scaffolds Based on Reverse Engineering

3.1 Integrative Design of Macro- and Microstructures in Biomimetic Bone Scaffolds

Considering the clinical needs, the artificial bone scaffolds were designed with macro- and microstructures, and 200–600 μm porous structures efficient for cell/tissue ingrowth were also involved [7]. According to the microstructural feature of cortical bone, methods for biomimetic artificial bone scaffold design and biofabrication were established, with microporous structure inside. The main process is shown in Fig. 13.20.

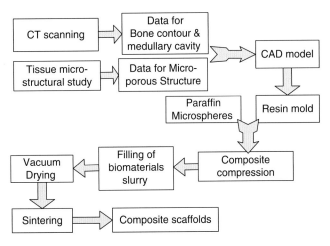

Fig. 13.20 Schematic for biomimetic artificial bone design and fabrication [6]

3.1.1 Biomimetic Microstructure Design
Based on the study of the Haversian canal system of cortical bone, representative microstructural features including the distribution of microtubules, angle, direction, etc. were extracted as the design guideline of internal microstructure based on biomimetic bone scaffolds.

Typical structures which would help cell attachment and neo-bone ingrowth were also considered in the internal structure design, including the size of the internal micro-canal, shape, direction, branch connectivity with each other, etc.

3.1.2 Biomimetic Macrostructure Design: CT Images Based on Customized External Contour Design
The shelling process was applied to obtain the external contour of marrow cavity from the distal femur solid model, and then the designed internal microstructure was added into the marrow cavity shell to create the integrative negative CAD model of biomimetic bone scaffolds (Fig. 13.21a), equipped with matched external contour and interconnected micro-canal internal structures.

3.1.3 Fabrication of Bone Scaffold
The negative CAD model of biomimetic bone scaffolds was input into rapid prototyping equipment to fabricate the negative resin moulds which was filled with biomaterials slurry, and bone scaffolds were obtained via solidification and sintering process, as shown in Fig. 13.21b.

As shown in Fig. 13.21c, the fabricated scaffolds are full of open interconnected porous structure, and the micro-canal structures are interconnected with the microporous structures with 1–10 connected pores between every two spherical pores; thus, the fabricated artificial bone scaffolds contain both canal and spherical pore systems.

The micro-canal is 220–250 μm in diameter, with pore size of 250–300 μm and connection pore size of 50–100 μm; these sized pore structures are proved to promote the mineralized bone formation.

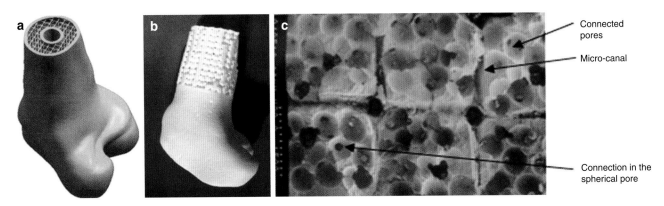

Fig. 13.21 Biomimetic macro- and microstructures of joint scaffolds [6]. (**a**) The negative CAD model of biomimetic bone scaffolds, (**b**) the ceramic femur scaffold, (**c**) internal microstructure inside of the composite scaffold

Based on reverse engineering techniques, methods for integrative artificial bone designs are developed. The biomimetic scaffolds could not only be designed with matched external contour but also reasonable three-dimensional microstructure for cell and tissue ingrowth. The biomimetic scaffolds provide the bone defect area with appropriate mechanical environment, which in turn would enhance neo-bone formation and mineralization process. Thus, the reverse engineering based on biomimetic bone fabrication techniques shows promising prospects for medical applications.

3.2 Metal/Ceramic Composite Artificial Joints and Its Clinical Applications

Currently, artificial joint prosthesis is made of metal and ultrahigh molecular weight polyethylene composite materials, of which the main problem is post-implant loosening caused by wear and tear. Moreover, there is no biological activity for the metal/polyethylene composite artificial joint, the mechanical integration between metal and soft tissues could be compromised over time, and then prosthesis failure might occur in the end. Thus, biological tissue engineering prosthesis becomes the development trend of artificial joints. On the basis of the existing techniques of prosthesis implantation, reverse engineering and artificial scaffold fabrication techniques are explored to develop composite ceramic prosthesis with metal articular surface, which has been successfully applied in clinic (as shown in Fig. 13.22). The composite artificial joints can not only improve the biological activity of artificial joints but also help to overcome the bioceramic limitation of high brittleness and low wear resistance.

3.3 Biomimetic Design and Fabrication of Osteochondral Scaffolds

3.3.1 Biomimetic Gradient Structural Design of Osteochondral Scaffolds

Osteochondral Scaffold in Cartilage and Bone Connection Interface Design

According to the morphological characteristics of the bone-cartilage interface, 3D model of the bone transitional phase was constructed with Pro/ENGINEERING software (Fig. 13.23), with interface hole diameter of 400 μm and hole area accounted for 10% of the total area of the interface. The structure of natural bone-cartilage interface parameters and the design of the bone-cartilage interface model are shown in Fig. 13.23, and the structure of the hole area accounts for 10 % of the total area of the interfaces. The diameter of the quadrature intermediate layer pipe is 400 μm.

There are three layers for osteochondral interface model. At the first layer, the canals were interconnected with each other in deeper layers to simulate gomphosis and interlocking structures of natural bone-cartilage transitional region. Some conoid ventages were designed to connect with the bone phase to simulate gomphosis and defects in subchondral bone plate. The width of conoid was equal to the depth based on the measured data. This structure can also permit limited blood vessel invasion and can transport some nutrition from the bone cavity to the cartilage. The porous structure was designed to mimic the bone trabecular structure: 1000 μm pore size, 500 μm interconnected pore size and fully interconnected. The pores and interconnected pores were useful for new bone growth, and to stabilize the osteochondral scaffold, the 3D channel network was designed to allow blood vessels to grow into the scaffold.

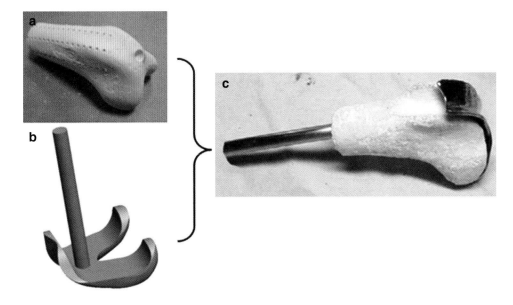

Fig. 13.22 Metal/ceramic composite artificial prosthesis [8]. (**a**) Prepared β-TCP joint scaffolds, (**b**) designed metal articular surface, (**c**) fabricated metal/ceramic composite artificial joint prosthesis

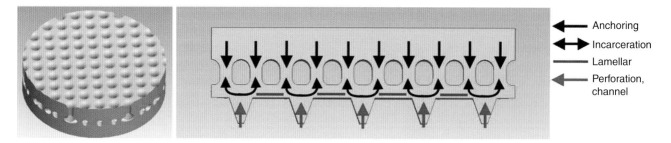

Fig. 13.23 Osteochondral interface CAD model [15, 16]

Fig. 13.24 Osteochondral scaffold [15, 16]. (**a**) Cross section of the entire bio-inspired osteochondral scaffold, (**b**) flow channel structures inside of the scaffold

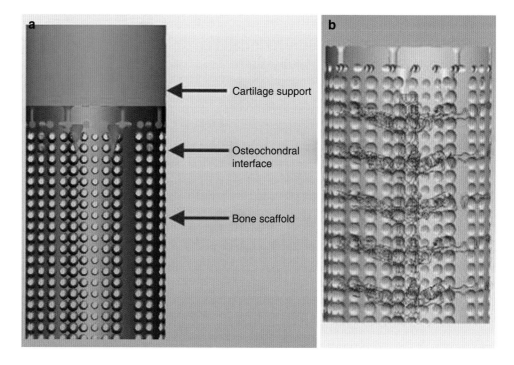

Gradient Osteochondral Scaffold Design

Based on the micro-canal study of the cortical bone [3, 6], the flow channel system in the subchondral bone part was designed, the angle between the main channel and the branch pipeline was 75°, the ratio of the diameter of the inlet and outlet pipes was 3:2 and the angle between the branch pipes was 72°. Boolean subtraction was applied to create the flow channels in the porous bone scaffold; these flow channels were interconnected with the porous structure (Fig. 13.24b). The biomimetic osteochondral scaffolds were dual biomimetic in biomaterials and structure design.

The proposed osteochondral scaffolds were fabricated with collagen as cartilage biomaterials and calcium phosphate ceramic as bone materials, and three parts were involved, including a cartilage phase, a transitional interface structure and a bone phase (Fig. 13.24a). The cartilage phase was added to the ceramic scaffold by gel casting and combined with the bone phase by mechanical forces that were created by the biomimetic structure designed within the transitional interface region (Fig. 13.24a).

3.3.2 Animal Experiments

Biomimetic osteochondral scaffolds were implanted in large-size osteochondral defects in canine and rabbit models. Animal experiment results showed that repaired cartilage integrated tightly with ceramic scaffolds, forming a native osteochondral interface-like integration. The neo-cartilage was highly similar with that of hyaline cartilage in gross appearance and histology levels. Meanwhile, the integration strength of osteochondral interface approached to 55 N, which was in the range of normal cartilage. The elastic modulus of repaired cartilage met the need of hyaline cartilage; thus, function of engineered cartilage could be preliminarily realized.

3.4 Reverse Engineering-Based Scaffolds for In Vivo Applications

Reverse engineering technique was applied in real-time monitoring of in vivo cartilage repair process. The repaired subchondral bone was scanned by micro-CT and 3D recon-

Fig. 13.25 Micro-CT reconstruction of repaired subchondral bone [17, 18]. (**a**) Area selection of interested subchondral bone on the two-dimensional CT image, (**b**) 3D reconstruction of repaired subchondral bone

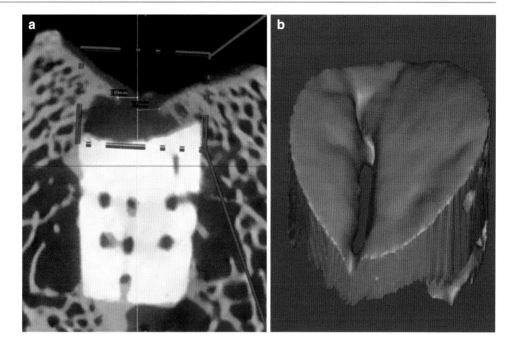

structed by Mimics software. Subchondral bone volume of interests was selected from the reconstructed 3D model using Boolean operations (Fig. 13.25), and then the total amount and microstructural parameters (such as bone volume fraction, trabecular thickness, number and separation, etc.) were obtained. The changes of subchondral bone remodelling and microstructural parameters were investigated during osteochondral repairing process, so the relationship between cartilage repair and subchondral bone remodelling was also studied to reveal the underlying repairing mechanism, which will provide enlightenment for developing targeted and effective therapeutic strategies to achieve functional osteochondral regeneration.

Conclusion

The porous structure is necessary for neo-bone ingrowth for large-size bone or cartilage defect repairing. It is a prerequisite for the construction of functionalized tissue and engineered bone or cartilage through fabrication of tissue engineering scaffolds with matched external bone contour and rational three-dimensional microstructure beneficial for cell and tissue ingrowth.

It has been widely applied in the experimental research and clinical repair using reverse engineering techniques to obtain tissue structural characters of bone and joint data from image data and computer-aided design for multi-tissue artificial scaffolds. In this section, existing reverse engineering technology, including medical CT scanning, histological staining, scanning electron microscopy, etc., is applied for bone and joint physiological structure acquisition, Haversian system reconstruction of the cortical bone and engineered structure model for bone and osteochondral interface.

Methods for bone and osteochondral tissue structure design are further proposed with characterized osteochondral interface structure and engineering model. The in vivo implantation experiments also show that artificial bone and joint scaffolds based on reverse engineering have good prospects for personalized medical applications.

References

1. Pallua N, Suscheck CV, Reichert JC, Hutmacher DW. Bone tissue engineering. Tissue engineering. Berlin Heidelberg: Springer; 2011. p. 431–56.
2. O'Keefe RJ, Mao J. Bone tissue engineering and regeneration: from discovery to the clinic — an overview. Tissue Eng B Rev. 2011;17:389–92.
3. Li X, Bian W, Li D, Lian Q, Jin Z. Fabrication of porous beta-tricalcium phosphate with microchannel and customized geometry based on gel-casting and rapid prototyping. Proc Inst Mech Eng H. 2011;225:315–23.
4. Xu S, Li D, Lu B, Lian Q. Study on two-phase flow of cell and cell suspension in artificial bone microtubules. China Mech Eng. 2006;17:67–70.
5. Xu S, Li D, Lu B, Tang Y, Wang C, Wang Z. Fabrication of a calcium phosphate scaffold with a three-dimensional channel network and its application to perfusion culture of stem cells. Rapid Prototyp J. 2007;13:99–106.
6. Li X, Li D, Lu B, Tang Y, Wang L, Wang Z. Design and fabrication of CAP scaffolds by indirect solid free form fabrication. Rapid Prototyp J. 2005;11:312–8.
7. Hollister SJ. Porous scaffold design for tissue engineering. Nat Mater. 2005;4:518–24.
8. He J, Li D, Lu B, Wang Z, Zhang T. Custom fabrication of a composite hemi-knee joint based on rapid prototyping. Rapid Prototyp J. 2006;12:198–205.
9. Roelofs AJ, Rocke JPJ, De Bari C. Cell-based approaches to joint surface repair: a research perspective. Osteoarthr Cartil. 2013;21:892–900.

10. Zaslav K, McAdams T, Scopp J, Theosadakis J, Mahajan V, Gobbi A. New frontiers for cartilage repair and protection. Cartilage. 2012;3:77S–86S.

11. Yang PJ, Temenoff JS. Engineering orthopedic tissue interfaces. Tissue Eng Part B Rev. 2009;15:127–41.

12. Bian W, Li D, Lian Q, Zhang W, Zhu L, Li X, et al. Design and fabrication of a novel porous implant with pre-set channels based on ceramic stereolithography for vascular implantation. Biofabrication. 2011;3:034103.

13. Hoemann CD, Lafantaisie-Favreau C-H, Lascau-Coman V, Chen G, Guzman-Morales J. The cartilage-bone interface. J Knee Surg. 2012;25:85–97.

14. Liu Y, Lian Q, He J, Zhao J, Jin Z, Li D. Study on the microstructure of human articular cartilage/bone Interface. J Bionic Eng. 2011;8:251–62.

15. Bian W, Lian Q, Li D, Zhang W, Jin Z Hierarchical Structure of Articular Bone-Cartilage Interface and Its Potential Application for Osteochondral Tissue Engineering. Proceedings of the 9th International Conference on Frontiers of Design and Manufacturing July 17 ~ 19, 2010, Changsha, China.

16. Bian W, Li D, Lian Q, Li X, Zhang W, Wang K, et al. Fabrication of a bio-inspired beta-Tricalcium phosphate/collagen scaffold based on ceramic stereolithography and gel casting for osteochondral tissue engineering. Rapid Prototyp J. 2012;18:68–80.

17. Zhang W, Lian Q, Bian W, Wang K, Jin Z, Li D. Critical-size Defect Repair Using Osteochondral Composite by Additive Manufacturing. Proceedings of the 11th International Conference on Frontiers of Design and Manufacturing May 23 ~ 25, 2014, Nanjing, China.

18. Zhang W, Lian Q, Li D, Wang K, Hao D, Bian W, et al. Cartilage repair and subchondral bone migration using 3D printing osteochondral composites: a one-year-period study in rabbit trochlea. Biomed Res Int. 2014;2014:746138.

Computer-Aided Preoperative Planning and Virtual Simulation in Orthopedic Surgery

14

Jiing-Yih Lai, Zhang Yuanzhi, and Y. Z. Zhang

1 Computer-Aided Preoperative Planning

1.1 Significance of Computer-Aided Three-Dimensional (3D) Preoperative Planning

Two-dimensional (2D) X-ray and CT images are conventionally used for the evaluation and planning in orthopedic surgery. Although CT images can provide more information than X-ray images, current 2D imaging platform faces many difficulties. The first one is that the surgeon must rebuild the 3D status of the bone structure and imagine its fracture in mind, which may not be easy for junior surgeons. The second difficulty is that the preoperative planning is generally implemented by freehand sketch because the surgeon almost can do nothing but look at the 2D images slice by slice. Substantial estimation must be done as it is difficult to perform surgical simulation in 2D imaging platform. With the development of 3D medical technologies, more and more studies have been conducted to explore and develop computer-aided 3D preoperative planning for orthopedic surgery.

For surgeons to benefit from 3D medical images in orthopedic surgery, the following four issues must be considered. Firstly, when the CT images are input, they must be displayed both on 2D and 3D viewports simultaneously. It is usually difficult to imagine the relationship of the plots on 2D and 3D viewports because the data on both kinds of viewports are displayed independently. Specific user interface

could be provided in order to manipulate the same region of interest on all viewports. Moreover, 3D bone segmentation is required because further visualization, manipulation, analysis, and simulation must be done in terms of each of the bone segments.

Secondly, virtual bone reduction and bone resection in a 3D environment provide the capability of simulating the bone reduction process in real surgery. In traditional 2D imaging platform, it is difficult to analyze the status of the fracture for serious orthopedic trauma. The virtual bone reduction technology enables the recovery of the displaced or dislocated bone fragments. In serious injury where multiple fractures occurred, manual bone reduction may not be sufficient enough for clinic applications. It is necessary to develop semiautomatic bone reduction technology to speed up this process. Bone resection may sometimes be necessary in real surgery to cut partially broken bones. The virtual bone resection can provide similar function.

Thirdly, fixation simulation is also necessary to help the selection, shape determination, and simulation of the plates and screws during the surgical planning. For ready-made plates and screws, various types of lengths are available in stock and must be determined case by case. Although this work can be done in a trial-and-error method during surgery, a presurgical simulation can offer the information needed for the size selection of the implant. Moreover, some bone reduction surgeries require the bending of the reconstruction plate so the plate can fit for the bone surface as much as possible. The development of a computer-assisted pre-bending process can shorten the trial-and-error work required in plate bending.

Finally, assistive data output is necessary to help the surgeon for making decision. The form of the output data can be varied in terms of the need. In particular, it can provide dimensional measurement in 3D space, enabling more accurate judgment and evaluation of the real situation. Moreover, with the 3D bone model available, various CAD models can be output for further applications, such as the fabrication of RP templates for surgical evaluation, planning, and the pre-bending of the reconstruction plates.

J. -Y. Lai (✉)
Mechanical Engineering Department,
National Central University, Taoyuan, Taiwan
e-mail: jylai@ncu.edu.tw

Z. Yuanzhi
Department of Orthopedics, Affiliated Hospital of Inner Mongolia Medical University, Hohhot, China

Y. Z. Zhang
The Affiliated Hospital of Inner Mongolia Medical University, Hohhot, China

Many investigators have addressed the issues of 3D computer-aided preoperative planning for various kinds of orthopedic traumas. Some of the studies are long bone fractures (Winkelbach et al. [1], Tockus et al. [2] and Koo et al. [3]), proximal femur fractures (Nakajima et al. [4] and Okada et al. [5]), proximal humerus fractures (Harders et al. [6] and Schweizer et al. [7]), and acetabular fractures (Munjal et al. [8], Citak et al. [9] and Brown et al. [10]). Most of them are related to partial issues of the following subjects: 3D modeling, visualization, segmentation, fracture reduction, and topics related to preoperative planning. In addition, 3D preoperative planning technologies are commonly applied in computer-assisted corrective osteotomy [11–13] and computer-assisted pedicle screw placement [14–16], in which various computational algorithms are developed in terms of 3D bone models and implant CAD models to evaluate appropriate parameters regarding the deformation of the bones or the motion of the surgical tools.

1.2 2D and 3D Bone Model Display and Manipulation

When CT images are input to a 3D medical imaging system, they are generally displayed both on 2D and 3D viewports simultaneously, where a 3D viewport is employed to visualize the isosurface of the anatomical structure, and three 2D viewports are employed to visualize coronal, sagittal, and transverse views of 2D images, respectively. With the setting of a threshold, the isosurface which displays on the 3D viewport can be set to the skin, muscle, bone, or organ. However, accurate display of bony structures is easier than soft tissues, because the former has a clearer boundary than the latter. Nevertheless, the display of 2D images is still necessary as it reveals sectional data of the tissue.

It is generally difficult to imagine the relationship of the plots on 2D and 3D viewports because the data on both kinds of viewports are displayed independently. To overcome such a problem, three reference axes, representing the normal axis to the coronal, sagittal, and transverse planes, respectively, are displayed both on 2D and 3D viewports simultaneously. As Fig. 14.1 depicts, the blue, green, and red lines represent the normal axis to the coronal, sagittal, and transverse planes, respectively, which give a relationship of the viewing direction between the 3D model and 2D images. Whenever the mouse is moved to a 2D viewport, an active plane is appeared on the 3D viewport, indicating the location of the current 2D viewport. All the above reference axes and planes are upgraded dynamically in accordance with the position of the mouse. In addition, the range of the data displayed on the 3D viewport can be operated through a range of setting on each of three 2D viewports. With the above interaction mechanism, the user can catch the same region of interest both on 3D and 2D viewports simultaneously.

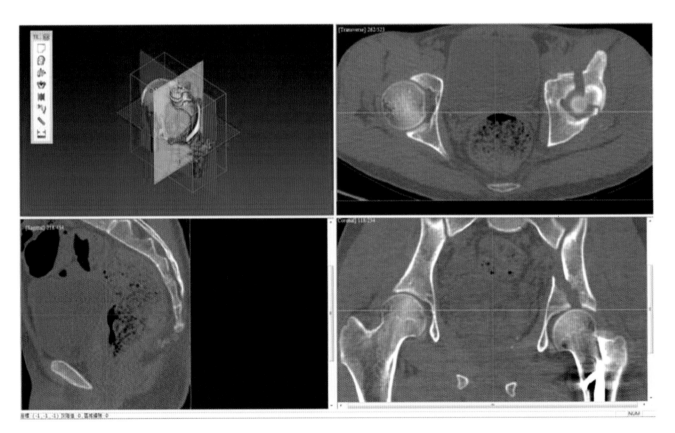

Fig. 14.1 2D images and 3D model are manipulated interactively through appropriate user interface

Bone segmentation enables the recognition and separation of different bone segments so that each of them can be displayed and manipulated individually. 2D slices of images are represented by a 3D array of volume elements or voxels for short. An image-processing procedure must firstly be proposed to separate the 3D images, where each group of the separated voxels is called a bone region. Various surface detection algorithms are then derived to detect the boundary facets on each bone region and then to connect the facets appropriately as triangular meshes. The separation of the bone regions is more difficult as it is affected by the complexity of the bone structure as well as the quality of the images. Once bone regions are acquired, they can easily be converted into triangular models by using the marching cube or modified marching cube method [17].

3D region growing is a common method for the segmentation of the bone regions on the 3D images. Starting from a seed point, voxels of the same region are grown along the six neighborhoods of each voxel on a front in accordance with a certain criteria. All new boundary voxels are added to the front, and each of them is checked one by one until the front is empty. Figure 14.2 depicts a procedure for the search of the seed points. Once all seed points are grown, separate bone regions can be obtained. Constant thresholding is typically employed for the growing of an isosurface. The model may not be very accurate yet good enough for the purpose of visualization. However, as far as the accuracy and completeness of the model are concerned, constant thresholding is still not good enough. In particular, Kwan et al. (2000) [18] and Kang et al. (2003) [19] emphasized on the methods for automatic extraction from bone boundaries. Zoroofi et al. (2003) [20] proposed several techniques for segmentation of the pelvis and the femur, in particular, segmentation of the acetabulum and the femoral head in the hip joint. Westin et al. (1998) [21] proposed a new solution to the problems due to constant thresholding based on 3D filtering techniques.

For the segmentation of multiple pieces of bones, the most difficult problem is the separation of the bones near the joint area. Ideally, adjacent bones are separated by a thin layer of soft tissue, and the intensity of the soft tissue is different from that of its adjacent bones such that a clear boundary can be recognized. However, in real CT images, the transition between the soft tissue and the bone may not be so clear, resulting in the vagueness of the boundary between adjacent bones. The gray levels on adjacent bones are generally so similar that none of the above threshold-determining techniques can deal with such a problem robustly. In addition, when multiple pieces of bones are considered, the seed points are conventionally assigned manually. Even if they are determined automatically, the available algorithms are usually not robust enough to deal with all kinds of problems. There are lots of examples that require automatic segmentation of multiple pieces of bones, such as knee joint, foot bones, spine bones, and neck bones. Figure 14.3 depicts a concept of simultaneous multiple regions growing to overcome the overflow of the regions near the joint area. It can achieve the segmentation of all kinds of bones from CT images accurately and efficiently (Huang et al. 2011 [22]).

1.3 Computer-Aided Preoperative Simulation

In orthopedic surgery for the trauma, computer-aided simulation tools, such as bone reduction and resection, fixation simulation, dimensional measurement, and analysis, are commonly required to provide additional information for the preoperative analysis and planning. Bone reduction enables the displacement of the fractured bones or bone fragments so that they can be recovered to their original positions and orientations. In general, bone reduction can be achieved by transforming each piece of bones one by one manually. But, it is generally difficult to align the fractured bone accurately and efficiently as the object must be adjusted along six degrees of freedom (three translations and three rotations). To enable the user to align the fractured fragments effectively, three operations with appropriate user interface on each of them are proposed. Figure 14.4 depicts the interface of moving a group of bone fragments simultaneously. The user interface is essentially composed of three circles, representing three rotational directions, and four arrows, representing four translational directions. The size of the circles is dependent on the overall bounding box of the bone fragments selected. All circles are concentric, with a center located on the center of the bounding box. When one of the circles is driven by the mouse, the group of bones can be rotated along the corresponding direction. Similarly, when the arrow is driven by the mouse, the group of bones can be moved with the mouse on the viewing plane. Manual positioning is easy for operation, but the final result must be judged visually.

The purpose of bone resection in orthopedic surgery simulation is to assist bone reduction. For example, in some serious pelvic injuries, the entire hip bone may be shifted due to the deformation or fracture on the sacrum, which results in the instability of the pelvic ring near the pubic symphysis. To recover the stabilization of the pelvic ring, the surgeon may cut the bones near the ilium, pubis, or ischium and then adjust the shape of the pelvic ring by adjusting the movable fragments. A bone resection interface, as depicted in Fig. 14.5, is explained as follows: The user first rotates the target bone so that the section to be cut is brought forward to the screen. He then draws a line across the bone to separate it into two regions, which represents two separate fragments. Such an operation is very strict and simple and can be performed easily. Multiple slices can also be done in a similar manner.

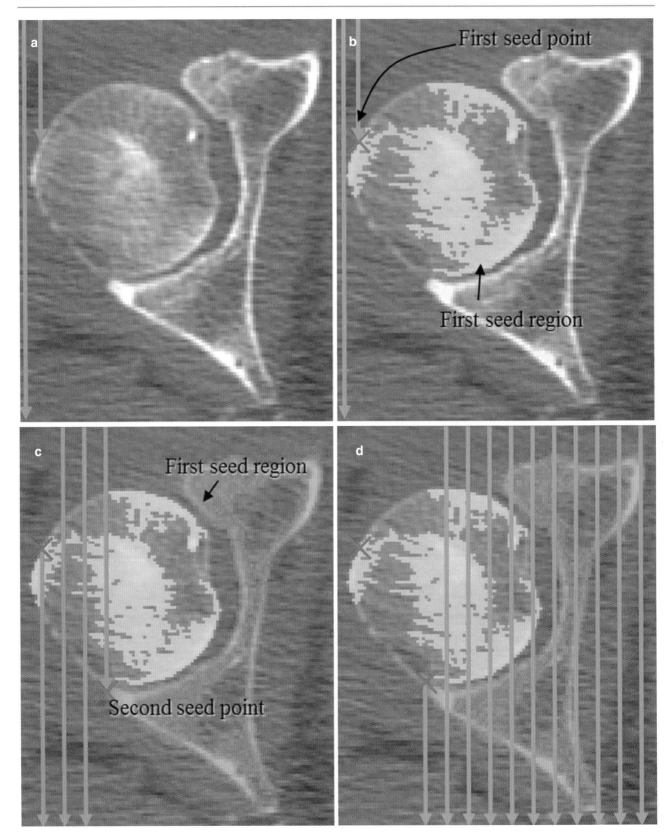

Fig. 14.2 Seed regions growing. (**a**) Scanning the first seed point, (**b**) generating the first seed region, (**c**) generating the second seed point, and seed region, (**d**) generating the last seed point and seed region

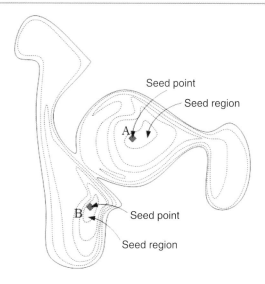

Fig. 14.3 Regions A and B are expanded in turn, with restriction in speed on the fronts, to yield appropriate boundary

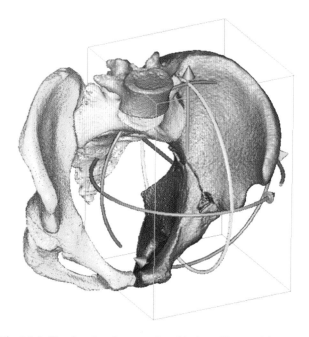

Fig. 14.4 User interface for manual positioning of fractured fragments

Fig. 14.5 Flowchart of bone resection

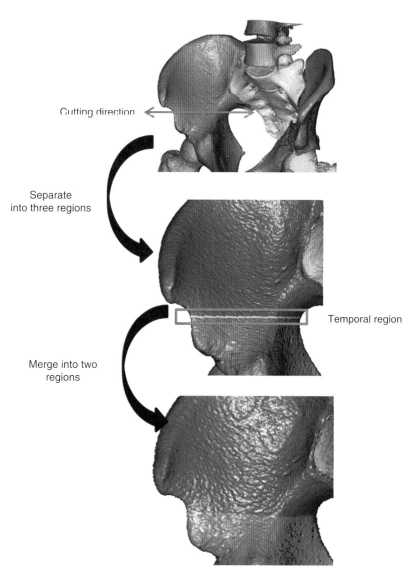

Fixation simulation provides a simulative placement of the plates and screws. With the 3D model available, not only the entire procedure of the implantable placement can be simulated, but also a detailed analysis of the plate type, its dimension, and possible interference become possible. In addition, the reconstruction plate must be bent during surgery as its shape is not fitted to the bone surface properly. Bending a plate is a crucial work because it is a trial-and-error work and cannot be done in advance. The shape of the reconstruction plate can be determined in accordance with the 3D bone structure extracted from 3D images.

The procedures to simulate the placement of a plate are as follows: A user interface is provided to determine the trajectory of the plate by specifying a series of points one by one on the bone surface. It allows the user to add or modify the points specified so that the trajectory can be more close to the user's wish. The trajectory is then projected onto the bone surface to yield another trajectory which is more close to bone surface. The plate model can be generated automatically in accordance with the projected trajectory. An RP part can be fabricated in accordance with the plate model for the pre-bending of the reconstruction plate in real surgery. The surface of the RP part to be referred must be equivalent to the bone surface. Therefore, a template model, an offset of the plate model, is generated for the fabrication of the RP part. Figure 14.6 depicts the basic units of the plate for the generation of the plate model and the relationship of the plate model and the template model.

For screws, the geometry of a screw is divided into three basic units so that any length of a screw in stock can be generated by using the combination of the basic units. All basic units are in a form of triangular meshes so that they can be integrated into a model and used later in the simulation. In screw insertion, a screw is initially perpendicular to the hole on the plate, and hence the insertion process can be simulated easily. However, actual screw may not necessarily be perpendicular to the hole of the plate. Therefore, a user interface is provided to adjust the orientation of the screw, as depicted in Fig. 14.7a. The importance of screw insertion is to check the possibility of penetration. If a screw is too long or too short, its length can be changed during the simulation. Checking the penetration of a screw in 3D model is essentially difficult. A graphic display of the sectional view is provided to evaluate the possibility of penetration. The sectional view is passed through the central axis of the screw, and it can be rotated along the central axis so that the user can have

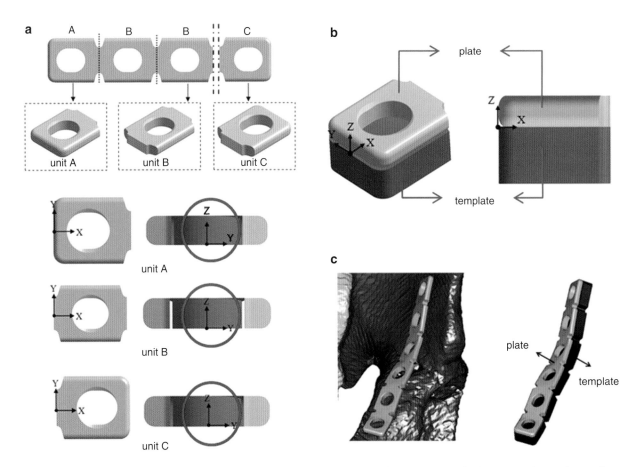

Fig. 14.6 Generation of reconstruction plate and plate template. (**a**) Basic units of a plate, (**b**) relation between a plate and a template, (**c**) plate and template models generation

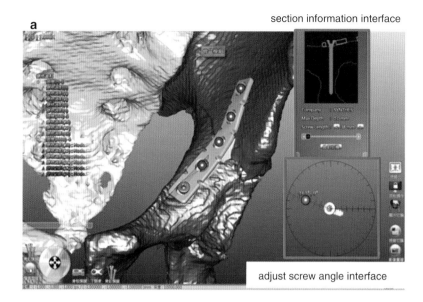
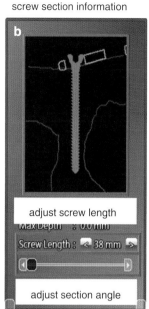

Fig. 14.7 Generation of screw models. (**a**) User interface for screws placement, (**b**) penetration analysis and adjustment

a visual feeling about the status of the screw. Figure 14.7b depicts the user interface of the screw adjustment mechanism, by which the length of the screw and the angle of the sectional view can be adjusted.

1.4   PhysiGuide: A Software Platform for Orthopedic Preoperative Planning

PhysiGuide is a software platform to provide 3D analysis and simulation for the preoperative planning of orthopedic surgical procedures. Both 3D medical images and implantable models can be displayed and manipulated simultaneously. It enables the user to view and manipulate the injured parts three dimensionally so that the user can catch more information than traditional 2D CT viewers. Moreover, it provides several simulation tools, in the form of different modules, to assist the planning of different orthopedic surgeries. In addition, it can output appropriate models for the fabrication of RP templates to assist the pre-bending of the reconstruction plate. Unlike other platforms which require the collaboration of several software programs, all functions are integrated into a software platform so that the surgeon can accomplish all simulation works easily.

Figure 14.8 depicts the overall structure of PhysiGuide, which can mainly be divided into five parts: (1) 2D and 3D display and manipulation of medical images, (2) dimensional measurement and labeling, (3) bone segmentation, (4) touch screen operating mode, and (5) surgical application modules. Each of them is briefly described below:

1. 2D and 3D display and manipulation of medical images: The X-ray and CT images are input as DICOM files. When CT images are input, both 2D and 3D viewports are activated simultaneously, by which the user can view and manipulate 2D and 3D images in an interactive way. Figure 14.9 shows several 3D visualization modes in PhysiGuide, which includes bone displayed alone, bone and skin displayed together, partial bone display, sectional display, and 2D/3D simultaneous display. A brief description for each of the functions is also shown in Fig. 14.9. With the abovementioned visualization utilities, the surgeons can recognize and analyze the type of the fracture more clearly. This is especially useful for comminuted fracture. Moreover, with the 3D images available, a virtual X-ray display module is developed for simulating X-ray and C-arm images. The virtual X-ray display can help to realize the inside of the 3D bone model, which is helpful for simulating the operation of surgical tool or implantable insertion.

2. Dimensional measurement and labeling: Enable distance and angle measurement in a 3D way and provide a series of functions to sketch and label on 2D and 3D viewports. Appropriate user interface is provided so the user can perform any kind of measurement on 2D and 3D plots. The measured data can be displayed graphically and recorded with the original images. In addition, the system provides a set of sketching and labeling modules, so the user can sketch or make notes on any of the images. The primary aim of these functions is to enable the surgeon to record what he observes in a digitized and graphical way so that the notes can go with the graphical data.

Fig. 14.8 Overall structure
of PhysiGuide

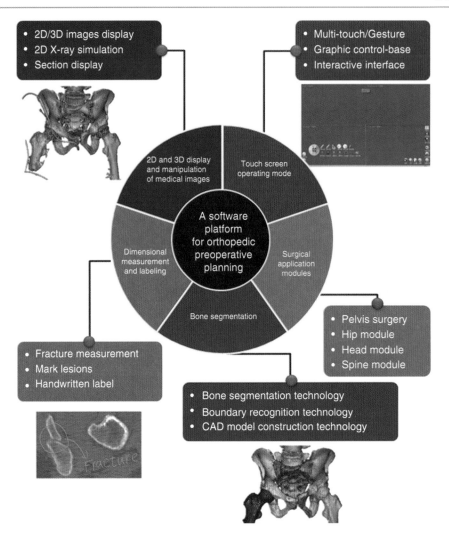

3. Bone segmentation: Provide a series of tools to extract and separate all fractured and normal bones efficiently. The bone segmentation algorithm is basically semiautomatic. A user interface is designed so that a primary threshold used to determine the segmentation result can be adjusted dynamically. The user can control the number of fragments to be generated while he adjusts the threshold continuously with a mouse. Bone re-segmentation and bone recombination modules are also designed in an easy operated way. With this bone segmentation module, bone segmentation becomes simple and efficient for any kind of CT images.

4. Touch screen operating mode: A touch screen operating mode is developed so that the entire program can be operated with a touch screen. The primary aim of touch screen operating mode is to simplify the operating procedures. Multiple-points control is developed so that several users can operate the same object on the screen simultaneously. Finally, a 1:1 touch screen platform is developed to import and display the virtual body in a more realistic way. The primary goal here is to provide a digitalized discussion environment so that the surgeons can analyze, simulate, and discuss the surgical plan in front of a realistic 3D model of individual patient.

5. Surgical application modules: Surgical application modules are varied in terms of the injured part of the surgery to be performed. Typical applications of PhysiGuide in orthopedic surgery are scapula, humerus, radius, spine, pelvis, femur, tibia, and calcaneus. Specific virtual simulation modules are also provided, such as bone reduction, bone resection, fixation simulation, plate placement, and RP template, for the preoperative evaluation, planning, and simulation in orthopedic surgery. Several examples will be provided in the next section to describe the applications of PhysiGuide.

1.5   X-Ray-Based Computer-Aided Preoperative Planning

X-ray-based computer-aided preoperative planning is performed two-dimensionally. The goal of this kind of preoperative planning is for sizing the implants as well as determining the position and dimension of the resection in orthopedic surgery. Several X-ray-based preoperative planning software systems are commercially available, such as

Fig. 14.9 3D visualization modules in PhysiGuide

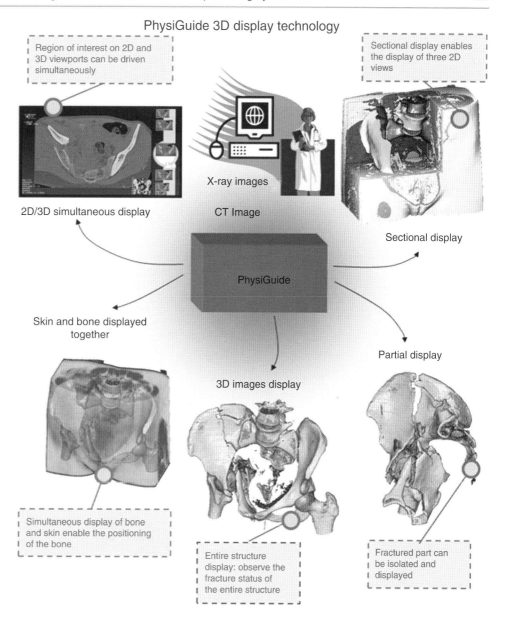

PhysiGuide 3D display technology

Region of interest on 2D and 3D viewports can be driven simultaneously

Sectional display enables the display of three 2D views

2D/3D simultaneous display

X-ray images

CT Image

Sectional display

PhysiGuide

Skin and bone displayed together

Partial display

3D images display

Simultaneous display of bone and skin enable the positioning of the bone

Entire structure display: observe the fracture status of the entire structure

Fractured part can be isolated and displayed

SECTRA [23], MediCAD [24], and TramaCAD [25]. Figure 14.10 lists typical functions involved in X-ray-based computer-aided preoperative planning. Typical application modules are the shoulder, spine, hip, knee, trauma, ankle, four limbs, and deformity. It is expected that this kind of systems can provide fast image information, quantitative tool for evaluation and hardware assistance to enhance the understanding of the disease site, surgical informing, and the understanding of the recovery status.

A preoperative assessment and planning system for hip fracture surgery and artificial joint replacement surgery are introduced below. The first example is a hip DHS surgery to demonstrate the process of X-ray-based preoperative planning. Fig. 14.11 depicts a fundamental user interface to help the positioning of the DHS implant, which includes a sphere tool and a ruler tool. As Fig. 14.11a depicts, with the sphere tool, a circle can be generated to simulate the femur head, by

which the directional axis of the dynamic screw can be determined, while with the ruler tool, the axis of the long bone and the position of the plate can be determined. As long as these two tools are defined, the position and orientation of the DHS implant can be determined, as shown in Fig. 14.11b.

Figure 14.12 depicts the process of the preoperative planning for a hip fracture case. This case belongs to 31-A2 in AO classification. The fracture occurred on the right lower limb, with two large fragments and a small fragment near the trochanter. In Fig. 14.12a, both the fractured bone and the normal bone are circled, with the position and orientation of the DHS implant defined on the normal bone by using the sphere tool and the ruler tool. Figure 14.12b depicts the input and display of the implant. The CAD models of the implant are drawn and saved beforehand. They are input and displayed simultaneously once the position and orientation of the sphere and the ruler tools are determined. Figure 14.12c

Fig. 14.10 Typical functions involved in X-ray based imaging platforms

Function	Description
2D Image	Browse 'Contrast ratio' Zoom-in and Zoom-out.
Measurement	Compute the angle among lines, length, direction, scale etc. and label them.
2D Osteotomy	Achieve the osteotomy by image cutting.
2D Reduction	Achieve the bone reduction by image cutting, then translating and rotating bones.
2D Implant	Simulating the placement of the implant by constructing the contour of the implant, then translating and rotating it on the image.
Information Export	State broken part, rotating angle, distance and picture of result.
Cloud System	By connecting with hospital system, uploading the information after operation. Simultaneously, discussing patient's condition with other doctors.

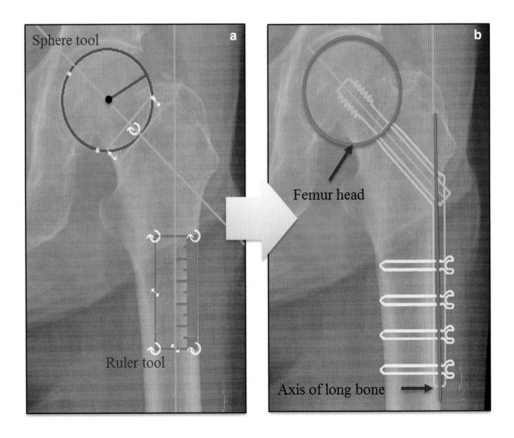

Fig. 14.11 Positioning of the DHS implant. (**a**) Sphere tool and ruler tool, (**b**) DHS implant placement

depicts the identification of the fracture fragments, where two large fragments are notified. A user interface in terms of a live-wire algorithm is provided to determine the outer profile of the fragment simply by pointing several points on the profile. The profiles of the broken fragments are mirrored onto the normal side, and a bone recovery simulation is implemented to adjust the position and orientation of the fragments, as depicted in Fig. 14.12d. The profiles of the aligned fragments and associated DHS implant are then mirrored onto the broken side, which show the final position and

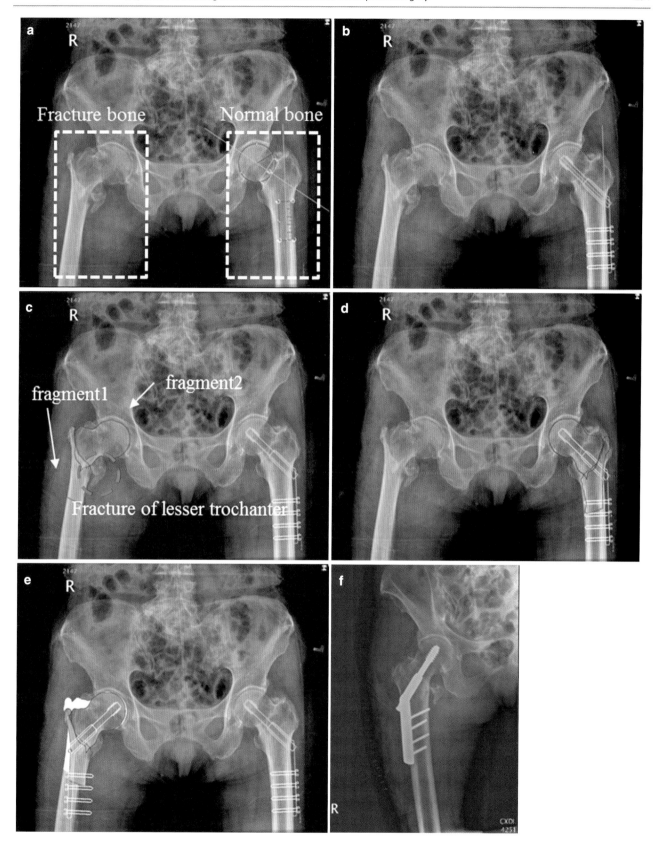

Fig. 14.12 Process of the preoperative planning. (**a**) Implant planning, (**b**) implant placement, (**c**) fractured fragment marking, (**d**) bone reduction simulation, (**e**) result of bone reduction, (**f**) X-ray image after surgery

orientation of the broken bones after surgery. Figure 14.12e depicts the X-ray image of the broken bone after surgery, indicating that this simulation can provide useful information for the preoperative planning.

For the second example, a computer-aided tool is developed to analyze the size and location of the resection for a knee replacement surgery. It employs two X-ray images, one from the front (AP view) and the other from the side (Lat. view), of the injured knee. Firstly, two profiles are obtained from the front view of the X-ray image, where one is on the femur and the other is on the tibia, as shown in Fig. 14.13a. Secondly, for each of the femur and the tibia, two reference points are determined manually, with which to determine two axial lines, one for the femur and the other for the tibia, respectively, as depicted in Fig. 14.13b. Once two axial lines are determined, the location and orientation of the resection can hence be determined. Two parameters can be adjusted during the computation of the resection data. One is the inclined angle, as shown in Fig. 14.13b, which is 5° in default; the other is a control point to determine the height of the tibia to be removed.

Once the resection data is obtained, a fixation simulation can be implemented, which utilizes the database of the knee implants. As Fig. 14.14a depicts, a set of default implants can be put on the front view automatically, while the location of the implants on the side view must be determined manually. The system provides a series of coordinate transformation functions to adjust the position and orientation of the implants on the side view. Once both objects on the front view and the side view are set, a set of virtual X-ray images can be generated to simulate the images of the knee after surgery, as shown in Fig. 14.14b. In summary, the computer-aided simulation tool not only provides digitized and graphical data to help the evaluation of the surgery but also provides virtual X-ray images to simulate the result after surgery. It provides more delicate information than those generated by using templates traditionally.

1.6   CT Image-Based Computer-Aided Preoperative Planning

When CT images are available, it is possible to perform the preoperative planning in a 3D environment, where various presurgical analysis and simulation can be carried out in terms of the 3D bone model of individual patient. Such a method is especially suitable for the trauma near the joints or on the pelvis, where 2D images are not sufficient enough to reveal the information needed for surgery. With the 3D bone models and associated simulation tools available, the surgeon can analyze the 3D status of the trauma freely and can even perform presurgical evaluation and simulation to realize the situation that might happen in real surgery. Figure 14.15 gives the possible applications of 3D preoperative planning on various bony parts of a human body.

Fig. 14.13 Osteotomy analysis of knee replacement surgery. (a) Contour marking, (b) dimensional analysis

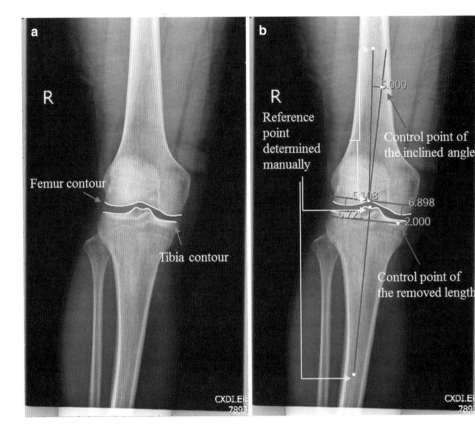

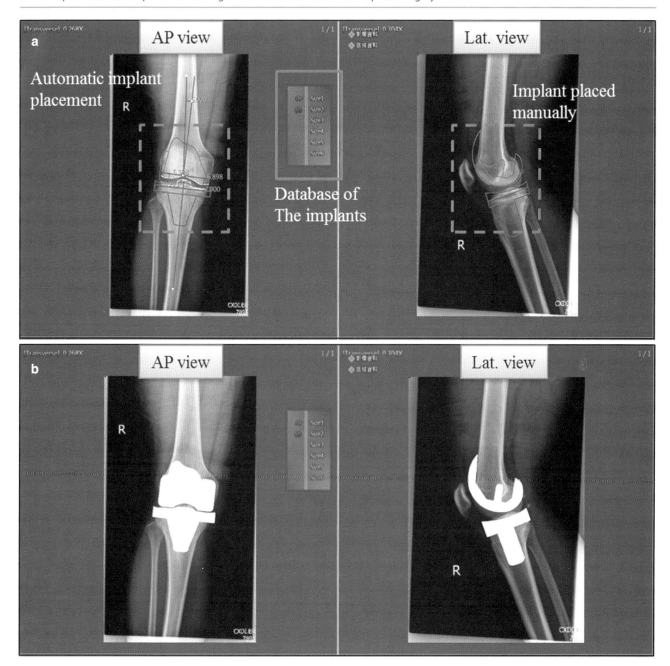

Fig. 14.14   Preoperative planning for knee replacement surgery model. (**a**) Implant placement, (**b**) virtual X-ray simulation

Pelvic disruption is among the most complex injuries in orthopedic surgery. It is not only because the fracture pattern is complex and diverse but also because conceptualizing the pelvic structure three-dimensionally is difficult. Two pelvic cases are employed to demonstrate how 3D preoperative planning can be implemented [26]. Other bone fractures shown in Fig. 14.15 can be processed with the same method. For the first example, the pelvic ring is seriously deformed due to fractures on the ilium, pubis, and acetabulum of the right pelvis. The right hip joint is also dislocated due to the fracture on the acetabulum. The surgery was performed

twice. Figure 14.16a depicts the X-ray image of the injured part after the first surgery, in which three reconstruction plates were fixed to maintain the stability of the right pelvic ring. Figure 14.16b depicts the X-ray image of the injured part after the second surgery, in which an acetabulum plate was fixed to maintain the stability of the right hip joint.

The simulation of the proposed system for this case is as follows: Figure 14.17a depicts the input of the CT images, where both 2D images and 3D bone model are displayed simultaneously. Three abnormal regions are found on the 3D representation, as indicated by the circles on the plot of

294

J.-Y. Lai et al.

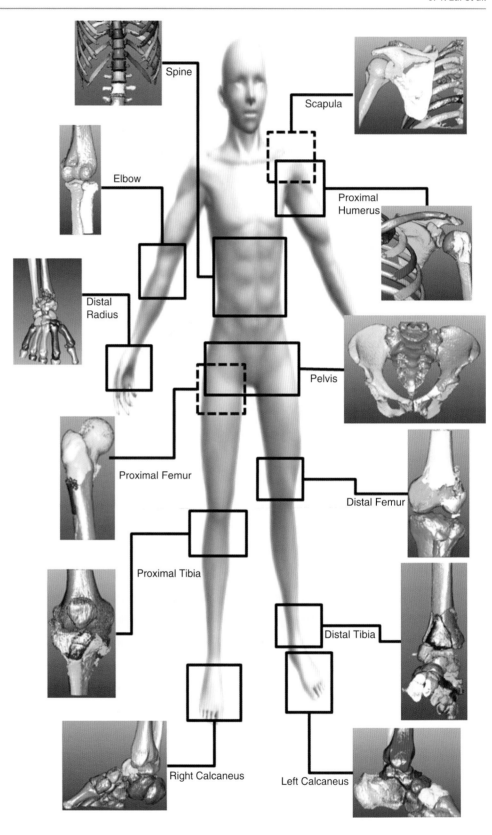

Fig. 14.15 Applications of 3D preoperative planning on various parts of a human body

Fig. 14.17b. Figure 14.17c–f depict the intermediate results of the preoperative planning process. Figure 14.17c shows the result of bone segmentation, with each bone region represented by different colors. It is noted that the regular number of regions for a pelvis is 5. However, ten separated regions are found in this case, indicating that several bones are completely broken. Figure 14.17d depicts the result after bone reduction, in which the integrity of the pelvic ring is primarily concerned. During the adjustment, the broken fragment of the pubis is aligned along its broken line and the

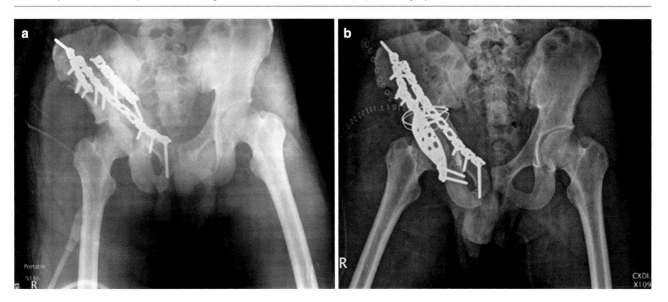

Fig. 14.16   X-ray images for the first case. (**a**) After the first surgery, (**b**) after the second surgery

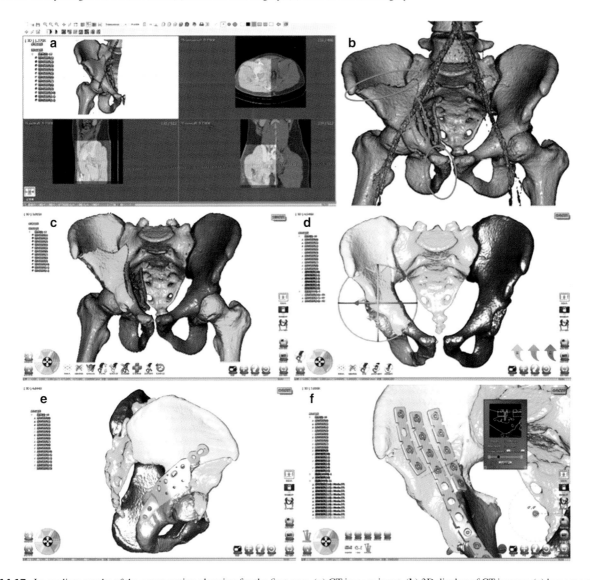

Fig. 14.17   Immediate results of the preoperative planning for the first case. (**a**) CT images input, (**b**) 3D display of CT images, (**c**) bone segmentation, (**d**) bone reduction, (**e**) placement of acetabular plate, (**f**) placement of reconstruction plates

right hip bone is aligned to reach a symmetric status with the left hip bone. Figure 14.17e depicts the fixation of the acetabulum plate. The CAD model of the acetabulum plate was generated beforehand with a CAD system. It was imported and positioned manually to the current position. Figure 14.17f depicts the fixation of three reconstruction plates and the corresponding screws, with each plate defined by specifying several points on the bone model. A cross-sectional view of each screw and the corresponding soft tissue can be shown to verify the appropriateness of the fixation. The plate model can be converted into a template model, by which a template can be fabricated by the RP technology.

For the second example, the proposed system is employed in a clinical case to demonstrate its practical application. In this case, the pelvis is seriously injured, as depicted by the X-ray image and 3D representation in Fig. 14.18a, b. The fractures occurred on both sacroiliac joints of the sacrum, which result in the dislocation of both ilia. In addition, both pubes are completely broken. As a result, both sides of the pelvis ring near the pubic symphysis are deformed too. The surgery is performed twice in this case. Figure 14.18c depicts the X-ray image after the first surgery, in which four standard SI screws and external fixation are implemented to stabilize the sacroiliac joints on both sides of the sacrum. Figure 14.18d

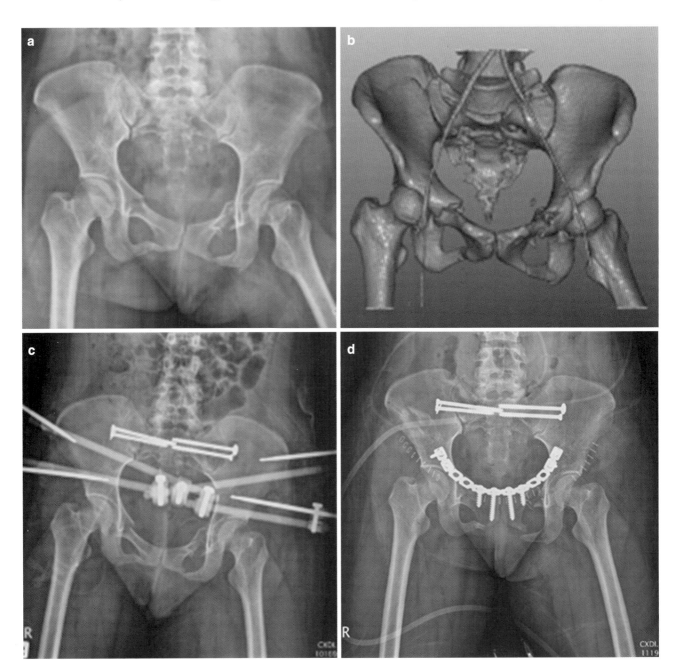

Fig. 14.18 Real surgery for the third case. (**a**) X-ray image of the fracture, (**b**) 3D display of CT images, (**c**) X-ray image after the first surgery, (**d**) X-ray image after the second surgery

depicts the X-ray image after the second surgery, in which both pubes are recovered and a reconstruction plate is applied to stabilize the pelvic ring. The external fixation is also removed here. The shape of the reconstruction plate was designed by using the proposed system, and the real reconstruction plate was bent in terms of a template fabricated through the proposed technology.

The overall process of the proposed system for bone reduction and implantable fixation for the second example is as follows: The CT images of this case are input and represented as a 3D model, by which the fracture status can be displayed and evaluated more clearly. Bone segmentation is implemented to separate each fragment, each of which is represented as a different color, as depicted in Fig. 14.19a. Bone reduction is then implemented to recover the position and orientation of the broken fragments, which are located on the sacrum, both ilia and both pubes. Figure 14.19b depicts the result of bone reduction. The reconstruction plate is employed here to stabilize the pel-

vic ring, and hence a long plate is implemented across both broken lines of the pubes, as depicted in Fig. 14.19c. In Fig. 14.19d, four SI screws are inserted one by one to test the best entry point and direction for each of them. As it is difficult to feel the relative condition between the SI screw and the bone model, a cross-sectional view right on the center of the screw must be provided, with appropriate user interface to rotate the view along the screw. Figure 14.19e depicts a more realistic display of the simulation, where the bone regions in Fig. 14.19d are replaced by 3D bone images. The bone model in this plot is much more realistic. Once the plate is determined, the plate model and the template model can be obtained from the simulation. Both models are fabricated by using an RP machine. The template part is employed for the bending of the stainless plate. A comparison between the RP plate and the stainless plate after bending is depicted in Fig. 14.19f. The stainless plate is directly used, without any further bending during surgery.

Fig. 14.19 Immediate results of the preoperative planning for the third case. (**a**) Bone segmentation, (**b**) bone reduction, (**c**) plate and template models generation, (**d**) one display mode for CAD models, (**e**) another display ode for CAD models, (**f**) RP template and real plate after bending

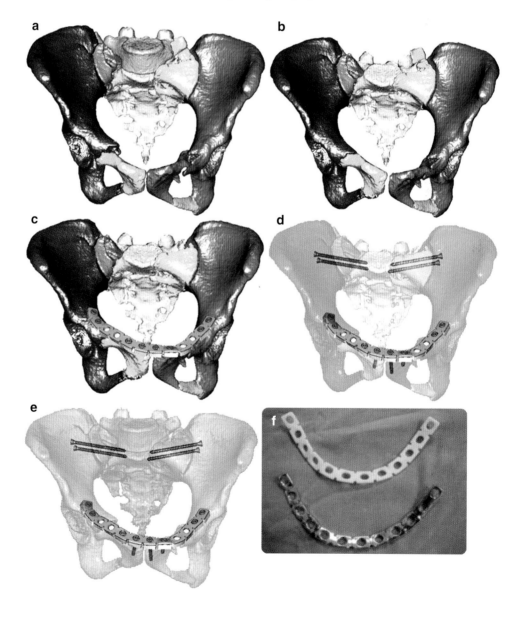

2 TraumaCad

Y. Z. Zhang

2.1 Introduction

TraumaCad is for assisting healthcare professionals in preoperative planning of orthopedic surgery. Clinical judgments and experience are required to properly use the software. TraumaCad allows surgeons to evaluate and manipulate digital images while performing various preoperative surgical planning and evaluation of images. TraumaCad enables increased productivity and improves patient safety. The program features full PACS integration and an extensive regularly updated library of digital templates from leading manufacturers.

The following provides a chronological overview of the process using TraumaCad:

```
┌─────────────────────────┐
│   Finding a Patient     │
└─────────────────────────┘
            │
            ▼
┌─────────────────────────┐
│ Selecting Patient Images│
└─────────────────────────┘
            │
            ▼
┌─────────────────────────┐
│  Selecting the Procedure│
└─────────────────────────┘
            │
            ▼
┌─────────────────────────┐
│    Defining the Image   │
└─────────────────────────┘
            │
            ▼
┌─────────────────────────┐
│ Performing Pre-operative│
│ Evaluation and Planning │
└─────────────────────────┘
            │
            ▼
┌─────────────────────────┐
│   Reporting and Saving  │
└─────────────────────────┘
```

View the list of patients from your local cache, PACS or OrthoWeb by clicking the applicable radio button at the top of the main view.

Select the image you want to evaluate by clicking its thumbnail. To select multiple images, click the images you want successively, one after another.

Select the relevant or analysis procedure to be performed to determine the specific templates and measurement tools that can be used in the application.

Calibration is a mandatory step that must be performed for each image.

TraumaCad offers a large and easily accessible templates library together with a suite of orthopedic tools and wizards for measuring the actual anatomy in an image.

Once the planning is completed, a full report is generated and can be stored together with the manipulated images in the patient's PACS file, locally or uploaded to OrthoWeb by saving the case.

2.2 Procedures

The TraumaCad application is procedure oriented. This means that you must select the relevant surgical or analysis procedure to be performed on the patient. Only the relevant templates and measurements for the procedure chosen are displayed. Click the icon corresponding to the surgical or analysis procedure to be performed (Fig. 14.20).

The procedures are divided into automatic procedures and manual procedures, as follows:

Automatic Procedures:

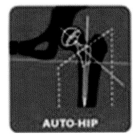 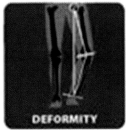

Manual Procedures:

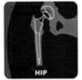   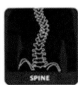 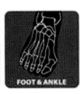

After you select a procedure, the patient's image is opened in the TraumaCad main window. After images are selected and defined and a procedure is determined, you are ready to perform the relevant procedure for the selected part of the anatomy (Fig. 14.21).

Templating is now the standard approach for preoperative planning of total joint replacement, fracture fixation, limb deformity repair, and pediatric skeletal disorders. The progression from standard celluloid films to digitalized technology in most medical centers led to new software programs to fulfill the needs of preoperative planning and to lessen the mismatch between the scanned or digitalized images and the transparent templates. TraumaCad software was developed to meet these requirements by enabling the import and export of all picture

Fig. 14.20 Procedure interface

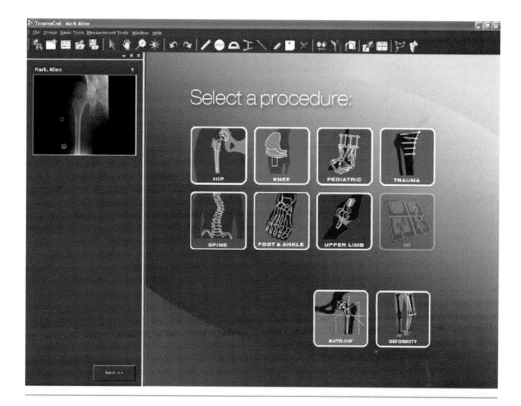

Fig. 14.21 This window consists of a series of tabs on the left and the main area on the right that displays the image(s)

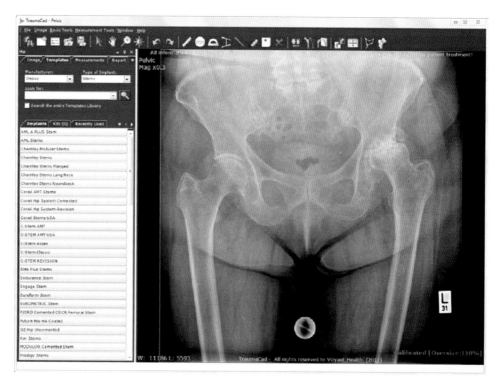

archiving communication system (PACS) files (i.e., X-rays, computed tomograms, magnetic resonance images) either from the local working station or from any remote PACS. TraumaCad optimizes templating for joint replacement procedures, trauma, and so on and is ideal for complex reconstructions and osteotomies, as well as for standard primary replacements. Surgeons can evaluate the postoperative anatomical alignment of various surgical scenarios (cutting, displacing, implanting) to create an optimal surgical plan. Incorporated into the patient file, this plan helps ensure the success of the procedure, while reducing operating time. TraumaCad offers a large and easily accessible template library.

2.3 Preoperative Planning of Joint Replacement

Preoperative planning for joint replacement in the hip, knee, shoulder, elbow, and ankle has become an integral stage of surgical preparation. It is an effective tool for training the surgeon by preoperatively deciding the type and size of the implant and probably reduces the intraoperative complication rate. In the past, preoperative radiological planning was performed by applying the transparent template onto standard film. Progression to digitalized technology led to the need for software that can perform digitalized templating (Fig. 14.22).

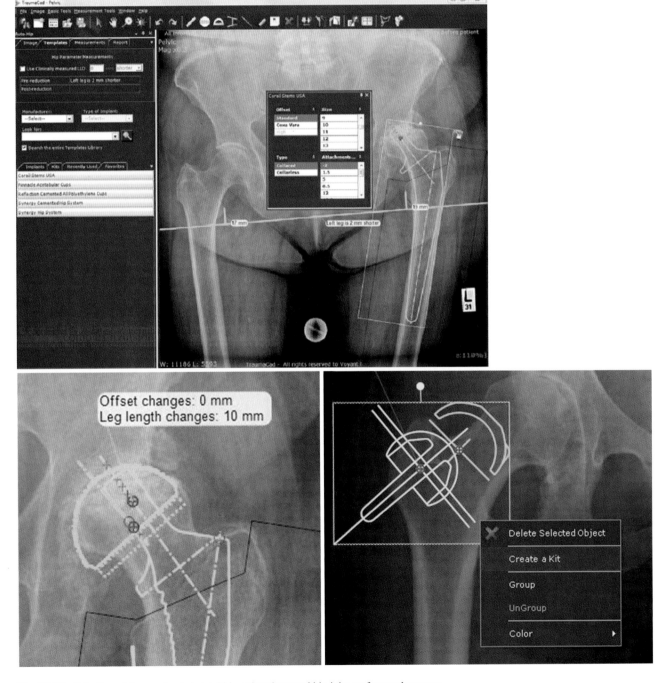

Fig. 14.22 Selection of the prosthesis in total hip arthroplasty and hip joint surface replacement

2.4   Trauma Procedures

Understanding the fracture pattern is a crucial step in the surgeon's preoperative planning of the proper approach and the type of hardware needed for fracture fixation. In addition to knowledge of the mechanism of a given injury, appropriate imaging modalities will be needed in order to correctly assess the fracture type.

TraumaCad enables you to define fracture or bone fragments and move, rotate, and copy fragments on the image and between images to reconstruct on the healthy side and accurately restore the anatomy on multi-view images prior to templating (Figs. 14.23 and 14.24).

2.5   Preoperative Planning for Limb Deformities

Limb deformities are mainly congenital or developmental and posttraumatic malunions. The first two etiologies will be discussed in the section of pediatric orthopedics below. Accurate estimations in the preoperative planning for the

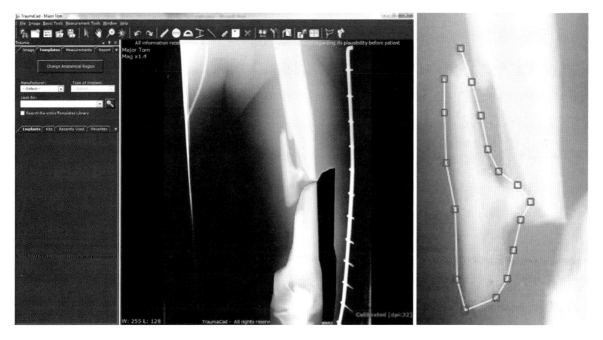

Fig. 14.23   Defining fragment

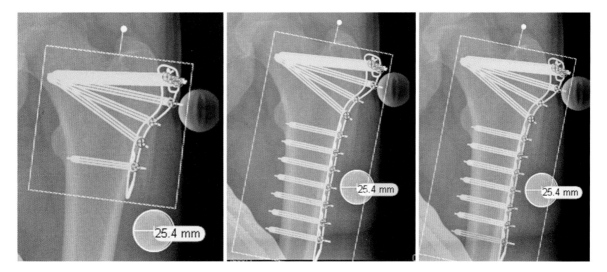

Fig. 14.24   Template contains both a plate and screws

correction of a malunion deformity require AP and lateral views of the bone, CT scans, or MRI studies, and 3D reconstruction in order to differentiate between a simple and a complex deformity. Specifically, a simple deformity is visible in only one plane while a complex deformity occurs in at least two planes (e.g., a shortening, angular, and rotational deformity). Images of both the normal and the deformed limb are needed to adjust the plan for performing the osteotomy, repositioning as close as possible to that of the normal limb. TraumaCad integrates all of the recorded images, and the preoperative planning is similar to that for fracture repair. The deformity outline is drawn and the bone is split into two fragments at the level of the desired osteotomy. The two fragments are then lined up to obtain the required corrected position. The TraumaCad archive is used in the ensu-

ing step for selecting the proper available fixation device (Fig. 14.25). When these steps are completed to the surgeon's satisfaction, the planned program is saved to be used at the time of the actual surgery (Fig. 14.26).

2.6   Opening a 3D Image

The series opened is shown initially with axial, coronal, and sagittal views. The yellow lines on the images represent the localizer lines, which help show the location of the image in relation to the other views. To change the location of each slice, scroll in the active window using the mouse wheel or click and drag with the mouse button on the yellow localizer lines (Fig. 14.27).

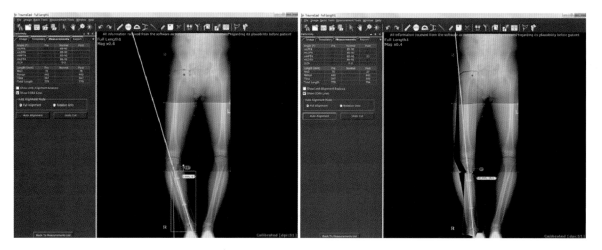

Fig. 14.25 Measurement of lower limb deformity

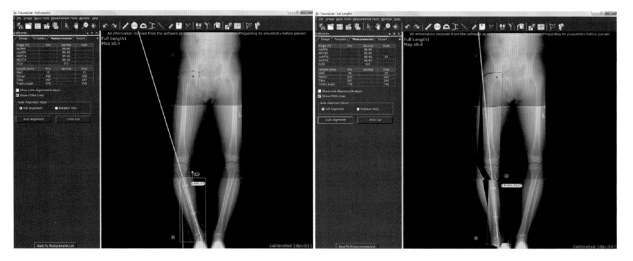

Fig. 14.26 Preoperative planning and osteotomy simulation

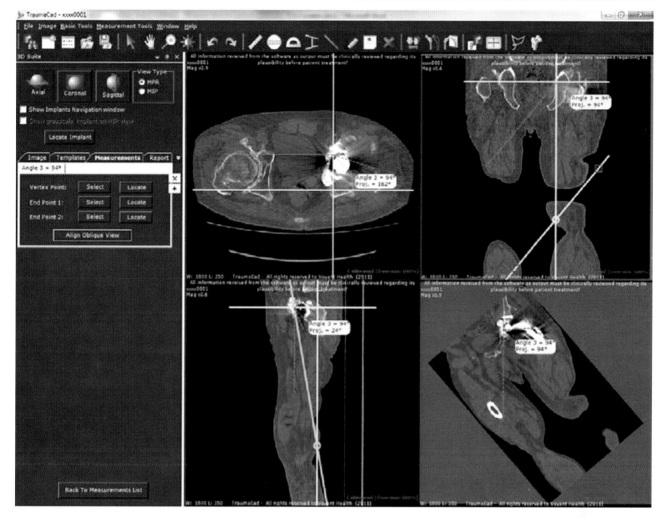

Fig. 14.27 MPR images

2.7   Generating Reports

A report consists of the selected images with templates or measurements that were added and textual information escribing the patient, the measurements, the surgical procedure to be performed and/or the implant to be used, and any text that the surgeon chooses to add.

TraumaCad
Pre Operative Planning Report

Patient Details:

Patient ID	Patient Name	Date of Birth	Gender	Accession
20495	Hip_With_Ball_1	9/23/1965	F	63507828

Referring MD Details:

Created by	Institution	Date	Procedure Planned	Side
ORTHOCRAT/yael	***	3/18/2011 10:44:22 AM	Hip	Right

Comments:

Implants Information:

Name	Manufacturer	Part No.	Quantity	Properties
Charnley Stems	Depuy	962369000	1	Offset : 35 Size : Standard Type : 3/4 Neck Comments : Please review the product IFU's for compatibility information.

AP View:

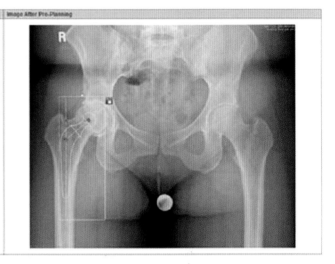

Original image   Image After Pre-Planning

Signature:

3 M3D Visualization Platform

3.1 Introduction

M3D visualization platform is Chinese interface software. To achieve the integration of the program, with a strong database from the individual files, you can carry out fast and diverse retrieval functions, greatly reduce the cost of the unit, and use all kinds of terminal remote access to the use of the tablet PC application. At the same time, with powerful remote medical treatment and teaching support, provide a new communication platform between doctors and patients.

Strong database management can save more than 100,000 data, rapid and diverse case preservation method, keyword search function, the establishment of the department of medical records, and medical personal case library.

M3D medical visualization platform has powerful image processing, optimal segmentation, 2D or 3D linkage measurement, simulation operation, and internal implant library, which can completely meet the needs of various departments, such as simulation, observation, research, and teaching work, and can be applied in various fields (Fig. 14.28).

M3D medical visualization platform can achieve remote diagnosis and treatment of the request, the two terminals at the same time to open a case, through the way of transmission of instructions for remote interaction (Fig. 14.29). It can rotate, zoom, section, and do other operations to show the other side of the observation site. By marking points, lines can be informed of the location of the other side to be noted, marking the important parameters of the needle point, pin.

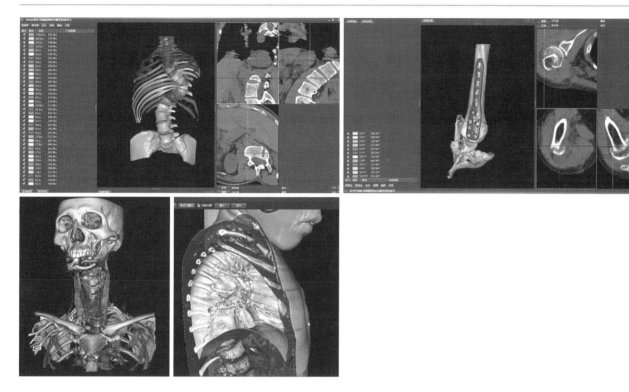

Fig. 14.28 3D visualization

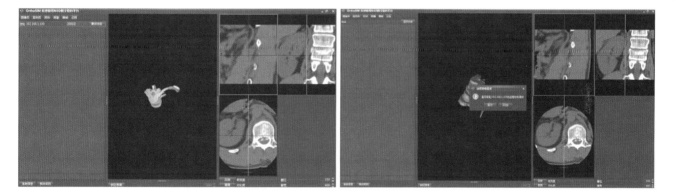

Fig. 14.29 Remote interaction

References

1. Winkelbach S, Westphal R, Goesling T. Pose estimation of cylindrical fragments for semi-automatic bone fracture reduction. Pattern Recogn. 2003:566–73.
2. Tockus L, Joskowicz L, Simkin A, et al. Computer-aided image-guided bone fracture surgery: modeling, visualization, and preoperative planning, Medical Image Computing and Computer-Assisted Interventation-MICCAI'98; 1998, p. 29–38.
3. Koo TK, Chao EY, Mak AF. Development and validation of a new approach for computer-aided long bone fracture reduction by using unilateral external fixator. J Biomech. 2006;39(11):2104–12.
4. Nakajima Y, Tashiro T, Okada T, et al. Computer-assisted fracture reduction of proximal femur by using preoperative CT data and intraoperative fluoroscopic images. Proc Comput Assist Radiol. 2004;1268:620.
5. Okada T, Iwasaki Y, Koyama T, et al. Computer-assisted preoperative planning for reduction of proximal femoral fracture by using 3-D-CT data. IEEE Trans Biomed Eng. 2009;56(3):749–59.
6. Harders M, Barlit A, Gerber C, Hodler J, et al. An optimized surgical planning environment for complex proximal humerus fractures, MICCAI workshop on interaction in medical image analysis and visualization; 2007.
7. Fornaro J, Keel M, Harders M, et al. An interactive surgical planning tool for acetabular fractures: initial results. J Orthop Surg Res. 2010;5:50.
8. Munjal S, Leopold SS, Kornreich D, et al. CT-generated 3-dimensional models for complex acetabular reconstruction. J Arthroplast. 2000;15:644.
9. Citak M, Gardner MJ, Kendoff D, et al. Virtual 3D planning of acetabular fracture reduction. J Orthop Res. 2008;26:547–52.
10. Brown GA, Firoozbakhsh K, Gehlert RJ. Three-dimensional CT modeling versus traditional radiology techniques in treatment of acetabular fractures. Iowa Orthop J. 2001;21:20–4.

11. Schweizer P, Fürnstahl M, Harders G, et al. Complex radius shaft malunion: osteotomy with computer-assisted planning. Hand. 2010;5(2):171–8.

12. Drapikowski P, Tyrakowski M, Czubak J, et al. Computer assisted SCFE osteotomy planning. Int J Cars. 2008;3:421–6.

13. Miyake J, Murase T, Ka KO, et al. Computer-assisted corrective osteotomy for malunited diaphyseal forearm fractures. J Bone Joint Surg. 2012;94(20):e150.1–11.

14. Briem D, Linhart W, Lehmann W, et al. Computer-assisted screw insertion into the first sacral vertebra using a three-dimensional image intensifier: results of a controlled experimental investigation. Eur Spine J. 2006;15:757–63.

15. Schlenzka D, Laine T, Lund T. Computer-assisted spine surgery. Eur Spine J. 2000;9(Suppl 1):57–64.

16. Iampreechakul P, Chongchokdee C, Tirakotai W. The accuracy of computer-assisted pedicle screw placement in degenerative lumbrosacral spine using single-time, paired point registration alone technique combined with the surgeon's experience. J Med Assoc Thail. 2011;94(3):337–45.

17. Huang CY, Luo LJ, Lee PY, et al. Efficient segmentation and construction of 3d bone models in medical images. J Med Biol Eng. 2011;31(6):375–86.

18. Kwan FY, Cheung KC, Gibson I. Automatic extraction of bone boundaries from CT scans using an intelligence-based approach. In: Proceedings of the 15th International Conference on Pattern Recognition, Washington, DC, USA; 2000.

19. Kang Y, Engelke K, Kalender WA. A new accurate and precise 3-D segmentation method for skeletal structures in volumetric CT data. IEEE Trans Med Imaging. 2003;22(5):586–98.

20. Zoroofi RA, Sato Y, Sasama T, et al. Automated segmentation of acetabulum and femoral head from 3-D CT images. IEEE Trans Inf Technol Biomed. 2003;7(4):329–42.

21. Westin CF, Warfield S, Bhalerao Q, et al. Tensor controlled local structure enhancement of CT images for bone segmentation. Proceedings of the first international conference on medical image computing and computer-assisted intervention, London, UK; 1998.

22. Huang CY, Lee PY, Lai JY, et al. Simultaneous segmentation of bone regions using multiple-level threshold. Comput Aid Design Appl. 2011;8(2):269–88.

23. Sectra's orthopaedic solutions. http://www.sectra.com/medical/orthopaedics/

24. MediCAD-The orthopaedic solution. http://www.hectec.de/content/

25. TramaCAD-Voyant Health. http://www.voyanthealth.com/index.jsp

26. Lee PY, Lai JY, Hu YS, et al. Virtual 3D planning of pelvic fracture reduction and implant placement. Biomed Eng. 2012;24(3):245–62.

Augmented Reality for Digital Orthopedic Applications

15

Min-Liang Wang, Yeoulin Ho,
Ramakanteswararao Beesetty, and Stephane Nicolau

1 Overview of Computer-Aided Surgery and Augmented Reality

Computer-aided surgery (CAS) is also known as computer-assisted surgery, a scientific method which covers all aspects of computer tools to help surgery. Computer-aided surgery is a surgical concept, a methodology, and a set of methods that apply computer technologies for preoperative planning, for simulation, and for guiding or performing surgical interventions [1]. For instance, minimally invasive surgery carried out by a video camera and a screen is a preliminary computer-aided surgery. The aim of computer-aided surgery is to increase and improve the utilization of computers in the development of new imaging technologies for medical services. This chapter of computer-aided surgery provides a basic knowledge for academic researchers, clinical scientists, caregivers, and industrial partners to expose new applications, techniques, and the latest solutions in this field. The chapter brings together research topics from all aspects related to medical visualization, simulation and modeling, virtual reality for computer-aided surgery, image-guided therapies, computer-aided surgery for minimally invasive intervention, surgical navigation, clinical application of computer-aided surgery, telemedicine, and telesurgery. This chapter helps readers to build a general concept of computer-aided sur-

gery and is a valuable resource for researchers and clinicians in the field. Figure 15.1 is divided in three main components that are described hereafter: three-dimensional (3D) modeling for data visualization, intervention planning and simulation, and intraoperative guidance.

1.1 Summary of Standard Process to Reach CAS System

The most important component for computer-aided surgery is the development processes of an accurate model of the patient. This can be conducted through a number of medical imaging techniques including CT, MRI, X-rays, ultrasound, PET-CT, and many more. After patient's image is acquired by modalities and saved into the computer database system, scientists organize and process volume data of these images into a patient-specific anatomical model to allow easy visualization of patient's organs, tissues, and specific properties when available. For instance, the flow of arteries and veins through the brain is visible in specific MRI modalities and can be added to the anatomical model. This first step one calls patient modeling creates a virtual image model of the patient. This approach allows assigning different colors to individual organ or functional area, which obviously helps clinical practitioners to analyze and distinguish safe tissue and sick area. Moreover, the surgeons can easily assess most of the surgical difficulties. They have a clear idea and maps of how to avoid risks and optimize the surgical approach and decrease surgical morbidity.

The second step is related to the development of computer tools with improved diagnostic and preoperative planning or surgical simulation (cf. Fig. 15.2). As we already mentioned, the gathered datasets can be rendered as a virtual 3D model of the patient. Firstly, this model can be easily manipulated by a surgeon to provide multiple views from any angle and at any depth within the volume. Thus, the surgeon can better

M.-L. Wang (✉)
Taiwan Chin Yi University of Science and Technology,
Taichung, Taiwan

Y. Ho
American MOST Company, New York, NY, USA

R. Beesetty
Dr. Rob Company, New York, NY, USA

S. Nicolau
Long Distance Minimally Invasive Surgery Center, Mokena, IL,
USA

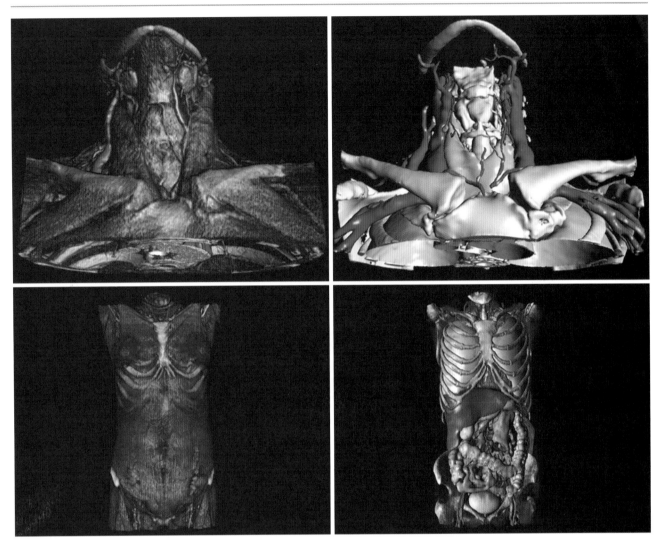

Fig. 15.1 Illustrations of the 3D model view and direct volume rendering

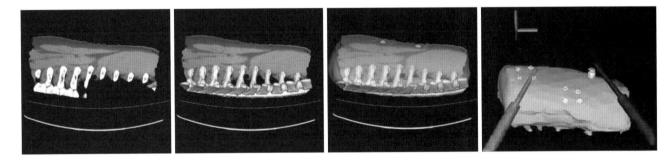

Fig. 15.2 The second step is image analysis and processing

plan and assess the case and establish a more accurate diagnostic. Secondly, surgical intervention can be virtually planned before actual surgery takes place. For instance, in the context of minimally invasive surgery, trocar insertion points can be planned on a 3D patient model and allow verification of optimal placement according to surgical standards.

The last step comprises all kinds of clinical intraoperative applications like surgical navigation, robotic surgery, computer-assisted orthopedic surgery (CAOS), computer-assisted radiosurgery, and computer-assisted oral and maxillofacial surgery. Computer-assisted surgery is the beginning of a revolution in surgery. It already makes a huge difference in high precision surgical domains, but it is also used in standard surgical operation procedures. During the operation, CAS system improves the geometrical accuracy of the surgical gestures and also reduces the redundancy of the surgeon's acts. This obviously improves ergonomic in the operating theater, minimizes the risk of surgical errors, and diminishes the operating time. There are two kinds of computer guiding systems: the first one is called augmented virtuality, displaying a virtual environment which is controlled by real information. Surgical navigation is an excellent example of augmented virtuality tool for guiding surgeon. Using a specific instrument, which is connected to the navigation system and tracked in real time, a software can simultaneously display its location relatively to a 3D or 2D image of the patient. The surgeon can thus use the instrument to "navigate" in the images of the patient by moving the instrument. The second one, called augmented reality (AR), is a live, direct, or indirect view of a physical and real-world environment, whose elements are augmented by computer-generated scenery with sound, video, graphics, or background data [2]. AR applies the existing sound, video, graphics, text, and other techniques to be integrated and improved, so that users can have "immersive" feeling and interact with an object. AR environment provides a comparison of the real scenery so that users can experience the feeling of a person or object in a scene anywhere. Xbox Kinect games of Microsoft are good examples of augmented reality application for large audience. It enables users to see computer-generated living scene and to control and interact with the Xbox 360 without needing to touch a game controller, through a natural user interface by using gestures and spoken commands. The most outstanding feature of the augmented reality system is its interactive and real-time response. Users or customers can follow the scenario and go through a game or a story and interact with the selected role in the game products. Computer-augmented reality techniques are the use of computer graphics or image synthesis technique and sound processing and touch and analog to construct a virtual world.

In medical applications, augmented reality is usually used to display virtual information on real images of the patient. More particularly, it seems practical to use AR technique in minimally invasive surgery to superimpose in either laparoscopic or endoscopic view structures, which is not visible by direct camera view but is visible in the preoperative image. In this practice, this means that the patient would be transparent for the surgeon's eyes, allowing localizing each important organs and tissues like tumors and vessels before reaching them, without needing to identify their positions with the sense of touch. It is worth emphasis that AR can also be used to show to junior surgeons the movement what should be done, by superimposing virtual instruments and sketching a specific task on the endoscopic view. Robotic surgery is named for correlated actions of a surgeon and a surgical robot, being programmed to carry out certain actions planned during the preoperative planning procedure [3]. A surgical robot is a mechanical device, generally like a robotic arm, that is controlled by a computer. Robotic surgery can be divided into three types, depending on the degree of surgeon interaction during the procedure: supervisory controlled, telesurgery, and shared control. In a supervisory-controlled system, Type I, the operation procedure is executed solely by the robot, which performs the preprogrammed action. A telesurgery system, Type II: remote surgery, demands a surgeon to manipulate robotic arms during the procedure rather than the robotic arms to work with a predetermined program. With shared-control systems, Type III, the surgeon implements the procedure with the use of a robot which offers steady-hand manipulations of the instrument. In most above robotic surgery, the working mode can be chosen for each separate intervention, depending on the surgical complexity and the particularities of the case [3]. It is interesting to notice that the current most used robotic system (da Vinci) can totally benefit from AR system for standard minimally invasive surgery since the surgeon performs its intervention by watching two screens in 3D. It is thus possible to superimpose any kind of information in the direct view of the surgeon. AR technique seems to be the most promising approach to guide surgeons and help them supervise a procedure in robotized telesurgery.

1.2   Superimposition of Information for Augmented Reality Surgery

The first step of developing an augmented reality system is to provide a 3D visualization of the preoperative patient imaging data. Two existing approaches to visualize the patient data in 3D are direct volume rendering from raw data and surface rendering from segmented data. 3D visualization which uses direct volume rendering is computed automatically from raw DICOM data of different modalities, like medical CT images. The method consists in visualizing simultaneously all voxels of the selected images through replacing their initial density by a color and a transparency defined through a transfer function [4]. This transparency allows thence to view or to hide contrasted anatomical or pathological structures in 3D pictures.

For clinic purpose, the main disadvantages of this 3D visualization are the lack of preprocessing and have no delineation being required to obtain useful results for diagnosis and surgical planning. In clinical routine, volume rendering is thus of great interest for all contrasted malformations in particular vascular ones, bones and all pathologies visible through an enhanced contrast, for example, blood vessel diseases (aneurysm, atheroma, atherosclerosis), contrasted tumors (in lungs, liver), or trauma (spine fracture, limb fracture). However, there are several limitations that can be prohibitive by depending on the medical application. Firstly, without manual interaction, users cannot visualize independently the organs they want to see if they have the same gray level in the DICOM data. Secondly, because independent structures are not delineated, to compute any organ volume is not possible. For the same reason, it is not possible to simulate an organ resection without cutting neighboring structures. Therefore, volume rendering still cannot be used for advanced surgical planning involving resection and associated volume. Finally, most software providing volume rendering functionality, such as the most known OsiriX [5], have been developed for radiologists and are not necessarily adapted to surgeons. Their user interface contains thus many complex options, so a long training is usually required to use properly the software.

Surface rendering is the second 3D visualization of a patient's medical images. This method needs firstly a structure of interest delineation followed by a mesh generation for processing and providing the surface of delineated structures. This preprocessing is the primary malpractice of the technique due to the possible obstacle and duration of such delineation. Once all important organs and pathologies have been segmented, it is able to visualize them in 3D, to adjust their surface transparency and to compute their volume. For the initial information of being reduced to important structures to be visualized only, the rendering is faster on a conventional computer. Moreover, for the meshes which are usually triangular meshes like in games, the rendering can be processed on any computer device, like notebook, tablet, or phone. Finally, the 3D models can be used in planning software for resection and preoperative simulation.

As you might know, the delineation step is a drawback of the surface rendering approach. More precisely, such delineations are a long and challenge task for radiologists/operators when using a software for allowing manual segmentation only. To overcome such a limitation, several commercial software have been developed and allow users to realize themselves the 3D patient model by using semiautomatic algorithms. The automated segmentation process is in practice and not guaranteed in clinical routine due to large variations in medical image quality: this means that an expert needs sometimes to check the segmentation quality by himself. This is why several companies offer updated online 3D modeling services from an uploaded DICOM image for dental, vascular, and digestive pathologies.

1.3 The Display Technologies of Augmented Reality

The existing display technologies for augmented reality have shown surgeons the additional information available from preoperative data. Three main categories of display devices are (1) the video-based display, (2) the see-through display, and (3) the projection-based device. Based on the medical applications, some displays are more adapted than others and require the addition in the operating room of a tracking system for head or camera position. This section describes the specificity, benefits, and drawback of each display system.

Video-based display method: Surgeons could see through a patient by augmented reality environment using one or several cameras in the operating room. The preoperative patient information will be superimposed on these video streams. In this context, the video image can be provided by an endoscopic camera [6–9] with external cameras located around the patient [6, 7, 10] or by video head-mounted camera which captures two videos that are displayed in front of the surgeon's eyes [11, 12]. External static cameras are certainly the cheapest and most effective solution for an external augmented reality view of patient internal organs. Indeed, although a camera-based head-mounted display has the benefit of providing an AR view directly along the surgeon's gaze, it is still uncomfortable for the surgeon, and it has to be tracked very accurately in the operating room, which increases dramatically its cost. In the case of laparoscopic surgery, it seems natural to provide augmented reality information directly on the laparoscopic image.

*See-through display is alternative: Vender*s have developed see-through devices that can superimpose the additional information onto the user's direct view since a camera cannot reproduce the quality of the human vision, which can be crucial in some augmented reality applications. This is a great solution to use a semitransparent mirror in front of the surgeon's gaze. While the surgeon can directly see the patient through the semitransparent mirror, a screen reflects the augmented reality information on the mirror [13]. Obviously those two small mirrors can be embedded on a head-mounted display (HMD) or a microscope as well and set directly in front of the user's eyes. In that case, the patient information is superimposed on both mirrors by using two tiny video projectors embedded on the HMD or microscope [14, 15]. Another way to provide see-through augmented reality is to use a semitransparent screen with autostereoscopic display [16, 17] or integral videography [18]. These screens, composed of micro-lenses, are special because they can display a 3D image with depth perception which allows at the same time to see through them. One of the major flaws of these technologies is their expensiveness. However, this drawback will be overcome. Thanks to the development of a large number of multimedia see-through glasses dedicated to entertainment, such as the Laster technologies Smart Vision system (www.laster.fr), the Optinvent clear-vuoptic system (www.optinvent.com), the Lumus system (www.lumus-optical.com), the Vuzix system Wrap 920 AR (www.vuzix.com), the scalar corporation T4-N glasses (www.scalar.co.jp), or the brother AirScouter system (www.brother.com). Another major flaw of this technology is the extreme challenge to provide an accurate augmented reality view superimposed onto the direct human vision. Indeed, to track in real time, pupil positions are essential when they move to ensure a proper registration in the surgeon view (the video-based head-mounted device needs head tracking only). Such a pupil tracking system already exists (for instance, Tobii IS-1 Eye Tracker from SMI) but needs better accuracy and a supplementary development to be embedded on the see-trough head-mounted device. Such an AR system will then be clearly more complex to develop and will increase the final integrated cost.

Project-based AR brings the preoperative information in the surgeon's field of view to directly project it on the patient's skin by using a video projector. Intraoperatively, the video projector is positioned in the operating room over the patient to obtain a direct visualization of the patient 3D model on the patient's skin. The outcome is so satisfied and very excellent because of a direct human vision and a real feeling of transparency of the patient. Although the video-projector visualization of the 3D patient model brings advantages to surgeons, its current result remains the most inaccurate techniques in terms of geometry point of view. Indeed, the projector projects deep internal organs on the skin surface after a registration phase by using only under skin bones (see registration section (Sect. 15.2)). Existing published work does not take the surgeon's head position into account with the surgeon's gaze of being variable from the video-projector optical center. This will create a notice-able error of perception for internal organs as illustrated. To compensate this phenomenon and project information on the skin so that surgeons do not make a depth estimation error, to track their head and the patient's skin is required. In such case, only one surgeon can be benefited from the aug-mented reality information. To provide this information to other surgeons, an additional head tracking is necessary to be associated with a synchronization projection system for each user. Such synchronization implies the addition of spe-cific glasses which are capable of hiding the images pro-jected for other users.

To conclude, the current projection system is not a perfect solution to give the feeling of a virtual transparency with pro-viding an erroneous deep structure location because of the lack of user head tracking. So, it should be used with limita-tion of under skin structure projection. By adding the track-ing of each user and an associated synchronized projection, the system will become extremely luxurious and complex which certainly explains why this approach is rarely applied.

1.4 Quick Review of Existing CAS Works

Augmented reality for intraoperative visualization has been a subject of particular research in the last decades [7, 19–25]. AR systems attempt to merge the real images and com-puter graphics (virtual view) into a single view for enhancing multimedia information around the user. The first medical application of AR technique was on neurosur-gery [26]. Parallel system [27] was developed indepen-dently, and AR had also been applied on otolaryngology [28]. These applications demand less of the AR system than laparoscopy for four reasons. The surgical field is small, the patient doesn't move, the view into the patient is from a single viewpoint and view direction, and this viewpoint is external to the patient. Frank et al. [29] have developed an AR image guidance system in which information derived from medical images was overlaid onto a video view of the patient. It simplifies the difficult task for building an enhanced visualization system.

For the contemporary high-tech advantages, laparoscopy and open and hybrid surgical systems are only capable of providing a 2D visualization through screens. Glossop et al. [30] have proposed a device which used scanned infrared and visible lasers to project computer-generated information such as surgical plans and entry points for probes directly onto the patient. Their device can be integrated with a 3D camera and is capable of measuring the location of projected infrared laser spots. It can be used on the display with a sur-prising degree of accuracy and apply corrections to the pro-jection path and to assist in registration.

To apply AR for spinal surgery, Paule et al. [31] have pro-posed a preoperative measurement technique that permits the matching between a patient and a virtual 3D medical image. Sauer et al. [29] also have developed an AR image for guiding system and adopting the head-mounted display for visualiza-tion. In 2007, Martin et al. [24] applied the AR for minimally invasive spine surgery. They used the HMD and preoperative CT images for stabilizing the spine without harming surround-ing tissue. Zein et al. [23] have introduced a prototypic add-on system for enhancing the intraoperative visualization within a navigated spine surgery by utilizing an extended reality approach. They also blended the spinal nerves or herniated disks and used image-based AR to superimpose the informa-tion on a dummy. In contrast to their approaches, our system adopts projector-based AR to develop a real-time landmark tracking, to transform the preoperative 3D model and to fit the body movement of clinical trials for demonstration.

Recently, a hybrid operating room [32–34] becomes widespread in the surgical field. Most of the hybrid operating rooms are with an agile mobile C-arm, laparoscopy, compact ultrasound system, intraoperative MRI, high-speed CT scan, automatic robot arm and latest gas insulation systems, etc. The design and implementation of hybrid operating rooms consume a complex multidisciplinary processes and signifi-cant investment. The advantages of these suites for the vas-cular surgeon are enormous in improving the spectrum, efficiency, and quality of care for complex patients.

Another application example is AR applied in minimally invasive surgery. Minimally invasive surgery represents one of the major evolutions of surgical techniques aimed at pro-viding a greatest care to the patient. However, minimally invasive surgery increases the operative challenges for surgeons because the depth perception is significantly diminished, the scope of view is minimized, and the sense of touch is substituted by instruments. However, these disadvantages can currently be reduced by AR guidance system. Indeed, from a patient's medical image of CT or MRI, AR remarkably enhances the surgeon's intraoperative vision by providing a virtual transparency of the patient. Imaging registration can be automatically performed interactively [ref Nicolau surgical oncology]. Several interactive systems have been developed and applied in medical centers, demonstrating the advantages and benefits of AR in surgical oncology. It also demonstrates the current limited interactivity because of soft organ movements and interaction between surgeon instruments and organs.

To conclude, existing systems are usually limited to real-time rigid registration or non-real-time rigid registration. Most commercial systems have been developed in neural and orthopedic surgery for hard tissues, although it is now admitted that soft tissue information (vessel and nerve positions, for instance, in orthopedic surgery) should be included in the current navigation system to provide an optimized guidance. On the opposite, existing works on soft organs remain limited with the main results having been obtained with a high level of interactivity or being limited to rigid registration. Thus there is no system which allows providing real-time automated augmented reality, which takes deformation and movement of soft organs into account.

1.5   AR for Orthopedic Surgery

We consider the problem of using augmented reality technologies for orthopedic surgery. The surgeons usually use the mobile C-arm with radiation for see-through and important organ or bone images of patient to decide the surgical steps in several clinical surgeries, such as brain, and orthopedics. Some research trends include using image-based technique instead of only traditional C-arm assisted by computer

screens, to solve the problems. The augmented reality is then considered as a hybrid of virtual and real environment spaces to register and simultaneously visualize the information of the patient in early reports for laparoscopic surgical procedures [21, 27].

To implement augmented reality (AR) for orthopedic surgery, the challenges are the pose deformation, body movement of patient, and lighting effect during surgical and operational gesture in progress. The pose deformation caused by the patient usually positions for C-arm X-ray, CT scan, and lie prone, supine, or lateral during surgery, and the body movement increases the difficulty of the registration between preoperative 3D model image and the backside surface of the patient in intraoperative spinal surgery. For the lighting effect, several healthcare workers and medical devices might change the rays of light sources or brightness and further impact the color of images captured by video camera. To overcome the challenges, researchers recommend that surgeons use the landmark detection and tracking methods for adapting and fitting the pose deformation and body movement, apply a projective method for registration, and process the image in a bit stable color space for avoiding the lighting effect [35].

The camera-projector system has been widely used for entertainment, industrial inspection, and education and training applications. It has been shown that using the mutual information of camera-projector system is calibrated quite accurately, such as planar-based calibration method [36]. The intrinsic and extrinsic parameters are easy to compute via the homography between the camera and the projector. For visualizing surgical information or operational plans directly onto the patient, a projector-based augmented reality system is used for cranio-maxillo-facial surgery. Kahrs et al. [37] proposed an evaluated prototype in the first clinical cases. Adding setup with a second video projector, to give additionally 3D information for localization and orientation (6DoF), is doable. With this method, the repositioning of a bone segment is intuitive and really applicable (Fig. 15.3).

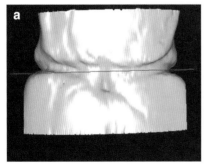 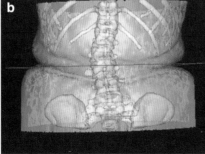 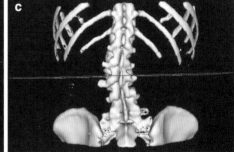

Fig. 15.3 The visible 3D patient model is used for constructing a 3D model of the patient for our ARCASS system. (**a**) It is the spinal 3D model of a patient with skin surface. (**b**) It is the spinal 3D model of a patient with 50% transparent skin surface. (**c**) It is the spinal 3D model without skin surface

2 Registration Methods for 3D Model and Intraoperative Scene

Registration can be defined as aligning two images into common coordinate system to monitor subtle changes; thus registration is the determination of a geometrical transformation that aligns points in one view of an object with corresponding points in another view of that object or another object. 3D images in medical field are generated by acquiring tomographic images, such as magnetic resonance (MR) imaging, computed tomography (CT), positron emission tomography (PET), and single-photon emission computed tomography (SPECT). In each of these image modalities, a contiguous set of 2D slices provides a 3D array voxels which are image intensity values. Typical 2D images may be X-ray projections captured on film or as a digital radiograph or projections of visible light captured as a photograph or a video frame or even 2D ultrasound images. In medical applications, the object, we focus in each view, will be some anatomical region of the body.

2.1 Introduction to Image Registration

Medical imaging techniques that help to see the inside of human body noninvasively and identify, locate, and diagnose the disease, with time image-guided treatment and surgeries, have evolved. Image registration can be defined as aligning two images of the same scene taken from two different viewpoints or taken at two different times or taken with two different sensors or image acquisition systems. Image registration is the backbone in image-guided radiotherapy [38, 39], image-guided radiosurgery [39, 40], image-guided minimally invasive therapy [41, 42] and surgery, endoscopic interventions [43], and interventional radiology [44]. Image registration is mapping of points in reference image also called pre-interventional image to sensed image and intra-interventional image [45, 46]. Usually pre-interventional images are 3D images constructed from CT or MRI images, and intra-interventional images are either 3D images from CT or MRI or SPECT or PET or 2D images from ultrasonography, fluoroscopy (projective X-ray), or X-ray images or mammograms.

Image registration helps in interventional techniques by reducing invasiveness and by increasing accuracy. In minimally invasive surgery, image registration of pre-interventional and intra-interventional images along with the instrument tracking help in locating the current position of the instrument with respect to the planned trajectory. Image registration helps in minimally invasive endoscopic surgeries by registering pre-interventional 3D images to intra-interventional endoscopic images for better visualization of

anatomy and pathology in real time which are hidden from direct view which provides augmented reality. In interventional radiology the pre-interventional data/images are registered to intra-interventional X-ray fluoroscopic or US images for 3D visualization of catheters or needles for better guidance. Image-guided radiotherapy like gamma rays focusing or radio isotope needed to be focused at site of tumor; hence, registration of pre-interventional CT images with daily pre-treatment images allows precise irradiation of pathological/cancerous tissue [47].

Wan Rui [48] in 2003 summarized medical image registration based on earlier research papers and proposed as following:

- Dimensionality: It is the dimension of images to be registered like 2D/2D, 2D/3D, and 3D/3D, and in general time is the fourth dimension.
- Domain of transformation: It could be global or local, which depends on whether the whole image or its part is to be registered.
- Type of transformation: The transformation could be rigid, affine, projective, or nonlinear.
- Tightness of feature coupling: The transformation can be interpolating (features of the objects in one image are exactly transferred into features in the other image) or approximating.
- Measure of registration quality: Various measures are applied, which depend on the data features or data itself.
- Method of parameter determination: The parameters of the transformation can be found out by using direct or search-oriented methods.
- Subject of registration: If the two images contain the same subject, it is intra-subject registration.
- If the subjects in the two images differ, it is intersubject registration.
- Type of data: It can be raw data, i.e., features extracted from data or introduced markers in data.
- Source of features: Features explicitly present in the data are called intrinsic features where as those introduced from outside are called as extrinsic features.
- Automatization level: This can be automatic or semiautomatic, which depends on user intervention level.

J. Michael Fitzpatrick [49] has suggested a classification which is slightly condensed than the above mentioned classification; they are image dimensionality, registration basis, geometrical transformation, degree of interaction, optimization procedure, modalities, subject, and object. Among these, registration basis has been discussed deeply and was classified mainly into three types: a. intensity-based methods, b. point-based methods, and c. surface-based methods. In this survey, we base on the previous registration methods and mainly classified them into two methods as follows:

- *Feature based*: Feature-based methods have three essential steps, which finally map the source and sensed image or model or scene:
  1. Feature detection. Salient and distinctive objects are manually, preferably, or automatically detected, and feature can be extrinsic objects like markers or stereotactic frames. For advanced processing in the literature, these features can be indicated by their point representatives, which are named control points (CPs).
  2. Feature matching. The correspondence between the features detected in the sensed image and those detected in the reference image is established in this step. Various feature descriptors and similarity measures along with spatial relationships among the features are used for that purpose.
  3. Transformation model estimation. Aligning the sensed image with the reference image is estimated. The parameters of the mapping functions are computed by methods of the established feature correspondence. The type and parameters of the so-called mapping functions.
- *Intensity based*: This method can be divided into two steps:
  1. Similarity measures. This method depends on the pixel or voxel values of registration for correspondence for matching rather than searching for features and then matching them.
  2. Transformation model estimation. In this method, transformation parameters are estimated by iteratively optimizing the similarity measures obtained from pixel or voxel values.

2.1.1   Feature-Based Method

Feature Detection

Feature detection is the first step of the image registration based on features. Features are salient structures or objects in an image, and they can be significant regions, lines, or points. They should be unique and easily distinguishable, circulate entire the image, and efficiently perceptible in both images. The features selected should be stable in time during the process of registration.

The comparability of feature set in the sensed and reference images is affirmed by the similarity and accuracy of the characteristic detector and by the overlap standard. In short, the number of common elements of the investigated sets of features should be plentifully high, regardless of the change of image geometry, radiometric conditions, and the presence of additive noise and of changes in the scanned scene. The features represent information on higher level. This property makes feature-based methods suitable for situations when

illumination changes are expected or multisensor analysis is demanded. Medical registration based on points, lines, and curves were reviewed by Peng Wen [50].

The surface or region features can be of regions with general high contrast, closed boundary, and appropriate size. In intraoperative scene or 3D images, the 3D surfaces of the body anatomy are easily characterized geometrical features. In surface-based registration, the correspondence between surfaces in 3D model and intraoperative scene is determined. The surfaces are skin air surface and cranial surfaces. Vertebral surfaces are used for CT/MR or image to physical registration. The surfaces are usually represented by point sets or finite elements or parametric surfaces. In intraoperative scene skin, surface points can be found by laser range finders [51], stereo video systems [52], and articulated mechanical, magnetic, optical (active and passive), and 3D ultrasound localizers. Figure 15.4 illustrates an example of surface-based registration.

To summarize, the use of feature-based methods is suggested if the images contain plenty of distinctive and easily detectable objects. This is usually the case of applications in remote sensing and computer vision. The typical images contain lots of details. On the contrary, medical images are not full of such details, and thus area-based methods are usually employed here. As always, the short of unique objects in medical images is solved by the interactive selection done by an expert or by introducing extrinsic features, rigidly positioned with respect to the patient.

Feature Matching

The detected features represented by control points (CPs) once detected in the reference and sensed images can be matched by means of the feature dimensional distribution or the feature symbolic description. While looking for the feature correspondence, some methods estimate the parameters of mapping functions at the same time and thus merge the second and third registration steps.

The relaxation method is one of the registration approaches for consistent labeling problem (CLP) which is to label the features from 3D model to intraoperative scene so that it is consistent with other feature pairs. In this method, the pair figure of merit is recalculated iteratively till a stable situation is reached considering matching quality of features and their neighbors. Feature descriptors are included in relaxation methods, and these methods are useful to handle translational and rotational distortions.

Transformation model estimation: The transformation model estimation is done after the feature correspondence is achieved. The task here is to calculate mapping function and its parameter estimation. Surface-based registration is of special interest in medical image registration as the 3D boundary surface of anatomy which is an easily characterized geometric feature (Fig. 15.5).

Fig. 15.4 Surface-based registration: selection of several femoral surface points by using digital probe for measuring position of points [53]

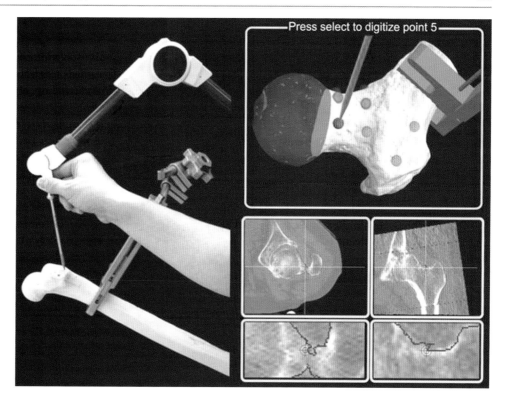

Fig. 15.5 Screws as fiducial marks for registration. Screws are inserted into the greater trochanter and femoral condyle before CT acquisition [53]

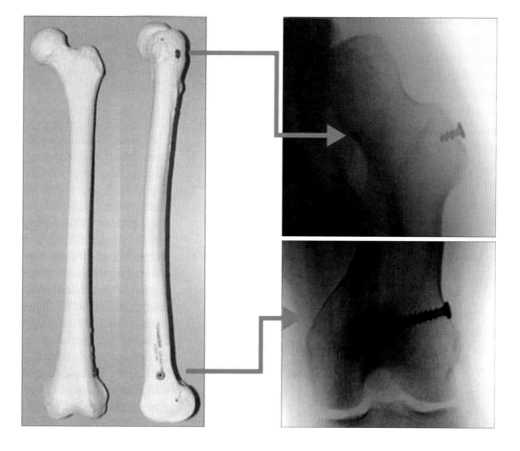

2.1.2 Intensity-Based Method

As for area-based or intensity-based method (see Fig. 15.6), the correspondence between images is based on pixel or voxel values. Transformation in area-based method or intensity-based method is determined by iteratively optimizing some similarity measures, and these are called voxel similarity measures. Similarity measures are mostly correlation-like methods, and the rest of the area-based methods are based on template matching. Area- or intensity-based method mostly merges the feature detection step with the matching part. These methods handle the images without attempting to detect notable objects. Windows of predefined size or even whole images are applied for the correspondence estimation during the second registration step [39, 45].

The limitations of the intensity-based method originate in their basic idea. Firstly, the rectangular window, which is most often used, suits the registration of images which locally differs only by a translation. If images are deformed by more complex transformations, this type of the window is not able to cover the same parts of the scene in the reference and sensed images (the rectangle can be transformed to some other shape). Several authors proposed to use circular shape of the window for mutually rotated images. However, the comparability of such simple-shaped windows is violated too if more complicated geometric deformations (similarity, perspective transforms, etc.) are present between images.

Another drawback of the area based method refers to the "remarkableness" of the window content. That a window containing a smooth area without any prominent details will be probably matched incorrectly with other smooth areas in the reference image due to its non-saliency. The features for registration should be preferably detected in distinctive parts of the image. Windows, whose selection is often not based on their content evaluation, may not have this property. Classical area-based method like cross-correlation (CC) exploits for matching directly image intensities, without any structural analysis. Consequently, they are sensitive to the intensity changes such as varying illumination, introduced, for instance, by noise and/or by using divergent sensor types. For correlation-like methods, the classical representative of the area-based method is the normalized CC and its modifications:

$$cc(i,j) = \frac{\sum_{w}(W - E(W))\left(I_{(i,j)} - E\left(I_{(i,j)}\right)\right)}{\sum_{w}(W - E(W))^2 \sum_{I_{(i,j)}}\left(I_{(i,j)} - E\left(I_{(i,j)}\right)\right)^2} \quad (15.1)$$

In addition, there are many similar ways proposed, such as video subtracter, portion of the image uniformity, partition intensity uniformity, joint histogram and joint probability distribution, mutual information, and Fourier method. This section will not elaborate these related methods in details.

2.2 Geometric Transformations

For understanding the registration methods, the geometric transformations in which the images involved in registration belong to two different coordinate systems which should be known. Geometric transformation is mapping data points or feature points from space X to data points or feature points in space Y. The transformation T applied to points in X represented by column vector x produces a transformed point x':

$$x' = T(x) \quad (15.2)$$

If point y in Y corresponds to x in X, a successful registration will make x equal or approximately equal to y. Any nonzero displacement $T(x) - y$ will lead to registration error. The set of transformation T functions can be broadly classified into rigid and nonrigid transformations. The main aim of the registration usually would be to estimate the parameter of mapping or transformation function.

2.2.1 Rigid Transformation

Rigid transformation preserves all distances, straight lines, and all nonzero angles between straight lines. All rigid transformation methods contain two components, namely, translation and rotation. Translation, t, is a 3D vector specified by three coordinates t_x, t_y, t_z which are either Cartesian or polar coordinates. Rotational components can be specified by many ways like Euler angles, Cayley-Klein parameters, quaternions, axis and angle, and orthogonal matrices:

$$x' = Rx + t \quad (15.3)$$

where R is an orthogonal matrix, i.e., $RR^t = R^t R = I$ (identity matrix) thus $R - 1 = R^t$.

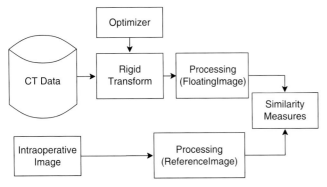

Fig. 15.6 Schematic view of 3D-2D registration intensity-based registration

2.2.2 Nonrigid Transformation

Nonrigid transformations are very important in medical image registration as most of the human anatomy is nonrigid and deformable. Nonrigid transformation also has importance when image distortions are imperative in image acquisition with intra-patient and inter-patient registration of the rigid anatomy.

Scaling Transformations

This transformation is most basic nonrigid transformation which almost seems like rigid but for scaling factor. This kind of transformation is helpful in compensating calibration errors during image acquisition systems. These transformations preserve straightness of lines and angles. This is defined as

$$x' = RSx + t \text{ or } x' = SRx + t \quad (15.4)$$

where S is a diagonal matrix (sx, sy, sz) whose elements represent scaling factors along three coordinate axes. If scaling is isotropic with $s_x = s_y = s_z = s$, the transformation is called similarity transformation:

$$x' = sRx + t \quad (15.5)$$

Affine Transformation

Affine transformation is defined by equation below in which matrix A has elements aij and can have any value:

$$x' = Ax + t \quad (15.6)$$

Affine transformation preserves straightness of lines, their parallelism, and planarity of surface, but angle between lines will change. Scaling transformation can be defined as a special case of affine transformation. In homogeneous coordinates, the above equation can be written as

$$\begin{bmatrix} u_1' \\ u_2' \\ u_3' \\ 1 \end{bmatrix} = \begin{bmatrix} a_{11} & a_{12} & a_{13} & t_1 \\ b_{21} & b_{22} & b_{23} & t_2 \\ c_{31} & c_{32} & c_{33} & t_3 \\ 0 & 0 & 0 & 1 \end{bmatrix} \begin{bmatrix} u_1 \\ u_2 \\ u_3 \\ 1 \end{bmatrix} \quad (15.7)$$

Projective Transformation

This transformation preserves straightness of lines and planarity of surfaces, but parallelism is not preserved unlike affine transformation. The projective transformation can be defined as

$$x' = (Ax + t) / (P.x + \alpha) \quad (15.8)$$

In homogeneous coordinates, this equation can be written as

$$\begin{bmatrix} u_1' \\ u_2' \\ u_3' \\ u_4' \end{bmatrix} = \begin{bmatrix} a_{11} & a_{12} & a_{13} & t_1 \\ b_{21} & b_{22} & b_{23} & t_2 \\ c_{31} & c_{32} & c_{33} & t_3 \\ P_1 & P_2 & P_3 & \alpha \end{bmatrix} \begin{bmatrix} u_1 \\ u_2 \\ u_3 \\ 1 \end{bmatrix} \quad (15.9)$$

Perspective Transformation

In medical imaging, the 3D scene is projected into a 2D plane, mostly camera sensor; this kind of projection is called perspective projection.

Assuming affine portion of the projective transformation as unity, $f = 1/|P|$, and unit vector along the direction of projection axis, P as p

$$x' = fx / (x.p + \alpha f) \quad (15.10)$$

This transformation equation represents formation of photograph of 3D scene acquired with a pinhole model camera where pinhole can be assumed as a substitute of lens system. Here x is the scene point, p is the axis of projection, and f is the distance of the screen which is perpendicular to projection axis from pinhole. In cameras with lens systems, a unique point is identified one equivalent to pinhole through which the light ray of traveling undeflected is called center of perspectivity. The above equations for lens systems and X-ray systems differ geometrically by $x.p + \alpha f$ greater f for lens systems and less than f for X-ray systems. Contrast with the curved transformation, this transformation does not preserve straightness of lines, and the simplest form of this transformation is polynomial in x:

$$x' = \sum_{i\ jk}^{IJK} C_{i\ jk} x^i y^j z^k \quad (15.11)$$

where $Ci\ jk$ is the three-element vector of coefficients for i, j, k term of polynomial expression for the three components x^i, y^j, z^k of x'. Curved transformations are rarely used with I, J, K values more than 2 or $M(i + j + kM)$ greater than 5 because of spurious oscillations associated with higher-order polynomials. To avoid this problem, peacewise polynomials and particularly splines are used for smoothening of edges. The most commonly used spline is cubic spline. Splines of degree m are often expressed in terms of a convenient basis set of polynomials with the same degree, called B-splines. Coordinates of every x must be to $ui \times (l + \alpha)$, $v j \times (m + \beta)$, $wk \times (n + \gamma)$, where l, m, n are integers and $0 \le \alpha, \beta, \gamma \le 1$. The cubic spline in terms of B-spline is expressed as

$$x'(l,,,,,m,,,,,n,,,,,\alpha,,,,,\beta,,,,,\gamma) = \sum_{i\ jk} B_{i-l}(\alpha) B_{j-m}(\beta) B_{k-n}(\gamma) c_{i\ jk} \quad (15.12)$$

Another most heavily used transformation for 2D problems is thin-plate spline. The Goshtasby's formula used in image registration is

$$x' = Ax + t + \sum_{i \to it}^{N} c_i \gamma_2 \ln \gamma_2 \qquad (15.13)$$

Thin-plate spline is one of the more general forms of radial basis functions, which for 2D and 3D spaces, the term $r2 \ln r2$ in the above equation is replaced by $f(ri)$.

2.3 3D Model to Intraoperative Scene Registration

In this section, we mainly discuss about 3D to intraoperative registration methods which use a 3D CT or MR pre-interventional image. The intraoperative or intra-interventional images will be one or more 2D X-ray projection images or 3D intra-interventional image like CBCT, CT, MR, or US image [54]. In 3D model to intraoperative registration, 3D/2D volume-to-slice [55–58] or (endoscopic) volume-to-video [59–61] registration are generally useful. The anatomic regions where 3D to intraoperative registration is frequently used are head (brain and skull), spine and vertebrae, pelvis (entire pelvis and perineum), limbs (knee joint, hip joint, femur, tibia, and patella), and thorax (heart, ribs). Most common surgical or interventional techniques where 3D to intraoperative registration is required are:

- Radiotherapy—for planning and treatment verification for patient positioning and motion tracking
- Radiosurgery—arteriovenous malformation
- Orthopedic surgery—total hip replacement and knee replacement
- Neurosurgery and interventional neuroradiology—head, neck, and spine minimally invasive surgeries [62]
- Vascular interventional radiology—angioplasty, stenting [63], and embolization
- Kinematic analysis

Radiotherapy and radiosurgery are two important branches which are beneficial because of image registration particularly 2D-3D registration. In radiotherapy, registration helps in aligning the anatomy to be treated with radiation beam. In radiotherapy and radiosurgery, intrinsic features or landmarks can be used for registration for treatment if they are close to bony landmarks like skull in case of brain tumors. For prostrate radiotherapy, the prostrate is aligned and tracked by using intrinsic marker-based 3D-2D registration by using pelvis as reference, and later extrinsic marker-based therapy by placing markers in prostrate had become a clinical method of choice. The marker-based registration method is also used for liver and pancreatic tumor treatment. In lung

tumor an optical tracking-based registration method is used for 3D-2D registration.

As for the spine surgeries, there are several spine surgeries which use image-guided intervention or surgery like percutaneous procedures, resection of tumors and arteriovenous malformations, treatment of spinal instability, and treatment of disk disease. Image-guided minimally invasive procedures where 3D image to intraoperative registration is required are pedicle screw fixation transarticular C1/C2 fixation, transoral odontoid resection, and anterior cervical corpectomy. In spine procedure, there are different methods of registration based on vertebra. Vertebra is the natural choice for registration for spine, abdominal, and thoracic surgeries because of its observed features on fluoroscopy. In spine surgeries, the intraoperative imaging is fluoroscopy or CT fluoroscopy or 3D ultrasound imaging. In image-based registration, algorithms require initial pose estimation of 3D model which will be done manually by selecting some anatomical landmarks preoperatively and intraoperatively [62]. There is a robust technique for initial pose estimation spectrum based on similarity measure for identifying the rotation of the 3D data, combined with phase correlation for the estimation of the in-plane translation, and this method was tested clinically with a success rate of 68.6%. In spine and orthopedic procedure, the registration between preoperative 3D and intraoperative scene for therapy, particularly radiotherapy, radiosurgery, or other tumor removals, images to physical registration transformation to track the surgical probe or to direct needle to surgical target. Imaging to physical registration is performed by using geometric features of spine. Fixing the spine in a frame is cumbersome, so external stereotactic frame that encloses the body has been used; however there is always an error around 2.5–10 mm due to patient movement. Anatomical landmarks or surfaces can be used for registration in open image-guided surgeries of spine and orthopedics. In point-based registration, the bony landmarks such as tip of the spinous or transverse process or a prominent facet or osteophyte are identified and marked in preoperative 3D model and in the physical world, and they are localized by using a tracking probe, and then the corresponding point pairs are aligned by using least square method. In surface-based registration, the bone surfaces extracted from the 3D model (CT images) are matched with the recorded surface points with tracking probe intraoperatively. The crucial step in surface-based registration is the surface segmentation which is often cumbersome computationally. The feature-based registration is more useful for open surgeries but not conducive for minimally invasive endoscope procedures or radiosurgery.

Alternative to image to physical is preoperative 3D model for intraoperative 2D image, mostly fluoroscopic image or X-ray image. Most common approach for 3D-2D registration is feature-based method particularly surface features. The object surfaces are segmented from the pre-operative image, and the contours are extracted from the intraoperative image, and then the registration is performed by minimizing the distance-based cost function. Selection of object contour is a tedious and time-consuming task with image-guided treatment for spinal lesion point-based alignment by using fiducial marks like metal pins and grids. Fiducial marker-based methods are fast, robust, and accurate; however the artificial and fiducial marks require surgical implantation, and that might involve some considerable risk particularly in cervical spine where the vertebral processes are small.

3 Clinical Trials of Real-Time Augmented Reality

Image-guided surgical and diagnostic intervention procedures have become popular in recent decades. This section addresses the clinical trials of applying AR to digestive surgical oncology and spinal surgery (vertebroplasty). The current automatic AR systems show the feasibility of such system, and it is relying on specific and expensive equipment which is not available in clinical routine. Moreover, they are not robust enough due to the high complexity of developing a real-time registration of taking organ deformation and human movement into account. The experiments demonstrate that the AR systems are extremely encouraging and show that it will become a standard requirement for future computer-assisted surgical oncology and spinal surgery.

3.1 AR for Minimally Invasive Surgery

Superimposing 3D model information in the endoscopic view is a dream for surgeons, and unfortunately, still a great challenge exists for augmented reality researchers. Preliminary works relied on a rigid registration of abdominal 3D patient model by using radiopaque landmarks that the surgeon stuck on the abdomen skin. This approach has been evaluated on phantoms [65], animals [9, 66–68], and humans [69], and experiments showed the potential benefits. However, it is still not used routinely in the OP room since it has too many drawbacks to be easily integrated in the surgical workflow. Indeed, not only the registration of the 3D models is not accurate enough (Marvik et al. [69] have reported a registration error above 7 mm), but also it becomes extremely inaccurate as soon as the patients or the organs are moved. In that case a new registration is necessary, which lengthen too much the surgical workflow.

In order to overcome this problem, one common approach is to acquire intraoperatively a 3D image of structures of interest. This strategy can thus take the organ motion into account. Some works have proposed direct superimposition of 2D US image in the endoscopic image [70, 71] and superimposition of liver tumor or vessel reconstruction from intraoperative 2D US [72]. In both cases, an endoscopic US probe provides the 2D US images, and its position is tracked in real time. The system in [70, 71] provides accurate registration of real-time information from US image; however, the user has to maintain the US probe on the organ surface at the proper location so that structures of interest are visible in the US image. The system in [72] firstly proposes to obtain a 3D model of the structures of interest by scanning the whole organ with the US probe. This idea is sufficiently fast due to a fast image analysis which allows to extract the liver vessel tree from the collected 2D US images. The resulting 3D model is then superimposed in the endoscopic view. This system finally provides an augmented reality that takes deformation into account once in a while. Practically, the registration becomes wrong when the liver is shifted by an instrument: a new 3D scanning that needs 3 min with the US probe has to be performed again. Although their system has been tested on patients, authors are trying to improve the scanning process so that it lasts much less time.

Shekhar et al. [73] have proposed to update the 3D liver model by using intraoperative low-dose CT image. The update is carried out by using a nonrigid intensity-based registration of the preoperative image on the intraoperative one. From the computed deformation field, a new 3D model can be obtained and then superimposes on the endoscopic view (the endoscopic camera being tracked by an optical tracking system). One could ask why they do not directly superimpose the information extracted from the intraoperative image. In fact, since CT acquisitions are low dose, many important details like organ vessel and tumor are not visible in the low-dose image. Finally, they manage to provide an updated augmented reality view of the liver after each low-dose CT acquisition. Currently, the main drawbacks of this system are the nonrigid registration computation time (about 1.5 min), the additional irradiation to the patient, and the cost of the procedure due to the CT scan device. It is worth mentioning that this strategy becomes more and more realistic due to rotational C-arm (like zeego from Siemens), allowing to acquire a 3D image of the patient in the interventional room with much less cumbersomeness [74].

The second classic approach to superimpose augmented information in the endoscopic view is to register a preoperative 3D model on real-time features extracted in the endoscopic image. Currently, all existing works focus on real-time organ surface reconstruction from endoscopic images, followed by a rigid or nonrigid surface registration with the preoperative 3D model. This approach has already been tested in open surgery conditions for breast [75] and liver [76], and experimental results were successful, as long as a large and relevant surface of the organ could be acquired, which corresponds to the main limitation of this approach, in addition to the supplementary surface acquisition system that has to be set in the OP room. Obviously, this strategy is much more difficult in the endoscopic surgery context since large surface acquisition is usually not possible in operative conditions: the nonrigid surface registration step will hardly be reliable since small surface cannot properly predict the real deformation of underlying structures. However, it is worth highlighting that clinically acceptable results have been obtained on uterus surgery by Malti et al. [77]. Indeed, in their context, an important part of the uterus can be obtained and thus registered with a small error with the preoperative model.

To tackle the organ surface acquisition, many approaches have been proposed, and they are properly reviewed in the recent following paper [78]. We briefly summarize them hereafter. Albitar et al. and Maurice et al. propose to use structured light projection on organs to acquire the organ surfaces in real time [79, 80]. They have validated their approach on in vivo organs, but miniaturization of their device is still mandatory so that it can be easily used with an endoscope. Penne et al. [81] and Mersmann et al. [64] have developed a time of flight (TOF) system devoted to endoscopic surgery, which allows recovering at 5 Hz on the surface in the camera field of view. A prototype system is already available for endoscope integration; however a better resolution seems necessary since the recovered surface has a resolution of 45×70 points only. Stoyanov et al. [82, 83], Mountney et al. [84, 85], Röhl [86], and Hu et al. [87] have proposed efficient approaches to acquire organ surface from stereo-endoscope by using disparity or camera motion. Although they reach real-time surface tracking, their method is restricted to stereo-endoscope which is used routinely by the robotic system da Vinci only. More recently, Hu et al. [88], Collins et al. [89], and Martinez-Herrera [90] have tackled surface reconstruction issue from monocular endoscope by using either motion or polarization and provided convincing results that are currently under validation. We highlight that all these works do not include the necessary registration step to provide an augmented reality view.

To our knowledge, Figl et al. [91], Su et al. [92], and Kim et al. [93] are the only ones to propose both organ surface reconstructions associated to a real-time (or almost) registration. Su et al. have registered a static 3D model of a kidney by using surface registration and shown the tumor position inside the kidney, and Figl et al. have registered a nonrigid 3D heart model to superimpose heart vessel position. Both systems rely on stereo-endoscope acquisition to acquire the 3D organ surface and thus cannot be easily adapted to standard mono-endoscope. Kim et al. instead use shape from shading to recover the organ surface and manage to superimpose in real-time augmented reality information following the organ motion. Unfortunately, the registration

accuracy could not be clinically evaluated because no ground truth data were available (an intraoperative CT scan, for instance).

3.2 AR for Spine Surgery

This section addresses an advance augmented reality method for seeking entry point of orthopedic surgery and be helpful for surgeons to simply coordinate transformations between several imaging displays. Based on landmark detection and tracking techniques and calibrated camera-projector system, a superimposed imaging system is developed and called ARCASS (Augmented Reality Computer-Assisted Spine Surgery) for assisting spinal surgery. The system is to rectify the images via the perspective projection model and projective registration of 3D model constructed by 3D visible patient. It then displays a merged real and synthetic image in the surgeon's natural point of view to see through the patient by camera-projector system. The proposed method not only simplifies the computation between surgical instruments and patient for surgeons but also reduces the intraoperative radiation exposure. Experimental results for the synthetic spinal image on dummy, two pieces of pork, and four clinical trial testing have demonstrated the feasibility of our approach, and the accuracy evaluation is also provided.

3.2.1 ARCASS System

We present an ARCASS system to construct superimposed display system by using a combination of the pinhole camera and projector (camera-projector system, refer to Fig. 15.7). The system is an implementation of a visualization system to assist with surgical procedures, especially in orthopedic surgery. In surgeries with open and minimally invasive surgeries, the physicians usually use personal experience and spend several years for side observation of the senior surgeons to learn the surgical skills. The major reason why taking a long learning curve is the complicated system coordinate transformation. The system coordinate includes the viewpoint of laparoscopy, surgeons' eyes, instrument positions, and several different display screens from different cameras. Physicians would image and predict all the system together and have to avoid the damage of any trouble, such as touch the aorta or nerves. For speeding up the workflow and reducing radiation times of a spinal surgery, the proposed ARCASS system directly projects merged virtual image, which extracted from the preoperative CT images or intraoperative C-arm device and convenient camera on the backside surface of the patient. It aims to reduce the radiation, training, and operating time of physicians to calculate the system coordinate transformation.

Fig. 15.7 The flowchart of AR technique via ARCASS system

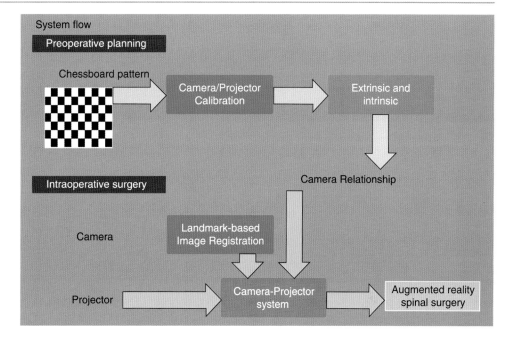

To project the bone image, the pre-captured CT images are required, and we construct the 3D model of being operated patient via using the visible patient [94], developed by IRCAD. The visible patient tool is automatic analysis of medical images and the geometrical, topological, and physical modeling of patients in 3D. It is designed for surgical planning and preoperative simulation guidance or augmented reality as intraoperative assistance. The proposed system would incrementally provide following contributions to the surgeon:

- First, it would allow merging images, an X-ray image or image extracted from the 3D model, with an external video view of the patient. C-arm/camera calibration and homography registration would be developed.
- Second, a real-time see-through body computer-assisted system (ARCASS) for showing the bone information during intraoperative surgery.
- Third, the system would provide an augmented reality view of a preoperative patient model in the video and X-ray view by automatic skin marker detection and tracking method for pose deformation and body movement of the patient.
- In the end, the system reduces the intraoperative radiation times and is robust under the varying lighting environment.

Not only would this approach simplify the procedure for the surgeon but also reduce risk during surgery to the patient. It would be shown how one of these incremental features allows reducing radiation exposure and providing higher accuracy, and particularly patient's safety is considerably increased. The techniques of the system can be divided into the following items: 3D modeling and calibration of camera-

projector system, image alignment, landmark detection, and tracking. In this section, we present the efficient 3D modeling tool "visible patient," and the rest sections detail the ARCASS system.

Providing a 3D visualization of the preoperative patient data is the first step to develop an augmented reality system. We adopt the tool which is called "visible patient" in this work for constructing 3D model of patients to visualize the patient data in 3D [95]. We are therefore based on the 3D model to generate a projection view for camera-projector system and discuss in the following subsections.

3.2.2   Calibration of Camera-Projector System

For using the camera-projector system in this work, it is very important to compute the geometry between projector and pinhole camera accurately. In our ARCASS system, there are three cameras which should be calibrated in advance. They are pinhole, projector, and C-arm (X-ray) cameras. The Tsai's calibration method [96] is used for calibrating the pinhole and C-arm cameras. For calibrating the camera-projector system, the planar-based calibration method [36] is adopted to compute the homography between the pinhole and projector, and the intrinsic, rotation, and translation vectors are obtained.

3.2.3   Intraoperative Projective Registration

To achieve spinal image projection on the surface of the patient, the image is first transferred from RGB to YCbCr color space. We then only extract the Cb and Cr channel images for landmark detection, due to the channel images which are insensitive to the environment lighting change [97]. For the landmark tracking, the double-Gaussian vector matching scheme [98] is adopted and processed on the Cb and Cr color space in a 30×30 square area segmented by manual for the landmarks. We then build the descriptor of each square area of landmarks. It is computed by applying the Gaussian mask twice to a processing area of pixels. The vectors are simple and easy to implement with acceptable tracking results for body movement.

We take the image projective registration into account after the landmarks have been detected. Suppose Ln_i is a 3D point and the coordinate center is located at the pinhole camera of the camera-projector system and Ln' is a point matched to Ln_i in preoperative 3D model (see Fig. 15.8). Thanks to LIBICP [99] and the correspondences, Ln_i and Ln' are matched by using the object function specifically

$$T = \arg\max_{R,t} \sum_{i=1}^{n}\sum_{j=1}^{m} \left\| Ln_i - R \times Ln' - t \right\|^2 \quad (15.14)$$

where $T = (R, t)$ is the estimated rotation and translation vector for transferring the preoperative 3D model to fit the intraoperative curved skin surface.

For intra-operation to project an X-ray image onto the backside surface of the patient, the 2D image registration of X-ray and pinhole images by using epipolar constraint [100] is adopted. The epipolar constraint is calculated via calibrated camera parameters, and the selected spinal image, which extracted from 3D model, and the images captured by pinhole and C-arm cameras are used for fusion. Suppose ix and ip are two images captured by X-ray and pinhole cameras. These two images are rectified by using calibration parameters, and then the rectified matrix is $R_{rect} = \begin{pmatrix} e_1^T \\ e_2^T \\ e_3^T \end{pmatrix}$, where $\begin{pmatrix} e_1^T \\ e_2^T \\ e_3^T \end{pmatrix}$ are the mutually orthogonal unit vectors [100]. The rec-

tified image pair is therefore can be applied on epipolar constraint to restrict a point in C-arm image pixel coordinate which should be presented in a horizontal line in pinhole image pixel coordinate. The mixing image is then generated from the rectified image pair to calculate the homography by utilizing four matching image points at least.

We have implemented the image rectification and explored the image fusion on the image pair (X-ray and pinhole images) through epipolar constraint. For projecting an X-ray spinal image on the back surface of the patient precisely, the transformation is as follows:

$$I_p = I_v \times H_{rv} \times H_{ps}^{-1} \quad (15.15)$$

where Ip is the last presented image on the backside surface of patient. Iv is a intraoperative C-arm image. The rest matrices are the calculation between projection area of projector and pinhole camera view. Hrv and H^{-1} are the homography of real-to-virtual and projector-to-pinhole transforms, respectively.

3.3   Clinical Experiment Results

To evaluate performance of the proposed ARCASS system, the human dummy, 2 pieces of pork, and several clinical trials are used. The system is a medical application of augmented reality for spinal surgery based on projective registration, landmark detection, tracking, and the epipolar-based image fusion for X-ray image, yet it can project the spinal image onto the backside surface of the being operated patient. All results are processed in the operating room of Show Chwan Memorial Hospital, and we also provide the precision analysis on pork and compare the accuracy of

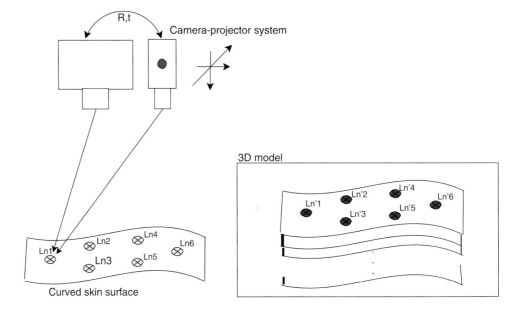

Fig. 15.8 It is the intraoperative projective registration method (ICP [92]) for converting the preoperative 3D model to fit the curved skin surface via the landmark detection and tracking. A projector and an industrial camera are used for demonstration.

insert and target positions. The proposed ARCASS system is equipped with six landmarks, a Ziehm 8000 C-arm camera, one Sony XCD-SX90CR industrial camera, and a BenQ DLP W7000 projector. The Sony XCD-SX90CR industrial camera is a CCD based that achieves a frame rate of up to 30 fps at 1280 × 960 (SXGA) resolution, and the image resolution is 1920 × 1080 (full HD) for the BenQ DLP W7000 projector (Fig. 15.9).

3.3.1 Human Dummy Simulation

In the simulated data, a dummy which contains four to six metal landmarks and a 3D model with spinal image is used to verify the proposed ARCASS. The world coordinate center is located at a pinhole camera and which also used as the video camera of camera-projector system. A dummy and a spinal image projected on the backside surface of the dummy (Fig. 15.10).

3.3.2 Pork Testing

We use two pieces of pork for the testing (Fig. 15.11), and the procedure is the same as surgery for a real patient. It is first to scan the CT images and use the visible patient tool for 3D modeling and labeling. We then apply the proposed projective registration method for the tested pork, and the ARCASS system is used for evaluating our results in the operating room.

3.3.3 Clinical Trials

There are two surgeons who had used the proposed ARCASS system for three spinal surgeries, and the C- arm times for guiding a needle toward an entry point to the target was shortened by 70%. The trials show that the system works perfectly in the operating room and provides the very useful information, especially for seeking the entry points for spinal surgery.

3.3.4 Accuracy Evaluation

For surgical accuracy evaluation of the proposed ARCASS, we apply the testing on a piece of pork for computing. We first preset a surgical planning for 20 entry and 16 target points in the 3D visible patient model and hit the nails into the piece of pork by using the projected information of ARCASS. The accuracy is then calculated by Euclidean distances between 3D positions of surgical planning of entry and target points, and the average errors are 4.4 ± 1.5 mm for entry points and 9.1 ± 3.4 mm for target points shown in Tables 15.1 and 15.2. As a consequence of the lack of angle information between entry and target points, the accuracy analysis results show that the proposed method is useful for searching entry points, however, not for target points. In our clinical trials, the surgeon could find the target points by utilizing a few times (less than eight times) of C-arm radiation exposures, and this much decreases the surgical time.

3.4 Conclusions and Future Works

The ARCASS system has shown the good performance of evaluating on simulated, pork, and clinical trials in the orthopedic surgery. For the real patient testing, the institutional review board (IRB 1010308) is proved for evaluating our method in advance. The surgeon's feedback to the proposed system for the experiments of spinal surgery is very positive and helpful. The major limitation of the system is the intrusion into the line of sight, it is caused by the image projected from a projector, and then the occlusion occurs on the projected area while the surgeon operates. The results show the proposed ARCASS system is compact and useful for spinal surgery, and the multiple camera-projector system will consider in the future (Figs. 15.12, 15.13, 15.14, and 15.15).

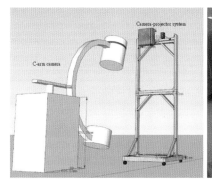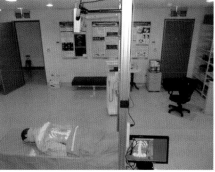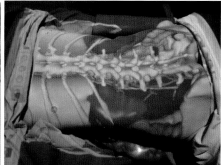

Fig. 15.9 The prototype of the proposed ARCASS system. A projector and an industrial camera are used for demonstration

Fig. 15.10 The first simulated augmented reality-assisted surgery of the pork. (**a**) The first pork experiment. The 3D visible images of the pork which are generated by the CT scans and visible patient tool. (**b**) The first augmented reality system setup and its corresponding pork testing simulation. The augmented reality system actually projects the preoperative CT scan imaging of the pork

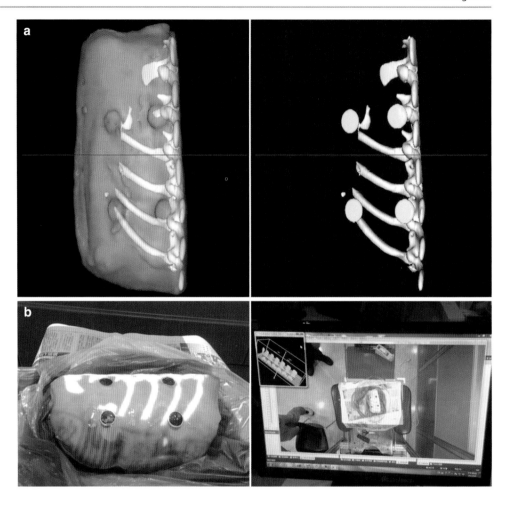

Fig. 15.11 The second piece of pork used for the simulated spinal surgery experiment. (**a**) The setup and 3D model of the second pork experiment. (**b**) The piece of pork and corresponding projection view of the 3D bone image on the piece of pork of the second pork experiment

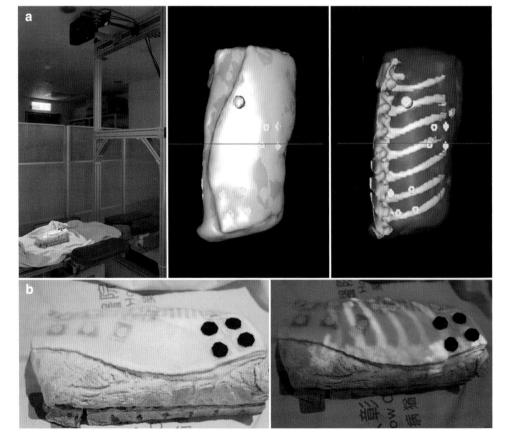

Table 15.1 The accuracy evaluation of 20 entry points of a piece of pork in 4 experiments

Points	The preoperative points (x, y, z)	After hitting nails (x, y, z)	Distance (mm)
Entry 1	89.7, 105.3, 169.9	91.3, 107.9, 169.7	3.1
Entry 2	102.4, 101.4, 223.4	105.9, 104.4, 219.5	6.1
Entry 3	128.5, 97.8, 175.7	130.0, 101.3, 174.6	3.8
Entry 4	154.7, 93.3, 206.1	151.8, 96.0, 205.8	3.9
Entry 5	189.3, 85.9, 215.6	183.1, 88.8, 216.3	6.9
Entry 6	205.1, 82.2, 206.2	198.7, 86.0, 206.7	7.4
Entry 7	218.9, 97.7, 232.8	216.6, 97.0, 231	3.0
Entry 8	191.0, 104.1, 204.3	190.2, 105.1, 208	3.9
Entry 9	218.2, 100.9, 202.6	214.4, 101.4, 207	5.7
Entry 10	247.5, 96.8, 205.9	243.7, 95.7, 211	6.4
Entry 11	220.4, 104.1, 179.1	218.5, 102.6, 184	5.3
Entry 12	72.7, 141.1, 133.7	71.9, 140.9, 131	2.9
Entry 13	118.0, 134.6, 136.7	118.3, 134.0, 140	3.2
Entry 14	103.2, 141.3, 117.1	102.1, 139.9, 121.9	5.1
Entry 15	73.4, 155.6, 91.0	75.0, 154.8, 88	3.5
Entry 16	117.3, 147.7, 98,9	120.2, 144.1, 98	4.7
Entry 17	160.8, 124.7, 150.7	157.9, 124.0, 149	3.4
Entry 18	141.8, 135.8, 120.3	141.5, 135.3, 119	1.4
Entry 19	160.5, 142.2, 101.0	158.8, 140, 98	4.1
Entry 20	186.0, 125.2, 132.7	182.7, 127.1, 129	5.3

The average mean of error distance is 4.4 ± 1.5 mm

Table 15.2 The accuracy evaluation of total 16 target points of the piece of pork in 3 experiments

Points	The preoperative points (x, y, z)	After hitting nails (x, y, z)	Distance (mm)
Target 1	92.5, 130.8, 150.2	94.6, 130.9, 152.9	3.4
Target 2	101.8, 143.8, 221.9	107.9, 151.6, 219.5	10.1
Target 3	128.3, 127.0, 160.4	127.4, 125.1, 169.0	8.7
Target 4	153.3, 123.0, 204.4	154.2, 126.8, 201.8	4.7
Target 5	191.4, 127.2, 191.5	180.3, 122.8, 192.3	12.0
Target 6	209.3, 113.3, 200.0	203.1, 124.8, 195.4	13.8
Target 7	147.3, 162.8, 107.2	141.6, 170.5, 112	10.6
Target 8	184.2, 150.5, 131.6	182.4, 160.4, 129	10.4
Target 9	212.1, 138.6, 199.9	213.2, 142.8, 195	6.6
Target 10	241.8, 136.6, 203.2	231.6, 142.8, 195	14.5
Target 11	157.9, 144.0, 152.9	157.6, 148.5, 153.0	4.4
Target 12	73.6, 155.4, 145.6	78.5, 166.1, 142	12.2
Target 13	121.3, 150.8, 138.1	118.3, 158.5, 140	8.5
Target 14	146.0, 159.3, 116.7	147.2, 164.2, 120	5.9
Target 15	66.3, 171.3, 107.5	64.0, 172.7, 115	7.9
Target 16	119.3, 168.2, 100.7	123.4, 179.2, 97	12.3

The average mean of error distance is 9.1 ± 3.4 mm

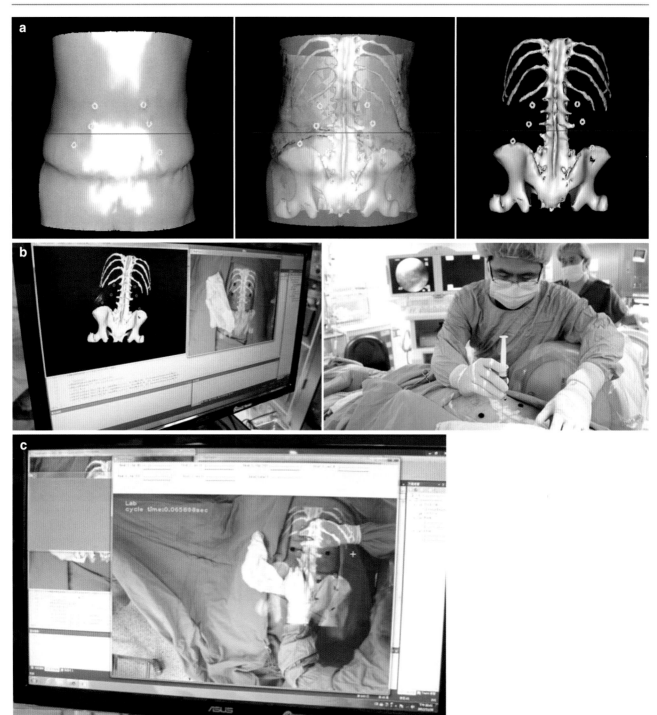

Fig. 15.12 The clinical testing of the spinal surgery by using the proposed ARCASS system. (**a**) The 3D visible images of the patient which are generated by the CT scans and the setup of the proposed ARCASS system in the operating room. (**b**) The screenshot of our intraoperative software of the first clinical experiment. (**c**) The surgeon used the projected information generated by the ARCASS system for a spinal surgery directly. (**d**) The camera view of the camera-projector system

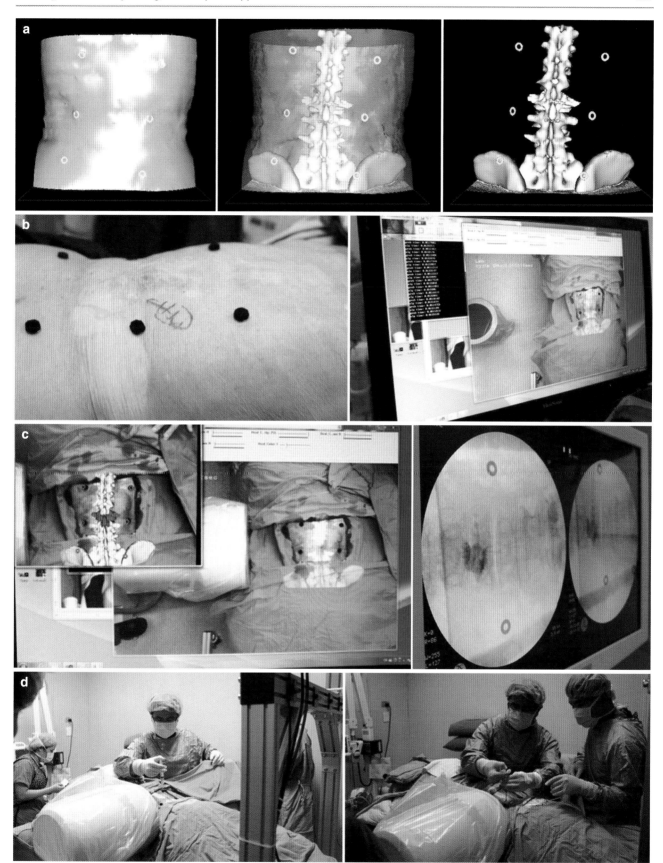

Fig. 15.13 The second clinical testing of the spinal surgery by using the proposed ARCASS system. (**a**) The 3D visible images of the patient which are generated by the visible patient tool. (**b**) The second patient experiment and the screenshot of our intraoperative software. (**c**) The screenshot of our intraoperative software and corresponding C-arm image of the second clinical experiment. (**d**) The surgeon used the projected information generated by the ARCASS system for a spinal surgery directly

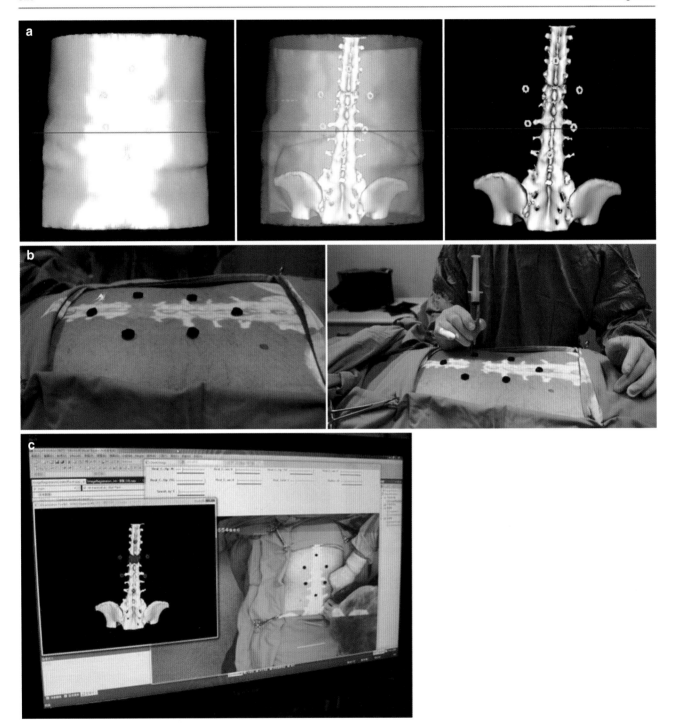

Fig. 15.14 The third clinical testing of the spinal surgery by using the proposed ARCASS system. (**a**) The 3D visible images of the patient which are generated by the visible patient tool. (**b**) The projected image and the surgeon used the projected information generated by the ARCASS system for a spinal surgery directly. (**c**) The screenshot of our intraoperative software and corresponding C-arm image of the second clinical experiment

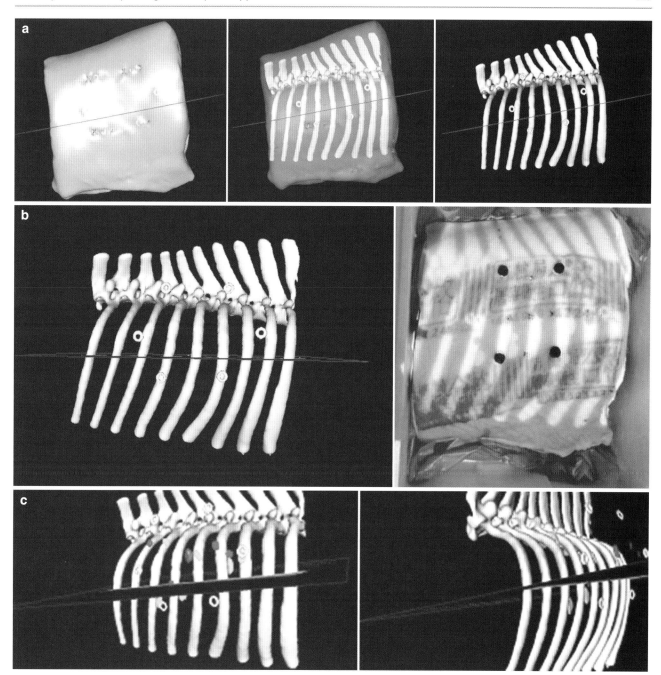

Fig. 15.15 The accuracy evaluation of the proposed ARCASS system. (**a**) The 3D visible images of the pork which are generated by the CT scans and visible patient tool. (**b**) The pork experiment is used to evaluate our accuracy. The circles with *yellow* color are the landmarks in the 3D model. (**c**) We first give a preoperative surgical plan which is to draw the entry (*red*) and target (*cyan*) points on the 3D model for hitting the nails. (**d**) We hit the nails with the hammer into the piece of pork (*left*) by using the preoperative entry and target points and its corresponding 3D model by using CT scan images (*right*)

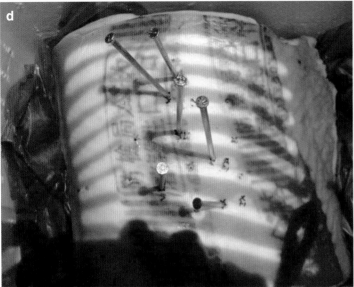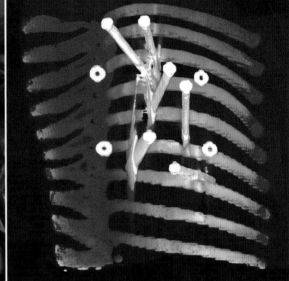

Fig. 15.15 (continued)

Acknowledgments The authors would like to thank Prof. Huei-Yung Lin for his useful discussion and Yeoulin Ho, Ramakanteswararao Beesetty, Stephane Nicolau, Ming-Hsien Hu, Jeng-Ren Wu, Kai-Che Liu, Luc Soler, and Pei-Yung Lee for their help of clinical trial and article writing. The work was supported by the National Science Council of Taiwan, R.O.C., under Grant NSC-101-2218-E-758-001- and NSC-100-2221-E-442-001 and is gratefully acknowledged.

References

1. Computer aided surgery definition from wikipedia. http://en.wikipedia.org/wiki/Computer-assisted_surgery.
2. Augmented reality. http://en.wikipedia.org/wiki/Augmented_reality.
3. Robotic surgery. http://en.wikipedia.org/wiki/Robotic_surgery.
4. Calhoun PS, Kuszyk BS, Heath DG, Carley JC, Fishman EK. Three-dimensional volume rendering of spiral ct data: Theory and method. Radiographics. 1999;19(3):745–64.
5. Osirix. http://www.osirix-viewer.com/AboutOsiriX.html.
6. Marescaux J, Rubino F, Arenas M, Mutter D, Soler L. Augmented-reality-assisted laparoscopic adrenalectomy. JAMA. 2004;292(18):2214–5.
7. Nicolau S, Garcia A, Pennec X, Soler L, Ayache N. An augmented reality system to guide radio- frequency tumour ablation. Comput Anim Virtual Worlds. 2005;16(1):1–10.
8. Bianchi G, Harders CWM, Cattin P, Székely G. Camera-marker alignment framework and comparison with hand-eye calibration for augmented reality applications. In: 2005. Proceedings. Fourth IEEE and ACM international symposium on mixed and augmented reality. IEEE; 2005. p. 188–9.
9. Feuerstein M, Mussack T, Heining SM, Navab N. Intraoperative laparoscope augmentation for port placement and resection planning in minimally invasive liver resection. IEEE Trans Med Imaging. 2008;27(3):355–69.
10. Paloc C, Carrasco E, Macia I, Gomez R, Barandiaran I, Jimenez JM, Rueda O, Ortiz de Urbina J, Valdivieso A, Sakas G. Computer-aided surgery based on auto-stereoscopic augmented reality. In: IV 2004. Proceedings. Eighth international conference on information visualisation. IEEE; 2004. p. 189–93.
11. Sauer F, Khamene A, Vogt S. An augmented reality navigation system with a single-camera tracker: system design and needle biopsy phantom trial. In: Medical image computing and computer-assisted intervention—MICCAI 2002. Berlin: Springer; 2002. p. 116–24.
12. Ferrari V, Megali G, Troia E, Pietrabissa A, Mosca F. A 3-d mixed-reality system for stereoscopic visualization of medical dataset. IEEE Trans Biomed Eng. 2009;56(11):2627–33.
13. Masamune K, Sato I, Liao H, Dohi T. Non-metal slice image overlay display system used inside the open type MRI. In: Medical imaging and augmented reality. Berlin: Springer; 2008. p. 385–92.
14. Birkfellner W, Figl M, Matula C, Hummel J, Hanel R, Imhof H, Wanschitz F, Wagner A, Watzinger F, Bergmann H. Computer-enhanced stereoscopic vision in a head-mounted operating binocular. Phys Med Biol. 2003;48(3):N49.
15. Birkfellner W, Figl M, Huber K, Watzinger F, Wanschitz F, Hummel J, Hanel R, Greimel W, Homolka P, Ewers R, et al. A head-mounted operating binocular for augmented reality visualization in medicine-design and initial evaluation. IEEE Trans Med Imaging. 2002;21(8):991–7.
16. Khan MF, Dogan S, Maataoui A, Gurung J, Schiemann M, Ackermann H, Wesarg S, Sakas G, Vogl TJ. Accuracy of biopsy needle navigation using the medarpa system—computed tomography reality superimposed on the site of intervention. Eur Radiol. 2005;15(11):2366–74.
17. Khan MF, Dogan S, Maataoui A, Wesarg S, Gurung J, Ackermann H, Schiemann M, Wimmer-Greinecker G, Vogl TJ. Navigation-based needle puncture of a cadaver using a hybrid tracking navigational system. Investig Radiol. 2006;41(10):713–20.
18. Liao H, Inomata T, Sakuma I, Dohi T. 3-D augmented reality for MRI-guided surgery using integral videography autostereoscopic image overlay. IEEE Trans Biomed Eng. 2010;57(6):1476–86.
19. Nicolau S, Soler L, Mutter D, Marescaux J. Augmented reality in laparoscopic surgical oncology. Surg Oncol. 2011;20(3):189–201.
20. Navab N, Traub J, Sielhorst T, Feuerstein M, Bichlmeier C. Action- and workflow-driven augmented reality for computer-aided medical procedures. IEEE Comput Graph Appl. 2007;27(5):10–4.
21. Fuchs H, Livingston M, Raskar R, Colucci D, Keller K, State A, Crawford J, Rademacher P, Drake S, Meyer A. Augmented reality visualization for laparoscopic surgery. In: Medical image computing and computer-assisted intervention. Berlin: Springer; 1998. p. 934–43.
22. Feuerstein M. Augmented reality in laparoscopic surgery. PhD thesis. 2007.
23. Salah Z, Preim B, Elolf E, Franke J, Rose G. Improved navigated spine surgery utilizing augmented reality visualization. In:

Bildverarbeitung für die Medizin 2011. Berlin: Springer; 2011. p. 319–23.

24. Schulze M. Interoperative guidance via medical augmented reality. Diploma thesis. 2007.

25. Marescaux J, Soler L, Rubino F. Augmented reality for surgery and interventional therapy. Oper Tech Gen Surg. 2005;7(4):182–7.

26. Kelly P, Kall B, Goerss S, Earnest F IV. Computer-assisted stereotaxic laser resection of intra-axial brain neoplasms. J Neurosurg. 1986;64(3):427–39.

27. Grimson W, Ettinger G, White S, Gleason P, Lozano-Pérez T, Wells W, Kikinis R. Evaluating and validating an automated registration system for enhanced reality visualization in surgery. In: Computer vision, virtual reality and robotics in medicine. Berlin: Springer; 1995. p. 1–12.

28. Edwards P, Hawkes D, Hill D, Jewell D, Spink R, Strong A, Gleeson M. Augmentation of reality using an operating microscope for otolaryngology and neurosurgical guidance. Comput Aided Surg. 1995;1(3):172–8.

29. Sauer F, Vogt S, Khamene A, Heining S, Euler E, Schneberger M, Zuerl K, Mutschler W. Augmented reality visualization for thoracoscopic spine surgery. In: Medical imaging. International Society for Optics and Photonics; 2006. p. 614106.

30. Glossop N, Wedlake C, Moore J, Peters T, Wang Z. Laser projection augmented reality system for computer assisted surgery. In: Medical image computing and computer-assisted intervention-MICCAI 2003. Berlin: Springer; 2003. p. 239–46.

31. Brodeur P, Dansereau J, De Guise J, Labelle H. A points-to-surfaces matching technique for the application of augmented reality during spine surgery. In: IEEE 17th annual conference on engineering in medicine and biology society, vol. 2. IEEE; 1995. p. 1197–8.

32. Nollert G, Hartkens T, Figel A, Bulitta C, Altenbeck F, Gerhard V. The hybrid operating room. 2011.

33. Van Breemen A, De Vries T. Design and implementation of a room thermostat using an agent-based approach. Control Eng Pract. 2001;9(3):233–48.

34. Nollert G, Wich S. Planning a cardiovascular hybrid operating room: the technical point of view. Heart Surg Forum. 2009;12:125–30.

35. Bailey J, et al. Ullmann's encyclopedia of industrial chemistry. New York: Wiley; 2001.

36. Park S, Park G. Active calibration of camera-projector systems based on planar homography. In: International conference on pattern recognition. IEEE; 2010. p. 320–3.

37. Kahrs L, Hoppe H, Eggers G, Raczkowsky J, Marmulla R, Worn H. Visualization of surgical 3d information with projector-based augmented reality. Stud Health Technol Inform. 2005;111:243–6.

38. Jaffray D, Kupelian P, Djemil T, Macklis RM. Review of image-guided radiation therapy. Expert Rev Anticancer Ther. 2007;7(1):89–103.

39. Peters TM, Cleary KR. Image-guided interventions: technology and applications. New York: Springer; 2008.

40. Romanelli P, Schweikard A, Schlaefer A, Adler J. Computer aided robotic radiosurgery. Comput Aided Surg. 2006;11(4):161–74.

41. Peters TM. Image-guidance for surgical procedures. Phys Med Biol. 2006;51(14):R505.

42. Mauro MA, Zollikofer CL. Image-guided interventions, vol. 1. Philadelphia: Saunders; 2008.

43. Mayberg MR, LaPresto E, Cunningham EJ. Image-guided endoscopy: description of technique and potential applications. Neurosurg Focus. 2005;19(1):1–5.

44. May GR. Image-guided interventions. Am J Roentgenol. 2010;194(3):W281.

45. DiMaio S, Kapur T, Cleary K, Aylward S, Kazanzides P, Vosburgh K, Ellis R, Duncan J, Farahani K, Lemke H, et al. Challenges in image-guided therapy system design. NeuroImage. 2007;37:S144–51.

46. Avanzo M, Romanelli P. Spinal radiosurgery: technology and clinical outcomes. Neurosurg Rev. 2009;32(1):1–13.

47. Markelj P, Tomaževiè D, Likar B, Pernuš F. A review of 3D/2D registration methods for image-guided interventions. Med Image Anal. 2012;16(3):642–61.

48. Rui W, Minglu L. An overview of medical image registration. In: Proceedings. Fifth international conference on computational intelligence and multimedia applications, 2003. ICCIMA 2003. IEEE; 2003. p. 385–90.

49. Fitzpatrick JM, Hill DL, Maurer CR Jr. Image registration. In: Handbook of medical imaging, vol. 2. Bellingham: SPIE; 2000. p. 447–513.

50. Wen P. Medical image registration based-on points, contour and curves. In: International conference on biomedical engineering and informatics, 2008. BMEI 2008, vol. 2. IEEE; 2008. p. 132–6.

51. Shamir RR, Freiman M, Joskowicz L, Spektor S, Shoshan Y. Surface-based facial scan registration in neuronavigation procedures: a clinical study. J Neurosurg. 2009;111(6):1201–6.

52. Lee J-D, Huang C-H, Wang S-T, Lin C-W, Lee S-T. Fast-micp for frameless image-guided surgery. Med Phys. 2010;37:4551.

53. Sugano N. Computer-assisted orthopaedic surgery and robotic surgery in total hip arthroplasty. Clin Orthop Surg. 2013;5:1–9.

54. Penney G, Barratt D, Chan C, Slomczykowski M, Carter T, Edwards P, Hawkes D. Cadaver validation of intensity-based ultrasound to ct registration. Med Image Anal. 2006; 10(3):385.

55. Micu R, Jakobs TF, Urschler M, Navab N. A new registration/visualization paradigm for CT-fluoroscopy guided RF liver ablation. In: Medical image computing and computer-assisted intervention–MICCAI 2006. Berlin: Springer; 2006. p. 882–90.

56. Birkfellner W, Figl M, Kettenbach J, Hummel J, Homolka P, Schernthaner R, Nau T, Bergmann H. Rigid 2D/3D slice-to-volume registration and its application on fluoroscopic CT images. Med Phys. 2007;34:246.

57. Frühwald L, Kettenbach J, Figl M, Hummel J, Bergmann H, Birkfellner W. A comparative study on manual and automatic slice-to-volume registration of ct images. Eur Radiol. 2009;19(11):2647–53.

58. Hummel J, Figl M, Bax M, Bergmann H, Birkfellner W. 2D/3D registration of endoscopic ultrasound to CT volume data. Phys Med Biol. 2008;53(16):4303.

59. Mori K, Deguchi D, Akiyama K, Kitasaka T, Maurer CR Jr, Suenaga Y, Takabatake H, Mori M, Natori H. Hybrid bronchoscope tracking using a magnetic tracking sensor and image registration. In: Medical image computing and computer-assisted intervention–MICCAI 2005. Berlin: Springer; 2005. p. 543–50.

60. Deligianni F, Chung AJ, Yang G-Z. Nonrigid 2-D/3-D registration for patient specific bronchoscopy simulation with statistical shape modeling: phantom validation. IEEE Trans Med Imaging. 2006;25(11):1462–71.

61. Burschka D, Li M, Ishii M, Taylor RH, Hager GD. Scale-invariant registration of monocular endoscopic images to CT-scans for sinus surgery. Med Image Anal. 2005;9(5):413–26.

62. Penney G, Varnavas A, Dastur N, Carrell T. An image-guided surgery system to aid endovascular treatment of complex aortic aneurysms: description and initial clinical experience. In: Information processing in computer-assisted interventions. Berlin: Springer; 2011. p. 13–24.

63. Russakoff DB, Rohlfing T, Adler JR Jr, Maurer CR Jr, et al. Acad Radiol. 2005;12(1):37–50.

64. Mersmann S, Müller M, Seitel A, Arnegger F, Tetzlaff R, Dinkel J, Baumhauer M, Schmied B, Meinzer H-P, Maier-Hein L. Time-of-flight camera technique for augmented reality in computer-assisted interventions. In: SPIE medical imaging. International Society for Optics and Photonics; 2011. p. 79642C.

65. Nicolau S, Goffin L, Soler L. A low cost and accurate guidance system for laparoscopic surgery: validation on an abdominal

phantom. In: Proceedings of the ACM symposium on virtual reality software and technology. New York: ACM; 2005. p. 124–133.

66. Scheuering M, Schenk A, Schneider A, Preim B, Greiner G. Intraoperative augmented reality for minimally invasive liver interventions. In: Medical imaging 2003. International Society for Optics and Photonics; 2003. p. 407–17.

67. Mourgues F, Vieville T, Falk V, Coste-Manière È. Interactive guidance by image overlay in robot assisted coronary artery bypass. In: Medical image computing and computer-assisted intervention-MICCAI 2003. Berlin: Springer; 2003. p. 173–81.

68. Coste-Manière È, Adhami L, Mourgues F, Bantiche O. Optimal planning of robotically assisted heart surgery: first results on the transfer precision in the operating room. Int J Rob Res. 2004;23(4-5):539–48.

69. Mårvik R, Langø T, Tangen G, Andersen J, Kaspersen J, Ystgaard B, Sjølie E, Fougner R, Fjøsne H, Hernes TN, et al. Surg Endosc. 2004;18(8):1242–8.

70. K. Konishi, M. Hashizume, M. Nakamoto, Y. Kakeji, I. Yoshino, A. Taketomi, Y. Sato, S. Tamura, and Y. Maehara, "Augmented Reality Navigation System for Endoscopic Surgery Based on Three-Dimensional Ultrasound and Computed Tomography: Application to 20 Clinical Cases," Int'l Congress Series, cARS 2005: Computer Assisted Radiology and Surgery. http://www.sciencedirect.com/science/article/B7581-4GFTP32-3N/2/fb6fb4fea-98d3ad4b823e59d3ae4b355, vol. 1281, pp. 537–542, 2005.

71. Feuerstein M, Reichl T, Vogel J, Traub J, Navab N. Magneto-optical tracking of flexible laparoscopic ultrasound: model-based online detection and correction of magnetic tracking errors. IEEE Trans Med Imaging. 2009;28(6):951–67.

72. Nakamoto M, Hirayama H, Sato Y, Konishi K, Kakeji Y, Hashizume M, Tamura S. Recovery of respiratory motion and deformation of the liver using laparoscopic freehand 3D ultrasound system. Med Image Anal. Amsterdam: Elsevier. 2007;11(5):429–42.

73. Hostettler A, George D, Rémond Y, Nicolau SA, Soler L, Marescaux J. Bulk modulus and volume variation measurement of the liver and the kidneys in vivo using abdominal kinetics during free breathing. Comput Methods Prog Biomed. 2010;100(2):149–57.

74. Soler L, Doignon C, Bano J, Nicolau S. Registration of preoperative liver model for laparoscopic surgery from intraoperative 3d acquisition. In: Medical image computing and computer-assisted intervention-MICCAI 2013. Berlin: Springer; 2013.

75. Carter T, Tanner C, Beechey-Newman N, Barratt D, Hawkes D. MR navigated breast surgery: method and initial clinical experience. In: Medical image computing and computer-assisted intervention–MICCAI 2008. Berlin: Springer; 2008. p. 356–63.

76. Rauth TP, Bao PQ, Galloway RL, Bieszczad J, Friets EM, Knaus DA, Kynor DB, Herline AJ. Laparoscopic surface scanning and subsurface targeting: implications for image-guided laparoscopic liver surgery. Surgery. 2007;142(2):207–14.

77. Malti A, Bartoli A, Collins T. Template-based conformal shape-from-motion-and-shading for laparoscopy. In: Information processing in computer-assisted interventions. Berlin: Springer; 2012. p. 1–10.

78. Maier-Hein L, Mountney P, Bartoli A, Elhawary H, Elson D, Groch A, Kolb A, Rodrigues M, Sorger J, Speidel S, et al. Optical techniques for 3d surface reconstruction in computer-assisted laparoscopic surgery. Med Image Anal. 2013;17:974.

79. Albitar I, Graebling P, Doignon C. Robust structured light coding for 3d reconstruction. In: IEEE 11th international conference on computer vision, 2007. ICCV 2007. IEEE; 2007. p. 1–6.

80. Maurice X, Graebling P, Doignon C. Real-time structured light patterns coding with subperfect submaps. In: SPIE photonics Europe. International Society for Optics and Photonics; 2010. p. 77240E.

81. Penne J, Höller K, Stürmer M, Schrauder T, Schneider A, Engelbrecht R, Feußner H, Schmauss B, Hornegger J. Time-of-flight 3-D endoscopy. In: Medical image computing and computer-assisted intervention–MICCAI 2009. Berlin: Springer; 2009. p. 467–74.

82. Stoyanov D, Scarzanella MV, Pratt P, Yang G-Z. Real-time stereo reconstruction in robotically assisted minimally invasive surgery. In: Medical image computing and computer-assisted intervention–MICCAI 2010. Berlin: Springer; 2010. p. 275–82.

83. Lo B, Chung AJ, Stoyanov D, Mylonas G, Yang G-Z. Real-time intra-operative 3d tissue deformation recovery. In: 5th IEEE international symposium on biomedical imaging: from nano to macro, 2008. ISBI 2008. IEEE; 2008. p. 1387–90.

84. Mountney P, Stoyanov D, Davison A, Yang G-Z. Simultaneous stereoscope localization and soft-tissue mapping for minimal invasive surgery. In: Medical image computing and computer-assisted intervention–MICCAI 2006. Berlin: Springer; 2006. p. 347–54.

85. Mountney P, Yang G-Z. Motion compensated slam for image guided surgery. In: Medical image computing and computer-assisted intervention–MICCAI 2010. Berlin: Springer; 2010. p. 496–504.

86. Röhl S, Bodenstedt S, Suwelack S, Kenngott H, Müller-Stich BP, Dillmann R, Speidel S. Dense GPU-enhanced surface reconstruction from stereo endoscopic images for intraoperative registration. Med Phys. 2012;39:1632.

87. Hu M, Penney GP, Rueckert D, Edwards PJ, Bello F, Casula R, Figl M, Hawkes DJ. Non-rigid reconstruction of the beating heart surface for minimally invasive cardiac surgery. In: Medical image computing and computer-assisted intervention–MICCAI 2009. Berlin: Springer; 2009. p. 34–42.

88. Hu M, Penney G, Figl M, Edwards P, Bello F, Casula R, Rueckert D, Hawkes D. Reconstruction of a 3D surface from video that is robust to missing data and outliers: application to minimally invasive surgery using stereo and mono endoscopes. Med Image Anal. 2012;16(3):597–611.

89. Collins T, Compte B, Bartoli A. Deformable shape-from-motion in laparoscopy using a rigid sliding window. In: Medical image understanding and analysis conference. 2011.

90. Herrera SEM, Malti A, Morel O, Bartoli A. Shape-from-polarization in laparoscopy. In: IEEE 10th international symposium on biomedical imaging (ISBI), 2013. IEEE; 2013.

91. Figl M, Rueckert D, Hawkes D, Casula R, Hu M, Pedro O, Zhang DP, Penney G, Bello F, Edwards P. Image guidance for robotic minimally invasive coronary artery bypass. Comput Med Imaging Graph. 2010;34(1):61–8.

92. Su L-M, Vagvolgyi BP, Agarwal R, Reiley CE, Taylor RH, Hager GD. Augmented reality during robot-assisted laparoscopic partial nephrectomy: toward real-time 3D-CT to stereoscopic video registration. Urology. 2009;73(4):896–900.

93. Kim J-H, Bartoli A, Collins T, Hartley R. Tracking by detection for interactive image augmentation in laparoscopy. In: Biomedical image registration. Berlin: Springer; 2012. p. 246–55.

94. IRCAD-France. The visible patient. http://visiblepatient.eu/links.html/.

95. IRCAD-France. Vr-med. http://www.ircad.fr/softwares/vr-render/Software.php/.

96. Tsai R. A versatile camera calibration technique for high-accuracy 3D machine vision metrology using off-the-shelf tv cameras and lenses. IEEE J Robot Autom. 1987;3(4):323–44.

97. D. Ghimire and J. Lee. A lighting insensitive face detection method on color images. In: 2012 spring congress on engineering and technology (S-CET). IEEE; 2012. p. 1–4.

98. Wang M-L, Wu H-S, He C-H, Huang W-T, Lin H-Y. Geometric constraints for robot navigation using omnidirectional camera. In: IEEE international conference on systems, man, and cybernetics (SMC). IEEE; 2012. p. 1724–9.

99. Geiger A, Lenz P, Urtasun R. Are we ready for autonomous driving? the KITTI vision benchmark suite. In: 2012 IEEE conference on computer vision and pattern recognition (CVPR), June 2012. IEEE; 2012.

100. Hartley R, Zisserman A, Ebrary I. Multiple view geometry in computer vision, vol. 2. New York: Cambridge University Press; 2003.

Hong Gao, Sang Hongxun, Cheng Bin, Wu Zixiang,
Fan Yong, Weihua Xu, Shuhua Yang, Ruoyu Wang,
Chen Yanxi, and Zhang Kun

1 Overview of Computer-Assisted Orthopedic Surgery (CAOS)

1.1 The History of Navigation Technology

1.1.1 The Early Stage of Navigation Technology

Surgical navigation technology was originally applied in some experiment research for small animals by Horsley and Clarke in 1907. With aid of some mechanical devices and anatomic landmarks, this technology was used to determine the surgical object inside the body. Due to poor precision, it was inappropriate for the human operation. With the discovery of X-ray images and rapid applications in medical field, X-ray fluoroscopy could provide doctors a lot of useful information, such as bone structures of the patient and locations of the surgical instruments within body, and the information was displayed and observed on the screen in real time. Mosher accurately inserted a probe into the frontal sinus with the help of X-ray photographic techniques in 1912. Cushing introduced some experiences of using the X-ray photographic techniques to locate sphenoid sinus and sella turcica during the operation of pituitary adenoma in 1914. Spiegel and

Wycis adopted "pneumoencephalography" to position spatially soft-tissue markers in 1947, and this new navigation technology was first applied to the human soft tissue [1]. Since then, Leksell, Riechert, and Talairach also respectively developed their own positioning systems based on the projection imaging techniques. During the 1950s and 1960s, navigation technology was extensively used for thalamotomy. However, the navigation systems in the period were still based on graphic images. Because of slow development of the imaging and the X-ray radiography technology, early framework navigation technologies had some inherent drawbacks, not only highly inaccurate but also quite traumatic in the aspect of positioning. In addition, the small visual field, a certain degree of geometric distortions of X-ray images, and long-term accumulations of radioactive radiation to damage surgeon also affected significantly the clinical application of this technology. Therefore, framework navigation surgery developed quite slowly for a long time.

1.1.2 The Later Stage of Navigation Technology

In the early 1970s, computer technology had rapidly developed and then applied in the medical field. Computed tomography (CT) scans could clearly show the anatomical structure of the human body, which raised the image-guided surgery (IGS). With the application of magnetic resonance imaging (MRI), it could further provide more clear view of anatomical structure. However, these sans from early CT and MRI could only provide two-dimensional (2-D) image information, and it was frequently necessary to reconstruct three-dimensional (3-D) images of anatomical structure in the mind of the surgeons based upon these 2-D data in order to make operation plans. With the rapid development of the computer, the radio, the signal, and other related disciplines, image-guided surgical techniques gained significant improvement, formed a truly interactive surgical planning and navigation tools, and contributed to the emergence of a

H. Gao (✉) · S. Hongxun · C. Yanxi · Z. Kun
Department of Orthopaedic Trauma, East Hospital,
Tongji University School of Medicine, Shanghai, China

C. Bin
The Fourth Military Medical University, Xi'an, China

W. Zixiang
Department of Orthopaedics, Xijing Hospital, The Air Force
Medical University, Xi An, China

F. Yong
Department of Orthopedics, Kunming General Hospital of
Chengdu Military Area Command, Kunming, China

W. Xu · S. Yang · R. Wang
Wuhan Union Hospital, Huazhong University of Science and
Technology, Wuhan, China

© Springer Nature B.V. and People's Medical Publishing House 2018
G. Pei (ed.), *Digital Orthopedics*, https://doi.org/10.1007/978-94-024-1076-1_16

new computer navigation system based on frameless stereo-tactic technique with more flexible use, more convenient manipulation, more accurate guide, and more extensive application, thus provided interactive 3-D images with which a certain operation could be carried out more excellently.

The emergence and development of CT technology has promoted improvements of navigation system, especially in the field of 3-D spatial orientation. Between 1986 and 1987, Watanabe and Roberts successfully developed the first CT interactive neurosurgery navigation system simultaneously, with the former using a mechanical arm to track objects, while the latter using an ultrasonic locating method [2, 3]. In the 1990s, a positioning system with mechanical joint arms amenable to be controlled was invented. Although remote control of mechanical joint arms was not be disturbed by line of sight, clumsy bulk of the mechanical arms obviously added inconvenience to the operation. On the other hand, a stereo-specific infrared camera system based on the principles of ternary and binocular machine vision had increased position accuracy, but positioning was easy to be interfered for problem of line of sight, that is, an unobstructed view between the optical camera and the tracked objects at all times.

Ultrasonic image can clearly and real timely display soft tissue and vascular constructs. Because the ultrasonic imaging equipment is relatively cheap and easy to carry, minimally invasive interventional surgery under ultrasound guide is a more common surgery manner for some soft-tissue tumors. After local anesthesia, puncture needles through the skin can be accurately inserted into the tumor tissue with the guide of real-time ultrasound imaging, and further treatment will be subsequently carried out. It is a typical application for liver tumor thermal ablation, including microwave ablation therapy and radiofrequency ablation therapy. In addition, ultrasound images can also help surgeons find some breast lumps which cannot be recognized through clinically physical examination during the operation of breast tumor. In the field of neurosurgery, ultrasonic image can be used to position lesions in real time, monitor focal extent, and determine the scope of the resection, which has obvious advantages to improve operation effect. However, compared with X-ray fluoroscopy images or CT scans, ultrasonic images of bone tissue are inferior; therefore, its applications in the field of joint surgery and orthopedic trauma are distinctly curtailed.

Among different types of medical imaging, MRI can display optimally soft-tissue structure. However, the MRI images themselves have a certain degree of geometric distortion and gray level distortion. Geometric distortion of MRI images is mainly attributed to inhomogeneity of the magnetic field of the equipments, which will increase the guide errors of operation. With the further progress of technology, a new type of MRI device has significantly decreased geometric distortion and increased image accuracy, which makes it possible to become a navigation equipment. Currently, the intraoperative MRI image-guided surgery does not get extensive application,

mainly because this technology has special requirements to MRI equipment and magnetic field environment. Compared with ordinary MRI images, low magnetic field environment reduces MRI quality and resolution. At present the PoleStar system (Medtronic Company) is a typically intraoperative MRI-guided equipment and works in a low magnetic field environment. In this system, magnetic field-generating equipment is placed in the bottom of operation bed and, if needed, ascended to the appropriate position. However, Magnetom Espree system (Siemens Company) works in a high magnetic field environment. The design of this intraoperative imaging guidance system is similar to that of conventional MRI devices.

Since the 1990s, different navigation concepts and techniques have been developed, realized, and evaluated throughout the world. Some of them have proven to be successful, while others appeared to be dead ends and have consequently been abandoned. There is now a wide variety of different navigation concepts and philosophies implemented by system manufacturers in the form of navigation products as well as those being developed by research groups as prototypes or experimental devices. Recently, FRACAS (fracture computer-aided surgery) navigation system has been developed to guide interlocking screws into the distal holes of intramedullary nail. This system improves the accuracy of screw fixation, and positioning error is less than 0.5 mm.

With the development of a new generation of medical imaging, image analysis, robotics, motion analysis, virtual reality, computational modeling, etc., computer-assisted surgery (CAS) is more and more frequently used in operating rooms all over the world. The role of CAS is that, on the one hand, it can help doctors make accurate diagnosis for the disease and, on the other hand, can guide surgeons to perform quick and accurate operation procedures.

1.1.3 The Application of Various Kinds of Surgery

As its efficiency and accuracy, CAS can help doctors reduce operation time, decrease surgical trauma, increase accuracy of the operation, and improve success rate of operation; therefore, this new technique has rapidly developed and been applied in a lot of surgical fields, including orthopedics, neurosurgery, urological surgery, laparoscopic surgery, etc.

In 1986, Roberts first reported a new method using acoustic digitizer to track surgical instruments or a microscope and applied this computer navigation technology to clinical practice, which created a frameless stereotactic neurosurgery (neuronavigator). At the same time, German researchers began a series of studies of image navigation systems in the application of otolaryngology and head and neck surgery and developed the first generation of robot C-arm-type navigation system. However, the movement range of the mechanical arms was so very limited and bulky that they could not meet the demands of operations of these departments. Then, based on further studies to this system, a new kind of computer system of six-joint visual encoder was designed with the accuracy of 1–2 mm. In 1991, researchers from the same institution introduced a new kind of image navigation system using light induction-type coordinate positioning technology. The system sensor can track infrared light from infrared-emitting diodes installed on the surgical instruments and position spatial location of the instrument tip.

Since the 1990s, minimally invasive technology in the field of tumor treatment has developed rapidly. Under medical imaging (including preoperative image and intraoperative real-time image) guidance, the special puncture needles and catheters are inserted into tumor body through the skin to implement treatment of local lesions. This technology has opened up a new type of effective treatment for many previously incurable diseases, especially unsuitable for operation of liver, lung, breast, kidney, and soft-tissue malignant tumor, with some advantages of less trauma and faster recovery.

1.2 The History of CAOS

Over the past few decades, with the rapid development of medical imaging technology, such as CT, MRI, DSA, and single-photon emission computed tomography (SPECT), human 3-D anatomical information has been able to be compressed into 2-D images for diagnosing disease, positioning pathological lesions, and making operation plans, which improves the safety and quality of operation. Despite the presence of the imaging which has a positive role to the development of orthopedics, it cannot provide enough information to meet the needs of the orthopedic surgery. In recent years, with the development of computer graphics, image, and computer graphics processing speed, reconstruction technology from 2-D to 3-D images in combination with tracking technology of surgical instrument has been used to make orthopedic surgical plan and simulation and navigation, which is called as CAOS [4, 5]. CAOS can thus be defined as the application of computer-based technology to assist the surgeon implement the basic orthopedic principle (BOP) in the operating room. The BOP is defined as the placement of an object (guide wire, screw, tube, or scope) at a specific site within a region, via a trajectory which is planned from X-ray-based 2-D images or other imaging modalities and governed by 3-D anatomical constraints [6].

Compared with the traditional concept of surgery, CAOS is in great progress. By virtue of the virtual image of the local anatomy and operation manipulation, it can improve operation visibility and precision and has a great benefit to doctors and patients. It has the following advantages: simplify operation, decrease time of surgery and anesthesia, greatly reduce physical suffering, shorten in-hospital time, and make the patients return to society as soon as possible (to avoid the old bedridden patients, reduce medical costs, etc.). It is safer, more accurate, and convenient than traditional orthopedic surgery. Also, it can greatly reduce patients and medical workers suffering from X-ray radiation.

Robot-assisted surgery is another important part of CAOS. Since RoboDoc system was applied clinically in 1994, the development of robot-assisted orthopedic surgery has been slow. At first, due to the robot huge volume, complex design, high price, and other shortcomings, it makes initial robot-assisted surgery not only prolong operation time and increase intraoperative hemorrhage but also improve insignificantly the surgical curative effect compared with the traditional technology. Today, the miniaturization of robot system and the combination with the other navigation technologies make it become a new research hotspot again.

1.2.1 The Applications in Subprofessional Surgery of Orthopedics

Trauma Surgery

Compared to the artificial joint surgery, spine surgery, and the other orthopedic areas, the application of CAOS in orthopedic trauma is relatively less. This is because the core technology of CAOS is medical image post-processing technology. It is the most suitable for this image processing technology if preoperative and intraoperative medical images have not changed. However, the significant changes of fracture images before and after fracture reduction and the difficult corresponding (registration) of preoperative and intraoperative images make navigation technology in application of orthopedic trauma field relatively slow. In addition, the treatment of orthopedic trauma is often emergency surgery or requires surgery as soon as possible to be completed, but in CAOS, intraoperative system setup, image acquisition, and registration are time-consuming than traditional surgery. In recent years, due to the rapid development of image processing technology and the improvement of the navigation tracking methods, rapid changes are being made, and experience is being gathered across a range of traumatically orthopedic procedures. It has brought new opportunities for CAOS application in orthopedic trauma.

Currently, the clinical indications for CAOS in orthopedic trauma have percutaneous screw fixation (pelvic ring fracture, acetabular fracture, femoral neck fracture, scaphoid fracture, etc.), percutaneous or minimally invasive plating, insertion of the distal interlocking screw into intramedullary nail, fracture reduction, preoperative planning, and hardware removal [7, 8]. Many experimental studies and clinical results have showed some obvious advantages of percutaneous internal fixation treatment of pelvis and acetabulum fracture with fluoroscopy-based computerized navigation. With percutaneous iliosacral screw fixation for the treatment of pelvic ring injuries, 96% of screws inserted with fluoroscopy-based navigation were well placed as assessed by postoperative radiographs and CT scans, and the mean deviation from the intended path was 1.9 mm at a drilling depth of 100 mm [9, 10]. Using percutaneous insertion of 45 cannulated screws in 29 patients, including sacroiliac screws, pubic ramus screws, posterior column screws, and a supra-acetabular transverse screw, Mosheiff et al. reported that the wire tip deviation was less than 2 mm and the maximum trajectory difference was less than 5° [11]. The average fluoroscopy time of 28.4–45 s and average operation time of 24.6–40 min were superior to that of conventional fluoroscopy alone with a mean fluoroscopic time of 62–73 s and a mean operation time of 30–75 min [12–16].

Navigation technology can be applied to treat long bone fractures. At the aspects of operation time, incision size, fluoroscopy time, and screw position, the internal fixation of intertrochanteric fracture under the guide of navigation system has obvious advantages over traditional operation method. The distal interlocking screw fixation of the long bone nail has the success rate of 97%. In order to achieve optimal guide wire placement of femoral neck fracture, computer-assisted percutaneous placement of cannulated hip screw can effectively reduce the attempt number of guide wire, fluoroscopy time, and X-ray radiation.

Using virtual images stored in a navigation system, femoral fractures can be indirectly reduced in sagittal and coronal plane, and rotational malalignment can also be corrected. Hofstetter reported a new surgical navigation system based on fluoroscopy to guide intraoperative reduction of femoral fractures and antetorsion correction in 2000 [17]. Some experimental researches showed an average displacement error of 1.2 mm and rotation error of 1.9° in simple fracture and an average displacement error of 1.7 mm and rotation error of 2.5° in comminuted fracture, both within clinical acceptable range [18]. For certain comminuted fractures unable to determine angulation and rotation degree rely on big bone segment relationship or cortical thickness change, navigation technology is particularly helpful to guide femur fracture reduction, to restore the length of the limb, and to prevent rotation deformity. Therefore, some scholars think that, in some specialized trauma centers, navigation guidance for treatment of femoral fractures may be integrated into clinical routine [19].

As the application of 3-D C-arm fluoroscopy in clinical practice, it makes possible to gain intraoperative 3-D imaging of surgical object in operating room environment. Three-dimensional fluoroscopy-based computerized navigation system is derived from combination of 3-D C-arm fluoroscopy with 2-D navigation technology, with the maximum system error of 1.18 mm and average error of 0.47 mm [20]. This new navigation technology particularly contributes to treat within or near joint fractures (especially acetabulum) using closed reduction and percutaneous screw fixation technique. The gathered image from 3-D fluoroscopy navigation system is slice image, while summation image from 2-D navigation system. The exact intraosseous path can be determined in each slice image independent of the complexity of the osseous structures, but limitations are observed for the 2-D summation images; thus it is indispensable to obtain multiple 2-D images to build a quasi-3-D visualization [21, 22]. Because this is not a 3-D image in a real sense, 3-D fluoroscopy-based navigation has theoretically higher accuracy in periacetabular screw placement compared to 2-D fluoroscopy-based navigation. In a study by Briem et al. for posterior pelvic ring injuries, the authors recommended 3-D navigation as a feasible and safe technique for iliosacral screw placement due to an increased precision and reduced fluoroscopy and procedure time compared with 2-D fluoroscopic navigation [23]. However, no differences were observed by Smith et al. reporting a 75% rate of screw misplacement independent of the used navigation procedures [24].

In a 3-D fluoroscopy-based navigation system, when a cannulated drill guide sleeve with a tool tracker is moved along the surface of the bone, the real-time position of the guide sleeve is displayed continuously and updated simultaneously on sagittal, coronal, and axial slice images on a computer screen. By means of an extended virtual line from sleeve at different tomogram images, the complete osseous corridor of planned screw can be assessed. However, in the clinical practice, this advantage is limited to a certain degree. Using 3-D fluoroscopy navigation, image acquisition is hindered due to the limited scan volume of 12 cm × 12 cm × 12 cm, unable to determine the complete trajectory of the planned screw. A study found that 10% posterior column screws and 20% anterior column screw had perforations of bony cortices or the articular surface using 3-D fluoroscopy navigation, which was mainly attributed to be unaccustomed to the 3-D fluoroscopy images for surgeons [25]. It is very important to generate preoperatively characteristic templates for each osseous corridor for an optimized screw placement. Intraoperatively, a virtual movement through the 3-D data cube along the planned screw axis in perpendicular slice images facilitates the secure evaluation of the complete intraosseous path, thus increasing the accuracy of the screw placement.

Spinal Surgery

Nolte initially introduced application of navigation system for pedicle screw placement in an experiment research, with the goal of improving the accuracy of pedicle screw insertion [26–28]. Since then, many clinical applications of this technology have been reported. In a study of comparison of pedicle screw implantation of 64 cases using traditional fluoroscopy and computer-assisted technology, deviation rate was 44% and 9%, respectively [29–31]. With the use of navigation technology for pedicle screw placement, a large incision to expose the spine is not generally needed, which is especially good for the patient with significant change of local anatomical constructs from multiply operations. In such a patient, the location of the pedicle screw can be determined preoperatively through 3-D reconstruction image technology, and the direction, location, and depth of the pedicle screw can be controlled intraoperatively through navigation screen. In vitro experiments showed that the precision of depth control could be up to 1 mm. Considering its safety and accuracy, navigation technology has been applied in scoliosis, spondylolisthesis, and spinal fracture.

Currently, the most common navigation systems used in spinal surgery are CT-based and fluoroscopy-based surgical navigation systems. CT-based navigation systems use a preoperative spine CT scan to provide intraoperative navigational feedback. Distinguishable landmarks (3–6) are defined preoperatively on the spine, such as the facet joints of vertebra. Paired-point matching is addressed intraoperatively using image devices. After that, the pedicle screws are inserted under the navigation guidance. Because of high accuracy and security of screw placement, it can be applied in cervical and upper thoracic vertebra. In contrast to CT-based surgical navigation, the use of a C-arm fluoroscope enables navigation based on intraoperatively acquired images. No manual matching between the patient and their virtual representation is required. Since the image data that is used by the CAOS system is generated during the intervention, the preoperative preparation time can be shortened. However, the drawback is unable to get 3-D reconstruction images, so it is mainly used for lumbar and lower thoracic vertebra. In recent years, with the emergence of 3-D fluoroscopy navigation system, it can also be applied in thoracic and cervical spine.

Although navigation technology is firstly applied in spine surgery, the more extensive application of navigation technology is in joint surgery. The key reason is cumbersome operation procedures and longer operation time. Recently, combining with the robot system to implement spine surgery, image navigation technology enhances itself advantages of high accuracy, visually preoperative simulation, and low fluoroscopy radiation. The typical product is SpineAssist system [32].

Joint Surgery

In 1993, image-free navigation was introduced into the surgical arena for knee joint operation. The first case of total knee arthroplasty (TKA) was carried out successfully under computer-assisted navigation guidance in 1997. Subsequently, this technology is widely used clinically.

Currently, image-free navigation technology is mainly applied to the placement of anterior cruciate ligament grafts and joint replacements in joint surgery. The key to anterior cruciate ligament reconstruction is determining accurately the location of bone tunnel in the distal femur and proximal tibia for ligament graft insertion. With the help of the navigation and image overlapping fusion technology, drilling bone holes can be achieved under intraoperative navigation. The tension of cruciate ligament graft can be adjusted through simulating kinematic knee joint.

Joint replacement includes hip and knee arthroplasty. The main problem of THA is to determine the prosthesis location and motion axis, which can be resolved using navigation technology. Compared with traditional technology, THA under navigation guidance has more accurate prosthesis placement and less dislocation.

The main factors affecting functional outcome of TKA include the location of the prosthesis, limb axis lines and length, soft-tissue balance, and joint mobility. The axis line error incidence of more than 3° is no less than 10% using the traditional method, while the position error is less than 1 mm and axis error less than 1° using navigation technology [33]. Compared with conventional surgery, navigation technology can obviously decrease axis line error and improve soft-tissue balance.

Because the virtual preoperative planning has been reported to have strong clinical relevance, the data stored in navigation system can be recommended as a useful educational tool. This is of great benefit to the young doctors also.

Bone Tumor Surgery

In tumor surgery, a differentiation of intact or infiltrated bony surface can be difficult but is necessary to define the resection line. CT-based navigation can use the information from the CT. With additional visualization, the resection line can be planned exactly and executed safely.

Using preoperative image information to reconstruct 3-D model and make plans, cervical vertebra giant cell tumor can be resected accurately under computer navigation intraoperatively. Navigation technology also is particularly helpful to position repeatedly lesions and to determine the boundary of surgical removal of the lesions. In contrast to other operation methods, such as CT-guided puncture and CT-guided radiofrequency ablation, the obvious advantage of navigation technique is able to determine the lesion's form and position atraumatically.

With the fusion of additional image modalities like MRI, CT-based navigation allows pelvic tumor resection with high precision. Preoperative CT scans are used to define the resection line, and the fusion of CT scans and MRI images can be used to determine the tumor boundary of the bone and soft tissue. For tumor resection, the reference points are defined within the operative area, and 15–20 points are acquired with the pointer to achieve surface matching. The matching procedure is easy to perform within the operative approach. After successful matching and verification, the navigated procedure can be started. Reports showed the tumor resection had been performed according to the preoperative planning with histologically safe resection areas [34, 35].

In addition, the computer navigation technology has overwhelming advantages over traditional methods in positioning bone and soft-tissue tumor and radiation therapy. It can make precise 3-D spatial radiotherapy plan for highly irregular tumor, provide appropriate treatment according to the actual tumor shape, distinguish clearly normal organs around the tumor, and determine the optimal projection angle and radiation field.

1.2.2 Robot-Assisted Surgery

In recent years, virtual surgery with surgical robot- and computer-aided surgery technology is becoming more and more popular among the scholars and research institutions. The purpose of the study is to utilize a variety of medical imaging data to build a simulation environment in the computer using virtual reality technology. With the help of the virtual information, the doctor can make surgical planning, operation exercises, surgery teaching, skills training, and postoperative rehabilitation.

The emergence of robot remote control system is a bridge of communication between the doctor and the robot and facilitates to solve the problem of the interaction of doctors and surgical robot. By means of the virtual system sound, image, and force sensing information, surgeons can observe the realistic human tissue structures, accurately determine the operation steps, control the appropriate operating force, and improve the quality of surgery in the process of operation by virtual reality technology. A lot of preoperative inspection information, through acquisition, integration, and processing, is manifested in a virtual surgery system, providing the most intuitive and comprehensive basis for doctors to diagnose. Using virtual surgical techniques can make preoperative surgical planning, optimizing the surgical programs. In addition, the virtual surgery system can be used as a surgeon trainer for the doctor's training, promote popularization and application of the new procedure, and improve the efficiency of modern medicine. Finally, because the virtual surgery is free of the restriction of the surgical equipment, virtual surgery and remote intervention technology will enable surgeons in the operating room to have real-time interactive consultation with remote experts; thus the expert skills are not restricted by space distance. As a result, the study of virtual surgery technology has become one of the hotspots worldwide.

As for surgical robot system, since PUMA560 system is used for CT-guided brain biopsy in 1985, it has been three decades of history. During this period, landmark systems mainly have PROBOT system for prostate surgery (1988), RoboDoc system (1992), AESOP (automated endoscopic system for optimal positioning) (1994), ZEUS, and da Vinci (2000). One of the most influential systems is da Vinci system.

Surgical robotic system is mainly composed of the console and multiple sets of mechanical arm. Console consists of computer system, operation manipulation monitor, robot control monitor, operating handle and input and output devices, etc. It can provide 3-D images in the operative field. At the same time, the system is equipped with force feedback device to back arm tip force to the operating lever. In addition, the built-in defibrillation function can filter out unconscious quiver manpower from surgeons by computer analysis. Compared with ordinary laparoscopic system, the mechanical arms of da Vinci system have an additional freedom degree to simulate the movement of the wrist, improving the operation flexibility. Meanwhile, the operating ends of the robot can enlarge proportionally surgeon's hand operation movement, and thus the robot system has higher stability and accuracy over hands. Despite the widespread application of the system, its application in orthopedics is still relatively limited. Because this system is master-slave surgical robot system designed for endoscopic system, the surgeon can carry out operation in robot system master end, and the surgical robot will complete the corresponding operation according to the surgeon's manipulation; thus, the system highlights its advantages in general surgery, hepatobiliary branch, urology, gynecology, and other department applications. However, it requires a lot of auxiliary imaging data to carry out an orthopedic operation, so da Vinci surgical robot system has not obviously advantage in orthopedics.

The typical representative of orthopedic surgery robot is RoboDoc system, mainly used to shape skeleton, orient, and implant prosthesis for joint replacement. It is an active system, which the robot with end effector holding the tool/implant positions and controls automatically the tool in accordance with the surgical plan. The system is equipped with a large database of joint surgery; can make preoperative plan, operation simulation, and evaluation according to preoperative individual data of the patients and joint surgery database; and perform automatically relevant surgical plans if intraoperative matching has been completed. Studies have shown that the operation effect supported by the RoboDoc system can achieve at least the level of traditional surgery, which does not require a long learning process and has advantages in preoperative planning [36]. However, at the same time, shortcomings of system failure and higher surgical complications hinder its wide clinical application [37]. CASPAR system (1997) is similar to that of RoboDoc system. The former can be used to process bone tunnel in cruciate ligament reconstruction and bone surface in TKA and THA. Clinical studies have shown that CASPAR system has obvious advantages over the traditional technology. Acrobot system (2001) is a semi-active robotic system, which the surgeon manipulates the end effector, but the robot only applies a constraining force that guides the surgeon to move the tool/implant as required by the plan and mainly used for TKA and minimally invasive single condyle knee replacement.

The fundamental reason of joint surgery robot enable to perform automatically surgical procedures according to the preoperative plan lies in the relative immobilization of the joint anatomic structures; thus establishing a complete database can solve thoroughly the problem of prosthesis positioning. However, it is not suitable to guide spinal operation according to the database of anatomical structure. This is the reason that joint surgical robot system like RoboDoc system cannot be applied in spine operations.

Currently, SpineAssist system (feasible pedicle screws surgery and the lamina articular process screw fixation surgery) is the only product enabling to be used in minimally invasive surgery of the spine and mainly provides accurate direction guidance of screw in the spinal fusion process. Although this system has higher precision of screw placement intraoperatively, its correction and registration time is very long, the positioning way of frame fixed to the patient also increases surgical trauma, and the working space of the system has certain degree limitation.

Modern surgical robot has binocular vision functions with at least six degrees of freedom. It can overcome some shortcomings of hand shake during operation, visual deviation, and fatigue, can clamp surgical instruments stably and lastingly, and can carry out surgical manipulation according to designed preoperative planning. More importantly, it can implement remote surgery by virtue of modern communication technology and network transmission means combining with navigation positioning system and remote sensing technique. At present, the binocular vision technology can ensure the robot has a pair of keen "eye"; tactile feedback and virtual reality technology can make the mechanical hand flexible like the surgeon's hands; precision machinery and automatic limit technology can guarantee the safety of operation. In the event of accidents, system can immediately get into the security program to terminate robot operation [38]. Developments in telecommunication will allow surgeons to communicate with colleagues and experts during the procedure virtually in any location around the world, which increases teaching possibilities and procedural safety. In 2001, using France telecom high-speed optical fiber digital network and asynchronous transfer mode (ATM), the surgeons in New York successfully performed laparoscopic gallbladder surgery by remotely controlling ZEUS in Strasbourg hospital operating room [39]. This is a milestone in remote surgery.

1.3   Problems and Prospect of Navigation Technology

Nowadays, the rapid development of the modern computer technology is not consistent with the traditional operating room setting and the technical level of the operation. Over 50 years, the main progress in orthopedic surgery is to introduce the X-ray fluoroscopy images into operating room, while the surgical technique has no significant changes. Because the bone is the main object in the process and a deformed tissue, orthopedic surgery is suitable for computer navigation by using preoperative and intraoperative fluoroscopy images. However, at the same time, the navigation technologies applied in orthopedic surgery have also produced many problems.

1.3.1   The Quality of Image and Type

Image quality is still one of the important limiting factors for fluoroscopy-based navigation. Although the resolution of the mobile X-ray device has great progresses, due to the limited unit volume and portability requirements of these devices in the operating room environment, image resolution and size are still relatively small.

If it is not able to gain high-quality image data from equipment limitations, navigation surgery, even for 2-D X-ray fluoroscopy navigation with low demand to image resolution, can't be performed. Image quality is still the limiting factor for fluoroscopy navigation. Iso-C 3-D offers the ability for axial and 2-D reconstructions, but image quality is clearly decreased compared to CT. In addition, a persistent problem of 3-D fluoroscopy navigation is the scan volume, only 12 cm × 12 cm × 12 cm. Although this scan volume is possible to be enough for the sacroiliac joint fixation, it can't meet the needs of fixing whole posterior pelvic ring. Big flat mobile fluoroscopy devices or navigation operating room equipped with fluoroscopy devices with high resolution and large volume is a possible direction to resolve this problem.

The image types also affect the implementation of the navigation surgery. Navigation systems may be categorized as fluoroscopy-based and CT-based navigation systems by imaging modalities [20]. The former includes 2-D- and 3-D fluoroscopy-based navigation system. Two-dimensional fluoroscopy-based navigation system can acquire intraoperatively real-time fluoroscopy image; provide feedback of local anatomical structures of operation site, surgical tools, and the C-arm fluoroscopy positions; and guide the manipulation of surgical tools. Three-dimensional fluoroscopy-based navigation technology is based on Iso-C 3-D arm (Siremobil®, Siemens Inc., Germany) and has been on the market since the beginning of 2003. First, a set of equally spaced 2-D fluoroscopy image is acquired. Then, a high-resolution 3-D image data set is reconstructed using a custom cone beam reconstruction algorithm. Finally, after calibration procedure, a set of accurate and reliable 3-D images are produced, automatically downloaded to the navigation computer and used to guide operation manipulation. However, its operative field is small, and image resolution is sometimes affected by the appearance of metallic implants. The first application of the CT-based technology was addressed at supporting the insertion of pedicle screws in the lumbar spine. Since then, this technology has been expended to other areas of the spinal column. This system requires preoperatively acquired CT scanning images with which surgical plans of different levels of complexity need to be performed. Then, these CT data are transferred to the workstation. After successful matching and verification, the navigated procedure can be started. The shortcomings of this navigation technology include the need of strict registration and reference to get high-resolution image, lack of image update in real time, and reduction of the navigation accuracy if having intraoperative registration errors.

1.3.2 The Working Process

Navigation systems rely on the interaction of multiple devices, including the tag in the surgical field, a few tracer sensors, a computer for data processing, and finally feedback to the surgeon after processing data. Although equipment manufacturers are very confident in their own tracking technology, positioning, and rotation accuracy, lack of unified standards makes the orthopedic surgeon unable to evaluate the pros and cons of different devices, and there are also certain difficulties to compare different clinical application results. In addition, the software and hardware of the CAOS is mostly developed by manufacturers of orthopedic surgical instruments, their products are usually designed for only one procedure and their software from this kind of closed system cannot fitted with different hardware from other orthopaedic implant companies. This is one important reason for the CAOS equipment to be expensive. Only to improve the level of light positioning technology, meanwhile, increasing the study of other positioning methods can improve the positioning accuracy. Using open architecture design, it makes software program of different navigation systems to be compatible with each other, and surgical instruments can be general, which can reduce the equipment cost [40, 41]. Wireless-type high-energy batteries can minimize the cable connection among intraoperative navigation equipments. Touch-sensitive screen man-machine interface operation, in accordance with the surgeon operating habits, can bring great convenience to operation manipulation.

Image quality, the accuracy of position markers, and changes of the tracer position all can interfere with navigation system to obtain accurate information, which affects the accuracy of the whole system. All of these factors are based on an inherent hypothesis through whole system workflows, that is, these factors are assumed to be in an optimal state at the time of image acquisition. Because this hypothesis is not verified automatically during the whole navigation procedure, errors may remain unnoticed and substantially impair the precision, particularly in the anatomically risk area [42].

Despite different navigation technologies, these navigation systems all use tracking system to locate the surgical instruments and the anatomic location of the surgical objects. Currently, two types of tracking technologies are available for medical application: optical and magnetic, with optical being by far the most commonly used tracking technology. Infrared light-emitting diode or reflective sphere is the most common marker. Some factors influence tracking accuracy in practice, such as blood covering the light-emitting diode or reflective sphere, surgical team accidentally blocking a direct line of sight between infrared camera and markers, and other strong light sources in the operating room environment.

In addition, it is very important to make a distinction between the virtual image displayed in CAOS in skeletal trauma procedures and a true view of the surgical site with an image intensifier. Because navigation system assumes that surgical instruments are inflexible, a perfect virtual position of a guide wire may be a false presentation of the real situation since the real guide wire may skip or bend and point to a wrong position during the insertion, without being detected or shown on the augmented image. A rigidly protective sleeve may contribute to preventing wire bending.

Intraoperatively, tool and bone tracking is achieved by rigidly attaching trackers to them with mounting hardware. It is important that the trackers should not move with respect to the attached tool or bone during surgery, since relative movement will increase system error. An undetected shift will result in inaccurate navigation images that might mislead the surgeon and lead to unwanted results and complications. Therefore, during the operation, in addition to the preset operation steps of the system software, an additional evaluation of surgical navigation accuracy, especially in some key steps, is very important in the early stages of the application of navigation technology; even a skilled navigation surgeon also needs to be fully aware of this point to avoid irreparable damage and consequences [42].

1.3.3 Preoperative Plan

Navigation is performed in a digital display model of the surgical field, which can display preoperative image data (CT or MRI) and intraoperative 2-D or 3-D fluoroscopy image. Bone imaging technology can completely change the preoperative plan of traditional orthopedic surgery. With the aid of computer navigation technology, preoperative planning can be made very intuitively and, specifically, used preoperatively to simulate operation manipulation and training. As a result, an additional plan can be made to aim to certain important operation details. A computer program has recently been developed to demonstrate virtually every step of pelvic and acetabular fracture operation procedures [43]. This program uses the preoperative CT data of the patients to build digital model of fracture site, then operation procedures are preoperatively designed by virtue of this model. A study showed that: in 26 cases of acetabular fractures, intraoperative operations are in complete accord with preoperative plan in 24 patients, intraoperative plate positions are in complete accord with preoperative plan in 14 patients, and intraoperative plate positions are in part accord with preoperative plan in 11 patients [44].

At present, the preoperative plan of navigation surgery mainly depends on combining of the patient preoperative imaging data and navigation software itself digital model. Based on the preoperative fusion of all kinds of medical images, it is convenient for displaying intraoperative image in real time. During image acquisition, important factors influencing the accuracy of the reconstruction image are image quality, resolution, and slice thickness. If CT and MRI scanning layer is too thick, bone signal strength will be low for soft tissue or air neutralization.

Some preliminary studies have been carried out to discuss how to place preoperatively navigation equipment more conveniently and more effectively and tried to establish a set of feasible navigation surgery workflow. Sufficient preoperative plan is made to facilitate the setup of navigation system in operating room in case of some inconvenient problems among surgical tool, camera, surgical bed, tracker, patient position, and the C-arm, such as the loss of line of sight.

1.3.4   Postoperative Testing and Assessment

In recent 20 years, intraoperative fluoroscopy and postoperative radiography have become the most common and important standard to detect and evaluate surgical effects during the operation. They include knowing the role of intraoperative diagnosis, displaying intraoperatively fracture reduction, determining surgical tools and drill position, and verifying implant placement. In CAOS, postoperatively routine use of radiography to evaluate position of internal fixation is less sensitive because its error is greater than that of CAOS itself.

1.3.5   Digital Modeling: The Clinical Application Through the Internet in the Future

Digital orthopedics is a new type of digital medical disciplines of digital computer technology integrated with clinical orthopedics closely on the basis of the bone with the auxiliary of computer image technology and also a cross discipline involving the human anatomy, 3-D geometry, biomechanics, materials science, informatics, electronics, and mechanical engineering fields. For now, the most important role of the digital modeling application in clinical orthopedics is to establish fracture model to improve the preoperative planning, guide the direction and depth of inserting screw intraoperatively, and measure limb axis to correct deformity.

With the acceleration development of computer navigation technology, the digital information is gradually enriching the whole process of orthopedic surgery. From preoperative imaging data, intraoperative bone and prosthesis positioning, and fracture reduction to postoperative evaluation (axis lines, angles, prosthesis position, etc.), all can be covered by digitalization. Such digitalization is not only the protection of information and storage but also extensive applications of computer navigation technology through the network in the future, including the use of digital imaging technology to remote control robot, the use of the Internet to public demonstrations of navigation operation, and education. It can eliminate the regional difference as much as possible and make more patients to get better medical resources (including experts in the field of academic, surgical tech-

nique, surgical equipment, etc.). All of these will make traditional orthopedic surgery faced with newer and bigger changes.

More powerful computers and software can automatically extract characteristic parameters or important geometric details from CT/MRI or virtual data to produce directly human bone and muscle tissue model through weight and simulation technology in the future. With the help of the computer, implants and prostheses can be designed individually using human-computer interaction technology. With the help of computer navigation, network, and surgical robot, remote operation can be carried out. Using automatic finite element technology, individual projections for stress distribution of implant can contribute to the selection of surgical procedures. With the development of navigation software module, the improvement of the image precision, and the progress of the navigation and positioning equipments, the computer navigation will play an increasingly important role in the orthopedic surgery.

2   Basic Working Theories and Application Principle of CAOS

The development of CAOS is based on the conversion and integration of many other advanced technologies, such as medical imaging, image processing and analysis, robotics, motion analysis, virtual reality, and computer simulation technology. Based on these technologies, different concepts and technologies of CAOS have been developed, implemented, and evaluated gradually for many years. With the development and improvement of related technology, every CAOS system will be constantly improved, while the basic principle of CAOS will become increasingly important. The basic principle of CAOS is to establish the association between the imaging and anatomical data by means of the registration process and to achieve accurate operation manipulation through the combination of the proprietary tools and surgical navigation images. Orthopedics doctors can make appropriate decisions targeting specific patients, hospitals, and surgeries, only if they know the goal, the scope of application, and limitations these systems can achieve.

2.1   Basic Theories and Application Principle

2.1.1   Navigation

Navigation technology is also known as a frameless stereotactic technology, using interactive image navigation form, to integrate the computer image processing and visualization technology with clinical surgery. Its working principle is establishing a series of tracking system with infrared light emitting and receiving device in the operating room and then using the camera which can recognize each of these optical signals to track the space position of the surgical site with the optical signal, surgery devices, and registered image; computer image processing workstation can digitally calculate spatial coordinates of each tracking target and store the data in the computer. Besides, computer can also put the virtual image and real surgical site to accurate overlaying and reflection, so that the surgeon can see the real-time position of surgical instruments and surgical site on the virtual images. According to the different operation procedures, the usage of corresponding operation software enables the surgeon to carry out accurate surgical manipulation according to the operation interface of the computer [20]. The surgeon's own clinical thinking will not combine with computer navigation interface very good until he or she has a correct understanding of the working theories.

Current clinical application of surgical navigation system can be divided into three major components:

- Surgical object (SO): It is the anatomical position of the operation. In orthopedics operation, the surgical object is limited to the bone, or bone fragments, and anatomical structure directly attached to the bone.
- Object virtual (VO): It is the virtual display of surgical object, according to which doctors can "really" plan and prepare the implementation of the surgical interventions and accurately implement the determined plan of operation without directly seeing the surgical site.
- Navigator (NAV): It is a device that can display the real-time position and orientation of the operating target and the end effector (end effector, EE) by establishing the coordinate system. The end effector usually refers to not only the passive operation devices but also semi-active or active equipment.

2.1.2 Registration

The aim of registration is to establish a relationship between surgical object and virtual object, so that the position of the object can be displayed on the virtual image. For plans created preoperatively, registration can be often point based where a number of fiducials are attached to the patient and then the position of these fiducials in the CT is registered by measuring the position of the fiducials on the patient on the operating table. This measurement is normally done using an optically tracked pointer. An alternative to the point to point registration technique is to use surface registration. Typically in this approach, one or more segmented surfaces from the volumetric CT images of the patient are intraoperatively matched with corresponding surfaces on the patient on the operating table. The latter surface information can be gathered by collecting a cloud of points using an optically tracked pointing probe or ultrasound [20, 45]. When using image

data acquired intraoperatively, through image transformation, registration is achieved automatically [45].

2.1.3 Tracing Technique

At present, the major tracking and locating methods used in clinic are optical positioning, acoustic positioning, electromagnetic positioning, and mechanical positioning. These methods have both advantages and disadvantages. According to the characteristics of orthopedics operation, optical positioning, especially infrared positioning technology, is the main tracking technology which CAOS has used.

- Optical positioning (infrared): It is currently the mainstream positioning method in the navigation system. The camera with 2–3 or more CCD receives infrared emitted (active) or reflexed (passive) by surgical instrument and then positions the instrument. Its advantages lie in high-accuracy positioning, up to 1 mm, flexible processing. But it is easy to be restricted by the infrared-receiving device and be obstructed by the object in the operation or influenced by the reflection of the surrounding light or metal objects. It can be divided into passive, active, and hybrid positioning system. Surgical instruments are installed with an infrared light-emitting tube. In the more advanced active positioning system, it can actively control the light with higher accuracy positioning, up to 0.1 mm.
- Electromagnetic positioning transmitter: It is used to generate the electromagnetic field, in which the electromagnetic induction signal is obtained by receiving sensor in the related position of the magnetic field, and then the signal can be converted into position and direction by the computer. The accuracy is high, generally 3 mm, which belongs to the noncontact positioning, and the system is simple and noninvasive. This positioning technique has obvious superiority in the catheter, endoscopic surgery, but it is less reliable in trauma surgery because of the distortion of the electromagnetic signal that may result from the complex operating room environment. It is very sensitive to metal objects in the work space, which is easy to affect the accuracy of positioning.
- Acoustic positioning: It mainly uses ultrasonic, applying at least three ultrasonic receivers and three acoustic emission units to get the space position information of at least six degrees of freedom. So the practical application needs at least three transmitters, sequential transmit, and the receiver is placed on the surgical instruments, receiving the acoustic signal of the transmitter in time. With the analysis of the time, space, location, signal intensity, and other data, the location information of the surgical instruments is then calculated and output. Its absolute accuracy is 2–4 mm, which can be influenced by temperature, noise, uneven air, and other disturbance.

- Mechanical positioning: It is the positioning device firstly used, which is composed of joints with angular sensor and rigid connecting rod. Sensor acquires the date of position and angle change, and the positioning is carried out by the mathematical model and computer processing. It is widely used in the operation of laparoscopic, oral, and department of neurosurgery. The advantage is that it is not easy to be blocked, and the surgical instruments can be placed in a specific position. However, the disadvantage is that it is clumsy, and the pressure exerted on the manipulator can change the data, and the positioning accuracy can reach 2–3 mm.

2.1.4   The Application of the Images

CAOS can be performed in different visual background based on the image source in combination with the navigation system. The most commonly used image sources in the fields of orthopedics and traumatology are CT, 2-D fluoroscopy, and 3-D fluoroscopy.

C-arm fluoroscopy is frequently used by trauma surgeons during percutaneous placement of screws in various trajectories around the pelvis, acetabulum, femur, etc. However, such imaging is generally available in only one plane at a time and exposes both the patient and the surgeon to radiation, particularly because of the increased soft-tissue mantle and the precise oblique projections necessary for adequate viewing.

CT is the first image modalities to be used for navigation surgery in the field of orthopedic, with relatively high-resolution images [27–29]. However, the preoperative CT images used for navigation cannot be altered after a closed reduction maneuver in the operating theater.

Over the past 20 years, there has been a significant evolution of imaging technology for the operating room. A mobile 3-D C-arm image intensifier has recently been developed that produces a comparable image quality and a CT-like 3-D image. The navigation system using this fluoroscopy image can allow the surgeon to update a virtual model of the patient in operating theater when intraoperative reduction or rearrangement of the patient's position is necessary. Using this unique imaging modality can help the surgeon assess some difficult area intraoperatively, such as the acetabulum and the posterior pelvic ring anatomy. The performance of the Iso-C 3-D system has been described with encouraging results. However, its main disadvantages are relatively inferior image quality and a limited image size of 12 cm × 12 cm × 12 cm, which may be sufficient for the sacroiliac joint but not for the entire posterior pelvic ring. Modification of the Iso-C 3-D has recently been introduced to offer superior image quality, increased field of view, higher spatial resolution, soft-tissue visibility, as well as eliminating the need to rotate around a fixed point.

MRI can provide high-quality images of soft tissue and clearly demonstrate the structure of the epiphyseal cartilage, ligaments, articular cartilage, and synovial membrane. It also improves the now universally used intraoperative navigation by real-time, interactive, near-real-time imaging, with frequent volumetric updates. The important limitations of MRI for procedural imaging are the presence of intense magnetic field and the presence of a large instrument usually surrounding the patient.

Ultrasound is nonionizing and is unique among other imaging modalities in that it depends not only on the various forms of electromagnetic radiation but on the vibration of physical media. Ultrasound is defined as acoustic waves. Modern clinical ultrasound systems use nonionizing energy while not requiring special environmental considerations. It can be used to implement pelvic surface registration.

2.2   Navigation Operation System Classification

CAOS system can be active or passive. Active navigation system can either perform surgical task or prohibit the surgeon from moving past a predefined zone. Passive navigation systems provide intraoperative information displayed on a monitor, but the surgeon is free to make any decisions he or she deems necessary. Based on the method of referencing image information, CAOS systems are further classified into CT based, fluoroscopy based, and image-free [8].

2.2.1   Image Guidance

CT-Based Surgical Navigation

The earliest navigation system clinically used in orthopedics is the operation navigation based on the CT, whose research began in the early 1990s [27, 29]. In concept, this kind of navigation system needs the preoperative CT scan image of the area of interest, so that it can carry out operation plan with different complexity. The CT scans are performed either pre- or intraoperatively with an O-arm and used to reconstruct 3-D images. Two working modes of guidance and real time can be chosen. In guidance mode, the operative steps and actions are planned preoperatively and are displayed on the monitor intraoperatively. The surgeons have to match the operative actions with the virtual ones. In real-time mode, the instruments and implants can be visualized and navigated as they are moved in the surgical field. This technique is mainly used to orientate prostheses, place pedicle screws, and correct fracture deformity and tumorectomy in the pelvic area. Basic operation procedures include preoperative data collection (usually thin layer CT); simulating surgical site, planning the operation, and selecting marks or anatomical landmarks for registration using 3-D images in the workstation (preoperative plan); intraoperative data collection; registration of surgical instruments and selected marker points to establish the space corresponding relationship of intraoperative images, surgical instruments, and surgical site (registration); and operation position in real time (navigation). CT-based navigation offers a precise representation of the surgical anatomy and allows for precise placements. However, the registration error may be ignored and lead to the reduction of navigation accuracy.

Two-Dimensional Fluoroscopy-Based Surgical Navigation

It is the most commonly used navigation system in the field of orthopedic trauma. Mobile fluoroscopy equipment (C-arm) has become a part of the standard configuration of operating room. They can provide real-time feedback on the location of bone and surgical instruments, whether by a constant or pulsed operation mode. Fluoroscopy-based navigation systems use several markers placed on specific anatomical landmark, which are captured by a small series of fluoroscopic images. A computer software program synthesizes these images to relate the surgical area of interest in space and identify the position of the instruments and implants. The main clinical indications are the placement of the sacral iliac screw, the percutaneous fixation of the pelvis and acetabulum fracture, the placement of pedicle screws, and the reduction of long bone fractures. Basic operating procedures include installing the C-arm tracking device and registering the surgical site, collecting intraoperative fluoroscopy images, and performing surgery under the guidance of its navigation. An advantage of this system is the virtual fluoroscopy, which allows surgeons to take arbitrary images intraoperatively and then choose the most appropriate position from the gallery of these images. In addition, 2-D fluoroscopy navigation can reduce radiation and improve the accuracy of operation.

Three-Dimensional Fluoroscopy-Based Surgical Navigation

In 1999, Siemens Medical Systems (Erlangen, Germany) presented the world's first mobile 3-D imaging equipment in C-arm operations, and later the official product was named Siremobil Iso-C 3-D. Through the improvement of the mechanical design, the deviation between the X-ray beam center and the rotation axis of the traditional C-arm machine is eliminated. In order to achieve 3-D imaging, a stepping motor is installed into the device to achieve the precise orbiting around the operation object with the total rotation angle of approximately 190°. This navigation system not only offers all of the benefits of virtual fluoroscopy but also permits virtualization in the axial plane, basically functioning as an intraoperative CT scanner. Using a computer software program, the 2-D images are converted into coronal, sagittal, and axial reconstruction, similar in appearance to CT images. Isocentric C-arm devices are able to produce 3-D CT-quality images. These devices can be combined with a computer

navigation unit to perform 3-D image-based navigation without the need for preoperative registration of the images. This system can automatically create the connection between the 3-D images and the operation object with the advantages of imaging in real time and automatic registration. Its major clinical indications include diagnostic or therapeutic drilling (such as tumor puncture) of osteochondritis dissecans, the placement of pedicle screw, and percutaneous screw fixation of pelvic ring and acetabulum fracture. The main drawbacks of this technique are relatively inferior image quality and a limited scan volume of 12 cm × 12 cm × 12 cm.

MRI-Based Surgical Navigation

Similar to preoperative CT, MRI can be obtained preoperatively and imported into the navigation system to position and navigate. The main clinical indications are the placement of the pedicle screws, the correction of the pelvis fracture deformity, and tumorectomy in the pelvic area. Its main advantage is that MRI, which has multirange imaging and good soft-tissue contrast degree, can show the structure of joints and muscles better and can clearly demonstrate the structure of the epiphyseal cartilage, ligaments, articular cartilage, and synovial membrane. The accuracy of navigation is mainly determined by the image quality of MRI; the higher the image quality, the higher the accuracy. Similarly, the registration error may decrease the navigation accuracy, so it still needs to be monitored in operation. At the same time, because MRI has special requirements of the operating room environment, inspection time and surgical instruments, using MRI to navigate in orthopedics operation has a certain degree of restriction.

Modality-Based Navigation

Modality-based navigation (MBN) means interactive tracking of instruments in a coordinate system defined by an imaging modality [46]. MBN relies on registration of the tracking system (an optical digitizer) with the imaging modality (CT, MRI, or a fluoroscopy). During the registration process, a transformation matrix between the two coordinate systems of digitizer and imaging modality is calculated. After this step, the tracking system knows where the images will be generated. This registration process is procedure-unrelated. As soon as the images have been acquired during an intervention, instruments with appropriate passive or active markers can be navigated immediately within the image volume without an intra-procedural registration. Navigation is performed on the basis of the CT data with the possibility of immediate CT control of the reduction and the navigation procedure as well, which is especially suitable for the treatment of percutaneous pelvic surgery. However, one has to take into account whether a special CT suite or an intervention operating room with CT is necessary for these procedures with some associated logistical problems.

2.2.2 Image-Free Guidance

For surgical procedures that can be fully exposed, image-free guidance navigation system can be used. That is, the dynamic reference coordinate system is installed on the undeformed anatomical structures near the surgical field, and the spatial location of the anatomical structures is determined by the spatial operation of the mark points. This kind of navigation system does not require preoperative or intraoperative radiological imaging, but the tracking system establishes the operating object virtual display of the characteristics parameters by determining the different anatomical structures and reference marks, which is also known as the CAS based on the anatomy defined by doctors. Image-free navigation systems consist of a computer platform, a tracking system (usually an optical camera), and a set of infrared markers. Depending on the planned operation, a predefined number of markers are positioned to specific anatomical bony landmarks using pointer probes with the method of triangulation. When needed, kinematics can also be used to determine the center of joint rotation. The referencing information is then processed by the computer software, which uses a large number of stored CT scans to construct a model that fits the registered surface points. The application of image-free-guided navigation in anterior cruciate ligament reconstruction and TKA has been a great success [47–50]. It mainly results from the relatively simple operation and work process with related advanced equipment. Recently, image-free guidance navigation technology has been applied in other knee and hip surgery, such as high tibial osteotomy and THA. The characteristics of these operations are minimally invasive, which leads to the difficulties in accurately getting all the anatomical landmarks using the concepts of anatomy defined by doctors. Therefore, image-free navigation relies mainly on surgeons' precision, experience, ability, and learning curve to mark the optimal anatomical bony landmarks for the application of the pointer probes. Its main advantage is the complete avoidance of radiation for the patient and surgeon.

2.2.3 Combined Application

The image-free navigation system is not able to provide anatomical details on the operation object. When the joints are severely deformed, it will be difficult to use an image-free navigation system to guide the operation. In this case, the navigation system using the image which can reflect the details of the joint anatomy is more advantageous to the operation, so the new navigation system combining both of them can determine which navigation operation to choose based on the amount of anatomical information. Combining the image-free navigation system with the surgical navigation systems based on 2-D and 3-D images enables to calculate the anterior pelvic plane by determining the pubic tubercle position in THA and identify lower extremity mechanical axis by skin digital anatomic landmarks in high tibial osteotomy.

Multimodal imaging is a method of augmenting guidance by combining different modalities into a single image. The goal is to provide the surgeon with complementary information about the anatomy that will serve to improve navigation selection. Examples of this type of image guidance include CT or MRI image overlay on the operative field for tumor surgery. In the surgical resection of bone tumors, the navigation operation combining MRI images and CT images will be more accurate to guide surgeons to determine the tumor boundaries in the soft tissue and bone and to remove completely the tumor tissue on the premise of retaining the normal tissue as far as possible [51].

3 The Components of CAOS System and Its Key Points in Application

3.1 The Components and Basic Equipment of CAOS

Normally, seven major components are involved in the clinical application of surgical navigation:

(1) The image processing computer unit, matching the virtual images with real images through calculation.
(2) Camera with receivers of optical as well as electrical signals, which can trace all kinds of trackers emitting or reflecting light or electrical signals.
(3) Patient tracker (reference array), which is a signal transmitter installed usually near the operative region and can be seen as the origin of system relative to which the positions in space are calculated.
(4) Tool tracker, which is mounted on the surgical instruments and helpful to track the spatial location of surgical instruments.
(5) C-arm, CT, MRI, or other devices acquiring image data in the operating room environment. C-arm of them is equipped with phantom and connected with a computer.
(6) Monitor, showing the location of the patients and surgical instruments.
(7) Tools with the navigation function, such as registration and calibration device.

3.1.1 Image Acquisition and Selection

The way of image acquisition can be classified as three different types. The first type is called preoperative imaging which is obtained preoperatively, such as CT and MRI images. It can provide anatomical shape of bones. The second type is called intraoperative image which is gathered directly from the navigated C-arm intensifier in the operating room. These image data can be automatically uploaded to the navigation computer to guide surgical procedures. The third type is called the non-perspective image, that is, the image simulated by software, which allows simultaneous representation of the surgeon-defined anatomy.

3.1.2 Hardware

The hardware is similar in most systems. The computer receives information from an infrared camera array. The camera emits infrared flashes which are reflected by passive marker spheres or communicated interactively with active markers. These markers are attached to the object that is to be navigated. This could be a bone fragment or a surgical tool. The position of the infrared camera is triangulated with both the infrared-emitting frame attached to the C-arm and the reference array at the surgical site. Through this triangulation, images from the surgical site are directly transferred to and processed in the computer unit, along with the precise location of the imaged structures in space. The images are displayed on the monitor. Tool trackers are attached to the surgical instruments. The infrared signals from tool tracker are received by the camera and are sent to the computer unit. The computer integrates the virtual images of the tracked surgical instruments into the image of the surgical site and provides a visual image of tracked objects relative to one another. This enables the surgeon to perform a navigation procedure in which a tracked instrument is manipulated in the actual surgical field while its image is simultaneously illustrated on the previously taken images of the surgical site.

3.1.3 Software

The software can rebuild the virtual operation model, save the image data, and filter and analyze the data, which further guides the operation process. For generally different operations such as TKA, THA, pedicular screw fixation, etc., completely different software programs are required. Sometimes an operation process could need several software packages, and different implants need to match with different software. In addition, the software is not compatible with each other between the manufacturers. Presently, there are two main product groups: closed system and open system. Closed system is composed of both hardware and software designed for only one procedure, and open system is designed such that common hardware may be fitted with different software, each of which is suitable for a different surgical procedure. The latter tends to have less impressive graphics but is simpler and more versatile in use.

3.1.4 Tools and Instruments

- Anchoring pins are used to fix the tracker in the bone.
- Universal tool/patient tracker.
- Surgical instruments.
- Adapter is used to attach the tool tracker to the surgical instrument.

- Calibration is used to register and calibrate surgical tools.
- Phantom can concentrate X-ray and calibrate the C-arm fluoroscopy images.

3.2 Key Points in the Computer-Assisted Orthopedic Surgery

The goal of navigation is to provide precise, real-time visual feedback about the spatial location of surgical instruments and anatomical structures that cannot be directly observed. Navigation requires tracking, registration, visualization, and validation. Tracking determines in real time the location of moving objects in space. Registration establishes a common reference frame between the moving objects and the images. Visualization creates navigation images showing the location of moving objects with respect to the anatomy at the orthopedic treatment site. Validation ensures that the navigation images match the true anatomical reality. Therefore, CAOS has the following characteristics.

3.2.1 Visibility

During a navigation operation, placing an implant in the correct position relative to the surgical site is generally achieved by the surgeon manipulating visually in the true reality of the situation. In CAOS, this manipulating at the treatment site is often via a virtual view that has been reconstructed by a computer where the view is close enough to reality. After image data are collected and stored in the navigator preoperatively and intraoperatively, navigation system can merge the preoperative and intraoperative images with the tools and bone location information to create navigation images. For fluoroscopy-based navigation, up to four fluoroscopy projections can be displaced simultaneously on the navigation screen. These images can show the tool movement with respect to the surgical site and update automatically. Therefore, the whole operation process can be performed under the guidance of the navigation image, that is, operating visualization.

3.2.2 Accuracy

The accuracy of CAOS system is determined in part by the quality of the information which is entered so that the quality of the image, the accuracy of localization of landmarks, and the stability of array all play an important part. At the same time, the accuracy will also be analyzed and evaluated by CAOS system. The latest software will reduce random error and system error to a great extent. Using surgical tools and placing implants are performed under the guidance of navigation so that the acceptable rate of the first pass of the guide wire and the accuracy of implant placement are improved greatly [15, 16]. As a result, the screw penetration into the joints and the unacceptable position of implants can be avoided. For a navigation system, the accuracy of the system should be at most 1 mm when the target is a single point, and when targeting a straight line trajectory or cutting plane, the error should be at most 1° [6]. There are many aspects at the interface between the patient, the surgeon, and the CAOS system that can affect accuracy of the clinical outcome. Therefore, the accuracy of the navigation system and the accuracy of the surgical results may not be consistent. A surgeon must have a good understanding of such issues and be ever vigilant of accuracy issues during surgery.

3.2.3 Repeatability

For navigation operation, if the position of guide wire or screw implant is not desirable, the second attempt of insertion of the implant still can be performed under the guidance of the same images and does not need another fluoroscopy for replacing the implant, which will ensure the manipulation repeatable if these images are acquired properly. Because the nonoperator accuracy for CAOS is generally precise with a standard deviation of 1 mm for position and a standard deviation of 1° for direction, the system error itself is very low [6]. This enables surgeons to place cannulated screw or implant a knee or hip prosthesis with high repeatability. Also, validation is an integral part of the surgical protocol for navigation. It is performed both before the surgery begins and at key points during surgery. System validation can guarantee further that accuracy performance of navigation operation is repeatable and reproducible. However, in CAOS, the operator error is a very significant factor that affects the overall accuracy of the surgery, and it is therefore important to minimize inter- and intra-operator error in order to make a repeatable activity of requisite precision.

3.2.4 Reliability

Due to the whole operation performed under the navigation guide, the success rate of operation can be greatly improved. Because images acquired intraoperatively can reflect faithfully the surgical site, the virtual guidance is generally reliable. However, it should be kept in mind that navigation image inaccuracy cannot automatically be detected. It is necessary to perform validation tests in some key steps during the operation.

3.2.5 Flexibility and Adaptability

CAOS is a minimally invasive surgery. When combined with the surgeries of other organs or the internal fixation of other fractures at the same time, CAOS can reduce secondary damage caused by excessive position changing and extensive incising. After using the navigation system, multiple fracture operation can be finished in the same body position, so that patients generally do not need to change position intraoperatively.

In the majority of the CAOS systems, the elements of the work flow specific for an image-guided operation are as fol-

lows: patient data acquisition, creation of surgical plan, intraoperative registration of this plan with the patient, and navigation of surgical tool/implant to implement the surgical plan. The key points of every step of navigation operation are described as follows.

- The setting of navigation system, including the placement of the C-arm, the aiming direction of trackers, and the location of navigation unit, should be preoperatively planned in order to avoid the blocking of navigation unit intraoperatively. Because an unobstructed view between the optical camera and the trackers at all times is the basic requirement of optical navigation, it is important to take preoperatively into account the positioning of the different navigation system components in the operating room in order to avoid loss of line of sight.
- The reference array is attached and maintained rigidly on the skeleton near the surgical site throughout the surgery to avoid shifting. Then the reference array is activated.
- Assemble tool tracker and calibrate it after activating. The calibration of surgical tools depends on the requirements of different operations. Calibration is usually done through calibrator with the ability to calibrate effectively various types of operation tools. Tool decalibration can be caused by tool wear and tear, such as tip bending, frame deformation due to repeated sterilization, or tool tracker shift. To avoid these situations, the surgeon should verify tool calibration before surgery, at key points during the surgery, and when in doubt.
- Install the phantom to the C-arm intensifier and activate it. The image acquired by the C-arm intensifier will be automatically uploaded into the navigation unit and processed distortion correction. Then these images will be stored into the navigation system and transferred into different image forms to be used. Images acquired for CAOS should be of high resolution and quality, sufficient to serve as the basis for intraoperative planning and execution.
- After activating all the equipments, adjust the infrared camera to track all these equipments. System can integrate them on the navigation images. Perform the operation under the guidance of navigation images.

3.3 The Advantages and Disadvantages of CAOS

3.3.1 Advantages

In spinal surgery, accurate positioning of the implants is a necessary element for operation success. Sometimes, it is hard to avoid some deviation even for some experienced doctors in performing this operation. However, an unobvious error is the possibility to do harm to important organs.

In order to avoid mistakes during operation and increase the success rate of operation, spinal surgery navigation system can be adopted to help the surgeon to know clearly the current operating status and the specific position of the implant. In the application of pedicle screw, navigation system can guarantee the accuracy of screw placement so as to avoid the complications related to the operation and reduce radiation damage and has some capacity to deal with anatomical variants, such as scoliosis, spinal congenital malformation, lateral curvature, and severe spinal degeneration [52, 53]. When comparing results between conventional and computer-assisted pedicle screw installation in the thoracic, lumbar, and sacral spine, Amiot et al. showed less neurological deficits and better alignment with image-guided surgery [54].

Traditionally radical tumor resection of pelvic malignant tumor requires extensive exposure, which may be complicated by infection, blood loss, wound healing problems, and nerve damage. Because most of these patients also have experienced other operations, radiotherapy and chemotherapy, as well as mutation and ambiguity of topography, the risks of surgical manipulation and the misjudgment of the tumor boundary may obviously increase. This means that the tumor sites have a high tendency for local recurrence and the surgery in itself can be very incapacitating for a patient especially when the malignant tumor invades adjacent structures [55]. Navigation based on the preoperative CT or MRI images can show the degree of the tumor invasion in the pelvis and the surrounding soft tissue well; thus, the tumor can be precisely resected along the boundary of the tumor, without extensive surgical exposure [51].

Intraoperative imaging with C-arm fluoroscopy is routinely used to assess fracture reduction and implant placement. Thus, standard trauma practice involves increased exposure of the surgeon and patient to ionizing radiation. For a fluoroscopy-based navigation, as up to four fluoroscopic projections can be displayed simultaneously on the navigation screen, no intraoperative reorientation of fluoroscope is needed so as to save fluoroscopic radiation exposure and reduce operation time. It can offer the advantage of the 3-D visualization of the drilling procedure and thus improve the precision of the procedure. This enables the surgeon to avoid neurovascular injury and the implant intra-articular penetration. Further, the patient who sustains a severe fracture, such as acetabular fracture, may have other associated injuries that require early assessment and simultaneous management. Multiple changes of patient's position and extensive surgical procedure of acetabular fracture and associated injuries can aggravate the adverse impact on a multiply injured patient who is at risk for multiple organ failure. Virtual fluoroscopic navigation provides potentially some advantages in a multiply injured patient over traditional surgical methods. The change of patient intraoperative position generally is unnec-

essary to percutaneous screw fixation of acetabular fractures, whether anterior column or posterior column fractures, with fluoroscopy-based computerized navigation. This technique may allow surgeons to manage other associated injuries and perform other surgical procedures simultaneously so as to reduce the whole operation time and improve functional recovery [15, 16].

Restoration of the axis line of lower limb is a key point in lower limb orthopedics surgery, such as high tibial osteotomy, knee arthroplasty, and ankle arthrodesis. It is a guarantee for high-quality surgery to understand accurately and dynamically the axis line of the lower limb. With the aid of computer navigation technology, the surgeon can intraoperatively observe the changes of the axis lines of the lower limb before and after osteotomy and make a relevant adjustment, which can contribute to placing accurately joint prostheses as well as controlling the correct angle and plane of osteotomy.

CAOS also benefits the education and training of clinicians. The educational potential of operating virtually by the use of 3-D CT-based preoperative planning software, particularly for pelvic and acetabular cases, may be beneficial for younger and less experienced surgeons. CAOS technology may also facilitate better performance and serve as a learning experience for the expert by providing real-time feedback [9]. In a randomized study of the training effect on the learning of surgical skills by trainees by comparing computer navigation with conventional methods that participants used to learn surgical skills related to total hip replacement, whether in 10 min (immediate) or 6 weeks (delayed) after the skill acquisition phase, the computer navigation group demonstrated similar or even better accuracy and precision than did the conventional group [56].

3.3.2 Disadvantages

First of all, the CAOS technology is complicated and involves additional steps which take both time and manpower. Many scholars have studied and put forward their own operational procedures and standards to achieve unhindered navigation manipulations. Next, navigation is a technically demanding procedure, and navigation technique has a long learning curve (which is considered to be the first 30 operations for TKAs) and may result in complications if any step of the navigation, from the image acquisition to implant placement, is not done with sufficient care. A senior surgeon who is confident in his or her operative techniques and results tends to be more hesitant in accepting the help of a computer in performing surgery. Moreover, the current indication of navigation operation is relatively narrow, and only a small part of patients can benefit from this technology. In addition, considering that the development of CAOS depends largely on the reform of computer and software technologies, medical software, especially the navigation software, is still far behind the development of industrial software, which limits the progress and development of navigation technology [41].

At present, a non-deformable tissue is suitable for computerized guidance based on preoperatively and intraoperatively obtained images. Despite the potential advantages of CAOS in the reduction of operation time and X-ray exposure by virtue of making preoperative plans and simulating surgical manipulation, the errors in registering and tracking process as well as soft-tissue deformation are likely to result in failure [57]. The reason of image registration failure or lack of accuracy may be that it is difficult to accurately identify the intraoperative anatomical marks which have been set up preoperatively, rending the acquired data unreliable. Even though it is easy to observe the markers stuck to the local skin near the surgical site, the skin movement relative to the local skeleton can result in malposition. Although fixing markers on the bone can improve the system accuracy, this produces minor but significant morbidity and risk, such as compartment hemorrhage, nerve injury, infection, and even intraoperatively iatrogenic fracture from improper insertion of anchoring pin at the sites [58, 59]. These problems may be solved by ultrasonic, X-ray, and laser registration technology via or on the skin, and a more direct and effective method is intraoperatively automatic registration of images. A more subtle effect can sometimes be observed for passively tracked instruments using reflective marker spheres. With increasing cycles of re-sterilization of tracking equipments or when the spheres are intraoperatively partially obscured or covered with blood, tracking accuracy may unnoticeably drop.

The discrepancy between what is visible to the camera and what is of interest for the surgeon also applies to the navigated instruments. The concept of remote object tracking relies on the rigid body principle, that is, each tracked object is assumed to be non-deformable. Especially for flexible tools, this principle may be difficult to achieve. Thin drill bits or K-wires are bent easily. When they are optoelectronically tracked during the operation, the resulting navigational feedback will be inaccurate because of the rigid body principle if extra-osseous guide wire or drill bit causes bending of the local soft tissues at the starting point. The use of a navigated rigid drill sleeve and predrilling the outer cortex of the bone at the desired entry point with a small drill bit can avoid deviation from the bone entry point [42, 60].

A reference array is used to track the operated skeletal structures. It is absolutely essential that this device is fixed to the bone in a very stable manner and remains in its initial position for the entire time of the navigated procedure. Any doubts about the consistency of the reference array position at any time must be verified immediately. Bad correspondence between the position of the tracked reference array and the real location of the bony structures can also result from an unstable anatomical situation, such as fracture segment displacement and osteoporosis. A reference array is

used to reference only one bone or bony fragment every time. This situation is especially boring and cumbersome for the treatment of multiple lumbar spinal fractures.

It also has to be mentioned that the total region of interest of the Iso-C 3-D imaging is limited to a cube of $12 \times 12 \times 12$ cm, due to the size of the image intensifier itself, which is sufficient for the sacroiliac joint but not for the complete posterior pelvic ring for bilateral sacroiliac screws or multi-segmental spinal instrumentation.

Image acquisition is affected by many factors in the registration chain. Sixty-five percent of the navigation operation time is taken by image acquisition. Due to the setup of the navigation system and the image acquisition, depending on different operations, an increase of operative time may be up to 33 min, even 60–90 min, which may increase the risk of local or systemic infection [61].

Due to expensive price of the whole equipment, as well as the cost of equipment maintenance, software upgrades, and the corresponding professional's fee, the development of navigation technology is restricted to a great extent. Furthermore, apart from bulky equipments and difficult handling, related navigation surgical equipment and surgical instruments are not completely versatile, so that the operation must be performed under the product of the same brand. So it is necessary to carry out the new research of CAOS system based on open system principles: open both to different procedures as well as to software upgrades. Same as other surgical instruments and methods, CAOS has shortcomings, limitations, and insufficiency, so the surgeon should keep a clear mind during operation and must not blindly trust the accuracy and security of CAOS.

4 The Clinical Application of CAOS

4.1 The Application of CAOS in the Traumatic Orthopedic Surgery

4.1.1 Application of Fluoroscopy-Based Navigation System in Pelvic and Acetabular Fractures

Percutaneous screw fixation has been extensively reported to treat nondisplaced, mild displaced, and displaced acetabular fractures. As a 3-D complex with susceptible structures crowded in a relatively small space, the pelvis provides only some narrow safe corridors for percutaneous screw fixation of acetabular fractures [62]. Inaccurate insertion of screw can jeopardize intrapelvic organ. To achieve good accuracy and avoid neural or vascular injury, the image intensifier is used most frequently in percutaneous acetabular fractures fixation in operation room environment. Because conventional fluoroscopy provides only a 2-D image and interpretability to radiographic image is explicitly limited by superimposition of anatomical structures, it requires multiple images in different projections to determine the correct point of entry and direction of the screw. Furthermore, using conventional fluoroscopy, imaging is available in only one projection at a time. Thus, its use lengthens the procedure and exposes the patient and the medical team to a prolonged radiation time. Moreover, as working around the complex anatomy of the acetabulum, initial screw placement with imaging in only one plane may result in an erroneous first pass of the guide wire, with potentially disastrous consequences. Recently, fluoroscopy-based computerized navigation for the placement of percutaneous screw across nondisplaced or minimally displaced acetabular fractures has attracted interest. With the use of stored patient-specific imaging data to provide real-time guidance in multiple image planes during implant placement, this technique not only potentially reduces operation time and radiation exposure to the patient and the surgeon significantly but also allows the surgeon to achieve maximum accuracy.

Indications:

- No displacement or only slight displacement of the fractures, including the pubic ramus, the anterior column, the posterior column, and the quadrilateral plate fracture.
- The displaced acetabular fractures can be reduced closely or through a limited open approach with the aid of reduction clamps.
- Supplementary fixation for anatomical reduction portions of complex both column fractures.
- The early stage of unstable injuries of pelvic ring.
- Patients with multiple injuries, which would be intolerant or prevent open techniques.
- Patients with burns or extensive closed degloving injuries.
- Elderly patients with severe comorbid conditions which put them at a greater surgical risk with an open technique.

Contraindications:

- Fractures of the posterior wall of the acetabulum
- Marginal impaction fracture
- The unstable fracture dislocation of the posterior wall

Provided that fractures of the superior pubic ramus can obtain satisfactory reduction, the percutaneous medullary screw can be inserted either in an antegrade fashion from the supra-acetabular area and directed medullary to the symphysis pubis or retrograde from the pubic tubercle and directed laterally above the acetabulum. When symphyseal disruption and fracture of the ramus coexist, a retrograde screw can be combined with plating of the symphysis. For fractures of the anterior or posterior column, percutaneous screws can be placed in either an antegrade (cephalad to caudad) or retro-

grade (caudad to cephalad) direction. For retrograde fixation of fractures of the posterior column, the hip and knee are held flexed to relax the sciatic nerve and to allow palpation of the tuberosity. A guide wire is passed through the center of the tuberosity and then behind the acetabulum to the brim of the true pelvis, taking into consideration the course of the sciatic nerve which lies lateral to the tuberosity. Magic screw is used to maintain reduction of the quadrilateral plate. The guide wire is inserted on the oblique surface of the wing of the ilium at a point cephalad and posterior to the acetabulum, passing toward the ischial spine and exiting the bone along the inner cortex of the quadrilateral plate at or near the ischial spine [63].

The Clinical Application of the Fluoroscopy-Based Navigation System Combined Minimally Invasive Reduction Technique in the Displaced Acetabular Fractures

With the further development of navigation technology, its application in the pelvic and acetabular fractures is no longer just limited to simple nondisplaced fracture. Navigation technology is preferred to the displaced pelvic and acetabular fractures, which can be reduced by closed reduction or a limited open approach with the aid of reduction clamps. The navigation technique avoids the risk and complication, which are caused by extensive open reduction. Then the indications for pelvis and acetabulum surgery under navigation technique are expanded. For displaced acetabular fracture, reduction is performed first via manipulation of the injured hip. The hip is manipulated in external and internal rotation, abduction, adduction, and longitudinal traction. Traction on the muscle is used to bring the fracture fragments into alignment. Schanz screws or external fixation, sometimes, is used to facilitate fracture reduction. If acetabular fracture alignment is not acceptable by closed reduction, reduction is performed through a limited open approach [14]. The clamp is placed through a small stab incision above the anterior-superior iliac spine or at the medial of iliacus muscle, down over to the pelvic brim, and is then seated against the displaced acetabular fracture. During the use of the clamp, the hip is flexed in order to relax the iliopsoas muscle complex. The outer tine of the clamp is passed through a small incision in the abductor muscles and is seated in the supra-acetabular region. Reduction is judged on fluoroscopy. If reduction is adequate, stabilization is performed with percutaneously placed cannulated screws under the fluoroscopy-based computerized navigation. Otherwise, it is advisable to attempt formal open reduction and internal fixation.

Operation steps:

- A 52-year-old male sustained a closed left acetabular fracture in a vehicle accident. Preoperative radiograph and CT scan images showed anterior column and quadrilateral plate fractures, central displacement of femoral head (Fig. 16.1).

• Under general anesthesia, the patient was placed in the supine position on a radiolucent operating table.

• Reduction was initially performed through a limited open approach with the aid of a specific reduction clamp (Fig. 16.2). After fracture reduction had been acceptable, stabilization was performed with percutaneously placed cannulated screws under the fluoroscopy-based computerized navigation.

• C-arm intensifier is located on the side of injured and the system platform with an infrared camera on the distal of the uninjured side.

• The patient tracker is generally fixed on the uninjured iliac spine, or on the injured side also, to allow tracking of the acetabular fractures during the procedure.

• Start the navigation system.

• Activate the patient tracker.

• Tool tracker was assembled to the sleeve. The navigation system registered the tool tracker after activating the tool tracker.

• Activate the calibration device to register the surgical tool and calibrate the apex of the tool and its long axis (Fig. 16.3).

• Active the C-arm tracker and then register the C-arm intensifier.

• Once the system registration is completed, position the C-arm in the fracture orientation.

• With the fracture end as the center, fluoroscopic images of the acetabulum, such as pelvic anteroposterior (AP), inlet, outlet, and obturator-outlet views, were obtained, corrected immediately for distortions, transferred, and stored on the

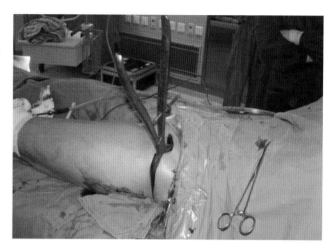

Fig. 16.2 Reduction of the acetabular fracture through a limited open approach with the aid of a special reduction clamp

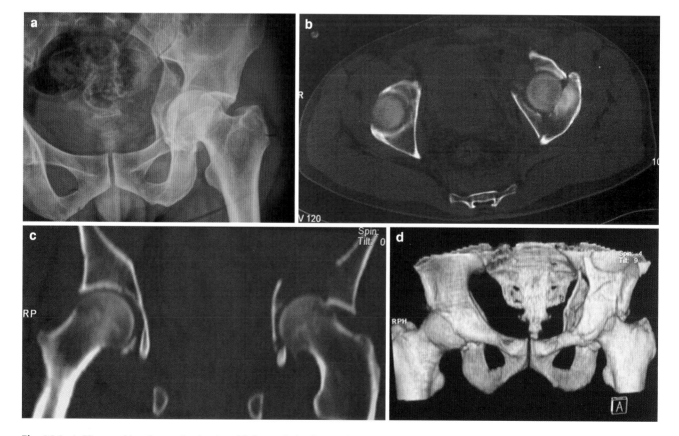

Fig. 16.1 A 52-year-old male sustained a closed left acetabular fracture in a vehicle accident. Preoperative radiograph (**a**) and CT scan images (**b–d**) showed anterior column and quadrilateral plate fractures, central displacement of femoral head

computer platform. As many as four standard fluoroscopic projections were displayed on the screen simultaneously (Fig. 16.4).

- Move the guide sleeve to determine accurately the entry point and direction of each screw by means of an extended virtual line from the planned screw. Do a 20 mm length incision at entrance point. Separate the tissue bluntly. Insert the sleeve to make sure the point and direction of the virtual cannulated screw.
- Drill a guide wire across acetabular fracture with continuous guidance by fluoroscopy images. Insert the first guide wire from the supra-acetabular area, through the anterior column fracture, to the pubic tubercle. After the position of the guiding wire was confirmed by the C-arm,

measuring the length of the planned screw in these virtual images and the first cannulated screw was driven through the guide wire (Fig. 16.5).

- Insert the second guide wire from the supra-acetabular area to quadrilateral plate using the same way. Place the second cannulated screw through the guide wire (Fig. 16.6).
- Insert the third guide wire from the anterior of the acetabular to quadrilateral plate through the small incision. Place the third cannulated screw through the guide wire (Fig. 16.7).
- Take out the guide wire and confirm the position of the screws by the C-arm (Fig. 16.8).
- Close the incision (Figs. 16.9, 16.10, and 16.11).

Fig. 16.3 Start of the navigation system and registration of the patient tracker, surgical tool and C-arm after fracture reduction

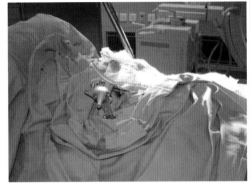
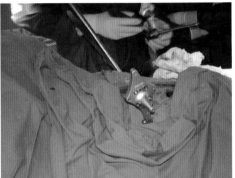

Fig. 16.4 Image acquisition. *Top left* pelvic AP view; *top right* outlet view; *bottom left* inlet view; *bottom right* obturator-outlet views

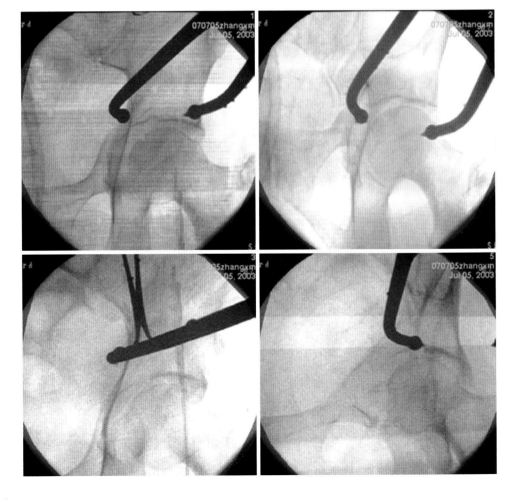

Fig. 16.5 Insertion of the first guide wire and the first cannulated screw from the supra-acetabular area to the pubic tubercle. *Top left* pelvic AP view; *top right* outlet view; *bottom left* inlet view; *bottom right* obturator-outlet views

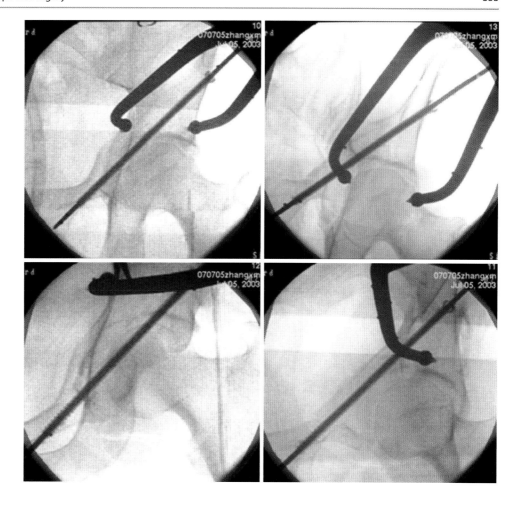

Pitfalls

Percutaneous screw fixation of acetabular fractures with fluoroscopy-based navigation can be applied not only to nondisplaced fractures but also to displaced fractures amenable to closed or limited open reduction. With the help of the fluoroscopy-based navigation technique, we can insert the screws safer and more accurate, decrease the operation time and radiation exposure chance, and promote the patient's early rehabilitation. Attention should be paid as follows: surgeons should be familiar with the principles and manipulation of the navigation system, the reasons of error and countermeasures, and accepted training systematically; acetabular fracture patients sometimes may have apparent intestinal pneumatosis which seriously affects the quality of the acquired images, so we should give preoperatively the patients intestinal preparation; the position of patient tracker should be planned preoperatively to avoid the loss of line-of-sight phenomenon between the patient tracker and the camera; as the patient tracker is the only way by which the infrared camera can track acetabular fractures, this device should be fixed stably to the iliac crest and remained in its initial position during the operation.

Unnoticed manipulations of the tracker can lead to complete shift of the images. Thus, any doubts about the consistency of the tracker position at any time must be verified immediately. Due to plenty of muscles in the hip and the tendency of the long guide wire to bend, obviously, the use of a navigated rigid drill sleeve can prevent the extra-osseous guide wire bending by soft tissues and reduce the deviation at the starting point and thus is safer and more accurate.

4.1.2   The Application of the 3-D CAOS in the Pelvic and Acetabular Fractures

Presently, the 2-D fluoroscopy-based navigation technology has been widely used in trauma orthopedics. It can increase the precision of screw placement, decrease the complications, and reduce operation trauma, which has been accepted by more and more surgeons. With the help of the 3-D C-arm, it becomes possible to use the 3-D fluoroscopy-based navigation technique during the surgery. Applications include fractures of anterior and posterior columns, the pubic ramus fractures, even the acetabular fracture with quadrilateral plate.

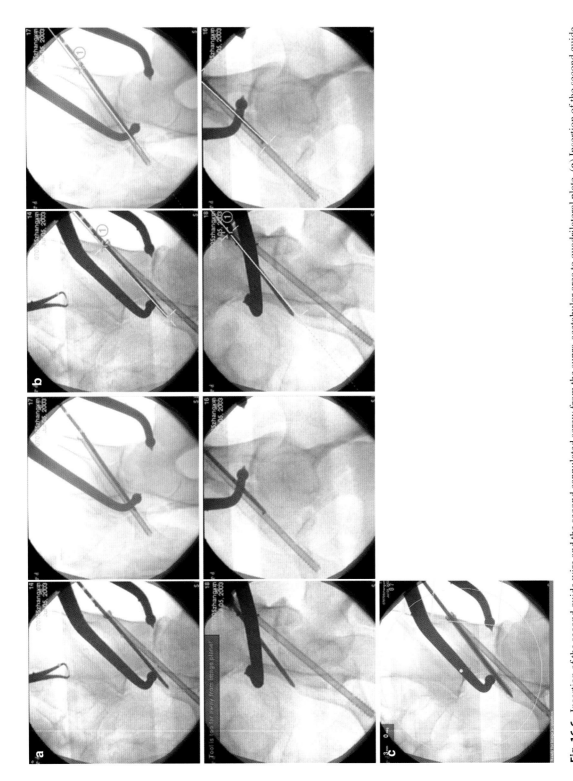

Fig. 16.6 Insertion of the second guide wire and the second cannulated screw from the supra-acetabular area to quadrilateral plate. (**a**) Insertion of the second guide wire; (**b**) measurement of the length of the guide wire; (**c**) placement of the second cannulated screw

Fig. 16.7 Insert the third guide wire from the anterior of the acetabular to quadrilateral plate through the small incision

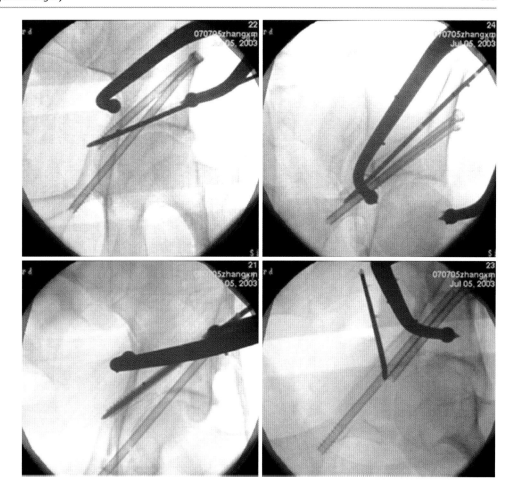

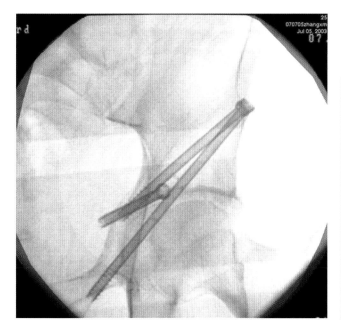

Fig. 16.8 Intraoperative fluoroscopy image

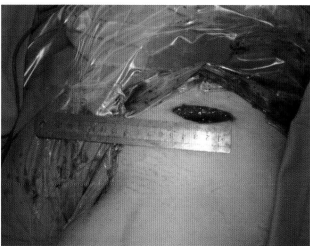

Fig. 16.9 The incision of about 5 cm

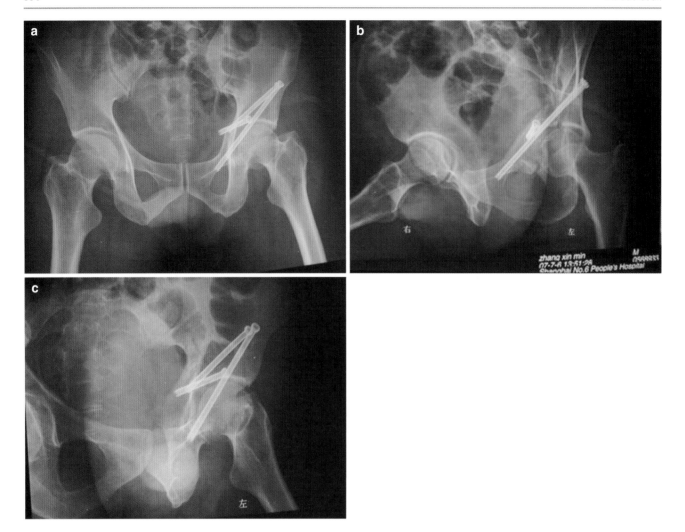

Fig. 16.10 A good fracture reduction determined by postoperative radiographs of pelvic AP (**a**), obturator oblique (**b**), and iliac oblique views (**c**)

Indications and contraindications are mentioned as above. Operation steps:

- A 55-year-old male sustained a right acetabular fracture. Preoperative radiograph and CT scan image showed a nondisplaced fracture of the posterior column of the right acetabulum (Fig. 16.12).
- Under general anesthesia, the patient was placed in the lateral position or float position on a radiolucent operating table.
- C-arm intensifier was located on the same side with the surgeon and the system platform with an infrared camera distal to the operation table.
- The patient tracker was fixed on the posterior iliac spine of the injured side.
- Start the navigation system.
- Activate the patient tracker.
- Tool tracker is assembled to the sleeve. The navigation system registers the tool tracker after activating the tool tracker.

- Activate the calibration device to register the surgical tool and calibrate the apex of the tool and its long axis.
- Activate the 3-D C-arm tracker and then register the 3-D C-arm intensifier according to the fluoroscopy-based navigation software procedure.
- Once the system registration was completed, position the C-arm in the fracture orientation.
- Using the infrared locator on the C-arm, the acetabular area which the screws would be inserted was centered on the AP and lateral fluoroscopy.
- It was guaranteed that there was no collision, and the reference trackers were always able to be traced by the camera during the rotation of the C-arm. The operative area was draped carefully for fear of possible contamination during the rotation of the C-arm. The 100 fluoroscopy images were created during the 190° rotation of the 3-D C-arm, and the image set was sent to the navigation system automatically and reconstructed to images like 3-D CT. Only 12 cm × 12 cm × 12 cm anatomical area

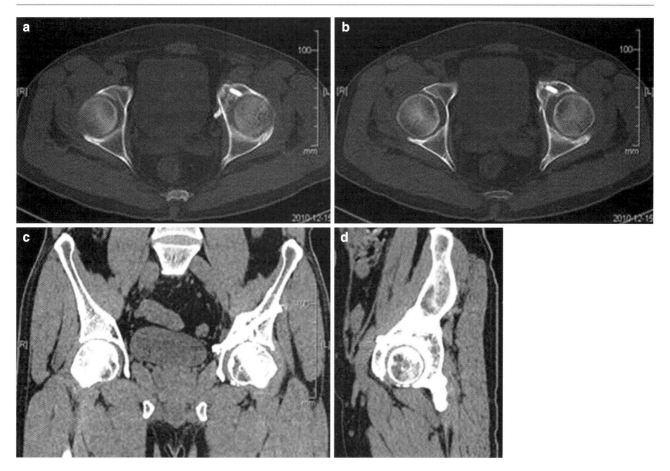

Fig. 16.11 A good fracture reduction without intra-articular penetration on the CT scan images at postoperative 42 months. Transverse (**a**, **b**), coronal (**c**), and sagittal planes (**d**)

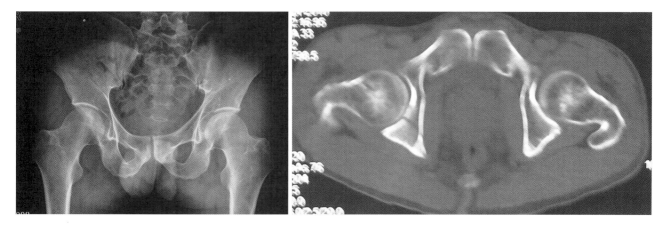

Fig. 16.12 A 55 year old male sustained a nondisplaced fracture of the posterior column of the right acetabulum

information was provided. These DICOM were transferred to the computer platform, corrected immediately for distortions, and displayed simultaneously axial, coronal, and sagittal images on the screen.

- With the help of these virtual images, the entry point and direction of the guide wire were ensured under the navi-

gation monitoring. Do a 20 mm length incision. Dissect soft tissue bluntly, and insert the drill sleeve tool to the outer cortex surface of the pelvis. When sliding the drill sleeve tool on the right acetabulum bone cortex, the multi-planar images were automatically altered correspondingly according to the alteration of the drill sleeve.

- Adjust the angle and position of the drill sleeve tool to ensure the best direction and position of the virtual guide wire on the monitor (Fig. 16.13). Insert the first guide wires across the fracture line, confirm the position of the guide wire by the C-arm, measure the length of the planned screw, and twist the first cannulated screws, through the fracture, into the posterior column of acetabulum (Fig. 16.14). Insert the second screw with the same method. After all the cannulated screws were inserted, the screw positions were confirmed again by the C-arm (Fig. 16.15). Take out the guide wires.

- Close the incision.
- Postoperative radiography (Fig. 16.16).

This was another case of applying the 3-D CAOS in the treatment of acetabular fractures (Figs. 16.17, 16.18, 16.19, 16.20, and 16.21). A 42-year-old male sustained right acetabular and femoral fractures in a vehicle accident. Preoperative radiograph and CT image showed a right acetabular fracture of the anterior column and an ipsilateral femoral neck fracture. The right femoral neck fracture was initially treated by open reduction and internal fixation with a dynamic hip screw

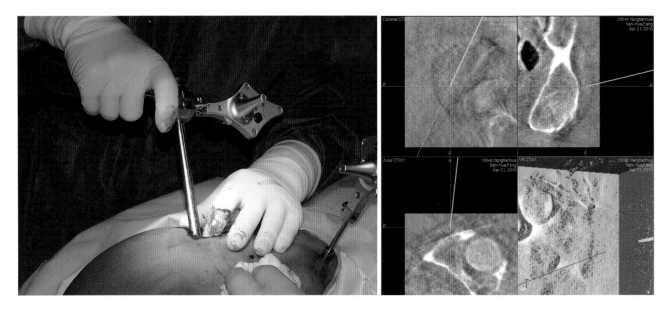

Fig. 16.13 Intraoperative determination by surgeon of the entry point and the direction of the guide wire according to the axial, coronal, and sagittal position and 3-D reconstruction images

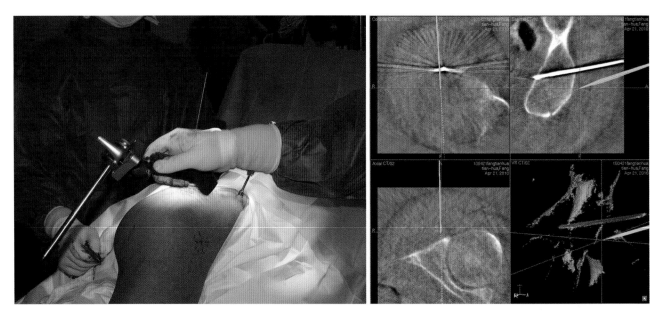

Fig. 16.14 Insertion of the first guide wire

Fig. 16.15 Confirmation of the positions of the two cannulated screws

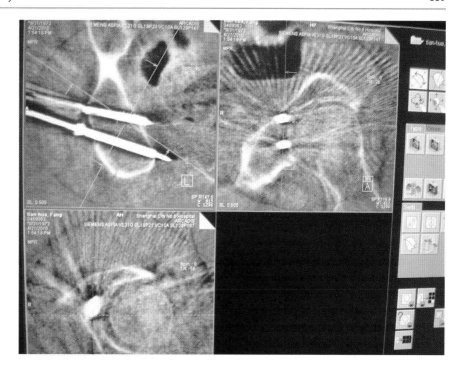

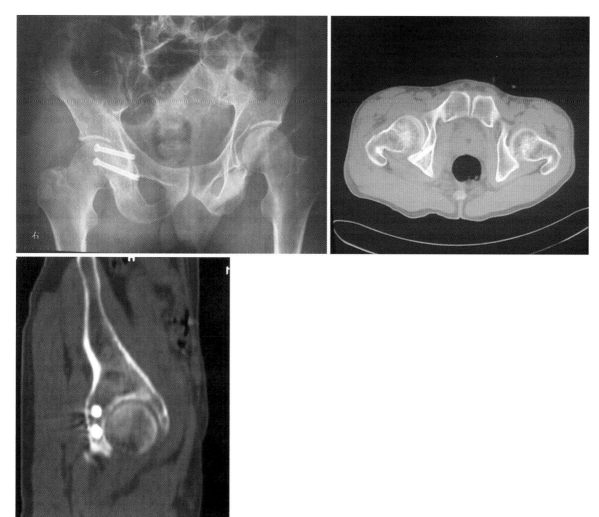

Fig. 16.16 The good positions of the screws on the postoperative radiograph and CT scan images

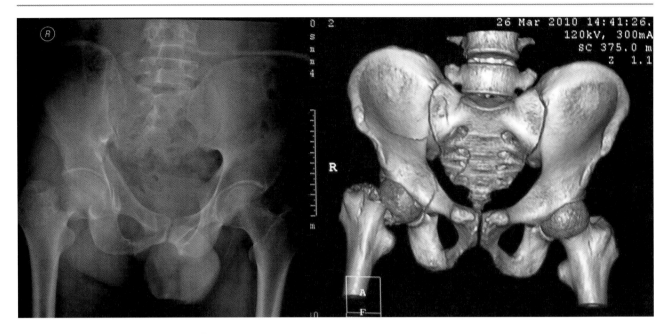

Fig. 16.17 Preoperative radiograph and CT scan

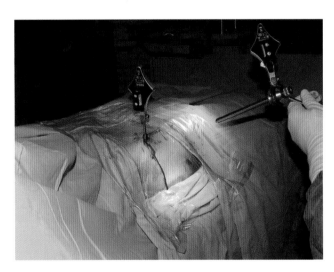

Fig. 16.18 Start of navigation system

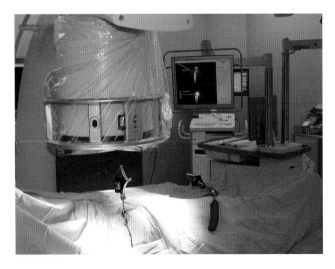

Fig. 16.19 Registration of the patient tracker, surgical tool, and C-arm to acquire the 3-D CT images of the right acetabulum

and a cannulated screw. Then the acetabular fracture is reduced with closed techniques. After fracture reduction was adequate, start the navigation system, register the patient tracker, surgical tool, and C-arm, and acquire the 3-D CT images of the right acetabulum. Ensure the guide wire of the cannulated screw across the fracture line under the guidance of axial, coronal, sagittal, and reconstruction images on the screen. After two cannulated screws were inserted, the images were acquired again to confirm the positions of the two screws. Intraoperative coronal and sagittal images showed a good reduction of fracture and a perfect placement of screws without intra-articular penetration.

Advantages and Disadvantages of 3-D and 2-D Fluoroscopy-Based Navigation System in the Clinical Application

The advantages of the 3-D fluoroscopy-based navigation technique:

- Using the 3-D fluoroscopy during the operation, the axial, sagittal, and coronal views of acetabulum can be displayed simultaneously on the screen. The surgeon can monitor the position of the screw based on the above three views and judge whether the screw penetrates into hip joint.
- The 3-D fluoroscopy image similar to the CT scan can clearly show the fracture line and spatial relationship between the screw and bone.
- The surgeon can insert the screw more intuitively and graphically under the virtual guide wire by the 3-D reconstruction images.
- Acetabular fracture line is often irregular. Under the guidance of 3-D fluoroscopy images, the screw enables to be crossed vertically over the fracture line as closely as possible, which benefits compression fixation between the fractures.

Fig. 16.20 Intraoperative determination of the entry point and the direction of the guide wire according to the axial, coronal, and sagittal position and 3-D reconstruction images

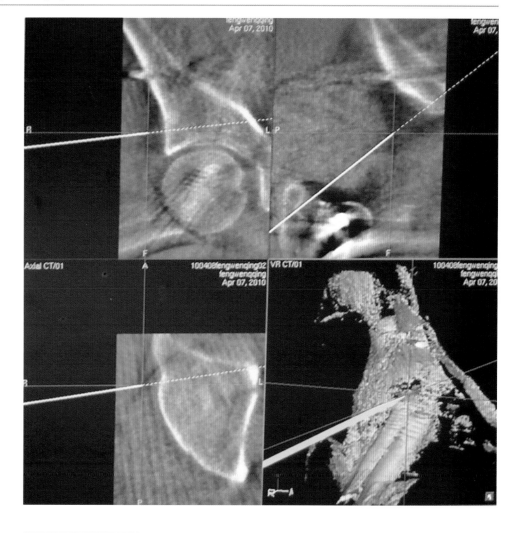

Fig. 16.21 Insertion of the two cannulated screws

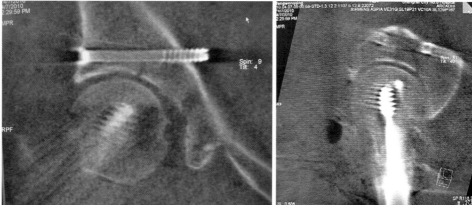

The advantages of 2-D fluoroscopy-based navigation technique:

- Multi-plane and multi-angle image guidance may reduce fluoroscopy time and radiation exposure to the patient and the surgeon significantly.
- The surgical area can be monitored real time during the operation so as to avoid neural or vascular injury and achieve good accuracy. Virtual fluoroscopic navigation

also provides advantages in a multiply injured patient. As the change of patient's intraoperative position generally is unnecessary, it may allow the surgeon to manage other associated injuries and perform other surgical procedures simultaneously.

- The skin incision can be determined more accurately using the virtual extended line from the planned screw, which may greatly reduce soft-tissue dissection and the "secondary damage" to the patients.

The disadvantages of 3-D fluoroscopy-based navigation technique:

- The operation field is relatively small. Using the 3-D fluoroscopy-based navigation system, image acquisition is hindered due to the limited scan volume of 12 cm × 12 cm × 12 cm. Unlike the 2-D fluoroscopy-based navigation system, the surgeons cannot observe visually the whole osseous corridor passed through by the guide wire during the operation using the 3-D fluoroscopy-based navigation system.
- Because the scanning area is narrow, it is not easy to identify the specific anatomical marks from these acquired images and find the specific anatomical relationship among three views (axial, sagittal, and coronal). This may affect the accuracy of the guide wire insertion [25].

The disadvantages of 2-D fluoroscopy-based navigation technique:

- Because the acquired images by the 2-D fluoroscopy-based navigation system are summation images, it is unable to accurately distinguish the real space relationship of different anatomical constructions on a summation image, which is difficult to display periarticular fractures [22].
- 2-D images cannot provide the real 3-D space structure to the surgeon to guide the operation manipulation.
- For intra-articular fractures, it is difficult to judge whether the screws penetrate into the joint gap for the surgeon.

Compared with the 2-D fluoroscopy-based navigation system, the 3-D fluoroscopy-based navigation system has similar or even higher accurate radiation exposure to the patient and the surgeon and more convergent of the entry point of the guide wires [22]. Thus, the experienced surgeons had better choose the 3-D fluoroscopy-based navigation system to do the navigation surgery in clinical practice. When the main treatment goals of acetabular intra-articular fractures lie in obtaining anatomic or near-anatomic reduction of articular surface and avoid screw intra-articular penetration, or when the different areas of the acetabulum need insertion of several cannulated screws, the use of 3-D fluoroscopy-based navigation system is better. If only one or two screws are inserted, or the surgeon is not familiar with the image acquired by the 3-D C-arm, it's best to use the 2-D fluoroscopy-based navigation system.

4.1.3 The Clinical Application of the Fluoroscopy-Based Navigation System in the Fracture and Dislocation of the Sacroiliac Joint

Sacroiliac joint plays a very important role in stability of the pelvic ring. Since Routtet et al. first reported the percutaneously sacroiliac screw technique in 1993, it has won more and more doctors' attention. Presently, clinical and biomechanical studies have shown that sacroiliac screw is a superior internal fixation method for pelvic ring injury. Due to the complex structures of sacroiliac joint and its neighboring tissues, the sacroiliac screw if improperly inserted can penetrate into the sacral canal or sacral hole or out of the vertebral anterior edge to damage the iliac vessels, lumbosacral nerve, and even internal organs. This may cause iatrogenic damage and serious surgical complications. To achieve accurately screw fixation, various types of computer-assisted techniques, including 2-D- or 3-D fluoroscopy-based navigation system as well as Ct-based navigation system, have been developed. This is an example of percutaneous sacroiliac screw fixation under the guidance of 2-D fluoroscopy-based navigation system (Figs. 16.22, 16.23, 16.24, 16.25, 16.26, and 16.27).

Pitfalls

The guide wire as a navigation tool must be rigid enough so as to monitor the direction and the position of the guide wire in real time during the operation. It is generally recommended to use guide wire of 3.2 mm in diameter. The sleeve is also used as the navigation tool. The advantages of the sleeve are that it is not easy to deform and surgical accuracy is higher, while its disadvantage is that the surgeon cannot observe real-time changes of the direction and the position of the guide wire in the process of inserting it.

4.1.4 Fluoroscopy-Based Navigation for the Internal Fixation of Femoral Neck Fractures with Cannulated Screw

Percutaneous cannulated screw fixation is an accepted method for the surgical treatment of femoral neck fractures. Because routine fluoroscopy image is performed in only one plane at a time, accurate placement of cannulated screw often requires multiple uses of fluoroscopy before optimal position is attained in all planes. Fluoroscopy-based navigation enables the surgeon to place screws in a very precise manner under the guidance of simultaneous real-time multi-projection views of the osseous anatomy of the femoral neck of the patient. This can significantly improve the parallelism and spread of the cannulated screws, which will reduce the surgical complications and increase the fixation stability.

Fig. 16.22 Intraoperative screenshot for 2-D fluoroscopy-based navigation for two S1 screws. After pelvic fluoroscopy images are acquired, the real-time spatial position of the guide sleeve is simultaneously presented on four fluoroscopic projections. A *dotted line* is a virtual linear continuation presenting the track in which the guide wire is planned to be inserted. *Top left* pelvic AP view; *top right* inlet view; *bottom left* outlet view; *bottom right* lateral sacral view

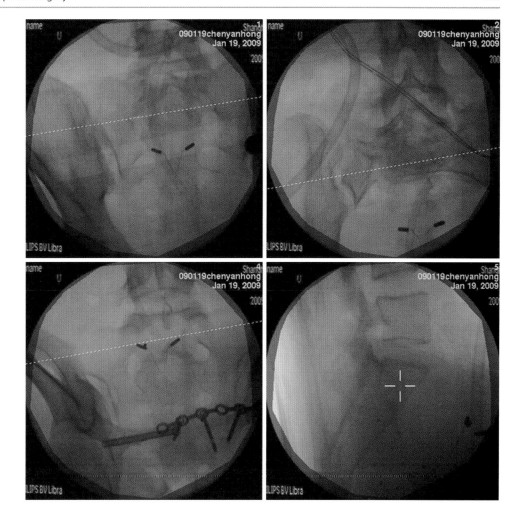

Fig. 16.23 Insertion of the first guide wire

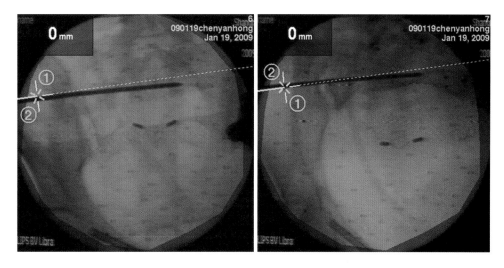

Fig. 16.23 (continued)

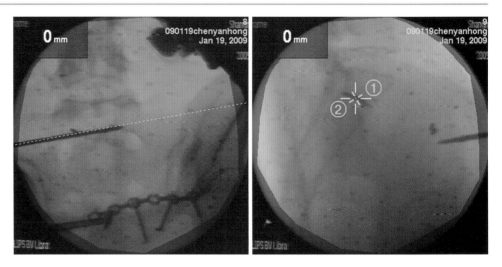

Fig. 16.24 Insertion of the first cannulated screw

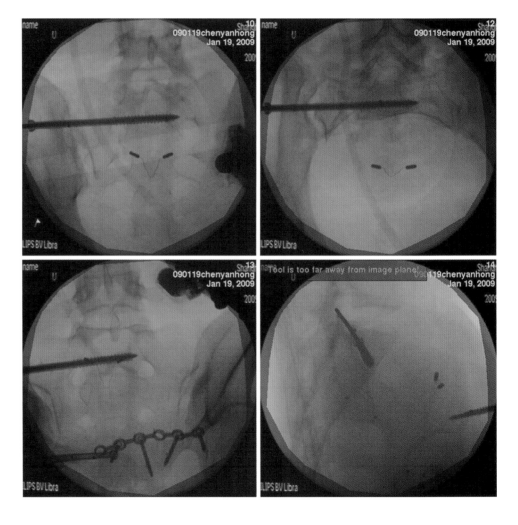

Fig. 16.25 Determination of the entry point and direction of the second guide wire under the navigation monitoring

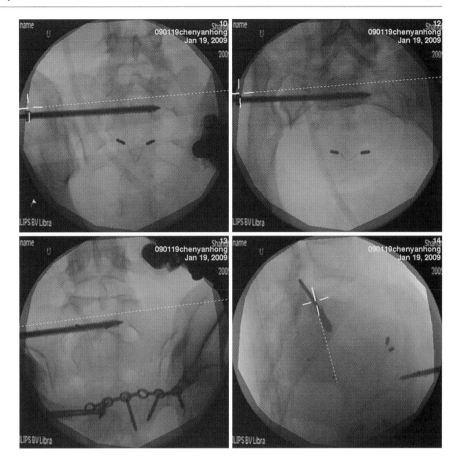

Fig. 16.26 Insertion of the second guide wire and cannulated screw

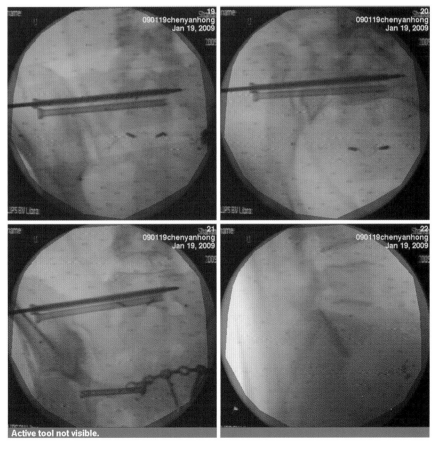

Fig. 16.27 Confirmation of the final position of the two screws

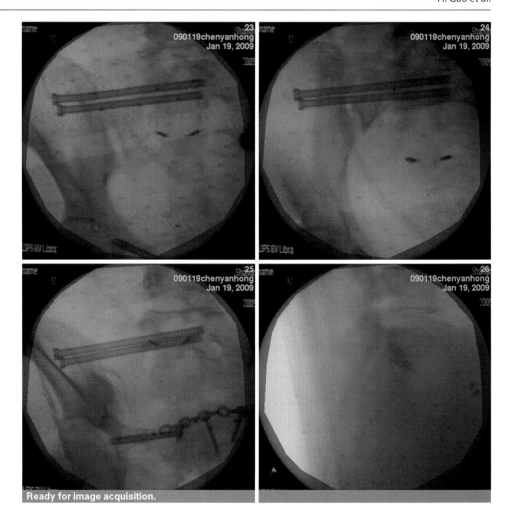

4.1.5 The Clinical Application of the Navigation System in the Femoral Intertrochanteric Fracture

Intramedullary interlocking nail has been widely used in the treatment of femoral intertrochanteric fracture. Computerized navigation has potential utility in various steps of intramedullary nail fixation. For compromising precision and accuracy of the insertion of the distal interlocking screw, it has been reported to carry out the insertion of the distal interlocking screw under the fluoroscopy-based navigation system.

Operation steps:

- After the setup and the insertion of a tracker into the bone, AP and lateral radiographs are taken and stored in the computer. Several images are used simultaneously to determine the precise location of the nail entry points through a minor incision with relative ease (Fig. 16.28).
- The real-time direction and position of the lag screw are displayed on the navigation image after the insertion of the intramedullary nail (Fig. 16.29). These images may also be used to determine the precise location of the lag screw.

- The surgeon can use the distal locking screw aiming device or the navigation system to place the distal locking screw. Change the position of the patient's tracker, and fix it on the proximal handle of the intramedullary nail. The tool tracker is installed on the sleeve of the distal locking screw. C-arm is located in the injured side and navigation platform at the uninjured side. Revalidate the trackers.
- Acquire the AP and lateral images of the distal locking screw. It is important to ensure the distal screw hole of the nail to be round enough on the lateral image. Transfer the images to the navigation unit (Fig. 16.30).
- Planning the position and the length of the locking screw on the navigation screen (Fig. 16.31). When the sleeve tool with tracker is moved in the distal femur, the best position and direction of the locking screw is that the virtual line of the sleeve comes to cross at the center of distal screw hole of the intramedullary nail on the lateral image. Drill bit into the distal locking hole along the sleeve and insert the suitable length locking screw. The length and position of the locking screw may be confirmed by the C-arm (Fig. 16.32).
- Insert another locking screw using the same method.

Fig. 16.28 Determination of the entry point of the intramedullary nail

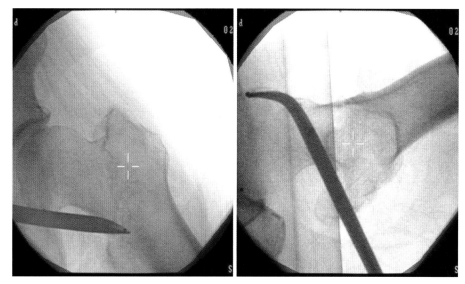

Fig. 16.29 Virtual direction of the lag screw guide wire on the AP and lateral view of the left hip

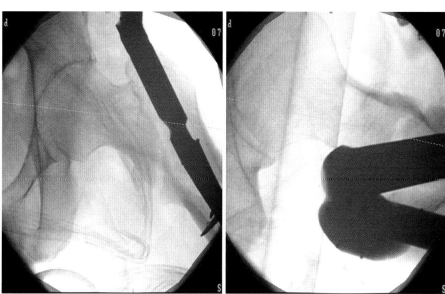

Fig. 16.30 Acquisition of the AP and lateral images of the distal femur

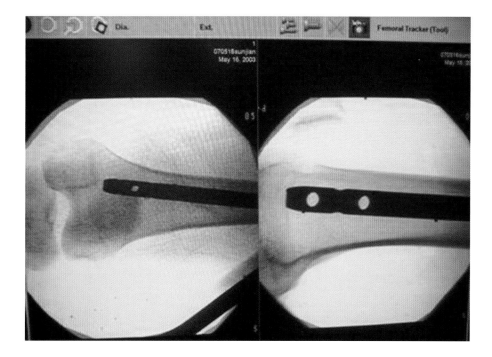

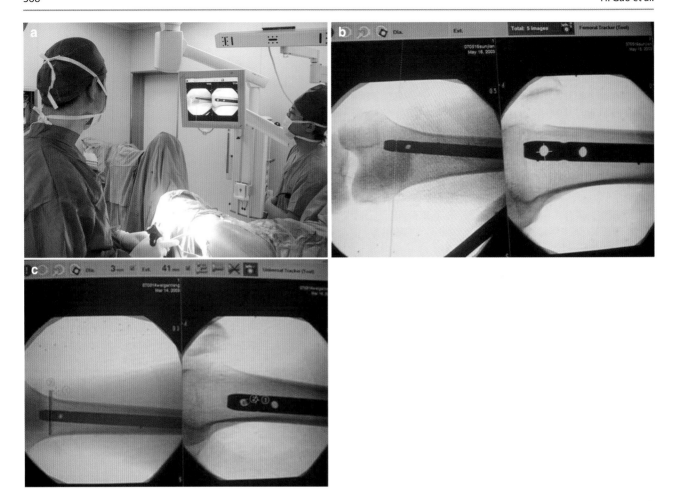

Fig. 16.31 Determination of the direction and entry point of the locking screw on the virtual images (**a**, **b**) and planning of the position and length of the locking screw (**c**)

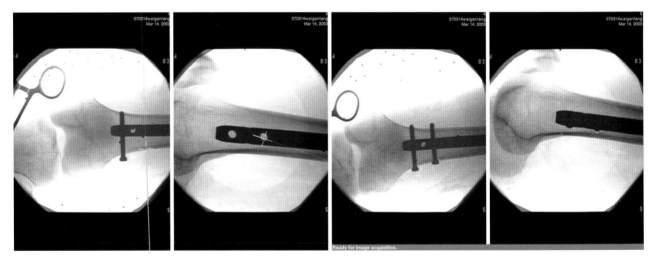

Fig. 16.32 Insertion of another locking screw proximal to the distal screw

Pitfalls

It is important to ensure the distal screw hole of nail to be round enough on the lateral image. If another screw hole on the lateral image that is acquired to verify the position of the first locking screw is not round enough, the previously stored lateral image with screw hole round enough can be used to guide the second locking screw insertion. When the drill touches the cortex, excessive sliding of the drill over the cortical surface should be avoided. Install the tool tracker on the rigid sleeve to avoid bending of the drill bit which can influence the accuracy of the operation.

4.1.6 The Clinical Application of the Navigation System in the Hip Fracture with Dynamic Hip Screw

Dynamic hip screw (DHS) is considered as a classical method for the treatment of hip fractures. As the AP and lateral images of the femoral neck are displayed simultaneously on the screen under the fluoroscopy-based navigation system, this can reduce the extent of radiation exposure.

During the procedure of the navigation surgery, the installation and stabilization of the patient tracker are a key point. The patient tracker should not be very close to the surgical site in case of interfering the surgical manipulation. The installation of the tracker must be secure, and the tracker should not be touched during the operation. Unnoticed manipulations of the tracker can lead to complete shift of the images. Thus, any doubts about the consistency of the tracker position at any time must be verified immediately, or restart a new navigation.

4.1.7 The Application of CAOS in the Pelvic Fractures with External Fixation

Indications:

- Unstable pelvic fractures with open limb injury or multiple traumas (Figs. 16.33, 16.34, and 16.35)
- As a temporary fixation in order to move the patients to get necessary examinations.
- As a decisional fixation method for the rotation unstable fracture, such as open book injury
- As one of the combined treatment for the unstable fractures, such as external fixation with lower limb traction or external fixation with open reduction and internal fixation

Fig. 16.33 Planning of entry point and direction of the fixator pin on the virtual images

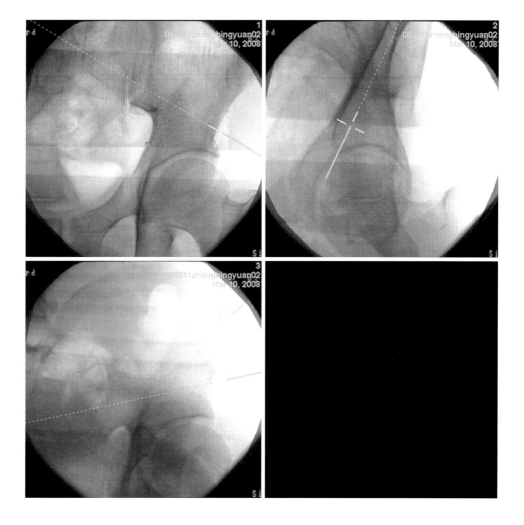

Fig. 16.34 Insert the left
fixator pin

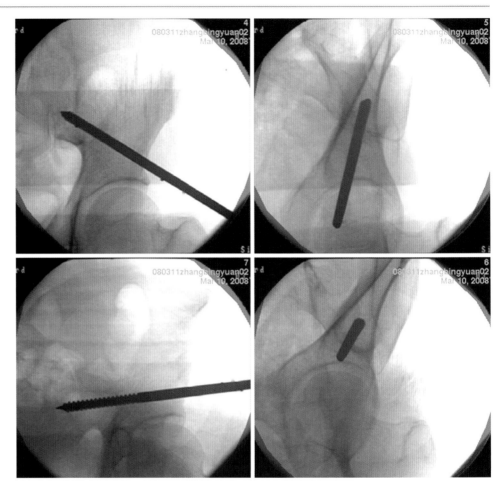

Fig. 16.35 The AP and
outlet view images of the
pelvic postoperatively

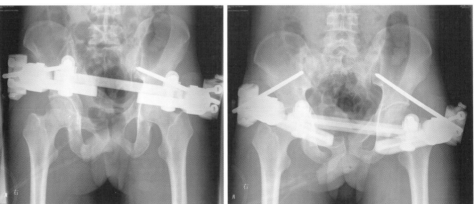

4.1.8   The Clinical Application of the Navigation System in the Long Bone Fracture

Although closed intramedullary interlocking nailing has been the current standard treatment for long bone shaft fractures, it is challengeable to assess intraoperatively rotational malalignment in long bone fracture, especially in femur shaft fracture, which is enveloped by surrounding abundant muscles and is closed reduction only by manual manipulation to adjust the distal and proximal fragments. Several conventional techniques of estimating and determining rotational malalignment intraoperatively have been described, including the radiopaque cables, a grid system, the lesser trochanter profile, and the cortical width sign. However, these techniques are qualitative and subjective, may fail to detect small deviation from the normal mechanical axis, and, thus, can require increased fluoroscopic radiation exposure. Some reports have demonstrated that, despite the use of established techniques for intraoperative torsion control, femoral antetorsion angle deviation above 15° following intramedullary nailing has still an incidence of 10–30% [64–66]. Moreover, during antegrade femoral intramedullary nailing, the common techniques of positioning the leg on the operating table (on an extension leg holder, using an abducted supine positioning of the contralateral leg, or the lateral positioning) do not allow a clinical correct comparison during the operation. Therefore, even today, postoperative malrotation still remains an unsolved problem [67].

The femoral anteversion (FAV) is usually used to express the femoral rotation angle. Although the difference of FAV from patient to patient is possibly large (−4–35°), the difference of bilateral FAV of the patient self is minimal [68]. The geometrical structure of the bilateral femur is symmetrical. As a result, the contralateral femoral FAV may be used to judge intraoperatively the rotation deformity of the injured femur.

With the development and application of the navigation technique in clinic, this new technique has been recently introduced to improve the alignment of diaphyseal fractures while reducing the amount of intraoperative radiation [17–19, 69]. In 2000, Hofstetter et al. initially introduced a surgical navigation system based on fluoroscopy that provides missing information for the procedure of femoral fracture fixation, and an in vitro study on computer-assisted measurement of femoral antetorsion demonstrated the high degree of precision of this technique [17]. In a study using a cadaveric femur to test the accuracy of a computerized navigation system to enhance multi-planar fracture reduction, the accuracy of restoration of femoral length was 1.2 mm for a simple fracture and 1.9 mm for a segmental fracture; rotational accuracy was 1.7° and 2.5°, respectively [18].

Operation steps:

- Under general anesthesia, the patient is placed in the supine position, and the injured leg is placed in traction with slight flexion and adduction.
- A "headband" with a reference array is fastened around the thigh of the uninjured leg. Activate reference array and the C-arm. Acquire fluoroscopy images of the proximal and distal femur and transfer these images to the navigation platform. The uninjured femoral FAV and length are provided automatically by the navigation software and displayed on the navigation screen.
- The patients' trackers are installed into the proximal and distal fragment of the injured femur and then validated (Fig. 16.36). The trackers are placed such that they do not interfere with nail insertion. Validate the patient tracker and surgical tool (the curved drill). Five fluoroscopic images of the injured side are necessary for initialization of the navigation system: an AP and a lateral view of both the femoral neck and the fracture site and a true lateral view of the condyles (ensure the medial and lateral posterior femoral condyles completely

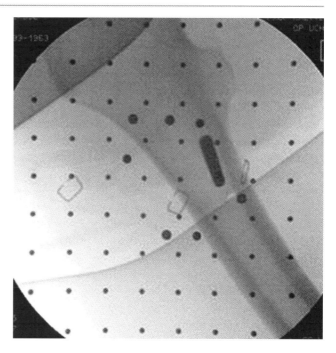

Fig. 16.36 Installment of the patient tracker on the proximal fragment

overlapping on the lateral view) (Fig. 16.37). The surgeon marks the point of interests on the images using the computers touch screen. The distal and proximal fragments are manually segmented on the navigation screen (Fig. 16.38). Alignment in the coronal and sagittal planes is defined manually by picking two points in each fragment that are the center of the medullary canal in the AP and lateral fluoroscopic images. Then the resultant anatomic axes are fine-tuned with a software tool that facilitates a best-fit line. A femoral neck axis line is defined as a line connecting the center of the femoral head and femoral neck. A point along the posterior condyles of the perfect overlapping medial and lateral femoral condyles is defined. The point defined the posterior condylar axis (Fig. 16.39).

- The C-arm then is removed from the field and fluoroscopic navigation is used. The calibration curved drill is inserted into the top of the greater trochanter and opens a hole for long guide wire insertion under the guide of the navigation.
- Real-time visual feedback from computer screen is used to reduce and stabilize the fracture in the desired position. While the bone is manipulated, the computer displays continuously updated and provided user with graphic information concerning the position of fragments relative to each other, in addition to numeric information regarding coronal alignment (varus/valgus), sagittal alignment (flexion/extension), length, and femoral anteversion. When the axes of the proximal and distal

Fig. 16.37 Acquisition of five standard images of the injured femur. (**a**, **b**) The AP and lateral view of the femoral neck, (**c**, **d**) the AP and lateral view of the fracture site, (**e**) a true lateral view of the condyles

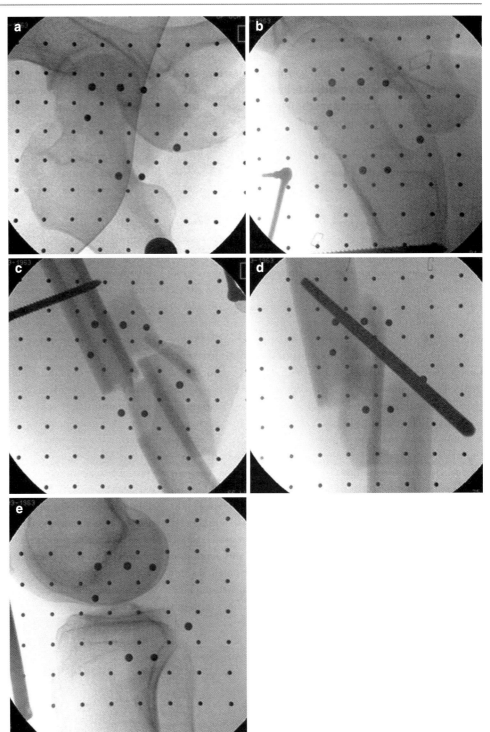

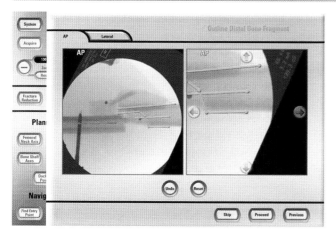

Fig. 16.38 Determination of axes of the distal and proximal fragments on the navigation screen. The resultant anatomic axes are fine-tuned with a software tool

fragments became a straight line on the AP and lateral virtual images, this means the reduction is good.
- The long guide wire is inserted into the top of the greater trochanter across the fracture site. Collect the images of proximal, distal femur and fracture site to confirm the position of the guide wire.
- After reaming, insert a suitable length intramedullary nail. Insert the distal locking screw (Fig. 16.40).
- Adjust the femoral rotation. The length and FAV of both the injured and uninjured femur can be displayed on the navigation screen in real time (Fig. 16.41). The length and FAV of the injured leg match the uninjured one. Insert the proximal locking screw until the length and FAV of the injured leg match the uninjured one.
- Finally confirm the fracture reduction and position of the locking screws by C-arm.

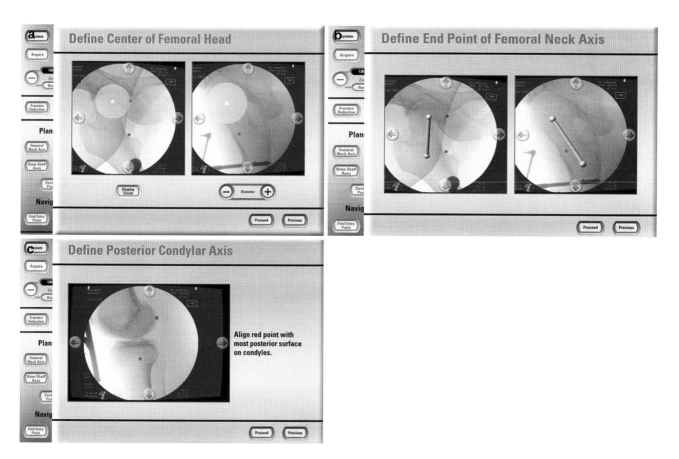

Fig. 16.39 Acquisition of landmarks for torsion control. *Top left* find the center of the femoral head; *top right* mark the axis of the femoral neck; *bottom left* mark the posterior condylar axis

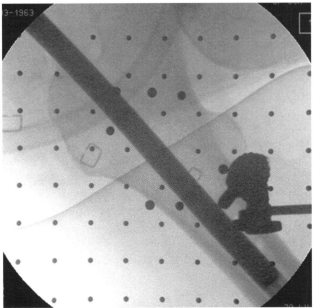

Fig. 16.40 Insertion of a intramedullary nail after fracture reduction

4.1.9 The Clinical Application of the Navigation System in the Periarticular Fracture

Indication:

- Nondisplaced fractures or fractures can be reduced by closed reduction or reduction through a limited open approach; also thesis fractures can be treated by compression screws.

Operation steps: (e.g., calcaneal and talus fracture)

A 42-year-old male sustained multiple fractures after car accident. Preoperative radiograph and CT scan images showed left calcaneal and talus nondisplaced fracture. Local soft tissue showed serious injury. Prepare to treat the calcaneal and talus fractures with cannulated screws under the 3-D fluoroscopy-based navigation system (Figs. 16.42, 16.43, 16.44, 16.45, 16.46, 16.47, and 16.48).

Fig. 16.41 Screenshot of navigation software during intraoperative reduction of the femoral shaft fracture. During navigation reduction, the *green* cylinder represents the distal fragment (*top half*), while alignment and rotation also are displayed (*bottom half*)

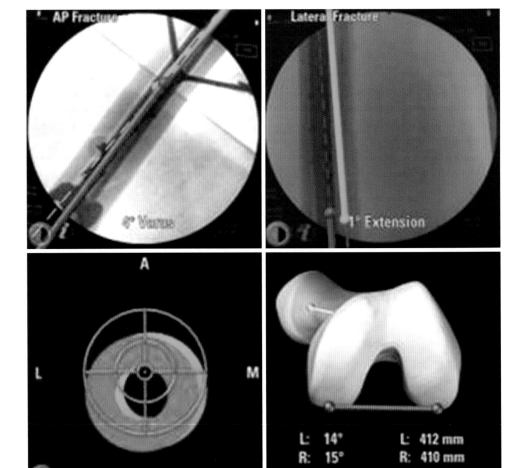

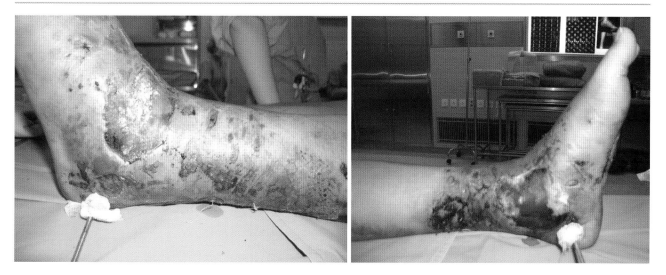

Fig. 16.42   Left heel with high-energy injury and poor soft-tissue condition

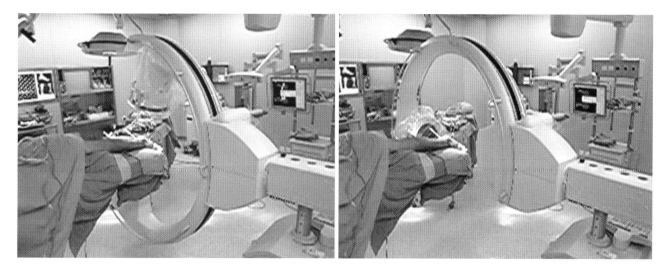

Fig. 16.43   Acquisition of the 3-D fluoroscopy images of the left calcaneal and talus during the operation

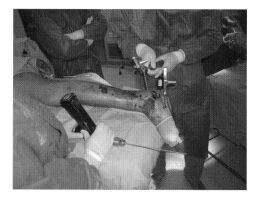

Fig. 16.44   Determination of the entry point and direction of cannulated screw guide wire on the virtual navigation images

Fig. 16.45 Insertion of a guide wire and a cannulated screw into the talus by the navigation image guidance

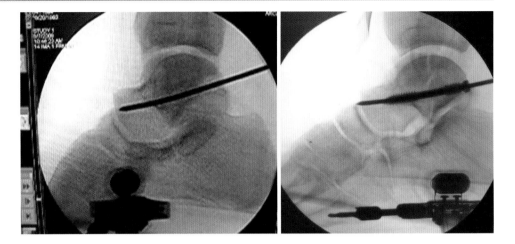

Fig. 16.46 The location of the talus screw on the sagittal and coronal images

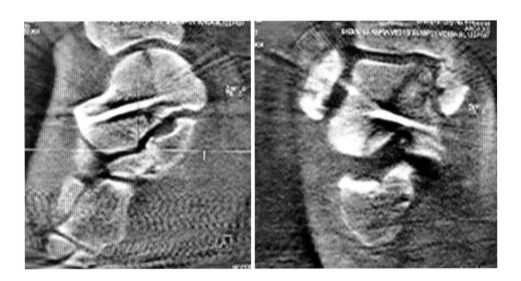

Fig. 16.47 Insertion of a guide wire and a cannulated screw into the calcaneus

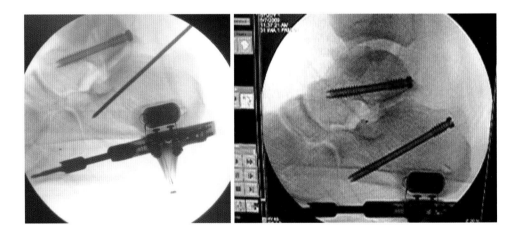

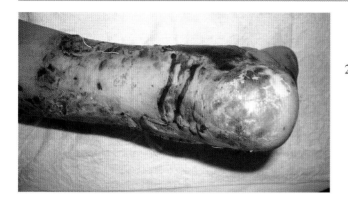

Fig. 16.48 The incision

Acknowledgments The author would like to thank Dr. Hao Ding and Dr. Xiao-Yan Huang for their useful discussion and Dr. Xin-Bin Fan, Dr. Kai-Hua Zhou, Dr. Ling Yao, and Dr. Wei Zhang for their help on clinical information and article writing.

5 Application of Navigation in Spinal Lesion Biopsy and Debridement

Sang Hongxun, Cheng Bin, Wu Zixiang, and Fan Yong

Spinal lesions, such as tuberculosis, cancer, etc., often require preoperative invasive biopsy for diagnosis. However, it is always difficult to get lesion tissues due to the deep-seated location of lesions. At the same time, it is often of concern that such lesions may not be fully removed during debridement or scraping. The application of navigation technology provides visible, precise positioning, and targeted biopsy and debridement may more thoroughly remove lesions, reduce unnecessary resection of normal bone tissues, and prevent loss to the anterior column.

5.1 Surgical Procedures

1. Preoperative: (1) Determine the position of the lesion and surgical plan after discussion based on preoperative CT, MRI, and other imaging data. (2) CT scan and then import the data into the computer navigation system for 3-D remodeling. Select the appropriate type of screw and specific surgical plan.
2. Intraoperative: (1) General anesthesia and position placement. (2) By posterior medium approach, fix the reference arc to the spinous process after exposure of the process and then start the registration after proper adjustment of the infrared camera: to register the reference points are set on the preoperative 3-D remodeling image in the navigation system as per the actual anatomical locations one by one, including point-plane registration and positioning after confirmation of registration, and the error must be controlled within 1 mm. (3) Implant the preoperative designed pedicle screws under the guidance of 3-D navigation technology and make an intraoperative confirmation that the pedicle screws are well positioned. Screw holder or open device and other instruments can also be registered when implanting the screws; after that, the positions of the screws or instruments can be seen on the computer screen and complete implantation under the guidance of the navigation.(4) Conduct temporary unilateral fixation to prevent vertebral displacement during debridement which may cause spinal cord injury. (5) Perform osteotomy via the pedicle of the affected pedicle to perform the debridement. Check the lesion in direct navigation display to verify whether the debridement meets preoperative design and whether it is thorough. (6) Perform implanted bone remodeling after thorough removal of the lesion.

5.2 Case 1

Male patient, 59 years old, diagnosis: T11–T12 vertebral tuberculosis and abscess accompanied by formation of partial paraplegia. Intraoperative 3-D navigation-guided debridement performed via bilateral pedicles of T12 and 3-D navigation displayed verification of thorough debridement or not (Figs. 16.49, 16.50, 16.51, 16.52, 16.53, 16.54, 16.55, 16.56, 16.57, 16.58, 16.59).

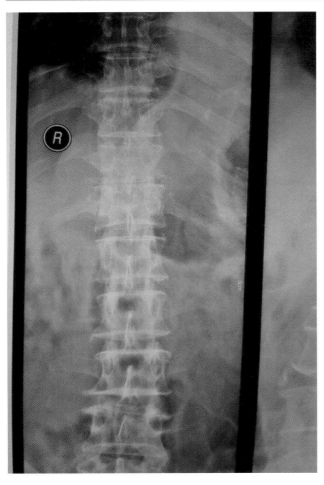

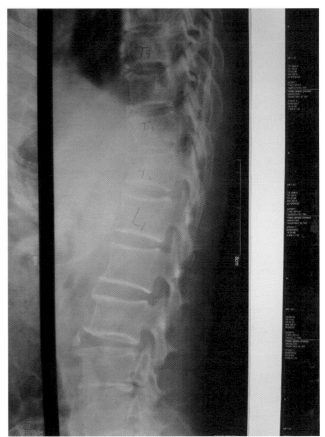

Fig. 16.50 Thoracolumbar lateral X-ray showed destruction of T11 and T12 vertebrae, collapsed disc space, and local kyphosis

Fig. 16.49 Thoracolumbar anteroposterior X-ray showed bone lesion of T11 and T12 vertebrae and collapsed disc space

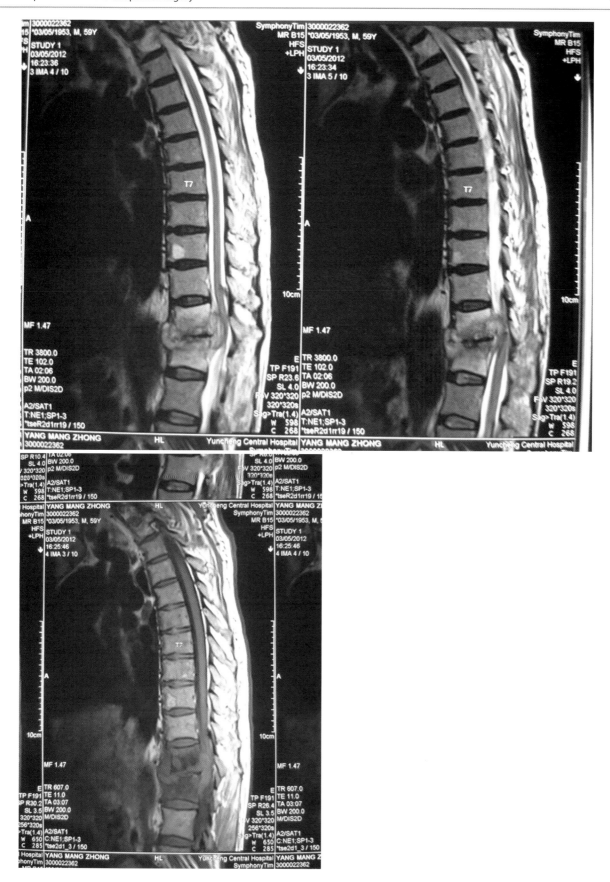

Fig. 16.51 Thoracolumbar MRI: destruction of T11 and T12 vertebrae, no destruction of appendixes, collapsed disc space, local fester fluid injected into the spinal canal, and severe spinal cord compression

Fig. 16.52 Thoracolumbar CT 3-D remodeling: destruction of T11 and T12 vertebrae, partial sequestration, no destruction of appendixes, and collapsed disc space

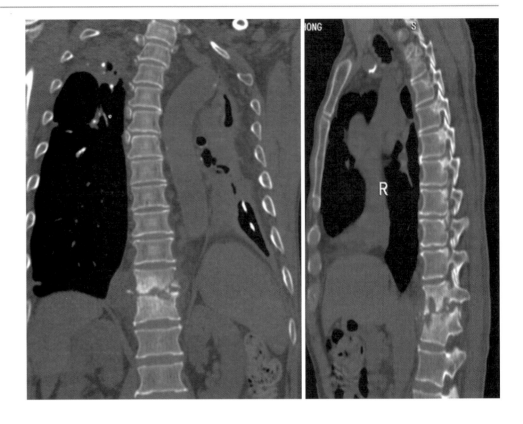

Fig. 16.53 Intraoperative point-plane registration under 3-D navigation

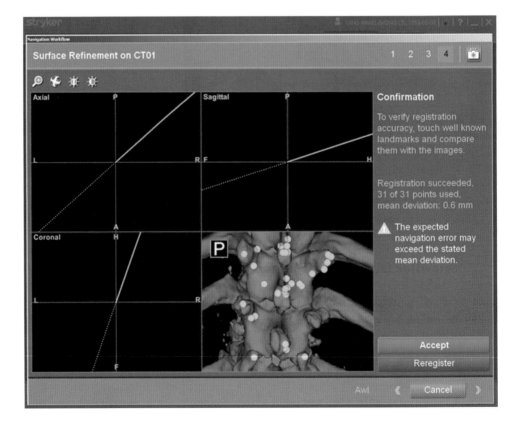

Fig. 16.54 3-D navigation-guided implantation of pedicle screws in the lesion to ensure the pedicle screws are implanted in normal bone substance and guide entry angle and length of pedicle screws

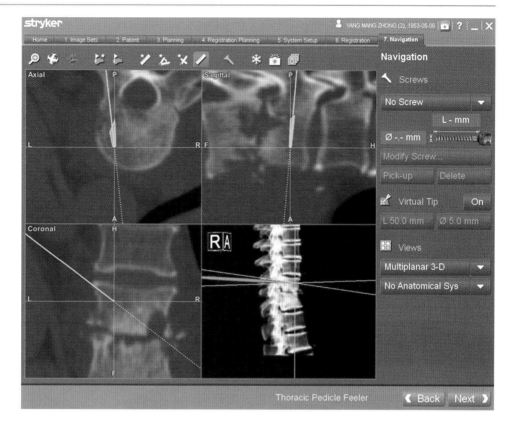

Fig. 16.55 3-D navigation-based design for position and length of each pedicle screw, in which the blue and yellow pedicle screws have smaller lengths

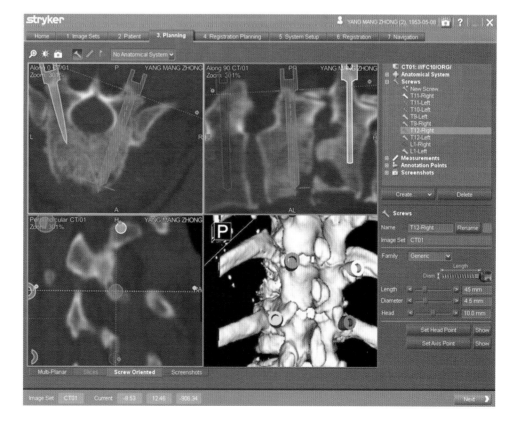

Fig. 16.56 Registered rongeur or probe entered into the space after debridement to verify whether a thorough debridement and to guide debridement position for the purpose of avoiding vital structures around the vertebral body

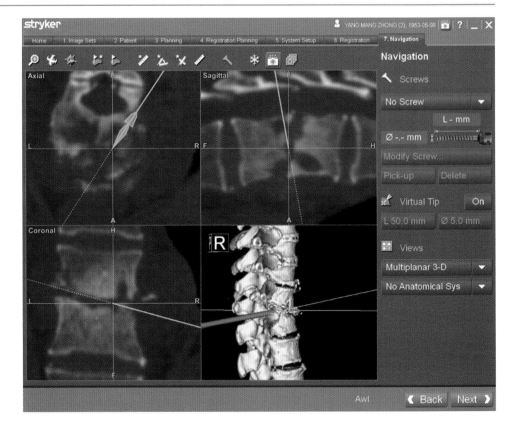

Fig. 16.57 Well positioning of internal fxation and satisfed correction of local kyphosis confirmed in postoperative X-ray

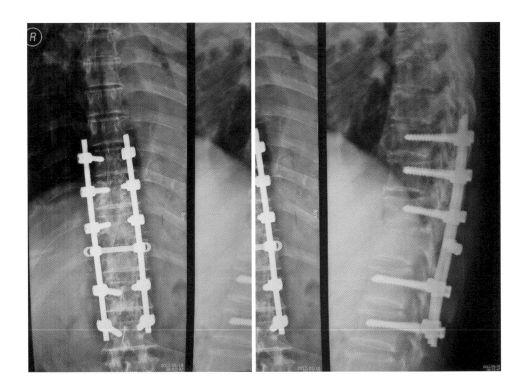

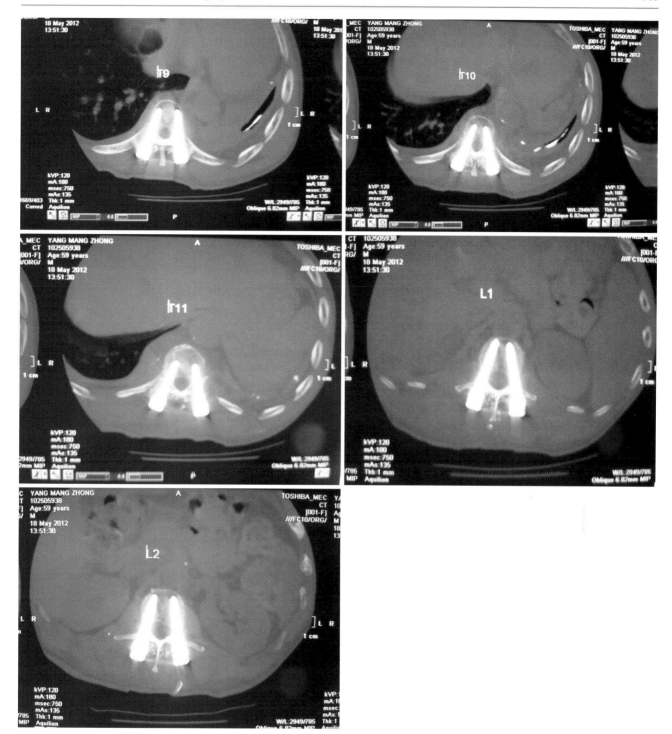

Fig. 16.58   CT scans of sagittal plane of each pedicle screw with satisfied position and length

Fig. 16.59 Follow-up after 1 year, fusion was achieved without screw loosening

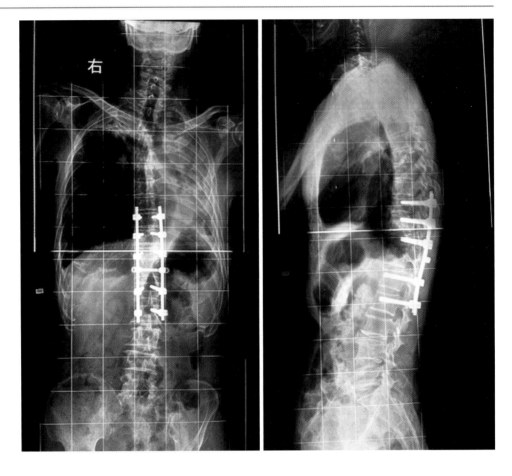

6 Application of Navigation in Spinal Osteotomy for Deformity

You may simulate the osteotomy with Mimics software before the surgery with a closed space after the osteotomy and deformity after kyphosis correction; measure the kyphosis angle after correction to minimize the kyphosis angle and obtain the optimal surgical plan, the final surgical location, methods, and range to guide the surgery; and it may also help find flaws and imperfections in surgical design so that you may improve surgical scheme immediately. It also avoids excessive or insufficient bone removing in surgery, affecting surgical outcomes, makes surgery more intuitive and precise, and indirectly reduces operative time and blood loss and lowers risk of surgery at the same time.

6.1 Methods of Surgery

After general anesthesia, the patient is in prone position with chest pad and waist bridge placed at thoracolumbar section and applied with intraoperative spinal cord monitoring system and autologous blood transfusion system. (1) By posterior medium approach, expose the vertebral plate, articular process, and transverse process layer by layer. (2) Position the apical vertebra by fluoroscopy, install intraoperative 3-D navigation system, adjust the position sensor, and register and calibrate intelligence tools. Point-plane matching error within 0.5 mm, and start with navigation-guided operation. In the nontargeted sections, implant pedicle screws of predetermined length and diameter in the predetermined vertebras above and below the apical vertebra with the assistance of

3-D navigation. (3) Expose the pedicle, transverse process, and upper and lower adjacent nerve roots of the apical vertebra; after proper protection of the nerve roots, perform osteotomy via the pedicle of the apical vertebra. Put 3-D navigation-based registered open cone into the space after osteotomy. You may find out whether you meet the preoperative designed range and amount by comparison. Install the opposite temporary fixation stick for osteotomy on the other side in the same way. (4) Push the bone cortex of vertebra posterior border to the ventral side with the rear wall bone knife for 360° decompression of spinal cord and nerve roots. (5) Pre-bending of final fixation stick based on physiological thoracolumbar curve, install the said pre-bent fixation stick after osteotomy, and extend the waist bridge to horizontal position with bilateral-alternately pressure to close the osteotomy and correct local kyphosis. (6) End of surgery, repeated washing, well-conceived hemostasis, and 360° graft of lateral

facet process and transverse process for the autologous bone generated after osteotomy.

6.2   Case 2

Male, 28 years old, postoperation of L1 fracture with progressive thoracolumbar kyphosis 9 years; local angular thoracolumbar kyphosis, Cobb angle 60°, Frankel Grade D. Preoperative Mimics software design of osteotomy location, range, bone cutting, and orthopedic operation simulation. Intraoperative 3-D navigation guided bilateral PSO via L1. 3-D navigation display verification of the conformance of local osteotomy space and amount; if conformance, gradually pressurized and closed the space of osteotomy; and correction of local angular kyphosis (Figs. 16.60, 16.61, 16.62, 16.63, 16.64, 16.65, and 16.66).

Fig. 16.60 Preoperative anteroposterior and lateral X-rays showed kyphosis Cobb angle was 60° and apical vertebra was L1

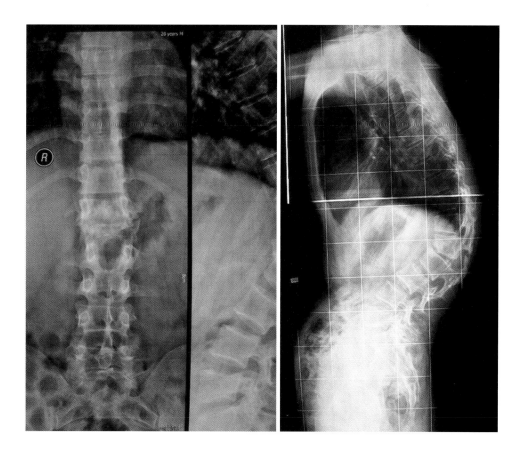

Fig. 16.61 3-D CT spine remodeling

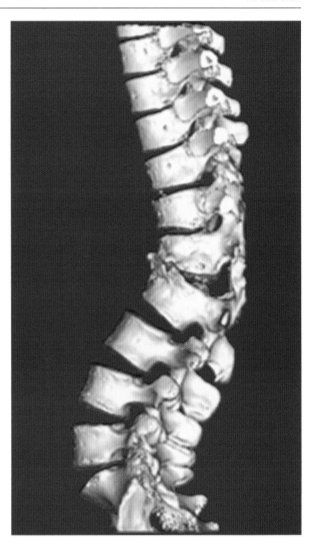

Fig. 16.62 Intraoperative
3-D point-plane registration

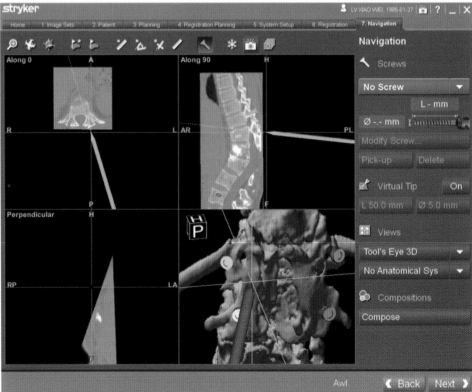

Fig. 16.63 Intraoperative 3-D navigation-guided implantations of pedicle screws

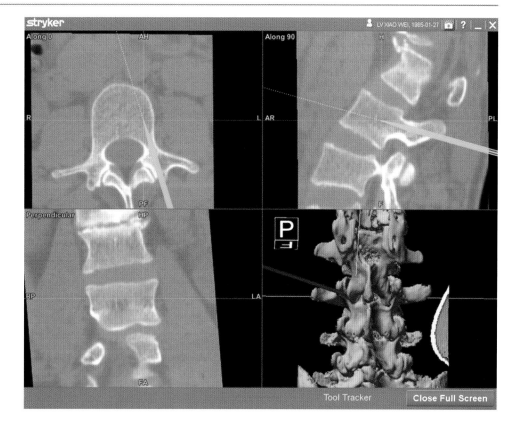

Fig. 16.64 Under Intraoperative 3-D navigation, put registered drill into the space after osteotomy to compare with preoperative 3-D CT image for verifcation that whether the amount and range of osteotomy is the same with the surgical plan. This fgure showed that the anterior 1/3 of vertebra was removed, which basically conformed to the surgical plan, and osteotomy was verifed

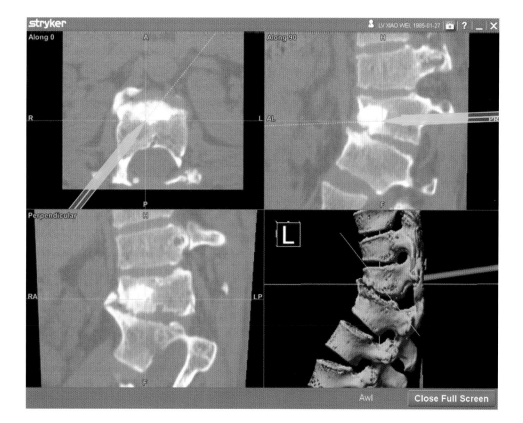

Fig. 16.65 Postoperative anteroposterior and lateral X-rays showed satisfied correction of local kyphosis with Cobb angle of 5°

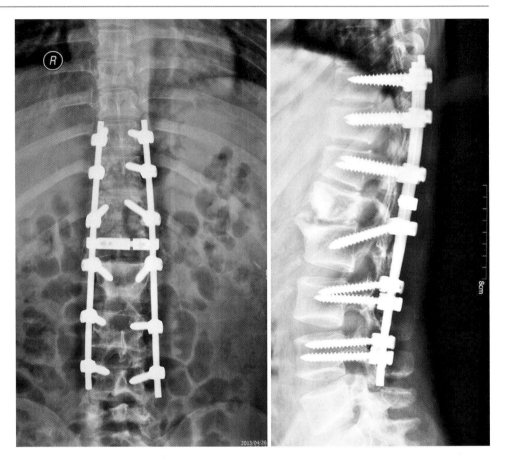

Fig. 16.66 Postoperative standing position, full-spine lateral X-ray showed Cobb angle was 60°; 1-week postoperative X-ray showed Cobb angle of kyphosis of 5°. Half a year after operation, X-ray showed Cobb angle was 6°, fusion was achieved, and kyphosis was not aggravated

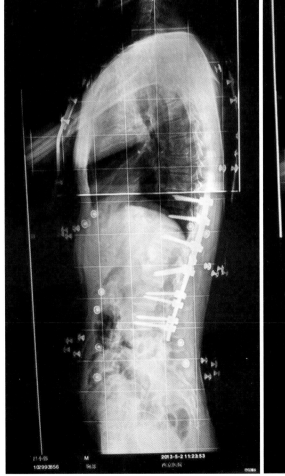
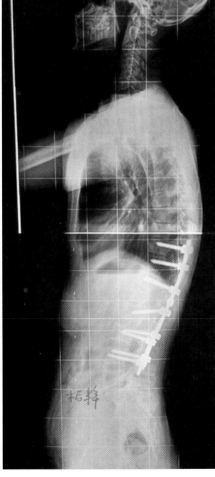

7 Application of Computer-Assisted Navigation Orthopedic Technology in Total Hip Arthroplasty and Total Knee Arthroplasty

Weihua Xu, Shuhua Yang, and Ruoyu Wang

Artificial joint replacement is one of the most successful orthopedic operations in the last century, by which numbers of patients impacted by joint dysfunction are treated and recovered to normal life. At present, total hip arthroplasty and total knee arthroplasty are of great common in joint replacement operations, whose success rates are beyond 90%. And the usage time limit of 80% patients can span over 20 years. Extension of life of artificial joints is due to improvement and consummation of joint design, usage of novel material, and accuracy of the operation.

Computer-assisted navigation technology (CANT) customizes suitable and unique operation plans for patients by bone three-dimensional rebuilding. During the operation, the navigation system tracks surgical instruments in real time and precisely decides the location of artificial joints to be fixed to approach an accurate angle and alignment. Navigation system supervises osteotomy and prosthesis and then detects subtle mistakes in time as well as corrects them, which makes the locating of arthroplasty more precise and process more controllable. The usage of CANT emancipates arthroplasty from naked eye measurement and manual operation and elevates fidelity from 0.1 to 0.2 mm far beyond the detection of naked eye. Thus, CANT helps to implant prosthesis in an ideal way, which extends the usage of prosthesis, reduces the rate of revision, and improves function after surgery. Admittedly, CANT cannot be widely used because it still has several drawbacks of high expansion, extension of time cost, etc. But we anticipate that usage of digital technology in arthroplasty is of great prosperity in the future.

CANT-based arthroplasty should build up a 3-D model of patient's bone, which has two sources. One is from data of CT or MRI scan of the patient, called CT-based navigation. Patients have to take a CT or MRI scan before surgery; after the data is transmitted into navigation system, computer rebuilds a 3-D model. The advantage of this method is the model having the same structure as the bones of the patient, while the drawbacks are extension expansion and preoperation time because of CT or MRI scan. The other one does not need a CT or MRI scan, called CT-free navigation. The computer has stored an advanced database containing numbers of 3-D models of normal and osteoarthritis. During the surgery, operators should define several important anatomic markers which a computer can compare to existing 3-D models and create a new one fitting to the patient. The advantage of this method is handy, without a CT or MRI scan, shortened time span, and reduced expansion. The limit

is that if important anatomic markers collected are not sufficient or incorrect, the model built is inconsistent with the bones of the patient, especially when the patient has apparent abnormal anatomic structures, for instance, fracture near the joints caused by malunion and severe acetabular dysplasia.

To accord the 3-D models with bone anatomic structures, operators should match the real anatomic structures with digital 3-D model, which is called registration. Two methods are provided for registration, one is pivoting and the other point acquisition. Pivoting involves rotating the femur in a circular manner until a sufficient number of points have been acquired. When navigation system acquires enough data of special position of pivoting movement, it then calculates the center of rotation of the femur head. The software uses pivoting to determine the rotational center of the femoral head, which then defines the starting point of the mechanical axis. Pointing acquisition includes two manners, one single landmark acquisition and the other multiple landmark acquisition. By single landmark acquisition, important landmarks are registered by holding the tip of the pointer to the relevant bone structure. On screen, points will be presented to indicate where the landmark should be acquired. Multiple landmark acquisition is used to register bone areas. Points acquired in this way are used to calculate the 3-D bone model.

Additionally, another method for registration is called fluoroscopic registration (Fig. 16.67), by using C-arm fluo-

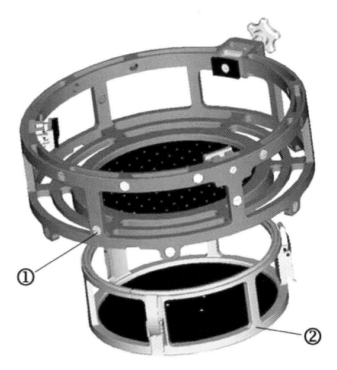

Fig. 16.67 Fluoroscopic registration. ① Reflective marker plate and ② calibration plate

roscopy instrument during surgery. It is mainly applied in CT-free navigation. Before registration, registration suite which contains a reflective marker plate and calibration plate should be firmly attached to fluoroscopic arm. The reflective marker plate is to record infrared to help navigation system to acquire spatial location. Wolfram element on the calibration plate is to decide location in fluoroscopic images. For fluoroscopic registration, every part of the bones should take two images in different directions.

7.1 Application of CANT in Total Hip Arthroplasty

Position of prosthesis is an important factor of short- and long-term success of total hip arthroplasty (THA) in both rigidity and function of artificial articulations. Severe poor cup position is associated with dislocation leading to failure of the operation. Slight poor cup position is related to accelerated polyethylene wear and dash in parts reducing the life of artificial joints. Saxler G applied THA for 105 patients with free hand, and the angles of inclination and anteversion of the cup were measured by CT scan. A safe position as defined by Lewinnek was only achieved in a minority of the cups that were implanted freehand. Lass R compared the acetabular component position when using the imageless navigation system compared to the freehand conventional technique for THA, and the result was published in a paper of randomized controlled trial. There was no significant difference for postoperative mean inclination, but a significant difference for mean postoperative acetabular component anteversion between the computer-assisted and the freehand-placement group. A smaller variation in the positioning of the acetabular component in the navigated group than in the non-navigated group was indicated by the lower standard deviations for the inclination and anteversion angles. In addition, the difference of postoperative leg discrepancy usually causes abnormal gait, back pain, and decline of satisfaction of patients, which is hardly avoided in free hand and mechanically guided techniques. Several papers have reported that CANT in arthroplasty acquires higher implantation accuracy and reduction deviation from the target position.

7.1.1 Process of CANT-Based THA

Pre-operation Preparation

Besides routine preparation, CANT-based THA requires to move the system into the desired position, connect cables correctly, input information of patients and image data, and open navigation software. Reference arrays should be fixed to the pelvic and femur firmly to trace the motion and location of bone structures in the entire operation. The position is usually transverse but the fix of reference arrays requires supine. In the process, sterilization should be considered in all the steps. The arrays are fixed where the operation process cannot be interfered, and they are usually attached beside the iliac crest. All the process should be under the camera scope of navigation system.

Registration

The pelvis can be registered after installation of the reference arrays. As the body's frontal plane is quite different with the position change, with computer-aided navigation, the plane where the anterior-superior iliac spine and pubic tubercle are located is set as the frontal pelvic plane. The navigation system can calculate the frontal plane of the pelvis and the median sagittal plane through a single point of registration of the above four points. Navigation system is with respect to the calculation of these two faces, inclination and anteversion, and other important indices of some of the acetabulum.

After pelvis registration is completed, replace the surgery position to one needed, perform routine disinfection, and fix femur reference arrays in the distal femur. Through pivoting movement operators should determine the center of rotation of the femoral head, by single-point registration method to determine the internal and external femoral condyle (Fig. 16.68). Only after cutting joint capsule to reveal hip and dislocated hip joint that trochanter vertex and pyriform can be registered. The operator should perform femoral neck osteotomy to reveal the acetabulum, and multiple landmark acquisition is used to determine the acetabular and articular surface and the rim. Navigation system can calculate the 3-D model of the femur and the acetabulum by the above registration point. The surgical operation can be displayed in real time on the screen of the system after then, and the system will also give important parameters of angle and distance.

If the acetabular prosthesis template is imported into the navigation system, the surgeon can also perform electronically surgical planning, and ideal size and location of the prosthesis will be displayed on the screen. If hip arthroplasty devices are equipped with navigation instruments in supporting navigation, operators need only to choose instruments with proper size, and the system can automatically identify and calculate the angle and distance; if not, instruments should be registered and adjusted by calibrator (Fig. 16.69) every time before operation.

Navigating the Operation

(1) Preparation of Acetabular

The purpose of reaming is to remove diseased bone and cartilage and to make room for a cup implant so that the center of the original acetabulum can be restored. In

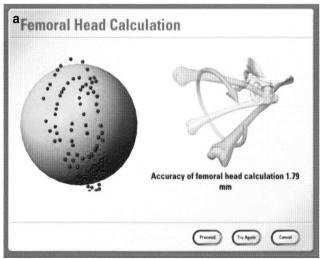
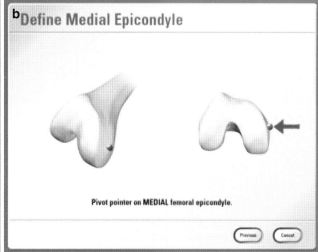

Fig. 16.68 (**a**) Pivoting movement to determine the center of rotation of the femoral head and (**b**) single-point registration

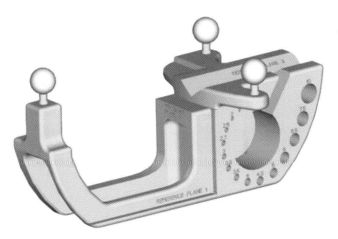

Fig. 16.69 Navigation calibrator

order to insert the cup implant at the desired angle, it is important to ream the bone at the same angle as the planned cup. Superiority of navigation lies in that during reaming, the cup operators can understand the angle directly from the system's screen including inclination and anteversion, so as to adjust to the desired cup angle. As the same with conventional hip arthroplasty operators should gradually increase the wear of reaming size until it fits the appropriate size. When implanting acetabular cup, operators should choose appropriate angle implants according to the angle displayed on the screen. After implantations, cup placement should be validated. The system can give the specific parameters of cup placement and angle for the operators to determine whether the cup position is appropriate.

(2) Preparation of the Femur

The incorrect size and location of the femoral stem often lead to unequal length of both legs, which often leads to patient poor satisfaction. Conventional methods of hip arthroplasty are difficult to completely avoid limb length. Operators have been plagued by the problem of how to restore patients' accurate leg length. In femoral preparation, computer navigation technology provides the conditions to restore limb length. Navigation femoral surgery often requires the use of customized handles and special adapters, whose sizes have been imported into the navigation system, so that handles and adapters need not to be calibrated. Operators should input the model of handles and adapters, and once completed, the system displays the deviations of location of canal reamer and the center of femoral head. As the position of the handle is calculated by the position of canal reamer, model of the reamer should be updated when cup reaming. Femoral implant can be validated by special verification tool. The system can calculate the height, eccentricity, and anteversion of the femoral stem, for surgery to determine whether the size and location of the handle are appropriate.

Navigation has no use in femoral side navigation if the branch of prosthesis does not have special tools. However, Renkawitz et al. created a method to use computer navigation technology to check the length of the lower limbs under the situation lack of special tools. After the trial of prosthetic, hip implant should be reset into the acetabular. Navigation system can measure the position of the screw in order to determine the length and eccentricity of lower limb after arthroplasty.

System Shutdown

A report of the operation parameters can be generated before shutdown for archiving and research.

7.2 Application of CANT in Total Knee Arthroplasty

Total knee arthroplasty (TKA) is regarded as the most reliable method to treat knee dysfunction, for instance, osteoarthritis, and it can effectively relieve pain and improve knee function. However, patient satisfaction after TKA is largely dependent on the axis of the lower extremities and balance of ligaments. It is reported that the incidence of aseptic loosening of prosthesis relatively increases as postoperative limb alignment deviation. It is reported that varus or valgus in frontal plane with a deviation less than 3° has better long-term follow-up results. Rand and Coventry found that patients with axial deviation less than 4° have the 10-year survival rate of 90%. Whereas, if the axis deviation is greater than 4°, 10-year survival of varus will be reduced to 73% and 71% in valgus. Hvid and Nielsen surveyed 138 cases of TKA limb alignment, and long-term follow-up of patients with femorotibial angle of 5–7° has better results. The results of 421 cases by Ritter analyze femorotibial angle of TKA patients (normal is 5–8°, inner turn less than 4°, eversion more than 9°), showing that an incidence rate of aseptic loosening of patients is the highest in patients with varus. Jeffrey analyzed the results of 115 cases of postoperative TKA patients, illustrating that patients whose postoperative limb alignment of varus or valgus deviation exceeded ± 3 degrees, had an incidence of aseptic loosening of 24%, while it is only 3% in patients with deviation within ± 3 degrees. Petersen and Engh report that lower limb alignment varus or valgus deviation of 19% patients exceeds ±3°. Mahaluxmivala reports the results of 673 cases of TKA and finds 25% of patients in the postoperative limb alignment varus or valgus deviation exceeds ±3°. Xu Weihua conducts a prospective comparative study of the line power cord and lower limb prosthesis position of the patient's knee replacement surgery using computer navigation and traditional methods finding that in traditional methods of knee surgery, 17% of patients' limb alignment has varus or valgus deviation exceeding ±3°, while it is only 7% in computer navigation surgery. Due to the precision of knee replacement surgery than hip prosthesis placed directly which affects the accuracy of the curative effect and the life of artificial joints, more doctors use the navigation line knee replacement surgery than hip replacement surgery.

7.2.1 Process of CANT-Based TKA

Preparation of Surgery

TKA has the same preparation with THA; navigation systems need to be placed in the appropriate location and connected with a cable to transfer data necessary for entering patient data and imaging data and the navigation procedures opened required for initial settings. Due to knee registration without changing position, routine disinfection and cover can be carried out with towels after completion.

Registration

Reference array can be installed after the skin incision and knee revealed. The reference array is usually placed in the distal femur and tibia in the lower section. During the installation, pay attention to avoiding the site of joint replacement surgical procedure, and ensure that the navigation system is located within the surgical procedure in the detection range of the camera. The purpose of registration is to determine the center of rotation of the femoral head and ankle center, as well as the anatomy of the distal femur and proximal tibia main parameters. After registering the computer navigation system, real-time monitoring the lower limbs and power lines as well as determining the thickness and angle of each knee osteotomy plane through modules can be achieved.

After the navigation system detects the femur and tibia reference arrays, system enters registration steps. The system automatically reminds the contents and methods of registration. Initially, the pivoting motion is determined by the rotational center of the femoral head, which is the starting point of the lower extremities and the force line of the femur. Then, after points of inside and outside malleolus are registered, the system can calculate the midpoint of the ankle joint which is the end of the lower extremities and alignment of tibia. Alignment of the end of the tibia and start of femur force is registered by direct pointregistration (Fig. 16.70). To rebuild

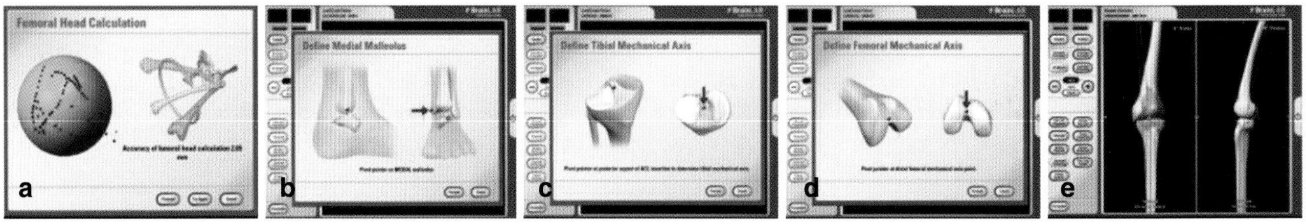

Fig. 16.70 (**a**) Determination of power line by registration and determination of rotation pivot by rotation of the femur head. (**b**) Point registration to determine the inside malleolus. (**c**) Point registration to determine the start of force starting line. (**d**) End of the tibia and femur force. (**e**) Power line displayed on the screen

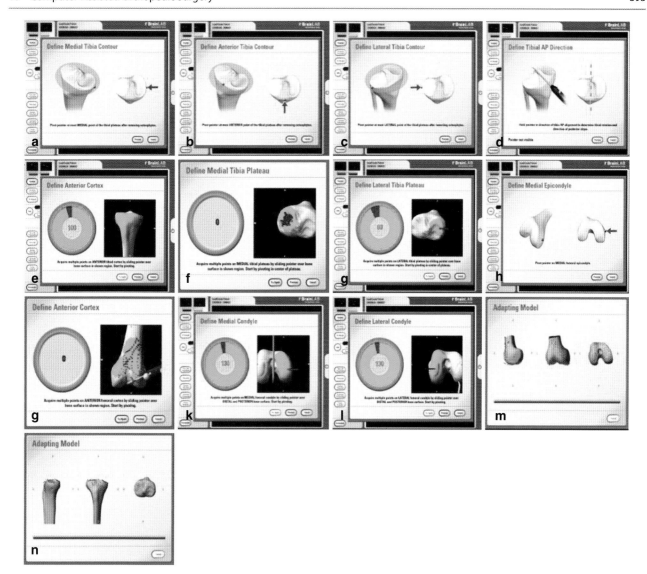

Fig. 16.71 Navigation system collecting anatomic landmarks and direction of proximal tibia and distal femur; boundary point around tibial outer and inner side (**a–c**). Longitudinal direction of the tibial plateau (**d**). Tibial anterior cortical bone surface (**e**). Articular surface of the lateral tibial platform (**f, g**). Inside and outside condylar (h). Front femoral cortical bone surface. Using registration navigation system to generate a 3-D digital model of the knee surgery (**g**). Articular surface of the femoral inside and outside condylar (**k, l**). 3-D digital model generated by computer system (**m, n**)

the bones around the form of a knee, the navigation system will in turn collect important anatomical marks and direction of proximal tibia and distal femur, including boundary point around tibial outer and inner side, the longitudinal direction of the tibial plateau, tibial anterior cortical bone surface, articular surface of the lateral tibial platform, femoral condyle, femoral osteotomy plane reference points, Whiteside line, articular surface of the femoral inside and outside condylar, front femoral cortical bone surface, etc. Using registration navigation system to generate a 3-D digital model of the knee surgery (Fig. 16.71), surgery can be performed after testing the accuracy of navigation.

Navigation Surgery

Preparation of Tibia
By selecting *Tibia Cut* button, operators can activate the navigation tibial osteotomy guide and insert the tibial osteotomy adapter into the osteotomy module slots. Once the adapter enters the range of the camera, the system displays the virtual osteotomy plane on the screen and prompts an angle and thickness of osteotomy. Operators should adjust the position of the tibial osteotomy module to the desired thickness and angle (Fig. 16.72). After completion of the osteotomy of the tibia, operator should select *Update the Tibia Cut*, and the

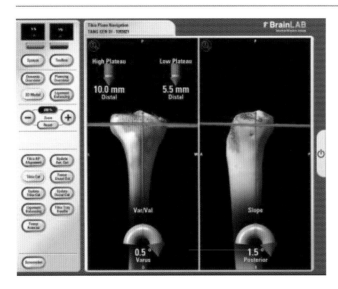

Fig. 16.72 Desired thickness and angle of tibial osteotomy displayed on screen

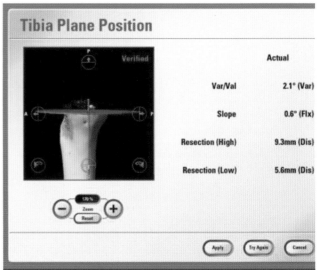

Fig. 16.73 The proximal of tibial osteotomy plane removed from the 3-D virtual model

osteotomy adapter should be placed on the surface of the tib-ial osteotomy for about 2 s. Thus, the system can automati-cally calculate the parameters of the osteotomy plane. If it is satisfied, click *Apply* button to update tibial osteotomy plane. Then, the proximity of tibial osteotomy plane will be removed from the 3-D virtual model (Fig. 16.73).

Two optimal methods can be chosen to locate rotation of the tibial plateau navigation. One is to use the navigation pointer on the tibial anteroposterior direction. The pointer and angle of tibia direction can be displayed on screen. Operator should adjust the direction of the pointer to overlap with the tibia forward and backward and then place the tibial plateau according to the direction of pointer. The other method is to place navigation adapters on the tibial plateau handle and then adjust the position and direction of the tibial plateau to the desired location.

Preparation of the Femur

By selecting distal *Femur Distal Cut* button to activate the navigation guidance distal femoral osteotomy, operator inserts the osteotomy plane adapter into the osteotomy module slot. As same as tibial osteotomy, once the adapter enters the range of the camera, the system displays the virtual osteotomy plane on the screen and prompts an angle and thickness of osteot-omy. Operators should adjust the position of the femur oste-otomy module to the desired thickness and angle (Fig. 16.74). After osteotomy, select *Update the Distal Femoral Cut button*. The osteotomy adapter should be placed on the surface of the femur osteotomy for about 2 s. Thus, the system can automati-cally calculate the parameters of osteotomy plane. If it is satis-fied, click *Apply* button to update femur osteotomy plane. Then, the distance of femur osteotomy plane will be removed from the 3-D pelvic model (Fig. 16.75).

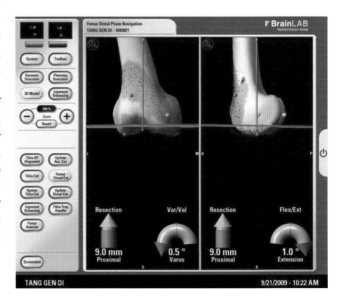

Fig. 16.74 Desired thickness and angle of femur osteotomy displayed on screen

Select Femur *FourInOne* button to enter the femoral osteotomy navigation. Osteotomy adapter should be inserted into the first slot of *FourInOne* module, and anterior femo-ral osteotomy plane is displayed on the screen as well as posterior femoral condyle line, Whiteside line, and inside rotation angle of condyle and epicondyle. Osteotomy mod-ule should be modified with property angle and height and operator should fix osteotomy module to perform osteotomy. To update the anterior femoral cut should be chosen to remove the front side of the femoral bone from the femur model.

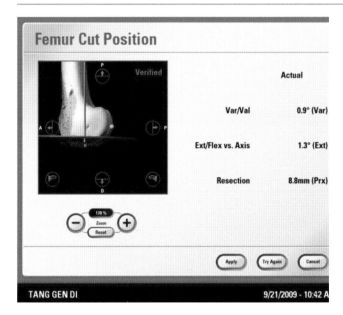

Fig. 16.75 Distance of femur osteotomy plane removed from the 3-D pelvic mode

Fixing Prosthesis

Operator should complete the osteotomy of the femur and tibia according to knee osteotomy mold, fix mold, move knee, and detect internal and external ligament flexion gap balance. Knee prosthesis should be placed finally.

System Shutdown

A report of the operation parameters can be generated before shutdown for archiving and research.

7.3 Prospect of THA and TKA by CANT

It is obvious that CANT has several advantages, making surgery more controllable and precise and promoting operation more intuitive of bone malformation diseases. However, CANT in THA and TKA is not widely performed, mainly because of high expense of devices. Only a small number of large medical institutions purchase such equipment. Moreover, preparation should be performed in navigation operations, extending the span of operation time. When installing reference arrays, holes are required to be drilled to increase bone trauma surgery.

The development of computer-aided surgical navigation in future has several directions. The first is to reduce the cost of equipment, making it lighter and smaller to carry, as well as improving the use experience and efficiency. More doctors and patients can benefit from high-quality effects from computer navigation surgery. There are already some portable devices, such as IASSIST Knee Navigation System of Zimmer. The second is to make operation easier, faster in registration, and less invasive in surgery. Holes are not

needed to fix reference array. Thirdly, in addition to precise navigation osteotomy, the balance of the soft tissue can be accurately assessable. Balance of ligaments around the joints at different angles will be calculated to achieve the best reconstruction and recovery. Fourthly, as improvement of surgical navigation technology, some or all of the process will be completed by computers. The development of these technologies will lead to the improvement of the accuracy of surgery which cannot be reached by naked eye and hand. CANT will improve human health.

8 Musculoskeletal Tumor Surgery Aided by Computer-Assisted Navigation System

In recent years, computer-assisted navigation system (CANS) is a novel rapidly developing technique in surgery, especially in orthopedic surgery. This technique can not only achieve human-computer interaction but also be used for operation planning, intervention, and evaluation by using multivariate data and system software quantitatively. This technique has some special advantages, including better 3-D image reconstruction, computer-aided imaging, computer simulation operation, and surgical robots. Thus, compared with traditional surgery technique, CANS has more unique advantages not only in benign bone tumor surgery but also in surgical treatment of malignant bone tumors.

Since 1999, the orthopedic surgical navigation system has been successfully applied in spine surgery, joint replacement, limb fractures, pelvic osteotomy, and other surgery. In 2004, Hufner reported cases treating pelvic malignancies assisted by CANS. In 2007, Kwok-Chuen Wong completed pelvic bone tumor resection and prosthesis reconstruction by using CANS. In the same year, Stockle reported pelvic tumor resection by using CT and MRI imaging navigation. In 2014, Cartiaux reported precise resection and reconstruction of the pelvic tumors with 3-D technology and navigation. After that, CANS has been widely applied in the field of bone tumors treatment.

Application of computer-aided techniques in orthopedic surgery was named as computer-aided orthopedic surgery (CAOS). CAOS has been proven to be an effective method in bone tumor resection and reconstruction. The greatest advantage is realizing the accurate location during the surgery, which enables the surgeon to know the exact location. Through continuous adjustment intraoperatively, CAOS can realize bone tumor resection and accurate installation prosthesis. In the meantime, it can supervise and verify surgeons' operating results. Many reports show that through navigation techniques, precise bone tumor resection and reconstruction can be achieved and thus ensure the surgical outcomes of bone tumor treatment.

8.1 Common Computer-Aided Navigation System and Working Principle

Depending on the navigation signal, computer-aided navigation can be classified into optical (infrared) positioning, magnetic (EMF) positioning, acoustic (ultrasonic signals) positioning, and mechanical positioning. From the initial CT interactive navigation to today's optical navigation and electromagnetic navigation, positioning accuracy and clinical usefulness have been improved.

In 1986, Japan, the United States, and Switzerland have developed almost simultaneously interactive navigation device consisting of CT machine, which is the first of CAOS technology. In 1990, Sofamor Company launched the world's first optical for orthopedic surgical navigation system and put into clinical use. A new generation of navigation system based on active optical navigation technology, with higher positioning accuracy, has been used widely. In addition, this technique is also the leading signal transduction in treatment of bone tumors. By using a camera as a sensor, the use of infrared space position and infrared light-emitting diode can determine the position and orientation of the surgical instrument, which guide doctors to complete the operation. Germany AESCULAP OrthoPilot navigation system uses the same principle, with the system accuracy of 1 mm. The advantages include easy to replace surgical instruments, small size, easy to operate, tracking multiple targets, and faster. The disadvantages are susceptible to interference by background light in operating room and other factors, like too expensive. At present, navigation system includes CLIPSS system developed by IBM Japan Tokyo Institute; FluoroNavTM orthopedic surgery navigation system developed by Medtronic, Switzerland Medvision system; and Germany OrthoPilot system. However, the active optical navigation system developed by Stryker is the most widely used nowadays. In China, Stryker surgical navigation system has been used since 2000. The company has also developed dedicated software modules including spine surgery, trauma surgery, joint surgery, neurosurgery, and ENT navigation. In recent years, bone tumor surgery software modules have been successfully developed (Fig. 16.76).

The computer-assisted navigation system is a three-dimensional (3-D) tracking system and works as Global Positioning System (GPS). In brief, the radiological data are obtained via preoperative CT or MRI scan and reformatted into coronal, axial, sagittal, and 3-D views of the bone using the navigation system, by image rectification and image fusion and marked virtual coordinates. The surgeon can complete the pre-operation plan such as tumor margin marking and special prosthesis design and simulate operation according to the virtual images. During the operation, the immediate position (the actual coordinates) between the operating instruments and patient's anatomical structure is

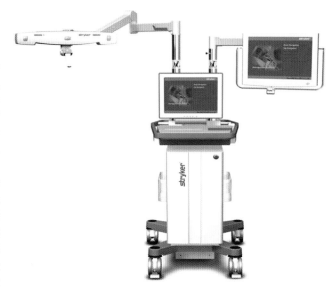

Fig. 16.76 Stryker Company's active optical navigation system

tracked by the infrared probe and displayed on the 2-D and 3-D digital images. Then, the surgeons could judge and debug the operative approach and the operative angle and depth, for avoiding the danger area, by matching the virtual and actual coordinates, and get the access to the aimed lesion area in short time.

The basic configuration of computer-assisted navigation system mainly consists of three parts, image workstation (image processing software, such as Simpleware and Mimics software), position detection device, and special surgical instruments and adapters.

8.2 The Applied Range of the Computer-Aided Surgical Navigation Technology in Bone Tumor Surgery

Based on the veracity and operability of this new technology, the clinical situations with the following criteria were considered eligible for navigational surgery:

1. To determine the tumor safety margin: the computer-assisted navigation could help define the area of the tumor invasion, by the fusion of the digital images such as CT, MRI, and PET-CT images.
2. To assist the micro-damage curettage of the benign bone tumor: the navigation system could guide the curettage of benign bone tumor such as osteoid osteoma and osteochondromatosis, especially in complex anatomical structure such as the proximal femur. The tumor can be precisely located and removed without the damage of the normal structure caused by the error of the traditional digital images, which benefits the postoperative functional excise.

3. To guide the joint preservation surgery and specially constructed prosthesis replacement for juxta-articular bone tumor: for this type of bone tumor including a tumor involving mostly the distal femur, proximal tibia, and proximal humerus, the traditional standard transverse osteotomies employed under intraoperative fluoroscopy surgery would jeopardize safe surgical margin and even the articular surface, thus necessitating osteoarticular resection and prosthesis replacement. The navigation system can spare the joint and preserve enough marked structure to special prosthesis reconstruction with less occurrence of prosthesis mismatch and loosing.

4. To enable the excising of tumors involving a complex anatomical structure: tumors in a complex anatomical structure such as the pelvic ring, with low sight of the lesion and its adjacent tissue, have been a challenge to excise the lesion and restore. With the navigation system, the preoperative fusion of CT and MRI could clear the lesion invasion of pelvic, especially in periacetabular (II pelvic area) and sacroiliac joint (IV pelvic area), assist the tumor excising according to the preoperative plan, and consequently salvage the loading bone for restoration.

5. To benefit the refining of allograft bone prosthesis and accurate reconstruction: the navigation system could assist the allograft bone replacement to restore the defect caused by the tumor excision, especially in children and adolescents. The technology could achieve the refinement and matching of bone prosthesis in accordance with the defect area, avoiding the articular surface irregularity.

8.3   The Navigation Surgery Procedure

A computer-assisted navigation surgery would include preoperative planning, prosthesis design and fabrication, intraoperative execution of surgical planning, and post-validation (Fig. 16.77).

8.3.1   Preoperative Planning and Manufacture of Implants

Determine the Tumor Safe Margin Based on Image Fusion

The ability to preoperatively define a resection on an imaging study and then precisely carry out that plan with an exact level of precision in the operating room can be considered as the primary benefit of navigation for orthopedic oncologists. The bone tumor resection would remove the bone tumor block and surrounding tissue. However, no single type of image completely manifests the complicated tis-

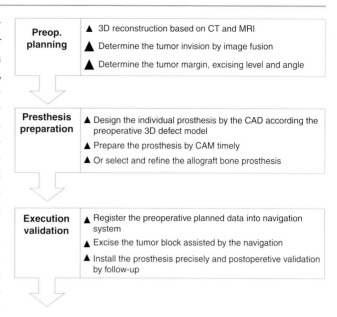

Fig. 16.77   A summary of a generic procedure for computer-assisted navigation in bone tumor surgery. (*CAD* computer-assisted design, *CAM* computer-assisted manufacture)

sue, necessitating the gathering of preoperative multiple forms of images including noninvasive X-ray, computed tomography (CT), magnetic resonance imaging (MRI), and positron emission tomography (PET-CT). X-ray reveals the lesion contour. CT is used primarily for evaluation of the bone cortex and provides detailed bony anatomy. MRI is preferred for soft-tissue anatomy and can better evaluate the extent of a pathologic process within the bone and bone marrow than a CT. PET-CT scans are a form of biologic imaging that demonstrates levels of labeled glucose uptake, which can help differentiate regions of tumor involvement from abnormal but nonneoplastic areas. Given the relative strengths and weaknesses of each modality, a fused image with multiple modalities represented on one screen could have significant benefit on the oncology surgeon during preoperative planning for tumor resection. With the fusion of images, mostly the CT and MRI images, and threshold image segmentation algorithm which is based on gradient (the bone cortex is about 2000), the surgeons could rebuild the 3-D fusing image and identify the structures containing muscle, nerve, blood vessel, and bone tumor, as well as the osseous component, soft tissue, and necrotic tissue in the tumor block. By analyzing the different levels of fusing image, the tumor spatial configuration and safe margin could be defined (Fig. 16.78). The surgeons could determine the tumor resection range according to the Enneking grade and mark it for the computer-assisted navigation surgery.

Digital Data Collection and Image Fusion

Preoperative CT and MRI examinations of the patients were performed. Axial CT images of the lesion and surrounding

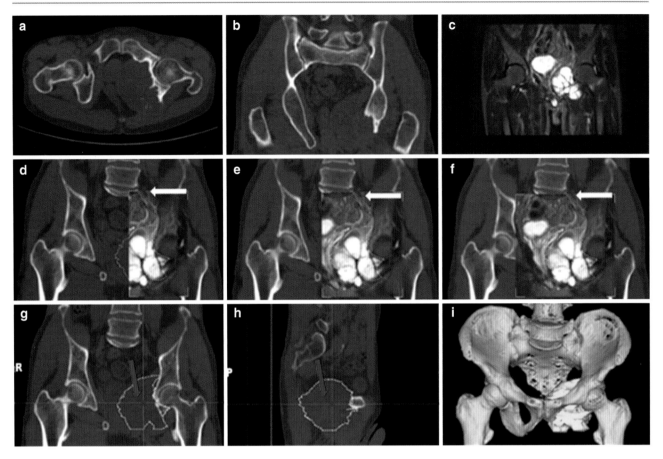

Fig. 16.78 The navigation-assisted preoperative planning: (**a**) the horizontal CT image of the pelvis. (**b**) The reconstructed image based on CT data. (**c**) The reconstructed image based on MRI data. (**d–f**) The process of the image fusion (the *white arrow* indicated the direction of the fusion). (**g, h**) The CT-based reconstructed image showed the tumor area (indicated by the *red arrow*). (**i**) The 3-D rendering image by image fusion (the *yellow arrow* indicated the tumor area)

area were acquired using a 16-detector scanner, and slices mostly with 0.625 mm (no more than 2 mm) were obtained, while MRI of the corresponding region was acquired using a 3 T unit, and the slice was more accurately thinner. The fusion of CT and MRI yields hybrid images that combine the key characteristics of each technique and enable better interpretation of each and accurate position of the lesion. Post-contrast T1-weighted axial images were used for fusion with CT images in view of better bone-soft tissue contrast. Image data sets would be saved in the format of DICOM 3.0 and imported into the Stryker navigation system for fusion. Because of the differences of slice thickness, image resolution, and stereotaxy despite the homology, the process is no single fusion and involved cross-sectional matching of the anatomic structures on the CT with those on the MRI image.

The system allowed CT and MRI images to be fused by matching segmented known structures in corresponding MRI and CT data sets manually. Firstly, the MRI data were input into the Simpleware software, and the MRI image processing requires the use of an interactive segmentation method, can be divided with a threshold segmentation tools

target area, and the threshold values used herein is not meaningful Hounsfield values, but only an MRI image is converted to a visible image on a display gray degree standard value, the human eye can distinguish gray to be displayed. Then, use brushes and seed filling and other segmentation tools in each 2-D image of a MRI flexible split out tumor invasion area. Save the tumor model MRI reconstruction of STL format for output, and select obvious sign point, and then import the data to the model CT reconstruction; with the use of the above sign point registration, adjust the spatial location of tumor models and complete the CT and MRI 3-D image fusion (Fig. 16.79). The fused image model must be kept in the same coordinate system without the resegmentation or reconstruction, in order to keep the unified coordinates when transferring into the navigation system. In the process of 3-D model, to ensure that the coordinate system of the original data remains unchanged, do not transform the 3-D coordinate system, and the volumetric data set cannot be recut or recombinant, because to convert the data in a variety of software and navigation systems or transmission model, there is a uniform 3-D coordinate reference.

The Design and Fabrication of Individual Prosthesis

For the reservation of limb function, accurate precision and reconstruction would attract the surgeon's attention. One of the potential benefits of navigation in orthopedic oncology is the ability to design complex individual prosthesis preoperatively according to the tumor site and lesion invasion, which need multiple department collaborations from different disciplines including surgeon, engineers of navigation, CAD, and CAM. The individual prosthesis is classified as basic ones and improved ones.

1. Basic individual prosthesis
   Based on the 3-D reconstructive image on the navigation system after image fusion, the tumor area was trimmed to get rid of the insignificant bony bumps according to the preoperative precision plan and exported in STL. It would be necessary to collect parameters of the contralateral

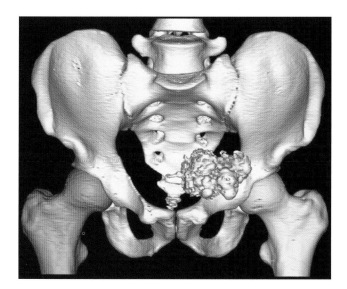

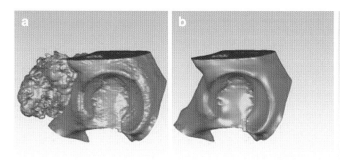

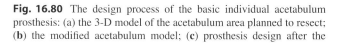

Fig. 16.79 The 3-D reconstruction renderings of the pelvis and tumor by CT data

bone when the bone was damaged badly. The STL data was input into the UG NX7.5 software (Siemens PLM Software, Germany), extracting and simplifying the excision level to achieve the tumor model parameterization. The design would be accomplished by the CAD engineer in the view of the surgeons' preoperative plan. Some accessory structures would be designed when necessary such as surrounding edge slot and mounting instruments for the acetabulum prosthesis (Fig. 16.80).

2. Improved individual prosthesis
   Unlike the basic prosthesis fully imitating the bony contour and its resulting difficulty in prosthesis design and manufacture, the improved individual prosthesis merely needs to retain and design the main bony structures. Take the acetabulum, for example, the parameters of precision level in the upper margin of acetabulum were collected, and the others were abandoned. Then, the structure of acetabulum was fitted as spherical surface and the acetabular lateral as flat surface. The parameters of the tip mounting the surface and the size and angle of the prosthesis were obtained and transformed. Consequently, the parameters were imported into UG software for prosthesis design by CAD engineer. Acetabular prosthesis wall thickness is 4 mm, establishing a spherical acetabular fitting concentric spherical 4 mm radius increases and the shear plane with the outer edge of the acetabulum both spherical, and the structure is formed semicircular acetabulum, the acetabular cup to complete design. The acetabular osteotomy plane on the edge of the contour lines extends outward 2 mm, to establish a new plane, and some distance down the stretch direction of the acetabulum, so that intersect with the acetabular cup, then trim, stitch, make faces, and other operations complete the overall appearance of the prosthesis design (Fig. 16.81).

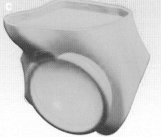

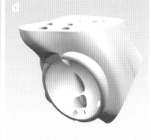

Fig. 16.80 The design process of the basic individual acetabulum prosthesis: (a) the 3-D model of the acetabulum area planned to resect; (b) the modified acetabulum model; (c) prosthesis design after the parameters was transformed; (d) the design of the accessory trajectory of the prosthesis

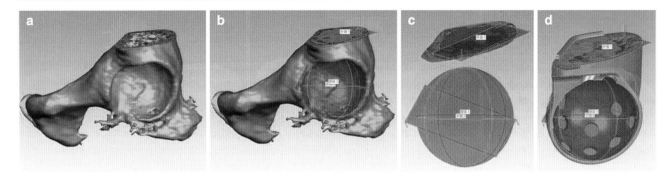

Fig. 16.81 The design process of the improved individual acetabulum prosthesis: (**a**) the 3-D model of the acetabulum area planned to resect. (**b**) The contour of acetabulum area was extracted and fitted as spherical surface and flat surface. (**c**) Parameterize the fitted structures. (**d**) Achieve the design of the prosthesis

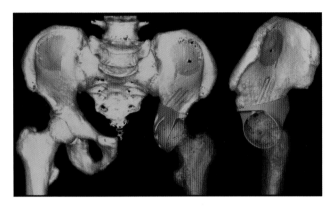

Fig. 16.82 The computer-imitating reconstruction of the improved individual acetabulum prosthesis

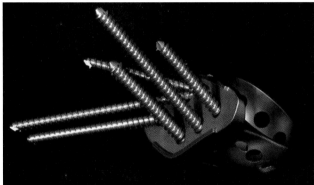

Fig. 16.83 Modified individual acetabular prosthesis

3. Prosthesis computer imitating or pre-installation
   Before the prosthesis was manufactured, it was necessary to implement the prosthesis computer-imitating installation for its validation. The designed prosthesis model was saved as STL and transferred into the Simpleware software after the preoperative CT-based reconstructive model was imported. Because of the 3-D coordinate system was consistent in all processing, the prosthesis model could be directly positioned in the prescheduled tumor excision site for validating without any rectification. The matching of the designed prosthesis and the reconstructed bone and the conformity of mounting instruments to the plan were verified, and the prosthesis model could be retransferred to the UG software for CAD further modification till it meets the requirements (Fig. 16.82).

In other way, the designed prosthesis could be fabricated by the rapid prototype (RP) using the jaffaite. According to planned precision range, the rapid prototyped prosthesis was pre-installed on an excised saw bone pelvic for the verification. After prosthesis simulated installation verification is satisfied, prosthetic material production preparation with CNC machining center, prosthesis and screws are mostly made of titanium. Accomplished by qualified equipment manufacturers, executors are CAM engineers. Because individual prosthesis has complex surface irregularities, production preparation requires special tools, fixtures, etc. on the manufacturer's manufacturing capacity and higher requirements (Fig. 16.83).

The Digital Bone Bank and Navigation-Assisted Allograft Reconstruction

Establishment of the digital bone bank is considered to significantly shorten the selection time of allograft osteoarticular materials before surgery and improve the selection accuracy compared with routine preparations of osteoarticular allograft, as well as reducing the risks of immunity rejection and disease transmission. Combining the navigation-assisted bone tumor resection and digitally selected allograft osteoarticular reconstruction, the surgeons could employ more accurate and individual operating and reconstructing program to patient with orthopedic oncology.

By using bone bank manage software, massive bone allografts can be classified by anatomical site, including the scapula, clavicle, proximal humerus, distal humerus, ulna, radius, pelvis, proximal femur, distal femur, proximal tibia, distal tibia, fibula, and calcaneus. Allografts were then scanned by 64-row computer tomography (CT) and analyzed. The 3-D information of each allograft, including length, width, and height, was saved in Digital Imaging and Communications in Medicine (DICOM) file format. Important data, such as articular surface and osseous mark, were also noted. All of the information related to the massive bone allografts were coded and saved to establish a digital system for the management and analysis of allografts; as choosing, firstly bone allografts were selected by the size of the bone and distance of osseous mark, and then the definite curve was matched. Before surgery, the digital data of patient including X-ray, CT, MRI, and SPET-CT were collected and processed for definition of the resection range. Then, the data were input into the digital bone bank manage software to match and select the most optimal massive allograft for further intraoperative cutting and trimming for the navigation-assisted reconstruction after the en bloc resection.

Allogeneic bone matching process: preoperative patient's X-ray acquisition, CT, MRI, bone scintigraphy and local SPET/CT and other imaging data, clear tumor boundaries, staging, and develop resection. The preoperative data import digital orthopedic management software on your computer, based on data developed tumors after imaging range, virtual surgery program tumor resection, using a large segment of allogeneic bone repair. After extracting the best match according to a large segment of allograft bone ends after resection of residual bone in the data repository, according to the 3-D shape of the defect after allogeneic bone osteotomy trimming, it can be used for allogeneic bone after tumor resection bone repair.

8.3.2 Navigation-Assisted Surgery

The Bone Tumor Resection
The preparation of navigation surgery was implemented 1 day before the surgery. The CT of lesion area and the preoperative planned parameters, including the resection ones such as resection range, level, and angle as well with the prosthesis mounting parameters such as the trajectory site and orientation, were transferred into the navigation system.

1. Navigation registration and tumor resection
   Registration is a process that correlates points on a patient's body with corresponding points on a navigation image. Several forms of registration exist, and the selection is currently a matter of surgeon's preference. Basically, there are two main registration methods: paired point registration and surface registration. After the appropriate exposure, a tracker was attached to the bone in which the tumor was located. The image-to-patient registration to match the corresponding points between

the patient's real anatomy and preoperative CT images was performed by paired points of four landmarks and surface matching of 50 points.
2. The tumor resection
   Real-time matching between the anatomy and the virtual images was assessed by putting the registration probe on the bone surface and by checking specific known and well-defined landmarks. Next, the navigation probe mounted with navigation trackers (drill and diathermy) were calibrated to the system. This allowed the real-time spatial location of these probes to be displayed in relation to the patient's anatomy. We marked the intended resection by diathermy. The diathermy marks were connected to form the resection plane. The tumor was removed en bloc. The gross margins from tumor to the resection surface were measured on the sectioned specimen. Microscopic examination of the margins then followed to confirm clearance of the tumor. When the gross margins were deemed close, multiple blocks were then obtained perpendicular to the resection plane, and the microscopic margins were measured. The closest microscopic margin was then recorded. Intraoperative error of image-to-patient registration and histologic evaluation of resection margins in all tumor specimens were recorded. The cross sections at the resection plane of the specimens were measured and compared with preoperative plans (Fig. 16.84).

3. Navigation-assisted prosthesis reconstruction
   After the tumor resection, the cross sections at the resection plane of the specimens were measured and compared with preoperative plans. The individual prosthesis was pre-installed and debugged with the aid of the navigation system till the preoperative schedule was achieved (Fig. 16.85).

Bony union was evaluated through plain radiographs. Surveillance for local and systemic relapse consisted of CT of the chest every 3 months. The functional result of the reconstructed limb was assessed with the relevant score system.

8.4 Postoperative Evaluation

All resection specimens underwent pathological examination. Adjuvant therapy was determined according to the different tumor treatments. Patients were followed up on 3, 6, and 12 months postoperatively and annually thereafter. Physical examination, X-ray, and CT were performed to observe the tumor recurrence and metastasis. The International Association of Bone Tumor MSTS functional scores were used for every patient. The clinical outcomes of navigation-assisted bone tube resection and reconstruction were evaluated.

Fig. 16.84 The navigation-assisted resection of recurrent Ewing's bone tumor in the left femur: (**a**) after the appropriate exposure, the tracker was mounted to register and rectification; (**b**) the tumor area was tracked and marked with the aid of navigation; (**c**) the unicondyle was removed; (**d**) show the removed unicondyle

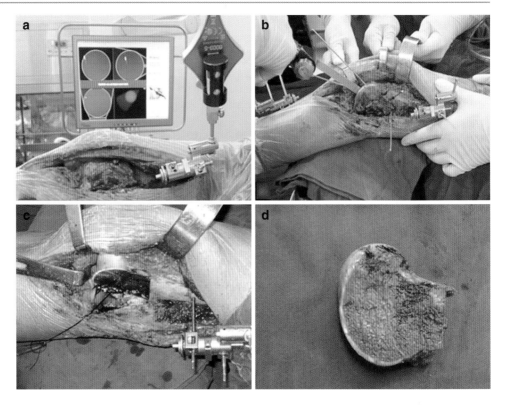

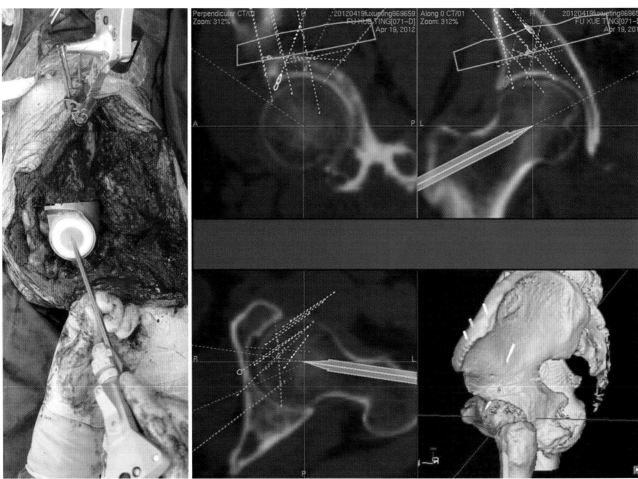

Fig. 16.85 Validation of the acetabulum prosthesis: one indicated the tracker located on the upper margin of the acetabulum (*left*); one indicated the real-time navigation imaging of the acetabulum prosthesis well matched with the upper margin (*right*)

8.5 Pelvic Tumor Resection and Reconstruction

8.5.1 Pelvic Tumor Accurate Resection and Customized Prosthesis Reconstruction

Patient Information: Male/30, Primary Osteosarcoma on the Left Acetabulum, Enneking IIB, with the Invasion of the Acetabulum and the Superior Ramus of the Pubis (Fig. 16.86)

Preoperative Plan

1. Put patient's CT and MRI imaging data into the software; image fusion and analog reconstruction to analyze the tumor resection security boundary and computer simulation reconstruction of tumor resection for intraoperative navigation guidance (Fig. 16.87).
2. Determine the boundaries of surgical resection, osteotomy plane, and angle analyzed according to the principles of tumor resection and pelvic biomechanics. Malignant tumor resection was mainly based on MRI examination outside the normal skeleton shown at the osteotomy of 2–3 cm. Acetabular osteotomy tumor resection needs to determine the three planes (Fig. 16.88): acetabular osteotomy plane of the upper edge of the front side of the pubic ramus, osteotomy plane, and rear ischial support osteotomy plane. Determining the upper edge of the acetabular osteotomy plane is the key, and this plane is necessary to ensure reaching the safe tumor resection border but also to ensure providing the installation of the individual customized prosthesis sufficiently to normal bone bed.
3. After installation of verification simulation prosthesis satisfaction, according to the resection extent of tumor, reconstruct the pelvic bone defect model, in order to carry out individualized prosthetic design, and install computer simulation (Fig. 16.89) and RP prosthesis simulation

in vitro installation (Fig. 16.90) to verify the design of the prosthesis reasonably (Fig. 16.91).

Navigation Surgery

1. Navigation register: prepare the navigation before surgery. Complete routine anesthesia, and navigate registration area after draping and surgical exposure. In the rear of the iliac crest fixed navigation and positioning tracker, calibration, first performed 4:00 registration (generally choose the iliac tubercle on the iliac crest, anterior-superior iliac spine, and the pubic tubercle 4 points), again face registration (usually requiring continuous selection of 40–60 registration points), calculate the average error, and verify the accuracy of navigation after successful registration, and the accuracy of the verification is complete if the navigation is satisfied with the process of registration.

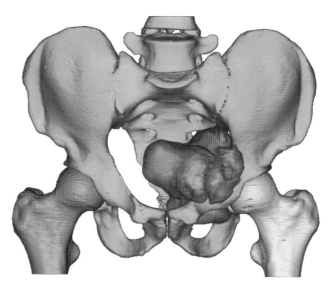

Fig. 16.87 The MRI-CT-based 3-D fused rendering sketch. The *red area* indicated the tumor invasion range based on MRI

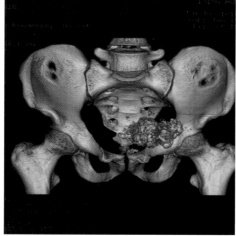
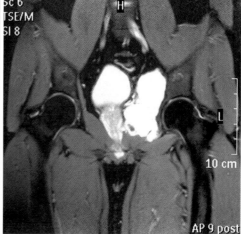

Fig. 16.86 Primary chondrosarcoma of the left pelvic in a 30-year-old male patient: the left indicated the CT-based 3-D tumor image in the inner acetabulum; the right indicated the tumor invasion range of MRI image

2. Tumor resection: according to the design of preoperative acetabular osteotomy plane, under the guidance of the navigation and the use of osteotomy positioning Kirschner wire positioning osteotomy range (Fig. 16.92), carry out osteotomy of acetabular in each osteotomy plane with oscillating saw along the positioning Kirschner wire. Pay

attention to protecting blood vessels and nerves. After completing the bony pelvic osteotomy, separate all directions of sharp dissection and blunt dissection of the tumor from the whole tumor resection.

3. Individualized prosthesis installation: test the individual prosthetic navigation and verify the accuracy of the prosthesis installed (Fig. 16.93).

The Postoperative Follow-Up

Resected specimens were sent for pathological examination, to understand whether the resection is complete. After routine prevention of infection, prevention and treatment of deep vein thrombosis systemic treatments and corresponding brake and functional exercise should be conducted. Patients were followed up on 3, 6, and 12 months postoperatively and annually thereafter. At follow-up of patients with clinical examination, routine pelvic X-ray, and selective pelvis and

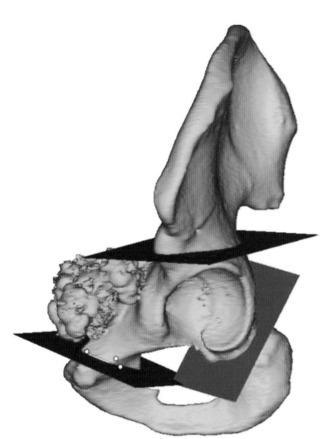

Fig. 16.88 The rendering sketch of the preoperative scheduled resection range of the pelvic chondrosarcoma

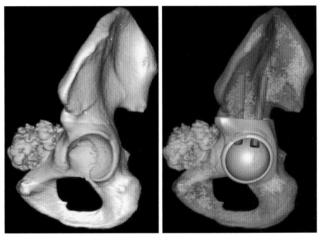

Fig. 16.89 The rendering of the preoperative planned tumor resection range (*left*) and the computer-imitating installation of the individual prosthesis (*right*)

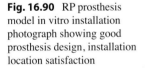

Fig. 16.90 RP prosthesis model in vitro installation photograph showing good prosthesis design, installation location satisfaction

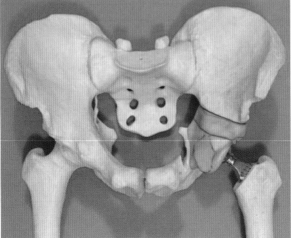
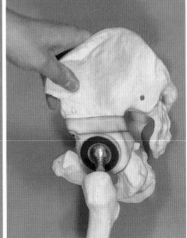

Fig. 16.91 The photo of the surface blast-treated prosthesis manufactured by the CAM engineer

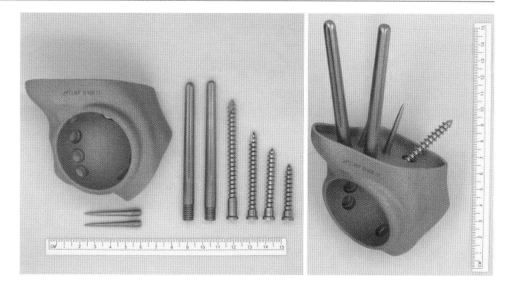

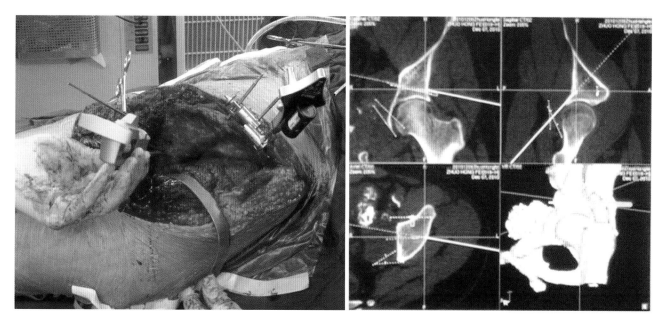

Fig. 16.92 The navigation-assisted tumor resection according to the preoperative plan: the *left* indicated the tracker located in the resection area; the *right* indicated the real-time navigation image while tracking

chest CT scan, observe the presence or absence of tumor recurrence and metastasis, with internationally accepted standard MSTS functional scores, and evaluate the pelvis and hip function reconstruction situation (Figs. 16.94, 16.95, and 16.96).

Semi-pelvic Tumor Accurate Resection and Assembly Prosthesis Reconstruction

Case

Male/32, Primary Chondrosarcoma on the Right Pelvis, Enneking IIB, with the Invasion of the Acetabulum and the Superior Ramus of Pubis Underwent Surgery, and Pathological Diagnosis was Chondrosarcoma

Preoperative Plan

1. Image fusion: preoperative X-ray, CT, MRI, ECT scanning, according to the above method, MRI, ECT fusion in CT imaging, shall be conducted to observe the tumor boundaries and decide the extent of resection with tumor staging. CT and MRI image fusion are the structure images (Fig. 16.97), and ECT fusion is functional image. To structure images (Fig. 16.98), use the same anatomical landmark corresponding method, and fuse CT and MRI

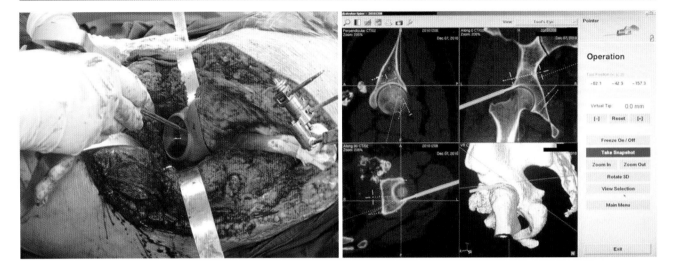

Fig. 16.93 The validation of the individual prosthesis reconstruction assisted by the navigation: the *left* indicated the tracker positioned on the superior border of acetabulum; the *right* indicated that the real-time navigation image showed the match of the superior border of the acetabulum with that of pre-operation

Fig. 16.94 21 months after surgery, 3-D CT image shows pelvic prosthesis in fine place

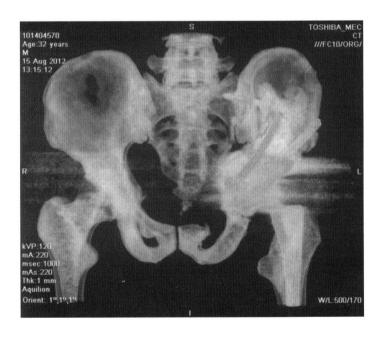

Fig. 16.95 The CT image of the pelvis 21 months after surgery: (**a**) the coronal view indicated the fine union of the prosthesis-bone surface, without loosening and dislocating. (**b**) The horizontal view indicated the four screws located well into the ilium

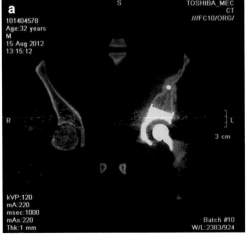
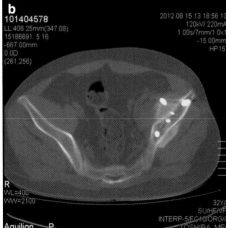

images. However, for the function of the image, it is difficult to find a clear anatomical landmark, and the data of image fusion is homologous equipment generation and uses the corresponding level to fuse.

2. Planning extent of tumor resection: determine the extent of disease with the fusion images, plan the parts and scope of osteotomy, and mark on a 3-D model of the pelvis (Fig. 16.99).

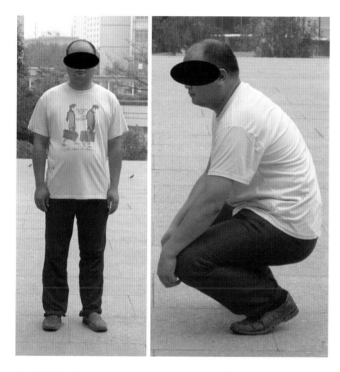

Fig. 16.96 2 years after surgery, patients with hip function well, MSTS score 28 points

Pelvic Tumor Resection and Reconstruction

Patients after routine anesthesia, sterilization, draping, exposed surgical area, install tracker in the area without affecting the operative site. After registration is completed, according to the preoperative plan, completed navigation guidance of tumor resection osteotomy screws the pedicle screws and puts pre-bent connection stick (spinal posterior pedicle screw fixation system). According to the original acetabular shape and size, select the matching acetabular support cup with connecting stick connected by a universal connector fixed to complete the reconstruction of the pelvis (Fig. 16.100).

Postoperative Follow-Up

According to the preoperative planning, the tumor excision and assembly prosthesis reconstruction were carried out using the navigation system. The patient was followed up (Fig. 16.101).

8.5.2 Application in Limb-Salvage Surgery

Limb-Salvage Surgery with Epiphyseal Preservation

Case

Female/16, Primary Osteosarcoma in the Proximal Tibia, Without the Invasion of the Epiphysis (Fig. 16.102)

Preoperative Planning and Surgical Implementation

1. Image fusion and tumor extent of resection planning: put the CT and MRI patient data into navigation system for image fusion and analysis to determine the security resection margin, and plan the reconstruction of tumor resection (Fig. 16.103).
2. Tumor resection, reconstruction of defects, and postoperative assessment: according to preoperative planning,

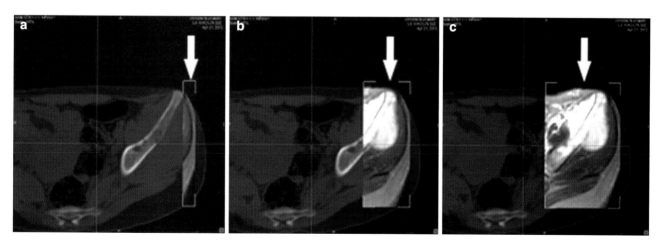

Fig. 16.97 The image fusing process of CT-MRI: (**a**) CT image showed the right ilium and the bone lesion area. (**b**) The partial fused image of CT-MRI image. The inner side showed the CT image, while the outside showed the MRI image. (**c**) The completely fused image indicated the rumor margin in soft tissue

Fig. 16.98 The fusion image
of the CT-ECT: (**a**) CT
showed the lobulated uneven
high density (the *white
arrow*); (**b**) CT and ECT
image fusion showed the
heavy radioactivity indicating
the tumor range (the *white
arrow*)

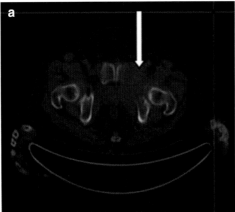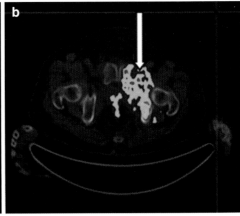

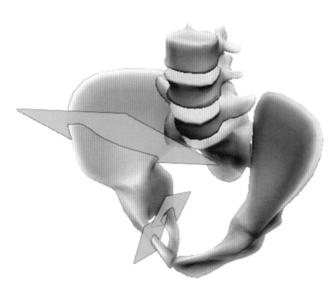

Fig. 16.99 3-D pelvic model marked the resection level and range

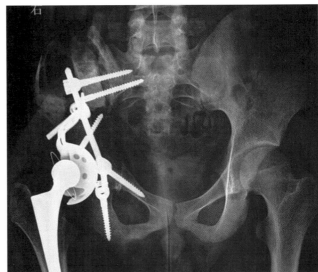

Fig. 16.101 Twelve months after operation, the X-ray showed that the semi-pelvic assembly prosthesis reconstructed was in good position. The rods, screws and shape, and prosthesis were stable with the MSTS scoring of 80%

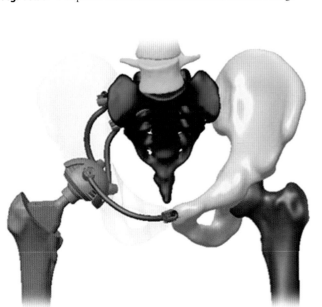

Fig. 16.100 The sketch map of the semi-pelvic assembly prosthesis reconstruction

under the guidance of the navigation system, retain the integrity of the knee joint, remove the lesion area (Fig. 16.104), and reconstruct with allograft.

The Postoperative Follow-Up
The patient received chemotherapy and followed up to evaluate the clinical outcomes. At the last follow-up, MSTS scores reached 80% without tumor recurrence or metastasis (Fig. 16.105).

Unicondylar Osteoallograft Prosthesis Composite in Tumor Limb-Salvage Surgery

Case
Male/25, Ewing's Sarcoma on the Left Distal Femur. The Tumor Involved Part of the Knee Joint (Fig. 16.106)

Fig. 16.102 A 16-year-old
girl with a high-grade tibia
osteosarcoma. (**a**) AP
radiograph, (**b**) CT scan, (**c**)
MR image

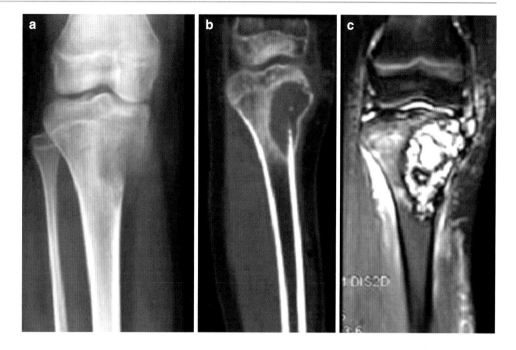

Fig. 16.103 Preoperative CT/MRI
fusion in sagittal line (**a**, **b**) and the
osteotomy line was marked with the aid
of navigation guidance (**c**, **d**)

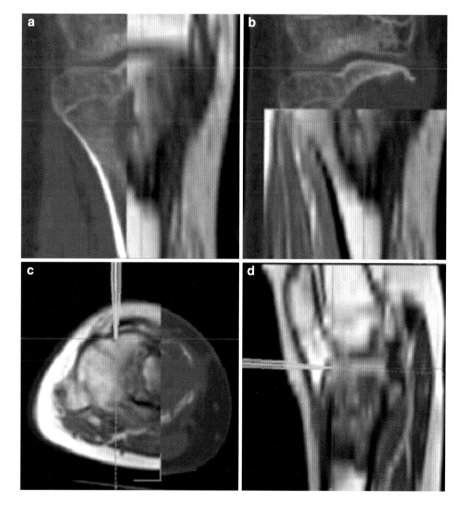

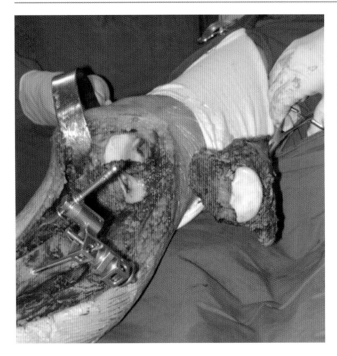

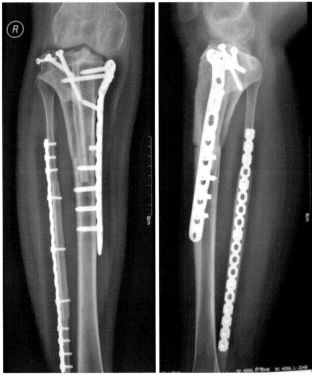

Fig. 16.104 An intraoperative photograph shows residual host bone after the irregular osteotomy making it possible to perform a part joint-sparing intercalary osteotomy. The osteotomy spares a portion of the lateral articular surface, cruciate ligament, lateral collateral ligament, and meniscus

Fig. 16.105 Anteroposterior and lateral radiographs obtained 2 years after surgery show united allograft to host bone

Fig. 16.106 The images illustrate the case of a 24-year-old man with a diagnosis of recurrent Ewing's sarcoma who received intralesional curettage and autogenous cancellous bone graft in his hometown hospital because of misdiagnosis. (**a**) Preoperative AP radiograph shows the extension of the tumor that compromised the lateral femoral condyle. (**b**) MRI scans determined tumor extension. (**c**) CT scan shows the area of bone destruction. (**d**) Bone scan shows increased uptake in the area of tumor invasion. These images were used to design the levels of tumor resection with the computer-assisted navigation system

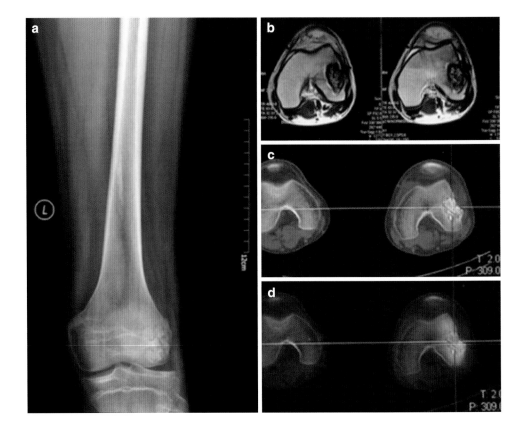

Fig. 16.107 The photographs show how the tumor resection was performed using computer-assisted navigation. (**a**) After appropriate exposure, a tracker was fixed to the femur to perform registration and calibration. This enabled the surgeons to match precisely the operative anatomy to the virtual image generated by the navigation system. (**b**)The anatomic position of the intended bone resection plane was marked with a K-wire by using navigated tools. (**c**) The lateral femoral condyle was removed using an oscillating saw. (**d**) The en bloc tumor resection had a wide margin

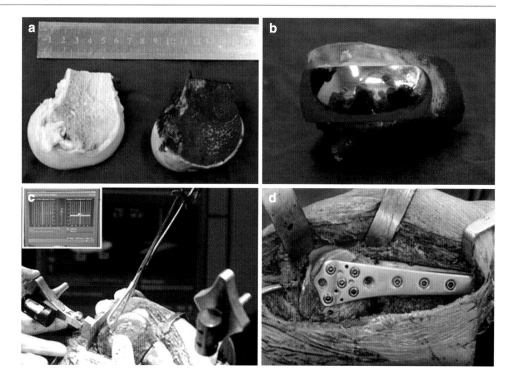

Preoperative Plan

With the same technique, CT/MRI images were fused, and the security resection margin and defect reconstruction plan were determined. During operation, bone tumor resection and reconstruction were performed under the navigation assistance (Fig. 16.107).

The Postoperative Follow-Up

Metastasis, recurrence, joint function and stability, allograft reconstruction, as well as joint degeneration were followed up. The MSTS scores were used to evaluate joint function (Figs. 16.108 and 16.109).

The Osteoallograft Reconstruction with the Aid of Combing the Navigation and the Digital Bone Bank

Case

Female/16, with Right Knee Pain for 9 Months, Exacerbation 1 Month. Preoperative CT and MRI Showed Soft-Tissue Mass Lesion on the Right Side of the Proximal Tibia Area. Biopsy Result Demonstrated Malignant Tumors. Digital Bone Bank and Navigation Aids Bone Tumor Resection and Reconstruction Was Used to Treat This Patient. Postoperative Pathological Diagnosis Was Osteosarcoma

Preoperative Plan

The preoperative CT and MRI imaging data were reconstruction. The resection area was determined by image fusion (Fig. 16.110). Platform parameter stored in the digital bone bank such as shape, length, and width of allograft tibia was matched with patient's tibia. The best allograft bone with same shape was chosen (Table 16.1).

Surgical Procedures and Postoperative Follow-Up

In the CT data of an involved limb, allograft bone was imported into computer-aided navigation system in DICOM format. By using navigation module, tumor resection and allograft trimming plan were shown in navigation system. After intraoperative registration and verification, tumor resection and allograft reconstruction were completed. The clinical outcomes were evaluated according to pathology and radiological and joint function (Figs. 16.111 and 16.112).

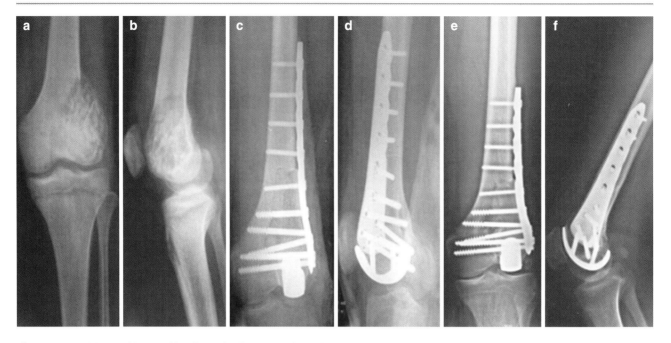

Fig. 16.108 A 25-year-old man with a diagnosis of recurrent giant cell tumor received a unicondylar osteoallograft prosthesis composite reconstruction after resection of the tumor. The preoperative (**a**) AP and (**b**) lateral radiographs show the extension of the tumor that compromised the lateral femoral condyle. The intraoperative (**c**) AP and (**d**) lateral radiographs show successful unicondylar osteoallograft prosthesis composite reconstruction. The (**e**) AP and (**f**) lateral radiographs show solid union of the osteotomy without obvious joint deterioration after 58 months of follow-up

Fig. 16.109 One year after surgery, the patient was satisfied with his knee function

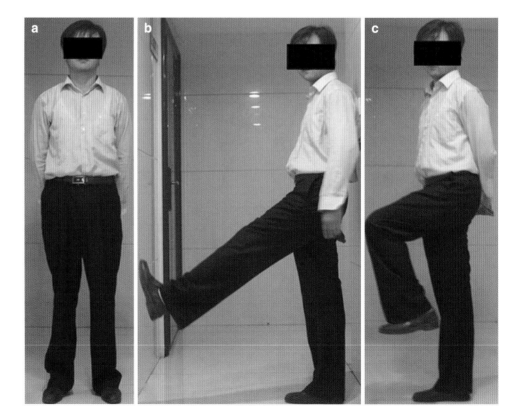

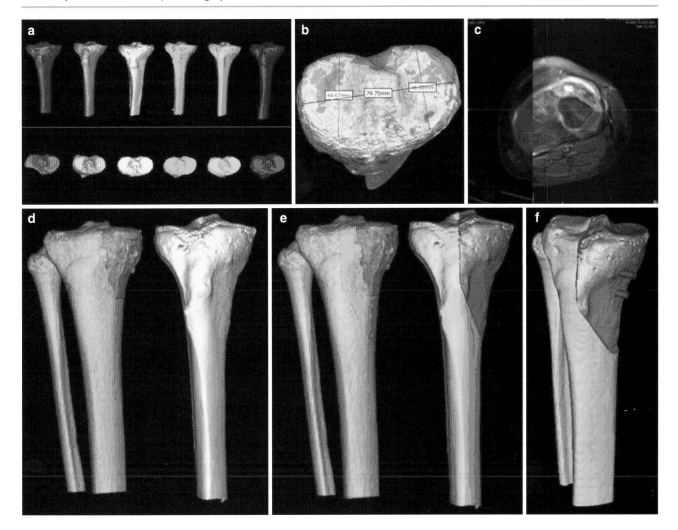

Fig. 16.110 (a) Measuring the right tibia allograft bone front view and a platform top view in digital bone bank. (b) Platform parameter measurement. (c) CT and MR image fusion techniques to determine tumor resection of bone and soft-tissue boundaries. (d) Marked tumor resection, optimal selection of the most suitable allogeneic bone segment. (e) Osteotomy line design. (f) Analog match allogeneic bone and fixation design

Table 16.1 Comparative data of right allogeneic tibia and the bone morphogenetic of limb

No.	Routing length between inner and outer platform	Routing length between front and back of inner platform	Routing length between front and back of outer platform	Difference value/ absolute value	Difference value/ absolute value	Difference value/ absolute value	Absolute value of difference value sum
1	78.22	47.23	45.56	1.61/1.61	−0.96/0.96	−0.98/0.98	3.55
2	78.02	45.35	43.29	1.81/1.81	0.92/0.92	1.29/1.29	4.02
3	79.75	46.08	44.67	0.08/0.08	0.19/0.19	−0.09/0.09	0.36
4	76.32	45.47	43.05	3.51/3.51	0.80/0.80	1.53/1.53	5.84
5	81.33	48.43	45.98	−1.50/1.50	−2.16/2.16	−1.40/1.40	5.06
6	80.03	47.25	44.83	−0.20/0.20	−0.98/0.98	−0.25/0.25	1.43
Injured limb	79.83	46.27	44.58	Select no. 3 (minimum absolute value of difference value sum = 0.36)			

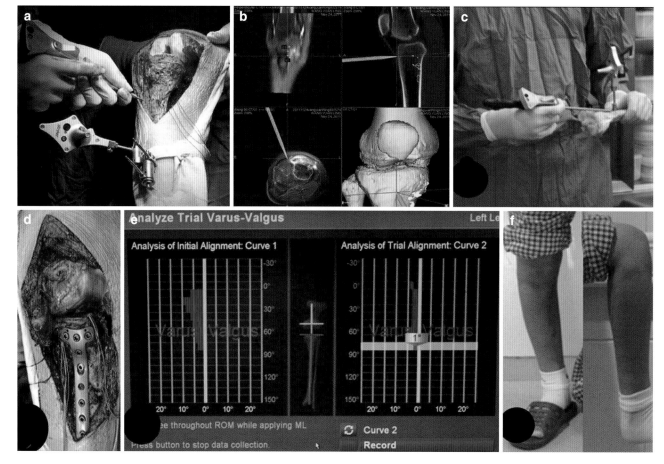

Fig. 16.111 Implementation process: (**a**) registration and verification and (**b**) real-time tracking tumor osteotomy range, angle. (**c**) Navigation aids allogeneic bone osteotomy. (**d**) Intraoperative findings, reconstruc-tion of allogeneic bone joint complex, and repaired ligaments and other soft tissues. (**e**) Limb alignment and varus angle normal after recon-struction. (**f**) Three months later, the joint function is good

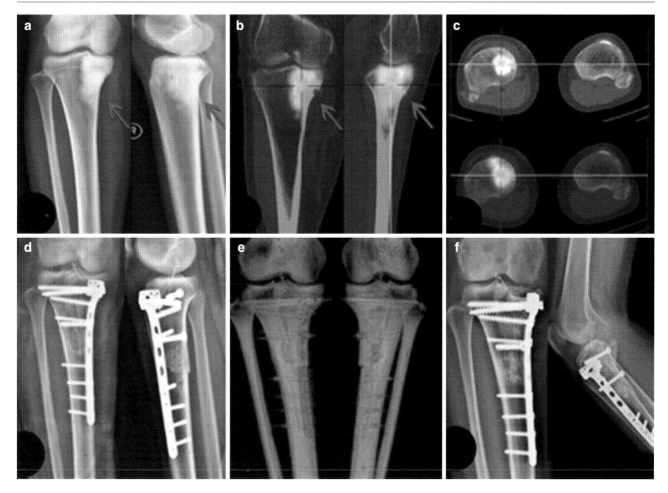

Fig. 16.112 Preoperative and postoperative radiographic: (**a**) preoperative X-rays, red arrows show bone tumor area. (**b**) Preoperative SPECT images (coronal plane). (**c**) Preoperative SPECT images (axial plane). (**d**) Postoperative X-rays show bone tumor resected. The joint alignment was good. (**e**) 3-D CT images show the resection area and the implanted allograft. (**f**) One and a half year after operation, X-rays show the bone union between the allograft and host bone. No joint degeneration occurs

8.5.3   Precise Location and Resection of the Benign Bone Tumors in the Complex Anatomical Structures

Case: Male/19, Giant Cell Tumor in the Proximal Tibia. It Was Scheduled to Carry Out the Navigation-Assisted Tumor Curettage and Allograft Reconstruction (Fig. 16.113).

Preoperative Planning

According to the above technique, radiological images were fused and reconstructed. The lesion area and resection area were determined by image fusion (Fig. 16.114). Bone defect area was matched with allograft in digital bone bank (Fig. 16.115). With navigation system assistance, tumor resection and allograft reconstruction were completed. The clinical outcomes were evaluated (Fig. 16.116).

Fig. 16.113 Preoperative CT image showed the area of bone destruction in the tibia

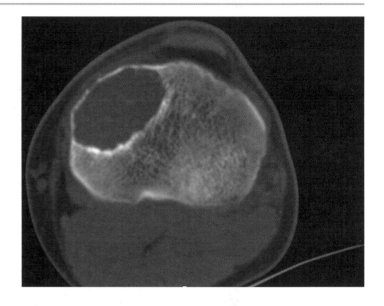

Fig. 16.114 Preoperative a b CT-based 3-D image: (**a**) CT reconstructed image showed the bone lesion in the proximal tibia. (**b**) The planned resection level was marked on the CT-based image

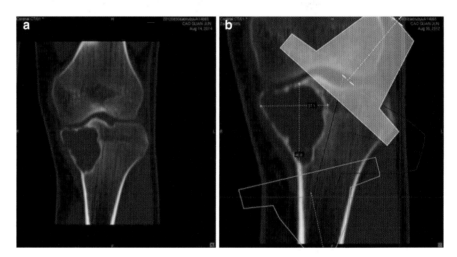

Fig. 16.115 The accurate excision curettage assisted by the navigation

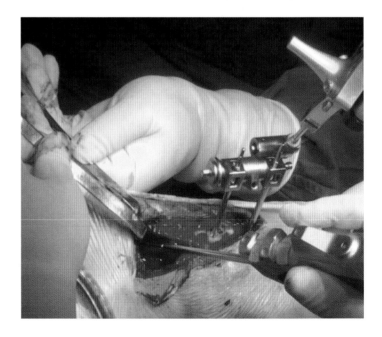

Fig. 16.116 The postoperative AP radiograph after 18 months showed the union of allograft to the host bone

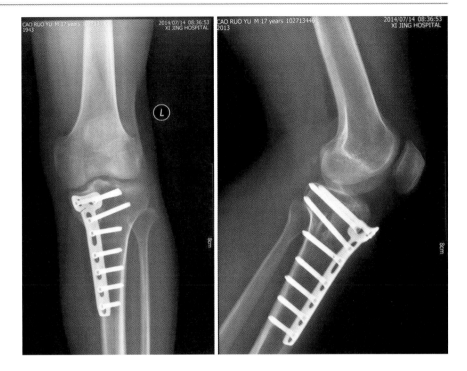

9 Summary

Computer-assisted navigation system in bone tumor resection and reconstruction is a novel technique in orthopedic surgery. By image information and fusion technique, the precise lesion area, safe resection margin, real-time displaying implants and instruments, and accurate prosthesis implantation can be realized intraoperatively. At the same time, this technique plays an important role in decreasing the radiation exposure, minimizing surgical risks and complications, shortening recovery duration, and improving clinical outcomes.

However, this technique has just started in China with some shortcomings to be solved: (1) The import of navigation system is expensive. New products with independent intellectual property rights need to be developed to lower the cost. (2) There is a learning curve to master computer-assisted navigation system. Surgeons need to pay massive enthusiasm and patience and cooperate with engineers to improve this technique. (3) In some area, the healthcare system does not cover the cost of this technique. The clinical application is limited. (4) Navigation drift needs to be solved when lesion zone is involved with soft tissue. New software should be developed. (5) Preoperative preparation is time-consuming (image input needs almost 1 h) especially for complex bone tumor surgery.

With the development of computer-assisted navigation system and software module in oncology, surgeons can improve the accuracy of bone tumor resection with the aid of navigation instead of personal experience. Computer-assisted navigation system has already been surgeons' right hand. It is helpful to make operation plan, guide surgical procedures, monitor tumor resection and reconstruction, and minimize complications. The potential benefits hold significant promise for application in tumor resections.

10 Clinical Application of Novel Computer-Assisted Orthopedic Surgery Pattern

Chen Yanxi and Zhang Kun
Department of Orthopaedic Trauma, East Hospital, Tongji University School of Medicine, Shanghai, 200120, China
cyxtongji@126.com

Since the computer-assisted equipment was imported into trauma surgery in the 1990s, computer navigation system has become a major part in the computer-assisted orthopedic surgery (CAOS). So far, 3-D navigation pattern based on radiography was the most widely used. Although some scholars suggested that 3-D navigation system could offer several medical images at the same time during the surgery, it real timely shows the position of surgical tools, target, and implant and thus reduces the frequency of use of X-ray during surgery. Other scholars believed that the equipment used in the CAOS would occupy extra space in the operation room, while its connection wires, position, and intraoperative adjustment could influence the original position of the image equipment, anesthesia machine, surgical bed, and patients; what is more, the extra time for building CAOS may gain the operating time and the procedure of the operation; since the CAOS requires high quality for medical image, it would lead to failure of the operation once it failed to sign in for the images. Compared with the traditional orthopedic surgery, the equipment at present for CAOS is quite expensive; given the cost for training doctors and updating software and hardware, it is hard for CAOS to be widely used in China. So we shouldn't simply evaluate CAOS in technical ways but combine it with the creative clinical thoughts of orthopedic surgeons and thus highly activate the subjective initiative of doctors and offer new theories and methods for clinical therapy. So building up a kind of digital platform equipped with high definition, editing, and dynamic observation function for skeletal structure imaging and combined with doctors' clinical experience and subjective initiative, thus coming up with the best therapy based on 3-D images and precisely preoperative planning at a low cost, should be the most valuable CAOS pattern, which we call the new CAOS pattern.

The clinical application of the new CAOS pattern should be based on a platform with advanced digital software and in which the clinical pathway (CP) acts as the key strategy. By integrating frontier interdisciplinary and great quantity of science research, a new multifunctional digital orthopedic clinical research platform, which is named "SuperImage" system, was invented by our scientific research team. The SuperImage system is a kind of viewable 3-D clinical research platform based on post-processing of clinical images, which is also the first digital system especially for orthopedic research in the world. By optimizing and taking full advantage of advanced software and hardware, the SuperImage system can operate on most computers with mainstream configuration with a high speed. By applying such intelligential zed system, more detail of the bone fracture can be observed omnibearing, which cannot only help with the operation plan but also make orthopedic surgeons compare the pathological difference between different patients more clearly to summarize more clinical experience, thus improving clinical therapeutic effect. CP is a new medical service pattern that was come up with by American medical institutions to conform to the changes inside and outside the hospital in the 1980s, which is a kind of standard therapy pattern and procedure for specific disease. According to the evidence and guide of evidence-based medicine, CP can standardize medical behavior and reduce regional variability and medical expenses, thus improving clinical therapeutic effect and evaluability of medical expenses. So far, it was pointed out by the Development Research Center of the State Council that advanced digital image technique should be developed without delay. The digital technique can bring the traditional qualitative diagnosis by doctors of radiology department into more detailed quantitate diagnosis by clinical doctors themselves. By offering a great quantity of data, digital technique lays the technical foundation for more innovative medical pattern and CP. The paragraph below is going to talk about the digital 3-D observation, preoperative planning, evaluation of reduction, and collection of clinical cases with the application of digital CP, so that its value of clinical use will be shown more clearly.

10.1   Digital 3-D Observation and Measurement

At present, multi-slice spiral CT and 3-D reconstruction technique have been widely used in orthopedic diagnosis and therapy. However, software that offers high-definition CT images and post-processing function can only run on professional workstation sold by image manufacturers with high prices. On the other hand, because of the lack of clinical cognition, the 3-D reconstruction images offered by radiologists, which should have been clearer than images taken by common X-rays, are still a kind of 2-D output other than the best view of images. Moreover, for some hospitals that have installed PACS system, the view point of reconstructed images is still fixed, which makes it hard for clinical doctors to choose view points by themselves. So far, all the developed digital orthopedic techniques are based on DICOM (Digital Imaging and Communications in Medicine) data of international standard. By reconstructing original data from CT, 3-D images with plotting scales that are of high definition and have abundant structures and multi-planar reconstruction (MPR) [70] with multiple pseudo-colors rendered are acquired, which can make it possible for pre-operating free viewing including free segmentation and section choosing, 2-D and 3-D viewing, right time rotating, moving, and zooming images, and any view of image for saving. In the SuperImage system, original thin slice CT data can be converted into high-accuracy 3-D images with multiple pseudo-colors and various structures within a few seconds of preprocessing, including volume rendering (VR) [71], surface-shaded display (SSD) [72], and hybrid rendering images, which can realize right time rotating, moving, and zooming images. By changing the transparency and colors of different kinds of tissue, the bone and the soft tissue around can be shown more distinctly. Compared with traditional CT which can only show images of the same transverse section, MPR imaging can show images of horizontal, coronal, and sagittal plane based on original CT data through post-processing imaging technique. In the orthopedic clinical works, images of coronal and sagittal plane can reduce some volume effect for images of horizontal plane, thus making it possible to view the surface of articular, and improving distinguishability of images is beneficial for observing details of the bone and joint. However, MPR imaging can't show the 3-D feature of bones, especially for flat bones, irregular bones, and some overlapping parts of bones such as the carpus and midfoot bones, which make it hard to recognize the exact position of injury. In the SuperImage system, MPR images of horizontal, coronal, and sagittal plane with multiple pseudo-colors are rendered and compared with SSD images of same colors. Therefore, the parameters can be measured precisely, and the position of tiny injury can be found out exactly [73].

The level and typing of fracture can be realized through digital 3-D viewing before operation. The typing of fractures is the most scientific, simple, and practical way to analyze the mechanism of injury, guide therapy, and judge prognosis. At the same time, typing of fractures has also become the basic language and foundation of exchanging therapy plans and summarizing clinical experience. In the past, the typing of fractures was based on regular radiograph. But because of the difference of view point of X-rays and the 2-D output of 3-D images, academic divergence occurred. Theoretically, the comparison of different therapy should be the same type of fracture strictly, so preoperative 3-D observation is quite important for typing of ankle fractures.

10.2 Digital Preoperative Planning

Because of the new interactive image segmentation package in SuperImage system, clinical doctors without professional image processing experience can easily segment 3-D images through simple and effective operation within several minutes on PC and then edit them freely like the virtual reduction of fractures. For reasonable surgical approach, proper exposure, precise reduction, and suitable and rapid placement of implant, precise operational design is necessary. Through the past decades, from methods of carefully X-ray image reading, hand drawing, and self-cutting in the early years to shooting by digital cameras, printing, cutting again, and implant comparing recently, scholars kept working on preoperative planning. However, because of the uncertain size of X-ray images, anamorphosis of digital images, and the error of manual operation, the accuracy of preoperative planning decreased. Digital preoperative planning is based on 3-D images with high definition and plotting scales reconstructed from the DICOM data of international standard. Highly intelligentized interactive operating pattern can make doctors without professional image processing experience finish a serious of virtual operation rapidly, such as the 3-D segmentation of fracture segments, virtual reduction, and virtual placement of implant, so that the best surgical approach, anatomic signs of reduction, and suitable implant can be found to reduce surgical injury, decrease operating time, and improve curative effect. What's more, MPR images of horizontal, coronal, sagittal, and free plane with multiple

pseudo-colors can also help to analyze the position of slight injury and the pathologic distribution in the marrow cavity. In a word, digital preoperative planning is a key part of the development of modern surgery and an important component of the new CAOS.

In the surgical therapy for ankle fracture, the fracture of distal fibula, malleolus medialis and posterior malleolus, and distal tibiofibular syndesmosis injury should be focused on. Among them, the key point which is also the first step is to recover the length of fibula and correct its rotation. For the fixation of distal fibula fracture, single screw, tension band wire, lateral protecting plate, or posterior antiskid plate can be chosen depending on the position, size, and number of fracture fragments viewed precisely before operation. As for posterior malleolus fracture, treating plan should be based on the type of fracture. When open reduction and internal fixation are operated, different surgical procedures can be chosen, such as internal fixation by two cannulated screws of 4.0 mm, rigid internal fixation by transverse screw from medial to lateral part of tibiotalar joint near the articular surface, construction plate, or locking plate at the medial side for antiskidding with screw fixing prominence of the lateral malleolus and rivet fixing fracture fragment to treat the injury of deltoid ligament at its ending on medial malleolus. In addition, close observation of the injury of articular surface can help with the planning of operation for ankle fracture of supination-adduction type II significantly. Once there are comminuted or compression fracture at the junction between the top of medial malleolar facet and tibiotalar joint facet, fractures should be fixed even bone grafting and fixed with lag screw. At present, the surgical indication for fractures of posterior malleolus is controversial [74–77]. The therapy plans are still based on a large amount of morphological quantified indexes, while any research including quantified indexes should be based on methodology with scientific and accurate measurement, without which the result would lose its reference value. In the past, traditional radiological measurement cannot offer the precise degree of posterior malleolus fracture such as the swelling of the soft tissue affecting the standard angle of X-ray. Ferries et al. [78] compared 25 regular X-ray images with their CT images of posterior malleolus fracture and found out 54% of result of measurements were not matched and thus believed the lateral radiographs for evaluation of posterior malleolus fracture were not reliable. Our team precisely evaluated the percentage of the surface of the fracture fragment of posterior malleolus fracture of the whole tibiotalar joint facet by the top digital technique combining with a large clinical sample analysis, which can help with the revision of the indication of posterior malleolus fracture. The diagnosis of distal tibiofibular syndesmosis injury is also controversial [79]. The integrity of distal tibiofibular syndesmosis has been a measurable indicator, while its method of measurement still lacks general acceptance. Syndesmotic injury may be difficult to diagnose by radiographs because of variations in the amount of rotation, the wide anatomic variability in the depth of the peroneal groove, and the shape of the tibial tubercles. CT scanning is more sensitive than radiography for detecting minor degrees of syndesmotic injury, but still relies mainly on 2-D axial imaging. Observation plane selection was still influenced by the positioning of the ankle. In the past the measurements of ankle-related anatomy indicators were based on 2-D methods, and these measurement methods could be roughly divided into two categories, including:

(1) Anatomical measurements of cadaveric ankle joints. It is difficult to carry out large sample prospective group studies because cadavers are scarce resources.
(2) Measurements based on X-ray films. Although there are numerous recommended ray angles, such as anteroposterior, lateral, ankle mortise, and external-rotation views, it is difficult to place the ankle on a standard and unified ray angle because of the posttraumatic peri-ankle swelling, pain, poor compliance, different projecting angles of the tube, and the errors of the manual measurement.

CT improves the ability to assess the injury and to formulate a preoperative plan before definitive fixation. Both conventional radiography and CT are considered low-dose exams. The introduction of 16-slice multidetector computed tomography has reduced ankle CT exam time to less than 10 s. It is important to minimize radiation exposure to the patient. Patient positioning is not as critical because of the ability to reformat the data. Beumer et al. [80] measured the indicator above on 12 ankles in different kinds of posture and found out that they didn't have consistency because of the influence of the rotation of ankle. As digital orthopedic technique develops, a measurement system based on reconstructed 3-D images has been built up, with which the normal anatomic relationship of distal tibiofibular syndesmosis can be viewed precisely. So far, the stress test during the operation to evaluate distal tibiofibular syndesmosis injury has been accepted in a certain extent, but tests like cotton test, squeeze test, external-rotation test, and fibula displacement test can only show the displacement on a certain plane. So the control of the direction and the capacity of load and the precise evaluation of space of distal tibiofibular syndesmosis should also be discussed deeply. In the SuperImage system, advanced reverse engineering technique is used to create implant with an accuracy of 0.1 mm for virtual operation, which can be used for virtual teaching, postoperative evaluation of the international implant, and analyses of the healing of fracture after the implant is removed or in case of bone union. The following is the flow path of the computer-assisted preoperative planning of fractures [81, 82]:

(1) Fracture fragment segmentation: 3-D images of the humeral shaft fractures were reconstructed by a surface-shaded display (SSD) algorithm with a reconstruction interval of 0.625–1.25 mm. The density threshold was 150H, and automatic removal of the image size was <500 mm^3. The 3-D interactive and automatic segmentation technique was applied, so the operator could distinguish all fracture fragments in the 3-D SSD image. Different colors may be assigned to different fracture fragments. (2). Simulated reduction: simulated reduction was obtained using a semiautomatic fragment reconstruction approach on the 3-D SSD image. Fracture fragments were reduced anatomically by selecting three characteristic points through manual operation. When the three anatomical points were selected, the "enter key" was clicked, and the system dragged and rotated the bones into correct anatomical positions automatically. Occasionally, the users had to do some additional fine adjusting of the positions. (3). Choice of internal fixation devices and simulated implantation: the appropriate plates were chosen from the internal fixation devices database of the system with the advanced AO principles and guidelines for clinical application of the relevant internal fixation devices. Implantation was simulated using a semiautomatic approach in the 3-D SSD image. The type of screws to be used (cortical bone screws or locking screws) is inserted into the plate or across the fracture. The length of the screws is measured accurately and recorded.

10.3 Digital Analysis and Evaluation for Reduction and Medical Document

The analysis and evaluation for reduction are usually proceeded 2 weeks after surgery through X-ray or CT, and then digital analysis is done afterward. When digital technique is used in the follow-up, the different patterns of extraction of implant can be combined with prospective or nonprospective 3-D volume rendering and free plane MPR technique to view the reduction and position of implant precisely, thus helping with guiding functional exercising afterward. The mid- and long-term follow-up includes two parts; the first part is the function scoring and the second part is the collection of original data (DICOM). Because of the complicated mechanism and various types of injury, the collection of image is very important. So the classification and storage of image documents should be done carefully for better indexing. What's more, standardized collection of digital medical documents can also offer basic technique and feasibility for multicenter orthopedic research [83, 84]. Limitations are inevitable when measuring using plain radiographs and original CT images. Errors may occur because the projection angle of the tube is incorrect ankle swelling and image overlap on plain films. The metal arti-facts generated by implants on axial CT images decrease the imaging quality and postoperative clinical application. In addition, residual surface steps and gaps in regions of the joint may be difficult to appreciate on routine axial CT images. SSD was the first 3-D rendering technique applied to medical imaging and was mainly applied in orthopedics because of its superiority for bony surface reconstructions [72]. The distinct surfaces under SSD mode facilitate distin-guishing all the component bones of the ankle joints. MPR images provide an additional perspective perpendicular to the fracture line, which can improve depiction of fracture reduction. MPR images can also reduce metal-induced arti-facts because of thicker reformats [70]. VR techniques pro-vide semitransparent and global views of bones and metal hardware. Various parameters, such as surface shading and opacity, can help to reveal both surface and internal detail. Surgeons and radiologists can clearly distinguish subcorti-cal lesions, minimally displaced fractures, and hidden areas of interest, such as multiple overlying structures and inter-nal features [71]. Therefore, the application of CT images can be extended widely [85].

Once advanced digital software platform is combined with the experience and subjective activity, digital technique-assisted operation based on 3-D image and precise preopera-tive planning can be built up, which is a new CAOS pattern with low cost and high value of popularizing.

References

1. Spiegel EA, Wycis HT, Marks M. Stereotaxic apparatus for opera-tions on the human brain. Science. 1947;106:349–50.
2. Watanabe E, Watanabe T, Manaka S, et al. Three-dimensional digitizer (neuronavigator): new equipment for computed tomog-raphy-guided stereotaxic surgery. Surg Neurol. 1987;27:543–7.
3. Roberts DW, Strohbehn JW, Hatch JF, et al. A frameless stereo-taxic integration of computerized tomographic imaging and the operating microscope. J Neurosurg. 1986;65:545–9.
4. Foley KT, Simon DA, Rampersaud YR. Virtual fluoros-copy: computer-assisted fluoroscopic navigation. Spine. 2001;26:347–51.
5. Simon DA, Lavallee S. Medical imaging and registration in com-puter assisted surgery. Clin Orthop Relat Res. 1998;354:17–27.
6. Phillips R. The accuracy of surgical navigation for orthopaedic surgery. Curr Orthop. 2007;21:180–92.
7. Atesok K, Schemitsch EH. Computer-assisted trauma surgery. J Am Acad Orthop Surg. 2010;18:247–58.
8. Mavrogenis AF, Savvidou OD, Mimidis G, et al. Computer-assisted navigation in orthopaedic surgery. Orthopedics. 2013;36:631–41.
9. Kahler DM. Image guidance. Clin Orthop Relat Res. 2004;421:70–6.
10. Stöckle U, König B, Dahne M, et al. Computer assisted pelvic and acetabular surgery: clinical experiences and indications. Unfallchirurg. 2002;105:886–92.
11. Mosheiff R, Khoury A, Weil Y, et al. First generation computer-ized fluoroscopic navigation in percutaneous pelvic surgery. J Orthop Trauma. 2004;18:106–11.
12. Crowl AC, Kathler DM. Closed reduction and percutaneous fixa-tion of anterior column acetabular fractures. Comput Aided Surg. 2002;7:169–78.
13. Mouhsine E, Garofalo R, Borens O, et al. Percutaneous retro-grade screwing for stabilisation of acetabular fractures. Injury. 2005;36:1330–6.
14. Starr AJ, Jones AL, Reinert CM, et al. Preliminary results and complications following limited open reduction and percutaneous screw fixation of displaced fractures of the acetabulum. Injury. 2001;32(Suppl 1):45–50.
15. Gao H, Luo CF, Hu CF, et al. Percutaneous screw fixation of ace-tabular fractures with 2-D fluoroscopy-based computerized navi-gation. Arch Orthop Trauma Surg. 2010;130:1177–83.
16. Gao H, Luo CF, Hu CF, et al. Minimally invasive fluoro-navigation screw fixation for the treatment of pelvic ring injuries. Surg Innov. 2011;18:279–84.
17. Hofstetter R, Slomczykowski M, Krettek C, et al. Computer-assisted fluoroscopy-based reduction of femoral fractures and anteversion correction. Comput Aided Surg. 2000;5:311–25.
18. Weil Y, Gardner M, Helfet D, et al. Accuracy of femoral shaft fracture reduction using fluoroscopy based computerized naviga-tion- a laboratory study. Clin Orthop Relat Res. 2007;460:185–91.
19. Wilharm A, Gras F, Rausch S, et al. Navigation in femoral-shaft fractures – from lab tests to clinical routine. Injury. 2011;42:1346–52.
20. Nolte LP, Beutler T. Basic principles of CAOS. Injury. 2004;35:SA6–SA16.
21. Ebraheim NA, Xu R, Biyani A, et al. Anatomic basis of lag screw placement in the anterior column of the acetabulum. Clin Orthop Relat Res. 1997;339:200–5.
22. Gras F, Marintschev I, Klos K, et al. Screw placement for ace-tabular fractures: which navigation modality (2-dimensional vs. 3-dimensional) should be used? An experimental study. J Orthop Trauma. 2012;26(8):466–73.
23. Briem D, Linhart W, Lehmann W, et al. Computer-assisted screw insertion into the first sacral vertebra using a three-dimensional image intensifier: results of a controlled experimental investiga-tion. Eur Spine J. 2006;15(6):757–63.
24. Smith HE, Yuan PS, Sasso R, et al. An evaluation of image-guided technologies in the place of percutaneous iliosacral screw. Spine. 2006;31(2):234–8.
25. Ochs BG, Gonser C, Shiozawa T, et al. Computer-assisted peri-acetabular screw placement: comparison of different fluoroscopy-based navigation procedures with conventional technique. Injury. 2010;41:1297–305.
26. Nolte LP, Zamorano L, Visarius H, et al. Clinical evaluation of a system for precision enhancement in spine surgery. Clin Biomech. 1995;10:293–303.
27. Nolte LP, Visarius H, Arm E. Computer-aided fixation of spinal implants. J Image Guid Surg. 1995;1:88–93.
28. Nolte LP, Zamorano L, Jiang Z, et al. Image-guided inser-tion of transpedicular screws: a laboratory set-up. Spine. 1995;20:497–500.
29. Merloz P, Tonetti J, Eid A. Computer assisted spine surgery. Clin Orthop Relat Res. 1997;337:86–96.
30. Merloz P, Tonetti J, Pittet L. Pedicle screw placement using image guided techniques. Clin Orthop Relat Res. 1998;354:39–48.
31. Merloz P, Lavallee S, Tonetti J. Image-guided spinal surgery: technology, operative technique, and clinical practice. Oper Tech Orthop. 2000;10:56–63.
32. Devito DP, Kaplan L, Dietl R, et al. Clinical acceptance and accu-racy assessment of spinal implants guided with SpineAssist surgi-cal robot: retrospective study. Spine. 2010;35:2109–15.
33. Mihalko WM, Krackow KA. Differences between extramedul-lary, intramedullary, and computer-aided surgery tibial align-ment techniques for total knee arthroplasty. J Knee Surg. 2006;19:33–6.

34. Wong KC, Kumta SM. Joint-preserving tumor resection and reconstruction using image-guided computer navigation. Clin Orthop Relat Res. 2013;471:762–73.

35. Fehlberg S, Eulenstein S, Lange T, et al. Computer-assisted pelvic tumor resection: fields of application, limits and perspectives. Recent Results Cancer Res. 2009;179:169–82.

36. Bach CM, Winter P, Nogler M, et al. No functional impairment after Robodoc total hip arthroplasty: gait analysis in 25 patients. Acta Orthop Scand. 2002;73:386–91.

37. Honl M, Dierk O, Gauck C, et al. Comparison of robotic-assisted and manual implantation of a primary total hip replacement. A prospective study. J Bone Joint Surg Am. 2003;85:1470–8.

38. Lanfranco AR, Castellanos AE, Desai JP, et al. Robotic surgery-a current perspective. Ann Surg. 2004;239:14–21.

39. Marescaux J, Leroy J, Gagner M, et al. Transatlantic robot-assisted telesurgery. Nature. 2001;413:379–80.

40. Sikorski JM, Chauhan S. Computer-assisted orthopaedic surgery: do we need CAOS? J Bone Joint Surg (Br). 2003;85:319–23.

41. Rivkin G, Liebergall M. Challenges of technology integration and computer-assisted surgery. J Bone Joint Surg Am. 2009;91:13–6.

42. Langlotz F. Potential pitfalls of computer aided orthopedic surgery. Injury. 2004;35:SA17–23.

43. Reddix RN Jr, Webb LX. Computer-assisted preoperative planning in the surgical treatment of acetabular fractures. J Surg Orthop Adv. 2007;16:138–43.

44. Cimerman M, Kristan A. Preoperative planning in pelvic and acetabular surgery: the value of advanced computerized planning modules. Injury. 2007;38:442–9.

45. Zheng GY, Kowal J, Ballester MAG, et al. Registration techniques for computer navigation. Curr Orthop. 2007;21:170–1179.

46. Messmer P, Gross T, Suhm N, et al. Modality-based navigation. Injury. 2004;35:SA24–9.

47. Dessenne V, Lavallee S, Julliard R, et al. Computer assisted knee anterior cruciate ligament reconstruction: first clinical tests. J Image Guid Surg. 1995;1:59–64.

48. Sati M, Staubli H, Bourquin Y, et al. Real-time computerized in situ guidance system for ACL graft placement. Comput Aided Surg. 2002;7:25–40.

49. Jenny JY, Boeri C. Unicompartmental knee prosthesis implantation with a non-image-based navigation system: rationale, technique, case-control comparative study with a conventional instrumented implantation. Knee Surg Sports Traumatol Arthrosc. 2003;11:40–5.

50. Sparmann M, Wolke B, Czupalla H, et al. Positioning of total knee arthroplasty with and without navigation support: a prospective, randomized study. J Bone Joint Surg (Br). 2003;85:830–5.

51. Wong KC, Kumta SM, Chiu KH, et al. Precision tumour resection and reconstruction using image-guided computer navigation. J Bone Joint Surg Br. 2007;89:943–7.

52. Villavicencio AT, Burneikiene S, Bulsara KR, et al. Utility of computerized isocentric fluoroscopy for minimally invasive spinal surgical technique. J Spinal Disord Tech. 2005;18:369–75.

53. Sasso RC, Best NM, Potts EA. Percutaneous computer assisted translaminar facet screw: an initial human cadaveric study. Spine J. 2005;5:515–9.

54. Amiot LP, Lang K, Putzier M, et al. Comparative results between conventional and computer-assisted pedicle screw installation in the thoracic, lumbar, and sacral spine. Spine. 2000;25:606–14.

55. Pring ME, Weber KL, Unni KK, et al. Chondrosarcoma of the pelvis. A review of sixty-four cases. J Bone Joint Surg Am. 2001;83:1630–42.

56. Gofton W, Dubrowski A, Tabloie F, et al. The effect of computer navigation on trainee learning of surgical skills. J Bone Joint Surg Am. 2007;89:2819–27.

57. Kendoff D, Bogojevic A, Citak M, et al. Experimental validation of noninvasive referencing in navigated procedures on long bones. J Orthop Res. 2005;25:201–7.

58. Gosling T, Oszwald M, Kendoff D, et al. Computer-assisted antetorsion control prevents malrotation in femoral nailing: an experimental study and preliminary clinical case series. Arch Orthop Trauma Surg. 2009;129:1521–6.

59. Bonutti P, Dethmers S, Stiehl JB. Case report: femoral shaft fracture resulting from femoral tracker placement in navigated TKA. Clin Orthop Relat Res. 2008;466:1499–502.

60. Stockle U, Krettek C, Pohlemann T, et al. Clinical application-pelvis. Injury. 2004;35(Suppl 1):46–56.

61. Hawi N, Haentjes J, Suero EM, et al. Navigated femoral shaft fracture treatment: current status. Technol Health Care. 2012;20:65–71.

62. Attias N, Lindsey RW, Starr AJ, et al. The use of a virtual three-dimensional model to evaluate the intraosseous space available for percutaneous screw fixation of acetabular fractures. J Bone Joint Surg Br. 2005;87:1520–3.

63. Giannoudis PV, Tzioupis CC, Pape HC, et al. Percutaneous fixation of the pelvic ring. J Bone Joint Surg Br. 2007;89:145–54.

64. Braten M, Terjesen T, Rossvoll I. Torsional deformity after intramedullary nailing of femoral shaft fractures: measurement of femoral anteversion in 110 patients. J Bone Joint Surg Br. 1993;75:799–803.

65. Jaarsma RL, Pakvis DF, Verdonschot N, et al. Rotational malalignment after intramedullary nailing of femoral fractures. J Orthop Trauma. 2004;18:403–9.

66. Yang KH, Han DY, Jahng JS, et al. Prevention of malrotation in femoral deformity in femoral shaft fracture. J Orthop Trauma. 1998;12:558–62.

67. Wick M, Muhr G. Ante- und retrograde marknagelung bei femurschaftfrakturen. Trauma Berufskr. 2005;7:103–6.

68. Hoaglund FT, Low WD. Anatomy of the femoral neck and head with comparative data from Caucasians and Hong Kong Chinese. Clin Orthop Relat Res. 1980;(152):10–6.

69. Kendoff D, Citak MC, Gardner MJ, et al. Navigated femoral nailing using noninvasive registration of the contralateral intact femur to restore anteversion. Technique and clinical use. J Orthop Trauma. 2007;21(10):725–30.

70. Stradiotti P, Curti A, Castellazzi G, Zerbi A. Metal-related artifacts in instrumented spine. Techniques for reducing artifacts in CT and MRI: state of the art. Eur Spine J. 2009;18(Suppl 1):102–8.

71. Calhoun PS, Kuszyk BS, Heath DG, Carley JC, Fishman EK. Three-dimensional volume rendering of spiral CT data: theory and method. Radiographics. 1999;19(3):745–64.

72. Kuszyk BS, Heath DG, Bliss DF, Fishman EK. Skeletal 3-D CT: advantages of volume rendering over surface rendering. Skelet Radiol. 1996;25(3):207–14.

73. Qiang M, Chen Y, Zhang K, Li H, Dai H. Measurement of three-dimensional morphological characteristics of the calcaneus using CT image post-processing. J Foot Ankle Res. 2014;7(1):19.

74. Michelsen JD, Ahn UM, Helgemo SL. Motion of the ankle in a simulated supination-external rotation fracture model. J Bone Joint Surg Am. 1996;78(7):1024–31.

75. Forberger J, Sabandal PV, Dietrich M, Gralla J, Lattmann T, Platz A. Posterolateral approach to the displaced posterior malleolus: functional outcome and local morbidity. Foot Ankle Int. 2009;30(4):309–14.

76. Tejwani NC, Pahk B, Egol KA. Effect of posterior malleolus fracture on outcome after unstable ankle fracture. J Trauma. 2010;69(3):666–9.

77. Abdelgawad AA, Kadous A, Kanlic E. Posterolateral approach for treatment of posterior malleolus fracture of the ankle. J Foot Ankle Surg. 2011;50(5):607–11.

78. Ferries JS, DeCoster TA, Firoozbakhsh KK, Garcia JF, Miller RA. Plain radiographic interpretation in trimalleolar ankle fractures poorly assesses posterior fragment size. J Orthop Trauma. 1994;8(4):328–31.
79. Chen Y, Qiang M, Zhang K, Li H, Dai H. A reliable radiographic measurement for evaluation of normal distal tibiofibular syndesmosis: a multi-detector computed tomography study in adults. J Foot Ankle Res. 2015;8:32.
80. Beumer A, van Hemert WL, Niesing R, et al. Radiographic measurement of the distal tibiofibular syndesmosis has limited use. Clin Orthop Relat Res. 2004;423:227–34.
81. Chen Y, Zhang K, Qiang M, Li H, Dai H. Computer-assisted preoperative planning for proximal humeral fractures by minimally invasive plate osteosynthesis. Chin Med J. 2014;127(18):3278–85.
82. Chen Y, Qiang M, Zhang K, Li H, Dai H. Novel computer-assisted preoperative planning system for humeral shaft fractures: report of 43 cases. Int J Med Rob Comput Assisted Surg. 2015;11(2):109–19.
83. Chen Y, Zhang K, Qiang M, Li H, Dai H. Comparison of plain radiography and CT in postoperative evaluation of ankle fractures. Clin Radiol. 2015;70(8):e74–82.
84. Qiang M, Chen Y, Zhang K, Li H, Dai H. Effect of sustentaculum screw placement on outcomes of intra-articular calcaneal fracture osteosynthesis: a prospective cohort study using 3D CT. Int J Surg. 2015;19:72–7.
85. Chen YX, Zhang K, Hao YN, Hu YC. Research status and application prospects of digital technology in orthopaedics. Orthop Surg. 2012;4(3):131–8.

Wu Zixiang, Sang Hongxun, Yue Zhou, and He Zhang

1 Basic Operational Principles of Robot

1.1 The Operational Principle of Robot-Assisted Orthopedic Surgery

Robot has many advantages, such as precisely implanting devices, stable maneuver, and working in a toxic environment or a special space by remote control, in which the physician fails or even cannot perform surgeries. Therefore, since the 1880s, many scholars focused on the basic researches to advanced robotics technology and attempted to apply it in orthopedic surgeries.

1.1.1 Working Principle and Basic Concepts

Modern orthopedic robot system usually works under the 3D (three-dimensional) navigation guidance and touch technology instead of simple robotic arm. The robot can cut the bone under the accurate guidance of 3D navigation technology on the basis of preoperative skeleton model. Compared with the image-based navigation, the touch-based navigation is more initiative, of which the interaction with the surgeon is better, guiding the surgical procedures, and correcting procedures in urgent situations to protect the patient.

The capacity of orthopedic surgical robot system includes the following aspects:

1. Data acquisition: Image plays an important role in navigation of surgical instruments. Image is absolutely essential

in pathological identification, displaying the instrument location as well as planning and correcting the tracking of surgical instruments. No matter the preoperative CT/MR or X-ray during operation, at least one should be obtained to use as the guidance image for the surgical robot.
2. Precise surgical instrument tracking: Precise position and measurement totally rely on the tracking of surgical instruments. Only based on the precise tracking of surgical instruments, the guidance of surgical navigation system for the surgical robot may be completed.
3. Spatial calibration and coordinate system conversion: For navigation surgical robot, the instruments should include at least the robot coordinate system, the patient coordinate system, and the image coordinate system. The conversion accuracy among these coordinate systems has a greater impact for the surgical robot to complete the surgery. Any coordinate system conversion error will be accumulated, leading to a larger surgery error, even surgery failure.

1.1.2 Navigation Mode of the Orthopedic Surgical Robot

Bone tissue and its features determine that the navigation mode based on endoscope and electromagnetic positioning is not suitable for orthopedic surgical robot. Currently, external landmark or landmark with optical properties is applied in the navigation mode of orthopedic surgical robot to conduct the calibration of surgical image and surgical space. According to the occurrence of proactive tracking for surgical instruments, the navigation of orthopedic surgical robot can be divided into active pattern and passive pattern.

1. Surgical robot based on passive navigation system
   After the initial space calibration, passive navigation system will not conduct relative positioning measurement of instrument and bone structure, just as an information-giving system in the surgery, not affecting the operation in the surgery. ACROBOT semiautonomous robotic system developed by the British Imperial College, adopting similar navigation technique with ROBODOC, conducts planning in the preop-

W. Zixiang
Department of Orthopaedics, Xijing Hospital, The Air Force Medical University, Xi An, China

S. Hongxun (✉)
Department of Orthopaedics, Shenzhen Hospital, Southern Medical University, Shenzhen, China
e-mail: hxsang@fmmu.edu.cn

Y. Zhou · H. Zhang
Xinqiao Hospital, Third Military University, Chongqing, China

erative CT image and needs to connect the clamp used for datum point fixation to femur and tibia, achieving the coordinate registration, which is mainly for total knee replacement and minimally invasive-single condylar knee arthroplasty. Currently, the only one commercial surgical robot system used in spine surgery, SPINEASSIST, adopted a more secure and reliable navigation and surgery assist method, providing a precise direction guidance in the process of pedicle screws artificial implant in the spinal fusion surgery.

2. Surgical robot based on active navigation system

Surgical navigation system based on active optical location tracking is used to assist physicians to complete some complex surgeries requiring precise positioning, such as minimally invasive neurosurgery and minimally invasive orthopedic surgery. However, GE, SIEMENS, Philips, Medtronic, and other large medical equipment companies have developed surgical navigation system, while these systems are not widely promoted, mainly due to the complicated procedures which affect accuracy. Thus, it is a trend to combining the optical navigation technology and robotics technology.

In recent years, O-ARM technology is well developed, and clinical equipment is produced and promoted. Since O-ARM can establish the real-time 3D model of the patient during surgery, the application integrated with optical tracking system can simplify the registration procedures, improve the usefulness of the navigation system, and provide a new way for the robotic optical navigation based on 3D images.

3. Touch-guided orthopedic robotic surgery

Touch technology is originated in perceptive technology. Touch instrument is able to integrate with visual environment, and then produce jumping, buffer, lag, and other physical effects. MAKO Surgical is the first to introduce touch-assisted orthopedic surgical navigation technology. The RiO system developed by them was approved by the FDA to apply in the orthopedic surgery in 2008.

Although widely used, even commercialized surgery based on touch navigation still has some drawbacks. Due to the different technical principles, tactile perception of equal volume cannot be obtained at the end effect or of the robot. This means that physicians will feel different resistance when cutting the bone, even in the free space. The other disadvantage is that the tactile perception with high rigidity cannot be provided by the end effector of the robot. The physical reason is that interaction of high rigidity means that end effector is required to exert a great force in a very short distance. When the end effector moves in a high speed, stress controller is required to get faster feedback information to obtain the desired rigidity, which cannot be provided by majority stress controllers, for which it will lead to instability of the system. Currently, this is still an unsolved technical problem.

Fig. 17.1 (**a**, **b**) Preoperative lumbar anteroposterior and lateral X-ray image

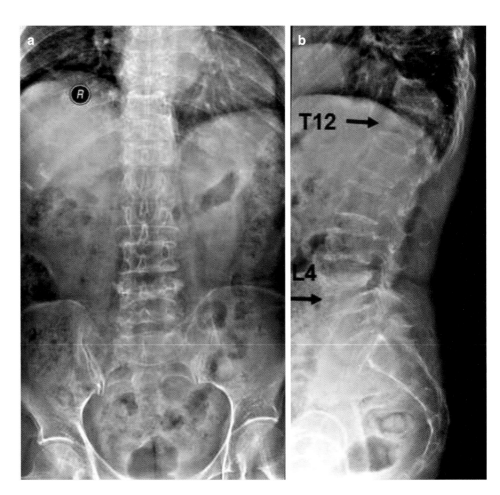

2   Demonstration of Robot-Assisted Spine Surgery

Wu Zixiang and Sang Hongxun

Patient, female, 58 years old, was admitted to the hospital due to severe back pain and difficulty in standing after slipping down for a week. According to the results of physical examination and imaging (Figs. 17.1 and 17.2), the patient was diagnosed as T12 and L4 osteoporotic vertebral compression fractures. Surgical plan: Renaissance spine robot-assisted T12, L4 percutaneous vertebral kyphoplasty.

2.1   Specific Steps

2.1.1   Step I: Surgical Design
Performed preoperative thoracolumbar CT scanning in prone position and imported DICOM format files into Renaissance software to reconstruct the thoracolumbar 3D image. Create a preoperative planning in a computer 3D environment, pre-designing the puncture angle and depth, and evaluate possible leakage position and risk of bone cement through dynamic playback software modules, to complete the designed operation.

2.1.2   Step II: Mounting Robot Directing Orbits and Positioning Device (Fig. 17.3)

2.1.3   Step III: 3D Sync

1. Transmitted the perspective data to the work station and conducted registration between anteroposterior and lateral X-ray images and CT image-based preoperative surgical planning, which was not dependent on the anatomical location.
2. The registration results showed that the accuracy between the X-ray and CT reached 0.07 mm.
3. Fixed the robot in the orbit, locate surgery trajectory automatically, and determine the working tunnel. It should be noted that, for some patients with severe osteoporosis, the low bone density would result in not enough clarity of X-ray image, which would lead to difficulties in registration, so we should carefully identify target vertebrae, in order to avoid surgical segment misjudgment.

2.1.4   Step IV: Start Surgical Procedure
1. According to the angle determined by the robot, after skin and subcutaneous tissue incision, put into the guide sleeve, using an electric drill to prepare a pedicle screw trajectory (Fig. 17.4).

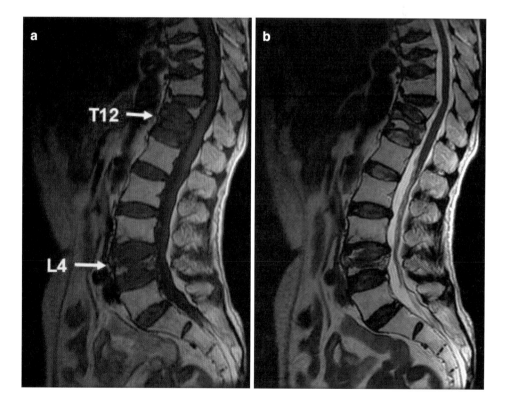

Fig. 17.2 (**a**, **b**) MR shows: multiple thoracolumbar vertebral compression fractures, including fresh compression fractures in T12, L4 vertebrae

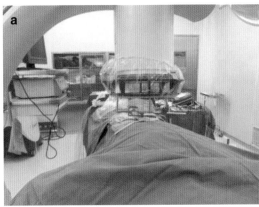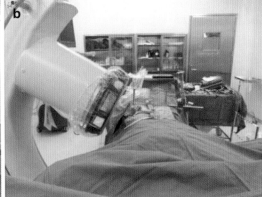

Fig. 17.3 Mount robot directing orbits, and preform anteroposterior, and 45° oblique X-ray fluoroscope

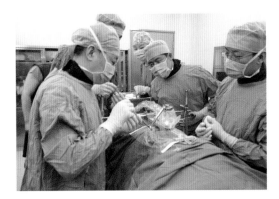

Fig. 17.4 Based on the angles determined by the robot, cut the skin

2. Put in the locating pins and conduct X-ray fluoroscopy to confirm the correct position (Fig. 17.5).
3. After completion of all surgical segment pedicle puncture, removed robots and obits, completing kyphoplasty under the X-ray monitoring. Postoperative 3D CT shows: the distribution of bone cement was good, without cement leakage (Fig. 17.6).

Conventional percutaneous vertebroplasty requires surgeons to conduct puncture by hand and injection of bone cement to strengthen the fractured vertebral body under multiple X-ray fluoroscopy, while the radiation exposure is much more for both surgeons and patients, and the puncture accuracy is insufficient and the repeated puncture are required. With the aid of Renaissance, through twice X-ray fluoroscopy during the surgery, completed the 3D registration of the preoperative CT and intraoperative spinal anatomical landmarks, and the positioning and puncture of two fractured vertebral bodies was finished in a short time. Compared with the current computer-assisted surgery navigation system, the robotic technology has the advantage of high precision, high speed, and accurate positioning, and the matching is more easy, which can reduce the suffering of patients, decrease the complications, and it can reduce the utilization rate of intraoperative radioscopy to the lowest, intraoperative radios-

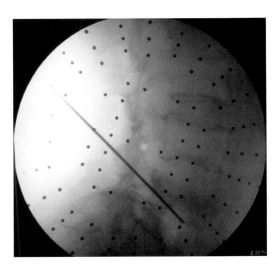

Fig. 17.5 Lateral fluoroscopic images after putting into the locating pins showed the good position of locating pins

copy utilization, especially for percutaneous vertebroplasty and other minimally invasive spine surgeries, and complex spinal deformity orthopedic surgery.

3   Trauma Surgery Robot

3.1   The Role of Robots in Trauma Surgery

Traumatic orthopedics is an important branch derived from orthopedics with the continuous development of medical science, which has been one of the three main orthopedic disciplines besides spine surgery and bone joint surgery. With the development of economy and society, the incidence of trauma, especially high-energy trauma increases year by year, which also contributes to the rapid development of traumatic orthopedic and puts forward higher requirements and new challenges to the basic knowledge and clinical operation of trauma.

In the study of surgical robots, surgical robots for trauma is one of the most rapidly developing branches, the reason of

Fig. 17.6 Postoperative 3D CT reconstruction image showed good position of bone cement, without bone cement leakage

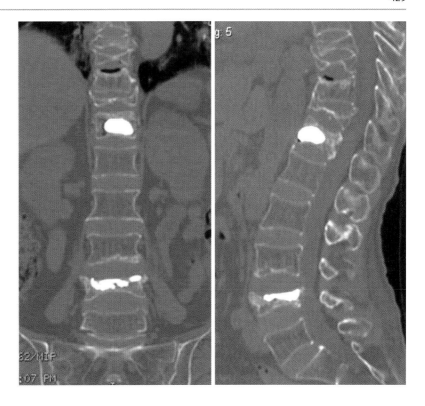

which has a direct relationship with the characteristics of trauma surgery. First of all, skeleton, as the operation target of trauma surgery, has good rigidity and a relative fixed position during the surgical procedure, so it is suitable for robot-assisted positioning and operation. Besides, in trauma surgery, especially minimally invasive surgery, surgeons mainly rely on the fluoroscopy images from C-arm X-ray machine to operate. To achieve better surgical results often requires repeated fluoroscopy images acquirement, and X-ray radiation will do harm to the surgeons and patients, so the introduction of robot in trauma surgery has the additional advantage—reducing intraoperative fluoroscopy times and decreasing the radiation damage to both surgeons and patients. For this reason, surgical robotics for trauma has become one of the hottest research fields of medical robotics research.

The purpose and significance of the introduction of robotics in trauma surgery can be summarized as follows:

1. Reducing surgical trauma

A major goal of surgical robotic system is to reduce surgical trauma, make the operation similar to the traditional surgical treatment, and minimize the negative impact caused by surgery, so as to contribute to the postoperational rehabilitation and significantly reduce the risk of complications.

2. Improving surgical precision

Surgical precision will greatly affect the success rate of trauma surgery. Introducing the robot during surgery can not

only precisely define surgical planning, which means quantitative consideration of the form and function of surgery, but also accurately perform the surgical planning, making the plan become the accurate surgical operation.

3. Reducing surgery time and intraoperative radiation

While the ultimate goal of surgical robot is to improve the quality of surgical intervention, in some cases, its clinical value lies on that it can greatly reduce the operation time of the surgery or some of the key steps. In addition, the introduction of robots can enable surgeons be away from the radiation devices such as C-arm to realize remote control, or significantly reduce the usage of intraoperative fluoroscopy, so as to reduce the radiation damage during trauma surgery.

4. Convenient for surgeons to operate

Introducing robots to assist the surgeon with positioning and operating in trauma surgery can effectively reduce the fatigue and mental stress of surgeons.

5. Becoming the basis for surgical simulator

Surgical simulation platform can be created by combining the surgical planning and the actual surgical robot systems, using the virtual human instead of corpse to conduct surgical training, which is very valuable for the information collection of clinical cases and the training of a large number of clinicians.

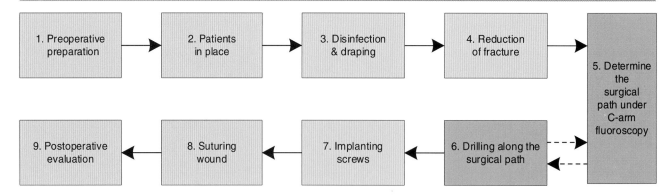

Fig. 17.7 Typical procedure of minimally invasive trauma surgery

3.2   The Procedure of Robot-Assisted Trauma Surgery

The typical surgical procedure of minimally invasive trauma surgery is shown below (Fig. 17.7).

As can be seen from the flowchart, the most important part, which is also the difficulty of the surgery, is the Step 5 and Step 6. In Step 5, the surgeon needs to determine a reasonable surgical path based on the intraoperative X-ray images with their own experience, which means the surgical path planning. Because the human brain cannot form quantitative spatial location from the images, the surgeon's planning cannot be converted into executable quantitative data. In this way, surgeons can only adjust the drilling position under fluoroscopy through their hand–eye coordination to realize the surgical path planning in mind. So in the actual surgical procedure, Steps 5 and 6 are a continuous cycle process, which cannot be strictly divided. Besides, because the C-arm can only provide two-dimensional fluoroscopy images, surgeons need to adjust the C-arm constantly during surgery, shooting images at different angles to determine the three-dimensional position of surgical path, which leads to time-consuming and long-time radiation exposure. In addition, it is difficult for surgeons to keep their hands steady for a long time due to the limitation of physiological conditions. Therefore, the surgical path will inevitably be changed during the repeatedly adjusting and drilling process, so it is difficult for the final result of the surgery to meet the surgeons' surgical planning accurately.

The introduction of robot navigation in minimally invasive trauma surgery could realize that using less intraoperative fluoroscopy images to get quantitative three-dimensional location of surgical path. Then, surgeons are guided to accomplish the operation along the planning path by the precise movement of the robot. So, the surgical accuracy was improved and the intraoperative radiation damage was reduced. Therefore, the core mission of trauma surgery robots can be summarized in two aspects: positioning and navigation. Positioning means: using a small amount of intraoperative X-ray images and the surgical path planning by surgeons, to get the spatial position of surgical path through space posi-

tioning algorithm. While navigation means: using the robot to fix the spatial position of the surgical path and guide the surgeons to operate according to this path. As we can see from the above definition, with the introduction of surgical robot, the process of surgical path adjustment by hand–eye coordination in traditional surgery is divided into two separate parts. The positioning part converts the original surgical planning in the surgeon's minds to the actual surgical path location, achieving a quantitative description of the experience of the surgeons; the navigation part cancels the original repeated adjustments, achieving accurate positioning through precise movements of the robot.

The procedure of robot-assisted minimally invasive trauma surgery is shown below.

3.3   Core Technology

3.3.1   Biplanar Positioning Algorithm Based on Intraoperative Fluoroscopy

The basic principle of biplanar positioning algorithm based on intraoperative fluoroscopy is as follows: first of all, using two X-ray intraoperative images containing scale marker information and surgery object information, we can get the coordinates of markers and surgical path points in the two-dimensional image coordinates by the surgeons' planning. Then, using projection transformation, we can get the coordinates of surgical path points in three-dimensional space coordinates. Finally, the coordinates are converted into the robot coordinates. The coordinates involved in the positioning algorithm include:

$O_W(x,y,z)$—Scale coordinates (world coordinates)
$O_R(x,y,z)$—Robot coordinates
$O_I(u,v)$—Fluoroscopy image coordinates

Therefore, the surgical spatial positioning algorithm based on fluoroscopy images is to establish the conversion between these three coordinates, while this conversion is accomplished by the scale as a reference and media. The entire calculation process of locating algorithm is as follows:

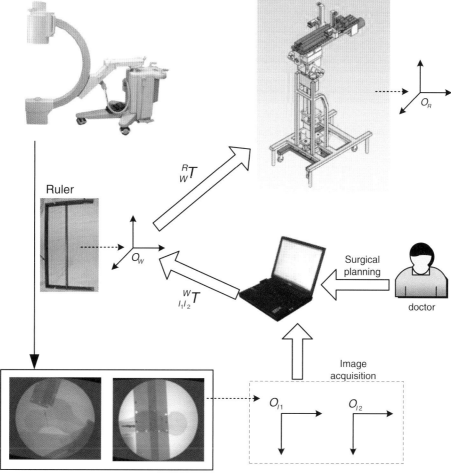

Fluoroscopic images

First of all, when a fluoroscopy image is acquired, using biplanar positioning algorithm, we can achieve a transformation from two fluoroscopy image coordinates to scale coordinate by the markers on the scale projected on the image. It can be defined: $_{I_1 I_2}^{W}T$, in which I_1 and I_2 represent the two-dimensional coordinates of the two fluoroscopy images.

Secondly, there is a fixed mechanical connection between the scale and the robot, leading to a fixed rigid transformation, which can be defined: $_{W}^{R}T$.

Thus, the positioning calculation process of orthopedic surgical navigation robot can be simplified as follows:

$$\left(x_W, y_W, z_W \right) = \left\{ \left(u_1, v_1 \right) \left(u_2, v_2 \right) \right\} \bullet {}_{I_1 I_2}^{W}T \qquad (17.1)$$

$$\left(x_R, y_R, z_R \right) = \left(x_W, y_W, z_W \right) \bullet {}_{W}^{R}T \qquad (17.2)$$

$$\left(x_R, y_R, z_R \right) = \left\{ \left(u_1, v_1 \right) \left(u_2, v_2 \right) \right\} \bullet {}_{I_1 I_2}^{W}T \bullet {}_{W}^{R}T \qquad (17.3)$$

$\{ (u_1, v_1), (u_2, v_2) \}$ represent the target point's coordinates in these two images; (x_W, y_W, z_W) represent the target point's coordinates in the world coordinates; (x_R, y_R, z_R) represent the target point's coordinates in the robot coordinates.

In the actual surgery positioning, the positioning of the final surgical path can be converted into the positioning of two points on the surgical path, which are called "in point" and "out point" in surgery. If $\left\{ \left(u_1^a, v_1^a \right), \left(u_2^a, v_2^a \right) \right\}$ represent the coordinates of "in point" in two fluoroscopic images, and $\left\{ \left(u_1^b, v_1^b \right), \left(u_2^b, v_2^b \right) \right\}$ represent the coordinates of "out point" in two fluoroscopic images, we can get as follows:

$$\left(x_R^a, y_R^a, z_R^a \right) = \left\{ \left(u_1^a, v_1^a \right), \left(u_2^a, v_2^a \right) \right\} \bullet {}_{I_1 I_2}^{W}T \bullet {}_{W}^{R}T$$

$$\left(x_R^b, y_R^b, z_R^b \right) = \left\{ \left(u_1^b, v_1^b \right), \left(u_2^b, v_2^b \right) \right\} \bullet {}_{I_1 I_2}^{W}T \bullet {}_{W}^{R}T$$

$\left(x_R^a, y_R^a, z_R^a \right)$ and $\left(x_R^b, y_R^b, z_R^b \right)$ represent the coordinates of "in point" and "out point" in the robot coordinates. The final surgical path outputted by robot is actually the spatial line composed of two points.

3.3.2   Workspace-Driven Design Method for Surgical Robot System

Workspace is one of the most important factors for trauma surgical robot. Because the work environment of trauma surgical robot is typical of unstructured space, not only each of the patient's physiological parameters and type of the

Fig. 17.8 Workflow of workspace-driven design method

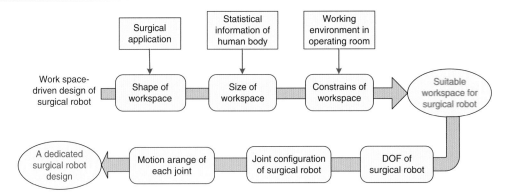

fracture site is different but also each of the operating room's physical space and the device configuration is not the same; besides, trauma surgical robot can only work close to the surgeons and patients, so its workspace is directly related to usability and safety of surgical robot systems. While the workspace of the robot is determined by the configuration of the robot, so configuration design is one of the most important technologies for the research of trauma surgical robot.

The basic idea of this workspace-driven design method is to get the requirements and constrains of surgical robot's workspace from orthopedic applications and then use this information to drive the process of surgical robot's design. The workflow of this method is illustrated in Fig. 17.8.

Such as minimally invasive trauma surgery (neck hollow nails, sacroiliac screw, etc.), the robot needs at least five DOFs, 3 for insert point's position and 2 for surgical path's orientation. Considering the complex working environment in operating room, 1 or 2 redundant DOFs for obstacle avoidance is recommended. To adapt to different requirements in different surgeries and have a bigger workspace with better dexterity, rotation joints are recommended. For the joint configuration of the surgical robot, a 3-DOF robot arm plus a 2-DOF robot wrist is suggested.

3.3.3 The Efficiency Evaluation of Robot Based on Data Envelopment Analysis

The research of trauma surgery robot has a history of more than 10 years and the overall technology and clinical application of surgical robot have a rapid development during these years. Some robotic systems have demonstrated its outstanding results in improving surgical results and reducing surgical trauma, and reducing labor intensity of surgeons when they are used in the clinical applications, which have been widely recognized in the field of engineering and medicine. However, the doubt about trauma surgery robots has never stopped in the past 10 years. One of the biggest doubts is the efficiency of the surgical robot, that is to say, to what extent will the robots help patients and surgeons and whether such help is efficient for the excessive consumption of resources needed by surgical robot. To answer these ques-

tions, we must solve the problem of efficiency evaluation of surgical robots, which is how to use a scientific and rational approach to evaluate the efficiency of surgical robot quantitatively. So, the efficiency evaluation of surgical robots has a great significance for its further development, especially for its clinical application.

Data Envelopment Analysis (DEA) is a new system analysis method developed based on the concept of "relative efficiency evaluation" by famous operation researchers A. Charnes and W. W. Cooper.

DEA is based on the "relative efficiency," which can evaluate the relative efficiency of a group of decision-making units (DMUs) having the same inputs and outputs, so the general procedure using DEA to evaluate the efficiency of surgical robots is as follows:

1. The establishment of DMU model

This step is the modeling of evaluation object. Usually, robot-assisted surgery and traditional surgery without robot assistance are modeled as DMU, respectively. Then, the inputs and outputs of surgery are analyzed. The inputs represent the resources consumed by surgery, including the medical staff, surgery time, and the usage of intraoperative fluoroscopy. The outputs represent the surgery's outcome, which are quantitative indicators of surgery's quality, such as the parallelism and dispersion of screws. To ensure the DEA evaluation, the DMUs involved in evaluation are demanded to have the same type of inputs and outputs. Moreover, these inputs and outputs must be described quantitatively.

2. Getting each DMU's input and output values

This step is to obtain the raw data used to calculate. That is, aiming to the surgery DMU model established in the above step, the specific input and output values are obtained of each DMU by experiments or clinical observation. Because these data are the basis of efficiency evaluation, the statistical data are usually chosen, which means the average of the corresponding data are chosen as the basis of calculation.

3. Selecting the model to calculate the efficiency

Using raw data obtained in the above step and substituting into corresponding DEA model and solving for each DMU, we can get the optimal solution for corresponding DEA model, and then we can judge the relative efficiency. At least one DEA is efficient in a group of DMUs involved in evaluating based on the existence theorem of DEA. The most common calculating model is C^2R. C^2R model is the initial and basic math model of DEA method and is also the most important and widely used one. The C^2R model is described below:

$$\left(C^2R\right)\begin{cases} \max \dfrac{\mathbf{u}^T\mathbf{Y}_0}{\mathbf{v}^T\mathbf{X}_0} = V_P \\[2mm] \dfrac{\mathbf{u}^T\mathbf{Y}_j}{\mathbf{v}^T\mathbf{X}_j} \leq 1, \quad j = 1,\cdots,n \\[2mm] \mathbf{u} \geq 0 \\[1mm] \mathbf{v} \geq 0 \end{cases} \qquad (17.4)$$

where $\mathbf{X}_j = (x_{1j}, x_{2j}, \cdots, x_{mj})^T$, $j = 1, \cdots, n$ represents the input vector of DMU_j, $\mathbf{Y}_j = (y_{1j}, y_{2j}, \cdots, y_{sj})^T$, $j = 1, \cdots, n$ represents the output vector of DMU_j, and $\mathbf{v} = (v_1, v_2, \cdots, v_m)^T$ and $\mathbf{u} = (u_1, u_2, \cdots, u_s)^T$ represent the weight vectors of inputs and outputs, respectively.

Because the initial C^2R is a fractional programming problem, in order to solve the problem conveniently, we can transform it into an equivalent linear programming problem using the C^2 transformation. The model is like this:

$$\left(D_{C^2R}\right)\begin{cases} \min \theta = V \\[2mm] \sum_{j=1}^{n}\mathbf{X}_j\lambda_j \leq \theta\mathbf{X}_0 \\[2mm] \sum_{j=1}^{n}\mathbf{Y}_j\lambda_j \geq \mathbf{Y}_0 \\[2mm] \lambda_j \geq 0, j = 1,\cdots,n \end{cases} \qquad (17.5)$$

The DEA relative efficiency is solved based on the model (Eq. (17.5)). If the minimum value V of a DMU equals 1, then this DMU is defined relatively efficient. On the contrary, if the minimum value V of a DMU is less than 1, then this DMU is defined relatively inefficient.

3.4 Typical Systems

3.4.1 Biplanar Surgical Robot System for Trauma Surgery

The biplanar surgical robot system for trauma surgery (described as below) invented by Beihang University and Jishuitan Hospital is the first trauma robot used in clinic in China. This system completes the first case of robot-assisted trauma surgery and the first case of remote trauma surgery in China between Beijing and Yanan (Fig. 17.9).

Fig. 17.9 Biplanar trauma surgical robot system

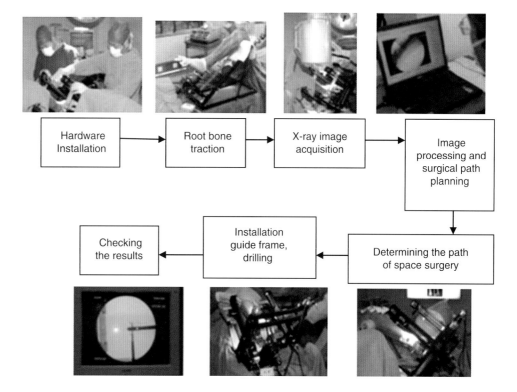

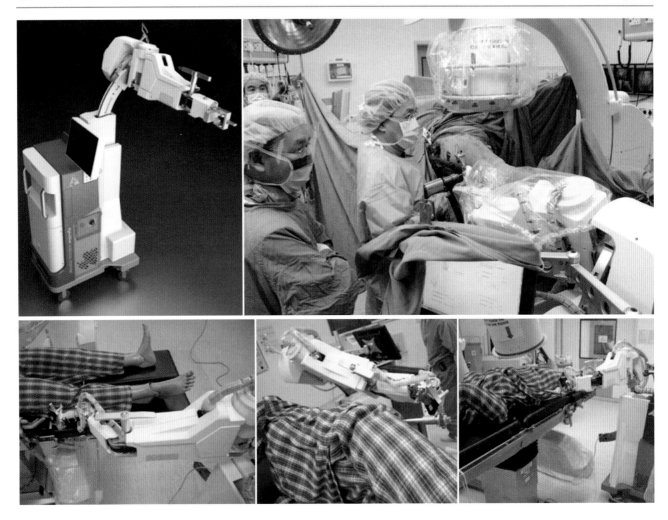

Fig. 17.10 Hybridot surgical robot system for trauma

The design and development of the robot system are based on the clinical environments and conditions in China. It adopts the compact and modular design ideas, having advantages of high accuracy, compact, easy to operate, safe, reliable, low cost, etc. Besides, the Tele-Planning mode based on narrowband is presented, reducing the data transmitted over the network and the pressure on the transmission bandwidth, avoiding the surgical safety problems caused by the instability of network transmission. So, it is suitable to promote the clinical application in remote areas and basic hospital environment.

The system also achieves a biplanar positioning method with independent intellectual property rights, which is simple and practical and will not cause additional damage to the patients. The small modular robot structure changes the traditional robot structure and can conduct different combinations depending on the different surgical environments, so as to assist surgeons to complete the surgical procedure safely and reliably. Considering the habits of medical staff in China and the surgical procedure, the system adopts human–computer interaction interface, so that surgeons can easily control the system to complete the operation. Based on the computer image processing and surgical planning techniques, the system reconstructs wide vision of surgical objects and assists the surgeons to complete preoperative planning, providing necessary surgical information for surgeons.

3.4.2 The Hybrid Surgical Robot System for Trauma: Hybridot

The hybrid surgical robot system for trauma—Hybridot invented by the Chinese University of Hong Kong and Beihang University—achieves an innovative 7-DOF robot configuration. The design of curved track joint can make robot rotate around the axis of the patient's body and provides suitable workspace and flexibility to meet the requirements of various trauma surgeries (Fig. 17.10).

In addition, the robot also achieved a free switch between active and passive control methods. The robot's active control, which means that robot acts autonomously under the control of the host computer's instruction, and has the advantages of high accuracy and good stability. However, due to the independent movement of the robot, there are safety risks that robot may mistakenly hit the surgeons and patients. Passive control, which means that robot acts following surgeons' manual traction, has the advantages of no independent movement for robot, so it is safe and can be completely controlled by surgeons, but the motion accuracy is difficult to improve.

The Hybridot system achieves the fusion of the respective advantages by the combination of two control methods. When surgery starts, surgeons lead the robot to the general location using the passive control methods, achieving preliminary positioning. Then, robot conducts the fine tuning of location under the automatic control mode, achieving accurate positioning. In this way, the system achieves high-precision surgery positioning under the premise of ensuring safety.

4 Robot-Assisted Spine Surgery

Yue Zhou and He Zhang

Spine-related trauma and diseases are common in orthopedics. The number of people who are suffering the disorders aforesaid is more than a 100 million and it is increasing ten million every year in China. And, about 60–70% of them need the operative interventions.

Due to the special anatomic structures, the pedicles have the ability of controlling the movement of spine, and to transmit the force to the anterior portion of the centrum. This means that besides the solid fusion, the transpedicular screws could also fix and correct the spine in three dimensions through controlling the whole centrum. And, that is why transpedicular fixation or vertebroplasty was accepted widely in clinic.

But, these procedures need to be extremely accurate because of the significant important surroundings of the pedicles. The misplacement of pedicle screws will lead to catastrophic damage of vertebral artery, nerve root, spinal nerves, or vital organs. In addition, transpedicular procedures are still facing such as fractures of pedicle, difficulty of surgical field exposure, and the long-time operating undergoing X-ray exposure.

Compared with the surgeons, robots have a higher accuracy and stability. And, they could assist the surgeons to complete the procedure undergoing the X-ray exposure repeatedly without decreasing their performance.

The robotic technique mainly applies with transpedicular fixation in spine surgery, and in addition, it is still used in biopsy, vertebroplasty, fact block, laminectomy, tumor ablation and resection, and the exploration in the subarachnoid space.

4.1 For Transpedicular Fixation

4.1.1 Robots Involves Retrofitting Industrialized Manipulators

PUMA 260

The earliest spinal robot was reported by Pascal Sautot and his research team in Grenoble, France. They designed an end effector, which holding a laser guide to point the drilling trajectories over the patient's vertebrae, to attach the industrial manipulator, PUMA 260.

The drilling trajectories were planned preoperatively by using the patient's segmented computed tomography scan result, which was registered to the intraoperative fluoroscopy images. The research team presented a drilling experiment on plastic vertebrae, and the accuracy reported was submillimeter.

PUMA 560

In 1995, Santos-Munné et al. proposed another robotic system for transpedicular fixation based on the research of Pascal Sautot and his team [1]. The system contained a drill guide end effector which was made of radiolucent material with embedded metal spheres.

Similarly with the first research, the drilling trajectories were planned preoperatively and registered with intraoperative fluoroscopic images. But, there is no accuracy or experimental results of this system reported by the authors (Fig. 17.11).

Stäubli

In 2008, a research team supported by the Third Military Medical University and the State Key Laboratory of Robotics (Shenyang Institute of Automation Chinese Academy of Sciences) designed a drill guide container for pneumatic drill connected with the manipulator named Stäubli.

Like the aforementioned systems, this one had the same planning and registration methods and almost the same compositions: manipulator, control plate for surgeons, and the surgery field camera. The system showed a fine accuracy result on spinal sawbones, cattle spine, and cadavers to meet the clinical needs (Fig. 17.12).

4.1.2 Robot with Optical Navigation System

VectorBot

To deal with the increasing cost and complexity of medical robotic systems, the Deutsches Zentrum für Luft- und Raumfahrt (German Aerospace Centre, DLR) had developed a series of lightweight robots for multiple surgical usages. BrainLab (Feldkirchen, Germany) named the transpedicular fixation robot, one of the DLR lightweight robots, as "VectorBot" and sponsored five million dollars. But unfortunately, they cancelled it before its industrialization.

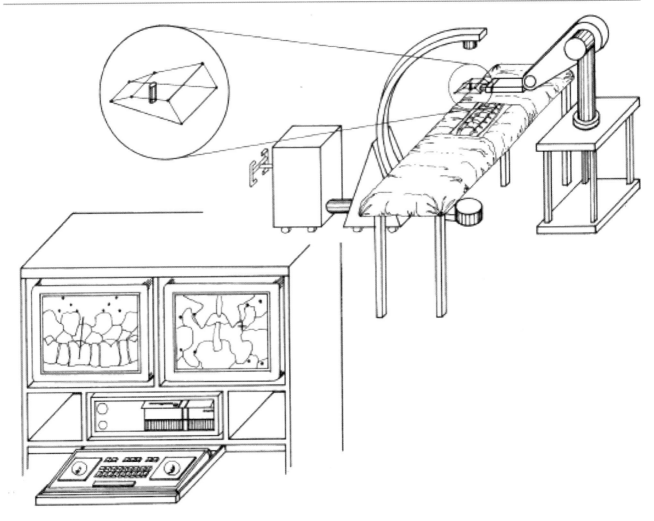

Fig. 17.11 Spinal pedicle screw implant system

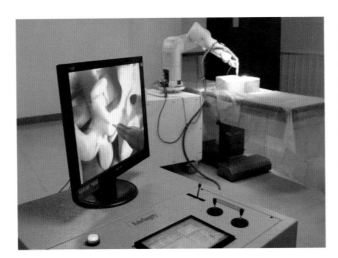

Fig. 17.12 Prototype of minimally invasive spinal surgery robotic system

The VectorBot consisted of the KineMedic robot, which was developed using Lightweight Robot II (LWR II) and

VectorVision optical tracking system developed by BrainLab. Different with the ones retrofitted by the industrial manipulator systems, the optical tracking system required no fluoroscopic images while tracking. The tracking process was achieved by the optical system tracking the markers attached to the patient's vertebrae. Although radiation was greatly reduced, the surgical incision was largely increased.

Ortmaier et al. published the results of a series of evaluation experiments about drilling and milling on the artificial bone and bovine spine [2]. The results showed that the milling process was superior to drilling on the deviation errors and reactive forces. In terms of control parameters, the optimum was reached with high proportional and integral gains, which led to higher robot stiffness, lower pose errors, reduced settling time, and decreased overshoot. They also claimed that the accuracy and latency of the optical tracking system were critical factors. But on the other hand, they admitted that they have not taken the preoperative image resolution, segmentation accuracy, and intraoperative registration errors, etc. in account (Fig. 17.13).

SPINEBOT, SPINEBOT v2, and CoRA

In 2005, a research team from the Hanyang University presented the SPINEBOT system, which consisted of its unique planning software (HexaView) and optical tracking system besides the manipulator. HexaView allowed the surgeons to plan the screw trajectory in six different views using preoperative CT or magnetic resonance (MR) scan results. The localization of the optical tracking system was based on spherical reflective markers fixed in surgical tools and patient's spine. And, the optical tracking system was commercialized by NDI (Waterloo, Ontario, Canada) and added a 30-Hz feedback for redundant position control of the robot in addition to its embedded encoders. The manipulator, which giving seven degrees of freedom (DoFs) in total, consisted of a Cartesian positioner, a gimbal, and a tool holder.

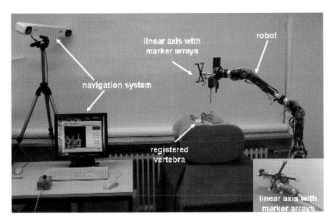

Fig. 17.13 VectorBot experimental setup for the navigated placement of pedicle screws with the new medical robot and the Brainlab VectorVision navigation system

The system applied two different types of working: assisted drilling as a positioning holder and autonomous drilling as an executor. In addition, the SPINEBOT system also contained a motion-correction system for correcting the patient's breathing motion based on the optical feedback. And, the result given by the authors showed a 3-mm amplitude in anteroposterior direction.

Relative experiments demonstrated that the error of optical tracking system was about 0.35 mm, and the error of motion-correction system was ±0.15 mm. Comparing with the assisted drilling of the system, the autonomous mode showed the better result, and both of the deviations observed were in the 1–2 mm range (Fig. 17.14).

In 2009, a research team from the Pohang University of Science and Technology (POSTECH) reported a robot system called cooperative robotic assistant (CoRA), which used HexaView system of SPINEBOT coupled with a robust prototype capable of automated screw insertion and haptic feedback. For withstanding larger reaction forces in the process of drilling and inserting, the research team designed a big robust frame which hindered the surgeon's access to the patient. In addition to the autonomous drilling and inserting mode, the CoRA still offered teleoperational control with realistic haptic feedback. By using the same planning and tracking system with SPINEBOT, the researchers expected CoRA to have similar error in screw placement. But, there was no further experiment result till now (Fig. 17.15).

In 2010, a cadaveric study was reported using SPINEBOT, which was totally redesigned and without the automatic drilling capabilities. The new manipulator just had five DoFs, one prismatic and four rotational joints, and replaced the original end effector by a simple tool holder. The planning software

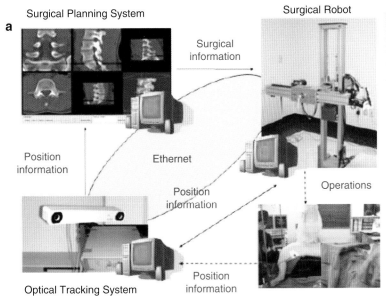
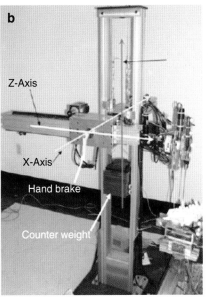

Fig. 17.14 SPINEBOT. (**a**) Systematic construction. (**b**) Manipulator

Fig. 17.15 CoRA. (**a**)
Systematic construction. (**b**)
Body structure of the CoRA.
(**c**) End effector of the CoRA

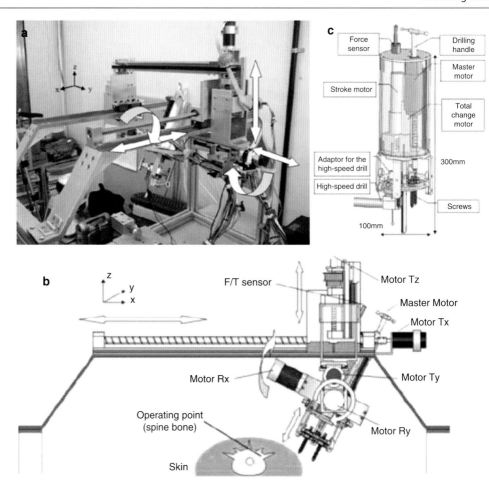

was also completed redesigned as the optical tracking system was replaced by biplanar continuous fluoroscopy.

The biplanar fluoroscopy, liked the G-arm, was "O" shape for more stability. Using this unique fluoroscopic instrument, SPINEBOT v2 could detect the relative position between the patient and the surgical tools by means of custom 2D–3D registration algorithms.

Lab experiment result showed that the overall positioning error of SPINEBOT v 2 was 1.38 ± 0.21 mm. And, the cadaver experiment in 14 different vertebrae of two cadavers showed that 26 of 28 screws were correctly positioned, with no observed perforations into the spinal canal. Average angular errors were 2.45 ± 2.56° and 0.71 ± 1.21°in the axial and lateral planes, respectively (Fig. 17.16).

Neuroglide

Neuroglide was proposed by Kostrzewski for cervical interbody fusion, especially for atlantoaxial fusion. The system consisted of parallel four-DoF mechanism manipulator which held a drill guide, infrared optical tracking system, joystick for the robot, and software for planning and navigation. The implant trajectory in each vertebra is planned preoperatively using fine-cut computerized tomography (CT) scans. The registration process was achieved

using point-to-point registration matching between the CT result and the patient's anatomy, and refined with a surface merge technique intraoperatively. While drilling positioning process was completed first approximately done passively by the surgeon, final precise instrument positioning was performed by the robot according to the planned trajectory through the target vertebra. And finally, implants (screws) are then placed through the robot-guided working channel.

The Neuroglide was evaluated by implanting ten screws in the upper two vertebrae of the human cervical spine with six cadavers. And, the implant placement accuracy was comparable with that achieved using freehand image-guided techniques by an experienced surgeon. The result showed that the mean translational error was 1.94 mm and the mean rotational error was 4.35°, although two screws were dropped from the statistical sample due to their abnormally large errors produced by drill slippage. As the system was kept improving during the experiments, so the results were not comparable directly. And, the authors gave a remarkable result after all their improvements were in place (0.41 mm and 2.56° for the last screw). In addition, comparing with the conventional image-guided procedure, the Neuroglide system assisted drilling only longer 3 min (Fig. 17.17).

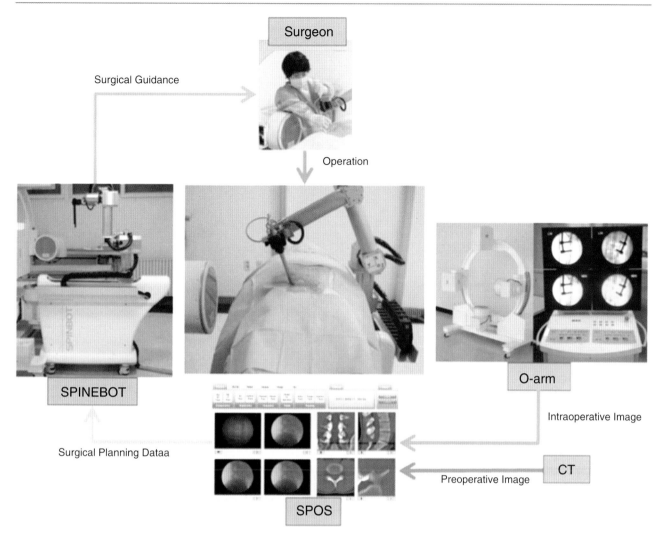

Fig. 17.16 SPINEBOT v2 experimental setup of the Biplane Fluoroscopy-Guided Robot System (BFRS). The BFRS consists of an O-shaped biplane fluoroscope (O-arm), a surgical planning and operat- ing system (SPOS), and an assistive robot with 5 degrees of freedom (SPINEBOT). CT indicates computed tomography

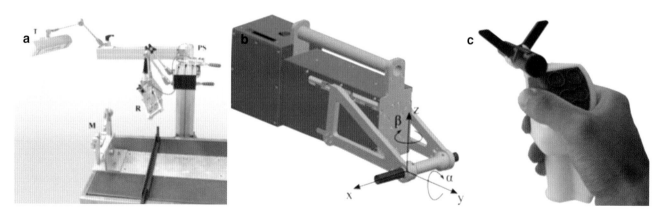

Fig. 17.17 Neuroglide. (**a**) System setup: R, robot; T, camera of the optical tracking system; PS, passive structure; M, Mayfield skull clamp. (**b**) Parallel four degrees of freedom robot. (**c**) New surgical input device

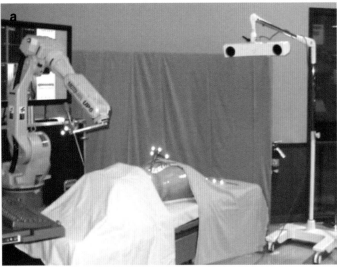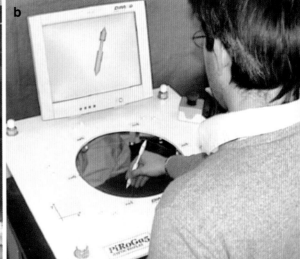

Fig. 17.18 RIME. (**a**) The surgical robotic system developed by the Wright State University, Wallace-Kettering Neuroscience Institute, and MotoMan Inc. As it shows, some optical markers are attached to the end effector of the robot and to a vertebra-mounted frame to perform a fully automated spine procedure. The stereo infrared sensor is shown on the right side of the figure. (**b**) The PiRoGa5 pen-based haptic display manipulated by an operator. On the screen, the 3D rendering of the end effector provided by the Crizia OpenGL-based software

RIME

In 2005, Boschetti et al. proposed a project named robot in medical environment (RIME) for drilling in transpedicular fixation [3]. The environment was made up of a haptic master, a slave robot, an optical tracking device, and a main control unit. The surgeon performed a drilling operation by using the telerobotic device of RIME, process of which was guided by haptic feedback: as soon as the vertebra moves, the optical tracking device measured vertebra pose, and a proper force was exerted on the operator's hand to let him/her adjust surgical tool position and orientation. Moreover, the haptic master produces the force feedback related to the teleoperation. There was a feasibility of haptic feedback teleoperation test experiment reported between two cities separated by 35 km. But, no publications about the experiments with cadavers or animals were found till now (Fig. 17.18).

RSSS

Jin et al. proposed a new robotic system for transpedicular fixation in 2011 and just named it as robotic spinal surgical system (RSSS), which consisted of haptic 5-DoF manipulator, infrared optical tracking system and a main control unit [4]. This system provided two control methods to not breakthrough the pedicle based on the force messages. One was the admittance control, and the other was a safety control during drilling process. The accuracy and safety experiments were completed using 32 screws with sheep spines. And, the results showed that the average deviations of the entry points in the axial and sagittal views were 0.50 ± 0.33 and 0.65 ± 0.40 mm, and the average deviations of the angles in the axial and sagittal views were $1.9 \pm 0.82°$ and $1.48 \pm 1.2°$ compared with the preoperative plans (Fig. 17.19).

4.1.3 The Commercialized Spine Robots

Evolution 1

In 2001, researchers from the Fraunhofer Institute developed the Evolution 1 surgical robot, which was commercialized by the Universal Robot Systems (URS) and deployed on several clinical institutions. Although Evolution 1 was designed for neurosurgery, someone still wanted to extend its application to spinal interventions under the project named "Robots and Manipulators for Medical Applications." However, with URS went bankrupt, the former users of this system have to stop using it due to the absence of the technical support.

SpineAssist/Renaissance

In 2003, a research team of Israel demonstrated a parallel robot named MARS, which was commercialized by the Mazor Robotics (Cesarea, Israel). The first generation of this system was named SpineAssist and the second generation with a total upgrade of the software and user interface named Renaissance. This system was designed for spinal interventions such as biopsies, transpedicular fixation, scoliotic back correction, and vertebroplasty. And, it passed the FDA and CE, and was the only robot available in the marker till October, 2014 (Fig. 17.20).

SpineAssist/Renaissance consisted of robotic device, workstation, outrigger arms, and registration and clamping devices. The robot device was a 6-DoF parallel manipulator with a dimension of 50 mm in diameter, 80 mm in height,

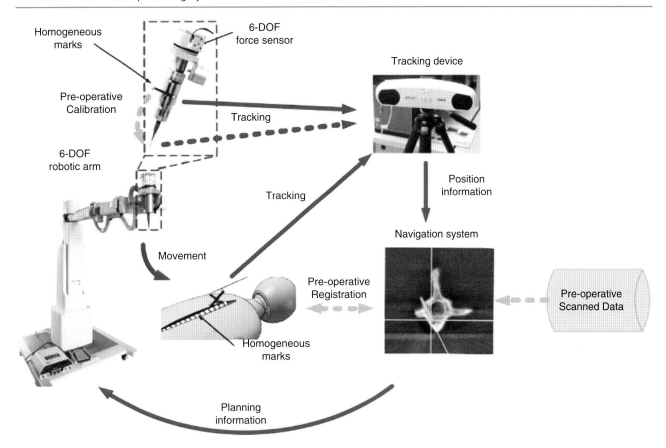

Fig. 17.19 RSSS architecture of the robotic spine-assisted surgery system

and 250 g in weight. And, its positional accuracy was less than 1 mm. The SpineAssist/Renaissance workstation contained specially designed graphic user interface software. This software enables the registration of the radiographic images, facilitates the preoperative plan for an optimal entry point and trajectory of the implant, and controls the robot device. Three different outrigger arms may be affixed to the upper moving platform of the robot device. Each arm accommodates a drill guide sleeve. The system determines which arm is to be used, based on the implants used and the relative location of the robot device to the predetermined entry point and implant trajectory. Pre-/intra-operation registration devices contained two parts, one was fixed on the patient's body using clamping devices and the other one was fixed on the fluoroscopic devices. Two different fixtures mounted the SpineAssist/Renaissance device to the bony anatomy of a patient: spinous process clamp and Hover-T frame. For open procedures, the robot device could be mounted directly over the spinous process using a clamp and bridge, while for minimally invasive interventions the fixation between the device and the spine would be completed with the Hover-T frame.

The surgical workflow with SpineAssist/Renaissance consists of four steps: (a) surgical planning—surgeon designing the optimal positions and dimensions of implants based on the preoperative CT scans; (b) mounting the platform attachment of the needed mounting platform to the patient's bony anatomy; (c) calibration and registration—fixing the registration device to the fluoroscopic device and patient's spine, and then acquisition of two X-ray images for automatically registering to the preoperative CT scan; (d) positioning and drilling for mounting of the robot on the platform, which latter aligns its arm with the planned screw (or tool) trajectory; and drilling through the guiding tube held by the robot's arm, followed by the insertion of the guide wire and screw.

After attainment of the FDA clearance, SpineAssist/Renaissance has been used by clinical teams worldwide. Until 2013, the system had been validated by more than 2500 procedures, on which over 15,000 implants had been placed without reported cases of nerve damage. Multiple publications reported the experiences of SpineAssist/Renaissance-assisted procedures demonstrated a better accuracy, less X-ray exposure for surgeons and nurses, and almost same operation time (no significant difference) comparing with the traditional technique. But, the deficits of this system are still obvious, such as: (a) working space limitation, (b) insecure robot device fixation

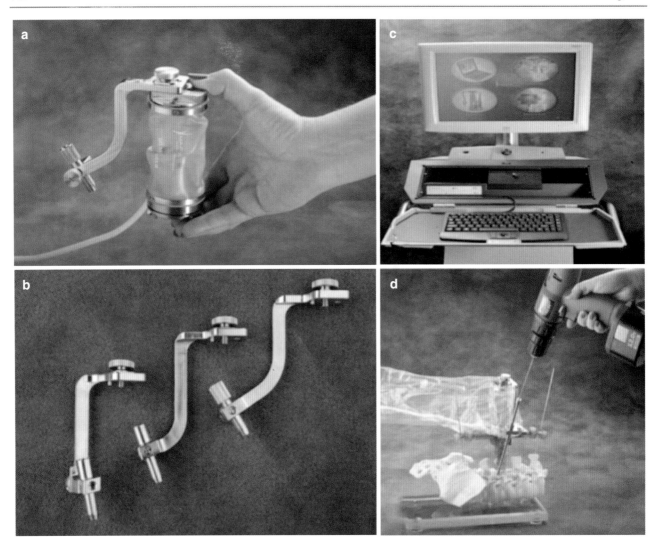

Fig. 17.20 SpineAssist. (**a**) SpineAssist device bone-mounted miniature robot. (**b**) SpineAssist workstation. (**c**) Three different types of arm (No. 1, 2, and 3 arms from the left). (**d**) Surgical setting of SpineAssist device for drilling

sometimes using bedside fixation, and (c) drill slippage caused by soft tissue stretch or insecure anchor point.

4.1.4 Other Robot Systems for Spine Surgery

Spine Bull's-Eye Robot

In 2012, Zhang et al. reported a robotic system for transpedicular fixation in thoracic and lumber spine, using a special view of fluoroscopy, pedicle standard axis view (PSAV) [5]. The system contained a seven-DoF hollow and radiolucent manipulator, base, console, and a main control unit. And, the surgeons could adjust the position of the manipulator remotely. After the PSAV was clearly acquired, the guide wire could insert into the "bull's eye" (the center of the pedicle circular projection) assisted by the special hollow manipulator, and then the drilling process could be started. By using the PSAV technique, the authors claimed that the guide wires were successfully inserted in all of the pedicles

whose PSAV were acquired clearly (203/209). And, there is no significant difference between drilling plans and actual results (postoperative CT) (Fig. 17.21).

4.2 For Vertebroplasty and Biopsy

4.2.1 AcuBot

In 2002, presented a plan for minimally invasive spinal surgery (MISS) system and led to the development of AcuBot system. The research team analyzed MISS and identified the main issues: unavailability of intraoperative axial images, difficult fusion of CT and MR data, lack of visualization of oblique trajectories, unavailability of spinal tracking systems, slow and difficult instrument insertion and lack of appropriate software. After that, to solve the aforementioned problems, they advocated a solution plan which included intraoperative CT, 3D visualization, optical tracking systems, robotic tool holders, and development of specialized software.

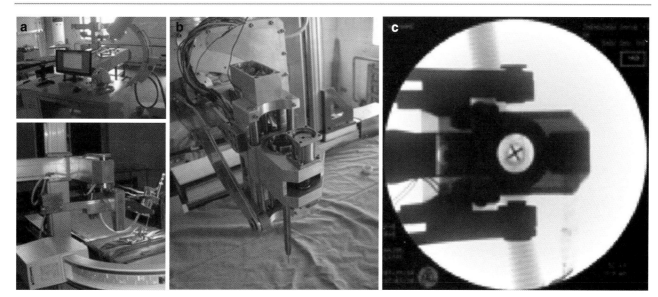

Fig. 17.21 Spine Bull's-Eye robot (**a**) the Spine Bull's-Eye Robot comprises a 7-df robot arm and base, console, control system, fluoroscope system, and hollow and radiolucent manipulator. (**b**) Close-up picture of the manipulator and guide wire. (**c**) "+" formed projection of the guide wire aimed at the bull's-eye

In 2003, the research team presented AcuBot which mainly consisted of manipulator, display, joystick, and the control unit. The system was used for assisting percutaneous biopsy and nerve root and facet blocks. The manipulator had six DoFs totally. Three of them composed a Cartesian manipulator, two of them supported a remote center of motion (RCM) mechanism, and the last one was the translational DoF along the instrument axis on the end effector of the manipulator. In addition, a seven-DoF passive mechanism was mounted between the Cartesian manipulator and the RCM mechanism, which was manually adjusted by the surgeon before the procedure, bringing the instrument close to the entry points. The joystick and the display were used to control the robot remotely. And, this system had already attained the FDA clearance.

In 2005, a randomized clinical trial was reported by Cleary et al. for image-guided nerve and facet blocks [6]. They divided the 20 patients into two groups, ten of whom underwent the conventional procedure and the remaining ten were operated with the assistance of the AcuBot. There was a similar result about needle insertion accuracy and pain relief between these two groups. But, the statistical sample was too small to draw significant conclusions. Currently, research with the AcuBot is focused on the development of a rotating needle holder for improved lesion targeting in soft organs, and giving less attention to spinal procedures according to the latest report (Fig. 17.22).

Innomotion

Because of superior soft tissue contrast and no radiation exposure, MR images have their special advantages for robotic and image-guided surgeries. However, the strong magnetic fields required compatible materials. And following special sensors, actuators and robotic designs were also the formidable challenges. But in 2003, presented a compatible manipulator, the manipulator for interventional radiology (MIRA). The system frame was built from polyether ether ketone (PEEK) and fiber-reinforced epoxy, and actuated using ultrasonic and pneumatic motors. Completely MR-compatible sensors were developed for positioning control.

In 2008, Melzer et al. presented the Innomotion system based on MIRA [7]. The new system was designed for MR-guided insertion of cannulae and probes for biopsy, drainage, drug delivery, and energetic tumor destruction. The five-DoF manipulator of Innomotion was attached to an orbiting ring mounted on the scanner's bed, linear pneumatic actuators, optical limit switches, and rotational and linear encoders. Innomotion's instrument holder was designed as a two-DoF RCM and was equipped with gadolinium-filled spheres for segmenting the intraoperative MR images to detect its position and orientation. The system obtained CE clearance and was introduced to the market by Innomedic GmbH (Herxheim, Germany), which was acquired by Synthes (Solothurn, Switzerland) in 2008. The Innomotion's commercialization was stopped in the early 2010 and was expected to be restarted in 2012 by the IBSmm Company (Brno, Czech Republic). For that propose, the research team is working on improvement of the system right now.

The phantom experiment inserted 25 needles and measured the deviation by hand using rulers. And, the result was 2.2 ± 0.7 mm. The robot's deviation of the animal test in the axial plane was estimated to be within the ± 1-mm range

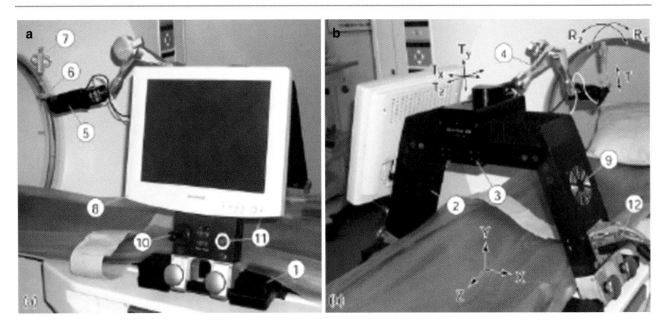

Fig. 17.22 AcuBot. (**a**) Front and (**b**) side views of the AcuBot mounted on a CT scanner

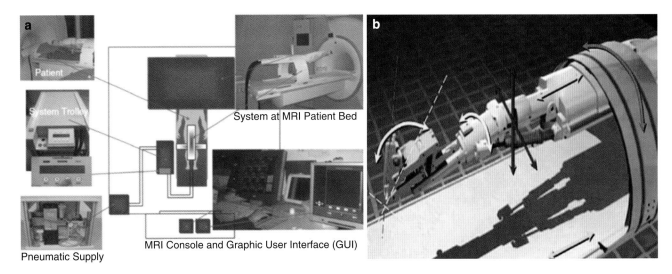

Fig. 17.23 Innomotion. (**a**) Setup for MRI-guided procedures as it has been evaluated for Siemens and Philips MRI platforms. (**b**) Schematic view of the INNOMOTION assistance system with five pneumatically driven DoFs and two manual adjustments for prepositioning at the orbit (red arrow) and at the patient bed (green arrow)

(minimum 0.5 mm and maximum 3 mm) and its angular deviation to be ±1° (minimum 0.5° and maximum 3°).Of the six reported clinical trials, two were carried out successfully around the spine: one was a bone biopsy in the iliac crest and one was an abscess aspiration in the L5–S1 region. No complications were observed in all six cases (Fig. 17.23).

LWR III

LWR III, the following version of LWR II (see VectorBot), was commercialized by KUKA and is increasingly being adopted for surgical robotics projects. The robotic system proposed by Tovar-Arriaga et al. for spine biopsies and ver-

tebroplasties just utilized this robot coupled with infrared optical tracking and intraoperative 3D radiography systems [8]. The errors of calibration between the tooltip positions measured by the optical system and the robot's controller had a mean of 0.23 mm and a maximum value of 0.47 mm. And, the errors of tooltip positions in a precisely manufactured phantom and 3D radiographies were to be in 1.2 ± 0.4 mm, with minimum and maximum values of 0.3 and 1.98 mm, respectively. Although the optical system's accuracy and low sampling rate still limiting the accuracy of this robotic system, it also satisfied the demands of spinal surgery (Fig. 17.24).

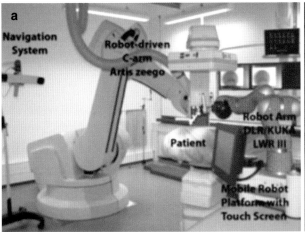
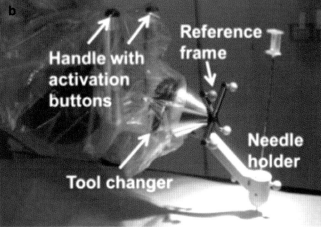

Fig. 17.24 LWRIII. (a) System setup in the interventional suite. The robotic needle holder is positioned inside the volume of measurement of the robot-driven C-arm. The navigation camera is used to measure the pose of the needle holder, which is then controlled in real time. (b) Robot arm including the interaction handle can be draped, and the autoclavable needle holder includes a DRF for the tracking by the navigation system and an exchangeable needle guide

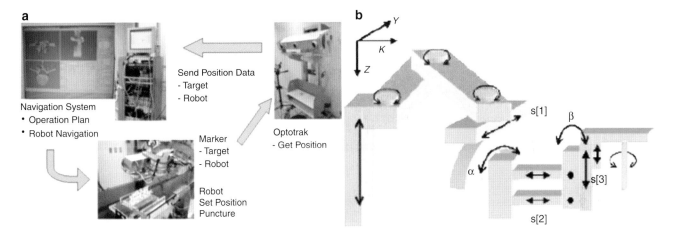

Fig. 17.25 Vertebroplasty robot of the Tokyo University. (a) Systematic construction. (b) Developed robot mechanism

Vertebroplasty Robot of Tokyo University

In 2005, developed a robotic system for vertebroplasty, based on a specially designed compact end-effector manipulator for inserting in the narrow space between the C-arm and patient on the operating table. The appropriate needle trajectory was planned based on the preoperative three-dimensional CT images. The needle holding part of the robot is X-ray lucent so that the needle insertion process can be monitored by fluoroscopy. The position of the needle during insertion process can be continuously monitored. In 2009, Onogi et al. reported the in vitro experiment result, which showed that the deviation in polyurethane phantoms of lumbar spines was 0.46 ± 0.80 mm and $1.49 \pm 0.64°$ (Fig. 17.25) [9].

SpineNav

In 2008, a research team supported by the Nankai University and Tianjin Medical University presented SpineNav system to insert needles autonomously for percutaneous vertebroplasty. This system consisted of a five-DoF manipulator mounted on the CT bed, a metal mask fixed on the CT scanner for segmenting from the CT images to estimate the robot's base position and orientation with respect to the patient, and a main control unit. The mean positioning error of this system was 0.89 mm, with a maximum of 1.14 mm. And till now, no cadavers or clinical trials results were reported (Fig. 17.26).

4.3 For Laminectomy

In 2010, Wang et al. proposed a robot to remove the lamina arcus vertebrae in laminectomy [10]. This procedure requires milling of the connective portion of the lamina and pedicle. With the possibility of injury in the spinal cord or nerve root, this kind of procedure required a very high precision. The robot device was a two-translational DoF manipulator, which could stop just before penetration into the spinal canal, leaving a very thin cortex for removing by the surgeon. The haptic sensor and custom algorithms provided the ability to identify whether the drill breaks into the spinal canal. The bovine spine experiments showed that the average value of thickness of the bone layer left was 1.1 mm. No breaching into the spinal canal was observed. And, the robot's recorded working times were 10–14 min similar to the traditional way (Fig. 17.27).

4.4   For Endoscopic Spinal Surgery

4.4.1   MINOSC

Ascari et al. developed a robot-assisted endoscope supported by the microneuro-endoscopy of spinal cord (MINOSC) project to intervene the spinal cord within the subarachnoid space (a few millimeters wide and full of delicate vulnerable structures) [11]. This system provided a direct view of spinal

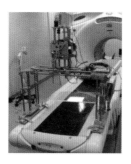

Fig. 17.26 SpineNav photograph of the testing environment

cord, blood vessels, and nerve roots and permitted localized electro-simulation. The system used image-processing techniques to analyze the surroundings and give feedback to its main control unit for avoiding damage that the obstacles even not be present in the endoscopic field of view. A series of experiments showed that the major implementation problems were already solved in its current stage; however, the prototype was still far from clinical usage.

4.4.2   Da Vinci

The da Vinci surgical robot (Intuitive Surgical, Sunnyvale, CA, USA) is the most successful robotic system, and applied widely in urology, general, and obstetrics and gynecology surgeries. As the manipulators and end effectors of Da Vinci system are primarily designed for the operations of soft tissue, which means that this system is not well suited for bone drilling, milling, or cutting and lacks appropriate tools for spinal operations. However, there are still several early stage successful experiments using it for spinal interventions, such as paravertebral tumor resections [12], transoral decompression of craniocervical junction [13], laminotomy, laminectomy, disc incision, dural-suturing procedures [14], and anterior lumbar interbody fusion [15].

4.5   For Radiosurgery

Radiosurgery was conceived as a treatment for deep seated intracranial tumors at first. But nowadays, it is still used for the treatment of neoplastic lesions and intramedullary arteriovenous malformations of spine. Current radiosurgical systems employed heavy-duty robots to move a linear accelerator (LINAC) around the patient, firing high-energy beams

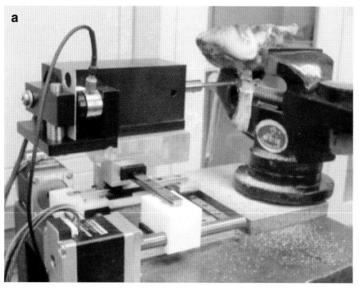
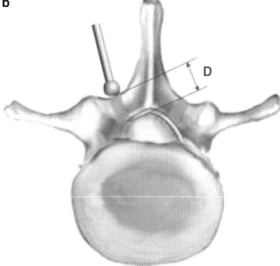

Fig. 17.27 Laminectomy robot. (**a**) Robot milling experiments. (**b**) Anatomical structure in laminectomy operation

according to a predefined plan, ablating internal tumors and minimizing damage to the surrounding healthy tissue. It was an effective and well-tolerated method. An observation followed 393 patients who showed a long-term pain control (86%) and a long-term tumor control (88%) with no cases of neurological damage induced by radiation.

The first commercialized robotic system was Gamma Knife (Elekta AB, Stockholm, Sweden), which gained worldwide acceptance since it had been introduced to the market. And nowadays, the dominators are the CyberKnife (Accuray Inc., Sunnyvale, CA, USA) and the Novalis (Brainlab, Heimstetten, Germany) because they permit interventions guided by intraoperative imaging directly without the need of stereotactical frames. Image-guidance systems had a high accuracy without the need of any type of marker. Studies showed that the mean accuracy of fiducial-based spinal radiosurgery was about 0.7 mm and image-based was about 0.5–0.6 mm.

4.6　Summary

In the field of spine surgery, as we could see, the highlight is transpedicular fixation. And right now, only SpineAssist/Renaissance attained the FDA and CE clearances. Although more than 20 robotic systems were researched and some of them were very interesting, most of the interested companies shrinked back at the sight of difficulties of the commercialization and attainment of the FDA and CE clearances.

In about two decades from 1992, when the spinal robotic system emerging first time, we could see, more and more attentions focus on the demands of spine surgery, and the transpedicular fixation is still the highlight of this area. And of course, comparing with autonomously drilling, robotic-assisted positioning is the appropriate position of the robotic system in spine surgery right now. With the development of spinal surgical robotic systems' relative techniques, we get better accuracy, less X-ray exposure, and possibility of subarachnoid space exploration. However, this field of technique is still facing two main issues. First, the accuracy of spinal robot-assisted surgery is located about 1–2 mm depending on the resolution of intraoperative images, accuracy of registration, and the slight movement of the spine. Which means that the submillimeter precision cannot be achieved yet. And second, facing the demands of the high accuracy, low invasiveness, low radiation, and high robustness, neither of the two main methods of tracking and registration (one

kind is based on the optical tracking technique and the other one is based on fluoroscopy or intraoperative and registrational algorithms) has the ability to satisfy them simultaneously. In addition, although the cost of robotic-assisted surgery is relative high, there is no publication that analyzed the costs and benefits of robotic spinal surgery, available.

References

1. Santos-Munné JJ, et al. A stereotactic/robotic system for pedicle screw placement. In: Morgan K, Satava R, Sieburg H, et al., editors. Proceedings of the medicine meets virtual reality III conference. San Diego, CA: IOS Press/Ohmsha; 1995. p. 326–33.
2. Ortmaier T, et al. A hands-on robot for accurate placement of pedicle screws. In: Proceedings, IEEE international conference on robotics and automation, 2006 (ICRA 2006). Orlando, Florida; 2006. p. 4179–4186.
3. Boschetti G, et al. A haptic system for robotic assisted spine surgery. In: Proceedings of IEEE conference on control applications (CCA 2005); 2005. p. 19–24.
4. Jin H, et al. Design and control strategy of robotic spinal surgical system. In: IEEE/ICME international conference on complex medical engineering. Harbin, China; 2011. p. 627–632.
5. Zhang C, Wang Z, Chen F, et al. Spine Bull's-Eye Robot guidewire placement with pedicle standard axis view for thoracic and lumbar pedicle screw fixation. J Spinal Disord Tech. 2012;25(7):E191–8.
6. Cleary K, Watson V, Lindisch D, et al. Precision placement of instruments for minimally invasive procedures using a 'needle driver' robot. Int J Med Robot. 2005;1(2):40–7.
7. Melzer A, Gutmann B, Remmele T, et al. INNOMOTION for percutaneous image-guided interventions: principles and evaluation of this MR- and CT-compatible robotic system. IEEE Eng Med Biol Mag. 2008;27(3):66–73.
8. Tovar-Arriaga S, Tita R, Pedraza-Ortega JC, et al. Development of a robotic FD-CT-guided navigation system for needle placement-preliminary accuracy tests. Int J Med Robot. 2011;7(2):225–36.
9. Onogi S, Gotoh M, Nakajima Y, et al. Vertebral robotic puncture for minimally invasive spinal surgery: puncture accuracy evaluation for vertebral model. Int J Comput Assist Radiol Surg. 2009;4(Suppl 1):121–2.
10. Wang T, Luan S, Hu L, et al. Force-based control of a compact spinal milling robot. Int J Med Robot. 2010;6(2):178–85.
11. Ascari L, Stefanini C, Bertocchi U, et al. Robot-assisted endoscopic exploration of the spinal cord. Proc Inst Mech Eng Part C J Mech Eng Sci. 2010;224(7):1515–29.
12. Yang MS, Jung JH, Kim JM, et al. Current and future of spinal robot surgery. Korean J Spine. 2010;7(2):61–5.
13. Lee JYK, O'Malley BW, Newman JG, et al. Transoral robotic surgery of craniocervical junction and atlantoaxial spine: a cadaveric study. J Neurosurg Spine. 2010;12(1):13–8.
14. Ponnusamy K, Chewning S, Mohr C. Robotic approaches to the posterior spine. Spine. 2009;34(19):2104–9.
15. Kim MJ, Ha Y, et al. Robot-assisted anterior lumbar interbody fusion (ALIF) using retroperitoneal approach. Acta Neurochir. 2010;152(4):675–9.